Third Edition

# Human Embryology and Developmental Biology

B r u c e   M .   C a r l s o n ,   M D ,   P h D

Professor, Department of Cell and Developmental Biology
Director, Institute of Gerontology
University of Michigan
Ann Arbor, Michigan

**Mosby**

*An Affiliate of Elsevier*

Mosby
*An Affiliate of Elsevier*

170 S Independence Mall W 300 E
Philadelphia, PA 19106-3399

HUMAN EMBRYOLOGY AND DEVELOPMENTAL BIOLOGY
Third Edition

Previous editions copyrighted 1999, 1994

**Library of Congress Cataloging-in-Publication Data**

Carlson, Bruce M.
  Human embryology and developmental biology / Bruce M. Carlson. — 3rd ed.
    p. ; cm.
  title: Human embryology & developmental biology.
  Rev. ed. of: Human embryology & developmental biology / Bruce M. Carlson. 2nd ed. c1999.
  Includes bibliographical references and index.
  ISBN-10: 0-323-03649-X
  ISBN-13: 978-0-323-03649-8
    1. Embryology, Human. 2. Developmental biology. 3. Human growth. I. Title: Human embryology &
  developmental biology. II. Carlson, Bruce M. Human embryology & developmental biology. III. Title.
    [DNLM: 1. Embryo and Fetal Development—physiology. WQ 210.5 C284h 2004]
  QM601.C29 2004
  612.6'4—dc22

                                                                                    2004040246

*Acquisitions Editor:* Inta Ozols
*Developmental Editor:* Joanie Milnes

ISBN-13: 978-0-323-03649-8
ISBN-10: 0-323-03649-X

Printed in China

Last digit is the print number:  9  8  7  6  5  4  3  2

# Human Embryology & Developmental Biology

# www.studentconsult.com

delivers **Human Embryology and Developmental Biology, Third Edition** online and more!

online access
+
interactive
extras
studentconsult.com

Thank you for purchasing the updated version of
## Human Embryology and Developmental Biology, Third Edition

**Your purchase entitles you to free online access.**

Find what you need to know, right now!
Access via your home computer,
the library, or the wards!

## Fully searchable text
- Access by keyword, subject, or index

## Link up
- Integration links give bonus content from other leading Elsevier titles

## Build your online library
- Search across all of your favorite textbooks
- View illustrations online and download for your own personal use

## POCKETConsult enabled
- Enables you to download excerpts to your handheld device

**BOOK CANNOT BE RETURNED ONCE PANEL IS SCRATCHED OFF**

## How to register

Scratch off the sticker below to get your **unique** PIN number. Connect to the internet and go to
**www.studentconsult.com**
for simple instructions on how to register – you'll need your PIN number for registration.

**Scratch off the sticker with care!** Use a hard plastic edge (rather than a coin), if possible, and don't scratch too vigorously to avoid smudging the PIN code.

**Important note:** Purchase of this book includes access to the online version of this edition for use exclusively by the individual purchaser from the launch of the site. This licence and access to the online version operates strictly on the basis of a single user per PIN number. *The sharing of passwords is strictly prohibited, and any attempt to do so will invalidate the password.* Access may not be shared, resold or otherwise circulated and will terminate on publication of the next edition of this book. Full details and terms of use are available upon registration and access will be subject to your acceptance of these terms of use.

**Scratch off Below**

C3R5MRK

*Also at studentconsult.com*
- Win great prizes in online games and competitions
- Sample chapters
- A full range of textbooks with online access
- Innovative PDA products
- *... and much more!*

*To Mom, Jean, Marty and Jim*

# Preface to the Third Edition

As was the case in the first two editions of this book, one of the main themes of the preface is the enormous amount of new knowledge that has accumulated in the previous four years and the difficulty of integrating it into a package that is digestible for students. If anything, the pace of new discovery in embryology and development has accelerated. Sometimes the new information has allowed the presentation of certain aspects of embryology to be simplified, whereas in others, connecting the links within new collections of individual data are less apparent. All this aside, these are exciting times in which to be writing an embryology text because it is increasingly possible to provide mechanistic explanations at a certain level for developmental phenomena that in former times could only be described.

Many parts of the text have been extensively rewritten for the third edition. A major change is the addition of a separate chapter intended to introduce the student to fundamental aspects of molecular mechanisms in development. Although many students have already had courses in molecular biology or biochemistry, it has been my experience as a teacher that they have often lost sight of the forest as they have worked at learning the molecular trees. This chapter is by no means comprehensive, but it does introduce the student to major families of important developmental molecules, such as the homeobox-containing genes, members of the transforming growth factor family, the fibroblast growth factor family, and *Pax* genes. Two developmentally important molecules, sonic hedgehog and retinoic acid, have been treated in some depth in order to give the student some appreciation of the kinds of molecular pathways that stimulate developmental processes.

Space does not permit a complete enumeration of all parts of the text that were extensively updated for the third edition, but some of the major ones include the basis for left-right asymmetry, major signaling centers in the early embryo, the cross-sectional organization of the central nervous system, the molecular organization of the gut, and the basis for early establishment of the vascular system.

As usual, I invite comments on the revised text, and I am especially appreciative when readers point out errors in the text or the figures. I can be readily reached by e-mail at *brcarl@umich.edu*. One mechanism that has proven to be exceptionally successful in getting students both to read the text and to realize that textbooks are not infallible is to offer one extra credit point for every new mistake found in the book. For this I credit my organic chemistry professor in college, Dr. Arne Langsjoen, who used to collect such mistakes in our text and then relay them to the appreciative author.

The production of any book involves far more people than just the author. I thank my editors, William Schmidt and Jason Malley, for their overall guidance of the project, the reviewers of early drafts of the text and the production staff, especially Joanie Milnes and Keith Roberts, for shepherding the transformation of the final manuscript into a real book. I am very grateful to Dr. Bradley R. Smith, Director of the Program in Medical and Biological Illustration at the University of Michigan, for providing one of his wonderful embryo images for use in the cover design. A book on embryology is especially dependent upon the quality of its artwork, and I want to extend my special thanks to Alexandra Baker of DNA Illustrations, Inc. for her superb translations of my chicken scratches into intelligible figures. Finally, my special thanks are due to my wife, Jean, for her usual forbearance of the general disruption that is involved in the birthing of yet another book.

Bruce M. Carlson

# Contents

## DEVELOPMENTAL TABLES

### Carnegie Stages of Early Human Embryonic Development (Weeks 1-8)

| Age (days) | External features | Carnegie stage | Crown-rump length (mm) | Pairs of somites |
|---|---|---|---|---|
| 1 | Fertilized oocyte | 1 | 0.1 | |
| 2-3 | Morula (4–16 cells) | 2 | 0.1 | |
| 4 | Free blastocyst | 3 | 0.1 | |
| 5-6 | Attachment of blastocyst to endometrium | 4 | 0.1 | |
| 7-12 | Implantation, bilaminar embryo with primary yolk sac | 5 | 0.1-0.2 | |
| 13-15 | Trilaminar embryo with primitive streak, chorionic villi | 6 | 0.2-0.3 | |
| 16 | Gastrulation, formation of notochordal process | 7 | 0.4 | |
| 18 | Hensen's node and primitive pit, notochord and neurenteric canal, appearance of neural plate, neural folds, and blood islands | 8 | 1.0-1.5 | |
| 20 | Appearance of first somites, deep neural groove, elevation of cranial neural folds, early heart tubes | 9 | 1.5-2.5 | 1-3 |
| 22 | Beginning of fusion of neural folds, formation of optic sulci, presence of first two pharyngeal arches, beginning heart beat, curving of embryo | 10 | 2.0-3.5 | 4-12 |
| 24 | Closure of cranial neuropore, formation of optic vesicles, rupture of oropharyngeal membrane | 11 | 2.5-4.5 | 13-20 |
| 26 | Closure of caudal neuropore, formation of pharyngeal arches 3 and 4, appearance of upper limb buds and tail bud, formation of otic vesicle | 12 | 3-5 | 21-29 |
| 28 | Appearance of lower limb buds, lens placode, separation of otic vesicle from surface ectoderm | 13 | 4-6 | 30↑ |
| 32 | Formation of lens vesicle, optic cup, and nasal pits | 14 | 5-7 | |
| 33 | Development of hand plates, primary urogenital sinus, prominent nasal pits, evidence of cerebral hemispheres | 15 | 7-9 | |
| 37 | Development of foot plates, visible retinal pigment, development of auricular hillocks, formation of upper lip | 16 | 8-11 | |
| 41 | Appearance of finger rays, rapid head enlargement, six auricular hillocks, formation of nasolacrimal groove | 17 | 11-14 | |
| 44 | Appearance of toe rays and elbow regions, beginning of formation of eyelids, tip of nose distinct, presence of nipples | 18 | 13-17 | |
| 48 | Elongation and straightening of trunk, beginning of herniation of midgut into umbilical cord | 19 | 16-18 | |
| 51 | Bending of arms at elbows, distinct but webbed fingers, appearance of scalp vascular plexus, degeneration of anal and urogenital membranes | 20 | 18-22 | |
| 52 | Longer and free fingers, distinct but webbed toes, indifferent external genitalia | 21 | 22-24 | |
| 54 | Longer and free toes, better development of eyelids and external ear | 22 | 23-28 | |
| 57 | More rounded head, fusion of eyelids | 23 | 27-31 | |

Data taken largely from O'Rahilly R, Müller F: Developmental stages in human embryos, Pub 637, Washington, DC, 1987, Carnegie Institution of Washington.

## Major Developmental Events During the Fetal Period

| External features | Internal features |
|---|---|
| **8 WEEKS**<br>Head is almost half the total length of fetus.<br>Cervical flexure is about 30 degrees.<br>Indifferent external genitalia are present.<br>Eyes are converging.<br>Eyelids are unfused.<br>Tail disappears.<br>Nostrils are closed by epithelial plugs. | Midgut herniation into umbilical cord occurs.<br>Extraembryonic portion of allantois has degenerated.<br>Ducts and alveoli of lacrimal glands form.<br>Paramesonephric ducts begin to regress in males.<br>Recanalization of lumen of gut tube occurs.<br>Lungs are becoming glandlike.<br>Diaphragm is completed.<br>First ossification begins in skeleton.<br>Definitive aortic arch system takes shape. |
| **9 WEEKS**<br>Neck develops and chin rises from thorax.<br>Cranial flexure is about 22 degrees.<br>Chorion is divided into chorion laeve and chorion frondosum.<br>Eyelids meet and fuse.<br>External genitalia begin to become gender specific. | Intestines are herniated into umbilical cord.<br>Early muscular movements occur.<br>ACTH and gonadotropins are produced by pituitary.<br>Corticosteroids are produced by adrenal cortex.<br>Semilunar valves in heart are completed.<br>Fused paramesonephric ducts join vaginal plate.<br>Urethral folds begin to fuse in males. |
| **10 WEEKS**<br>Cervical flexure is about 15 degrees.<br>Gender differences are apparent in external genitalia.<br>Fingernails appear.<br>Eyelids are fused. | Intestines return into body cavity from umbilical cord.<br>Bile is secreted.<br>Blood islands are established in spleen.<br>Thymus is infiltrated by lymphoid stem cells.<br>Prolactin production by pituitary occurs.<br>First permanent tooth buds form.<br>Deciduous teeth are in early bell stage.<br>Epidermis has three layers. |
| **11 WEEKS**<br>Cervical flexure is about 8 degrees.<br>Nose begins to develop bridge. | Urine is excreted into amniotic fluid.<br>Stomach musculature can contract.<br>T lymphocytes emigrate into bloodstream.<br>Colloid appears in thyroid follicles. |
| **12 WEEKS**<br>Head is erect.<br>Neck is almost straight and well defined.<br>External ear is taking form and has moved close to its definitive position in the head.<br>Yolk sac has shrunk.<br>Fetus swallows amniotic fluid.<br>Fetus can respond to skin stimulation. | Ovaries descend below pelvic rim.<br>Parathyroid hormone is produced.<br>Blood can coagulate. |
| **4 MONTHS**<br>Skin is thin; blood vessels can easily be seen through it.<br>Nostrils are almost formed.<br>Fetus may begin to suck its thumb.<br>Eyes have moved to front of face.<br>Legs are longer than arms.<br>Fine lanugo hairs appear on head.<br>Fingernails are well formed; toenails are forming.<br>Epidermal ridges appear on fingers and palms of hand.<br>Enough amniotic fluid is present to permit amniocentesis.<br>Mother can feel fetal movements. | Seminal vesicle forms.<br>Transverse grooves appear on dorsal surface of cerebellum.<br>Bile is produced by liver and stains meconium green.<br>Gastric glands bud off from gastric pits.<br>Brown fat begins to form.<br>Pyramidal tracts begin to form in brain.<br>Hematopoiesis begins in bone marrow.<br>Ovaries contain primordial follicles. |

## Major Developmental Events During the Fetal Period—cont'd

| External features | Internal features |
|---|---|
| **5 MONTHS** | |
| Epidermal ridges form on toes and soles of feet. | Myelination of spinal cord begins. |
| Vernix caseosa begins to be deposited on skin. | Sebaceous glands begin to function. |
| Abdomen begins to fill out. | Thyroid-stimulating hormone is released by pituitary. |
| Eyelids and eyebrows develop. | Testes begin to descend. |
| Lanugo hairs cover most of body. | |
| **6 MONTHS** | |
| Skin is wrinkled and red. | Surfactant begins to be secreted. |
| Decidua capsularis degenerates because of reduced blood supply. | Tip of spinal cord is at S1 level. |
| Lanugo hairs darken. | |
| **7 MONTHS** | |
| Eyelids begin to open. | Sulci and gyri begin to appear on brain. |
| Eyelashes are well developed. | Subcutaneous fat storage begins. |
| Scalp hairs are lengthening (longer than lanugo). | Testes are descending into scrotum. |
| Skin is slightly wrinkled. | Termination of splenic erythropoiesis occurs. |
| **8 MONTHS** | |
| Skin is pink and smooth. | Regression of hyaloid vessels from lens occurs. |
| Eyes are capable of pupillary light reflex. | Testes enter scrotum. |
| Fingernails have reached tip of fingers. | |
| **9 MONTHS** | |
| Toenails have reached tip of toes. | Larger amounts of pulmonary surfactant are secreted. |
| Most lanugo hairs are shed. | Ovaries are still above brim of pelvis. |
| Skin is covered with vernix caseosa. | Testes have descended into scrotum. |
| Attachment of umbilical cord becomes central in abdomen. | Tip of spinal cord is at L3. |
| About 1 L of amniotic fluid is present. | Myelination of brain begins. |
| Placenta weighs about 500 g. | |
| Fingernails extend beyond fingertips. | |
| Breasts protrude and secrete "witches' milk." | |

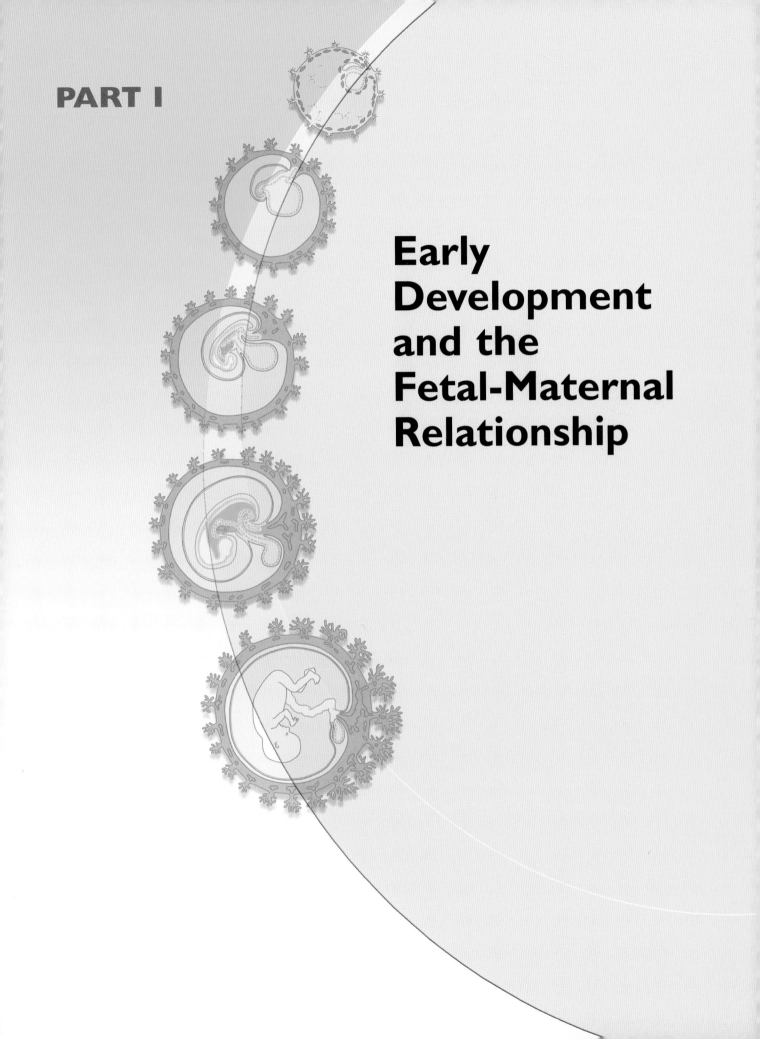

**PART I**

**Early Development and the Fetal-Maternal Relationship**

# CHAPTER 1

# Getting Ready for Pregnancy

Human pregnancy begins with the fusion of an egg and a sperm, but a great deal of preparation precedes this event. First, both male and female sex cells must pass through a long series of changes (**gametogenesis**) that convert them genetically and phenotypically into mature **gametes**, which are capable of participating in the process of fertilization. Next, the gametes must be released from the gonads and make their way to the upper part of the uterine tube, where fertilization normally takes place. Finally, the fertilized egg, now properly called an **embryo**, must enter the uterus, where it sinks into the uterine lining (**implantation**) to be nourished by the mother. All these events involve interactions between the gametes or embryo and the adult body in which they are housed, and most of them are mediated or influenced by parental hormones. This chapter focuses on gametogenesis and the hormonal modifications of the body that enable reproduction to occur.

## GAMETOGENESIS

Gametogenesis is typically divided into four phases: (1) the extraembryonic origin of the germ cells and their migration into the gonads, (2) an increase in the number of germ cells by mitosis, (3) a reduction in chromosomal number by meiosis, and (4) structural and functional maturation of the eggs and spermatozoa. The first phase of gametogenesis is identical in both males and females,

whereas distinct differences exist between the male and female patterns in the last three phases.

## Phase 1: Origin and Migration of Germ Cells

**Primordial germ cells**, the earliest recognizable precursors of gametes, arise outside the gonads and migrate into the gonads during early embryonic development. Human primordial germ cells first become readily recognizable at 24 days after fertilization in the endodermal layer of the yolk sac (Figure 1-1, *A*) by their large size and high content of the enzyme alkaline phosphatase. In the mouse, their origin has been traced even earlier in development (p. 408). Germ cells exit from the yolk sac into the hindgut epithelium and then migrate through the dorsal mesentery until they reach the primordia of the gonads (Figure 1-1, *B*). In the mouse, an estimated 100 cells leave the yolk sac, and through mitotic multiplication (six to seven rounds of cell division), about 4000 primordial germ cells enter the primitive gonads.

Misdirected primordial germ cells that lodge in extragonadal sites usually die, but if such cells survive, they may develop into **teratomas**. Teratomas are bizarre growths that contain scrambled mixtures of highly differentiated tissues, such as skin, hair, cartilage, and even teeth (Figure 1-2). They are found in the mediastinum, the sacrococcygeal region, and the oral region.

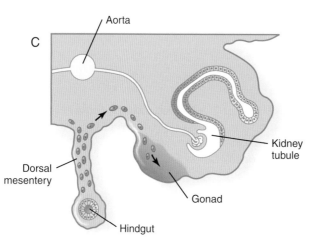

**FIGURE 1-1** Origin and migration of primordial germ cells in the human embryo. **A,** Location of primordial germ cells in the 16-somite human embryo (midsagittal view). **B,** Pathway of migration *(arrow)* through the dorsal mesentery. **C,** Cross section showing the pathway of migration *(arrows)* through the dorsal mesentery and into the gonad.

**FIGURE 1-2 A,** Sacrococcygeal teratoma in a fetus. **B,** Massive oropharyngeal teratoma. (Courtesy M. Barr, Ann Arbor, Michigan.)

## Phase 2: Increase in the Number of Germ Cells by Mitosis

Once they arrive in the gonads, the primordial germ cells begin a phase of rapid mitotic proliferation. In a mitotic division, each germ cell produces two **diploid** progeny that are genetically equal. Through several series of mitotic divisions, the number of primordial germ cells increases exponentially from hundreds to millions. The pattern of mitotic proliferation differs markedly between male and female germ cells. **Oogonia**, as mitotically active germ cells in the female are called, go through a period of intense mitotic activity in the embryonic ovary from the second through the fifth month of pregnancy in the human. During this period the population of germ cells increases from only a few thousand to nearly 7 million (Figure 1-3). This number represents the maximum number of germ cells that is ever found in the ovaries. Shortly thereafter, large numbers of oogonia undergo a natural degeneration called **atresia**. Atresia of germ cells is a continuing feature of the histological landscape of the human ovary until menopause.

**Spermatogonia**, which are the male counterparts of oogonia, follow a pattern of mitotic proliferation that differs greatly from that in the female. Mitosis also begins early in the embryonic testes, but in contrast to female germ cells, male germ cells maintain the ability to divide throughout life. The seminiferous tubules of the testes are lined with a germinative population of spermatogonia. Beginning at puberty, subpopulations of spermatogonia undergo periodic waves of mitosis. The progeny of these divisions enter meiosis as synchronous groups. This pattern of spermatogonial mitosis continues throughout life.

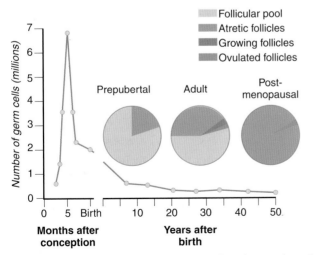

**FIGURE 1-3** Changes in the number of germ cells and proportions of follicle types in the human ovary with increasing age. (Based on studies by Baker TG. In Austin CR, Short RV: *Germ cells and fertilization (reproduction in mammals)*, vol 1, Cambridge, England, 1970, Cambridge University Press, p 20; and Goodman AL, Hodgen GD: *Recent Progr Hormone Res* 39:1–73, 1983.)

## Phase 3: Reduction in Chromosomal Number by Meiosis

### Stages of Meiosis

The biological significance of meiosis in the human is similar to that in other species. Of primary importance are (1) reduction of the number of chromosomes from the diploid (2n) to the **haploid** (1n) number so that the species number of chromosomes can be maintained from generation to generation, (2) independent reassortment of maternal and paternal chromosomes for better mixing of genetic characteristics, and (3) further redistribution of maternal and paternal genetic information through the process of crossing-over during the first meiotic division.

Meiosis involves two sets of divisions (Figure 1-4). Before the first meiotic division, deoxyribonucleic acid (DNA) replication has already occurred, so at the beginning of meiosis, the cell is 2n, 4c. (In this designation, **n** is the species number of chromosomes and **c** is the amount of DNA in a single set [n] of chromosomes before DNA replication has occurred.) The cell contains the normal number (2n) of chromosomes, but as the result of replication, its DNA content (4c) is double the normal amount (2c).

In the first meiotic division, often called the **reductional division**, a prolonged prophase (see Figure 1-4) results in the pairing of homologous chromosomes and frequent **crossing-over**, resulting in the exchange of segments between members of the paired chromosomes. During metaphase of the first meiotic division, the chromosome pairs (**tetrads**) line up at the metaphase (equatorial) plate so that at anaphase I, one chromosome of a homologous pair moves toward one pole of the spindle and the other chromosome moves toward the opposite pole. This represents one of the principal differences between a meiotic and mitotic division. In a mitotic anaphase, the centromere between the sister chromatids of each chromosome splits after the chromosomes have lined up at the metaphase plate, and one chromatid from each chromosome migrates to each pole of the mitotic spindle. This results in genetically equal daughter cells after a mitotic division, whereas the daughter cells are genetically unequal after the first meiotic division. Each daughter cell of the first meiotic division contains the haploid (1n) number of chromosomes, but each chromosome still consists of two chromatids (2c) connected by a centromere. No new duplication of chromosomal DNA is required between the first and second meiotic divisions because each haploid daughter cell resulting from the first meiotic division already contains chromosomes in the replicated state.

The second meiotic division, called the **equational division**, is similar to an ordinary mitotic division, except that before division the cell is haploid (1n, 2c). When the

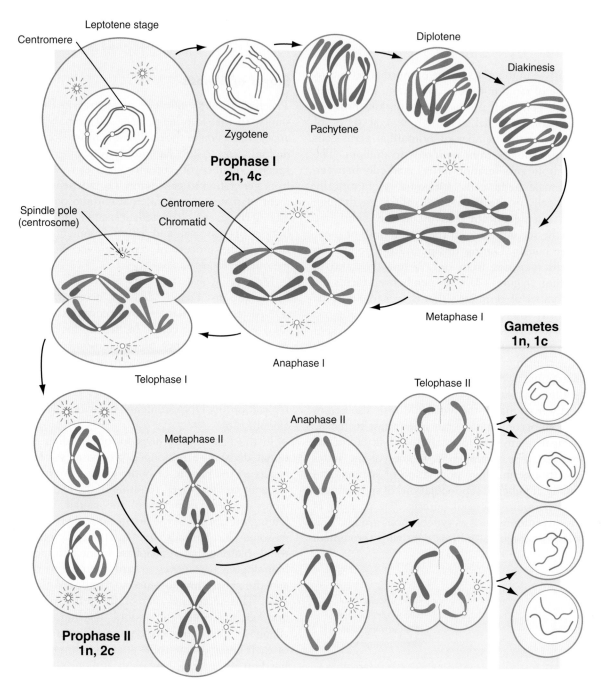

**FIGURE 1-4** Summary of the major stages of meiosis in a generalized germ cell.

chromosomes line up along the equatorial plate at metaphase II, the centromeres between sister chromatids divide, allowing the sister chromatids of each chromosome to migrate to opposite poles of the spindle apparatus during anaphase II. Each daughter cell of the second meiotic division is truly haploid (1n, 1c).

### Meiosis in Females

The period of meiosis involves other cellular activities in addition to the redistribution of chromosomal material.

As the oogonia enter the first meiotic division late in the fetal period, they are called **primary oocytes**.

Meiosis in the human female is a very leisurely process. As the primary oocytes enter the diplotene stage of the first meiotic division in the early months after birth, the first of two blocks in the meiotic process occurs (Figure 1-5). The suspended diplotene phase of meiosis is the period when the primary oocyte prepares for the needs of the embryo. In oocytes of amphibians and other lower vertebrates, which must develop outside the mother's body and often in a hostile environment, it is highly

| Age | Follicular histology | | Meiotic events in ovum | Chromosomal complement |
|---|---|---|---|---|
| Fetal period | No follicle | | Oogonium | **2n, 2c** |
| | | *Mitosis* | | |
| Before or at birth | Primordial follicle | | Primary oocyte | **2n, 4c** |
| | | *Meiosis in progress* | | |
| After birth | Primary follicle | | Primary oocyte | **2n, 4c** |
| | | *Arrested in diplotene stage of first meiotic division* | | |
| After puberty | Secondary follicle | | Primary oocyte | **2n, 4c** |
| | | *First meiotic division completed, start of second meiotic division* | | |
| Tertiary follicle | | | Secondary oocyte + Polar body I | **1n, 2c** |
| | | *Ovulation* | | |
| Ovulated ovum | | | Secondary oocyte + Polar body I | **1n, 2c** |
| | | *Arrested at metaphase II* | | |
| Fertilized ovum | | | Fertilized ovum + Polar body II | **1n, 1c + sperm** |
| | | *Fertilization—second meiotic division completed* | | |

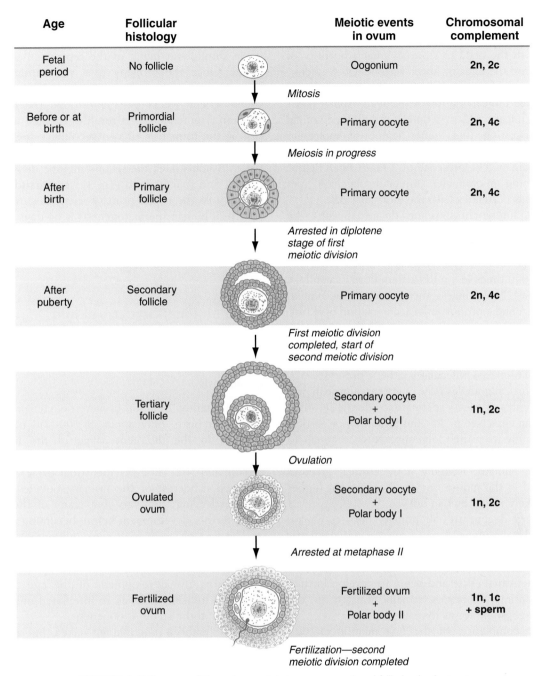

**FIGURE 1-5** Summary of the major events in human oogenesis and follicular development.

advantageous for the early stages of development to occur very rapidly so that the stage of independent locomotion and feeding is attained as soon as possible. These conditions necessitate a strategy of storing up the materials needed for early development well in advance of ovulation and fertilization because normal synthetic processes would not be rapid enough to produce the materials required for the rapidly cleaving embryo. In such species, yolk is accumulated, the genes for producing ribosomal ribonucleic acid (rRNA) are amplified, and many types of RNA molecules are synthesized and stored in an inactive form for later use.

Ribonucleic acid (RNA) synthesis in the amphibian oocyte occurs on the lampbrush chromosomes, which are characterized by many prominent loops of spread-out DNA on which messenger RNA (mRNA) molecules are synthesized. The amplified genes for producing rRNA are manifested by the presence of 600 to 1000 nucleoli within the nucleus. Primary oocytes also prepare for fertilization by producing several thousand cortical granules, which are of great importance during the fertilization process (see Chapter 2).

The mammalian oocyte prepares for an early embryonic period that is more prolonged than that of amphibians and that takes place in the nutritive environment of the maternal reproductive tract. Therefore it is not faced with the need to store as great a quantity of materials as are the eggs of lower vertebrates. As a consequence, the buildup of yolk is negligible. However, some evidence indicates a low level of ribosomal DNA (rDNA) amplification (2 to 3 times) in diplotene human oocytes, suggesting that some degree of molecular advance planning is also required to support early cleavage in the human. The presence of 2 to 40 small (2 μm) RNA-containing micronuclei (miniature nucleoli) per oocyte nucleus correlates with the molecular data.

Human diplotene chromosomes do not appear to be arranged in a true lampbrush configuration, and massive amounts of RNA synthesis seem unlikely. The developing mammalian (mouse) oocyte produces 10,000 times less rRNA and 1000 times less mRNA than does its amphibian counterpart. Nevertheless, there is a steady accumulation of mRNA and a proportional accumulation of rRNA. These amounts of maternally derived RNA seem to be enough to take the fertilized egg through the first couple of cleavage divisions, after which the embryonic genome takes control of macromolecular synthetic processes.

Because cortical granules play an important role in preventing the entry of excess spermatozoa during fertilization in human eggs (see p. 34), the formation of cortical granules (mainly from the Golgi apparatus) continues to be one of the functions of the diplotene stage that is preserved in humans. Roughly 4500 cortical granules are produced in the mouse oocyte. A somewhat higher number is likely in the human oocyte.

Unless they degenerate, all primary oocytes remain arrested in the diplotene stage of meiosis until puberty. During the reproductive years, small numbers (10 to 30) of primary oocytes complete the first meiotic division with each menstrual cycle and begin to develop further. The other primary oocytes remain arrested in the diplotene stage, some for as long as 50 years.

With the completion of the first meiotic division shortly before ovulation, two unequal cellular progeny result. One is a large cell, called the **secondary oocyte.** The other is a small cell called the **first polar body** (see Figure 1-5). The secondary oocytes begin the second meiotic division, but again the meiotic process is arrested, this time at metaphase. The stimulus for the release from this meiotic block is fertilization by a spermatozoon. Unfertilized secondary oocytes fail to complete the second meiotic division. The second meiotic division is also unequal; one of the daughter cells is relegated to becoming a second polar body. The first polar body may also divide during the second meiotic division.

### Meiosis in Males

Meiosis in the male does not begin until after puberty. In contrast to the primary oocytes in the female, not all spermatogonia enter meiosis at the same time. In fact, large numbers of spermatogonia remain in the mitotic cycle throughout much of the reproductive lifetime of males. Once the progeny of a spermatogonium have entered the meiotic cycle as **primary spermatocytes,** they spend several weeks passing through the first meiotic division (Figure 1-6). The result of the first meiotic division is the formation of two **secondary spermatocytes,** which immediately enter the second meiotic division. About 8 hours later, the second meiotic division is completed, and four haploid (1n, 1c) **spermatids** remain as progeny of the single primary spermatocyte. The total length of human spermatogenesis is 64 days.

Disturbances that can occur during meiosis and result in chromosomal aberrations are discussed in Clinical Correlation 1-1 and Figure 1-7.

## Phase 4: Final Structural and Functional Maturation of Eggs and Sperm

### Oogenesis

Of the roughly 2 million primary oocytes present in the ovaries at birth, only about 40,000—all of which are arrested in the diplotene stage of the first meiotic division—survive until puberty. From this number, approximately 400 (one per menstrual cycle) are actually ovulated. The rest of the primary oocytes degenerate without leaving the ovary, but many of them undergo some further development before becoming atretic.

The egg, along with its surrounding cells, is called a **follicle.** Maturation of the egg is intimately bound with the development of its cellular covering. Because of this, considering the development of the egg and its surrounding follicular cells as an integrated unit is a useful approach in the study of oogenesis.

In the embryo, oogonia are naked, but after meiosis begins, cells from the ovary partially surround the primary oocytes to form **primordial follicles** (see Figure 1-5). By birth, the primary oocytes are invested with one or two complete layers of follicular cells, and the complex of primary oocyte and the follicular (granulosa) cells is called a **primary follicle** (Figure 1-8). Both the oocyte and the surrounding follicular cells develop prominent microvilli and gap junctions that connect the two cell types.

The gap junctions permit the exchange of amino acids and glucose metabolites that are required for growth of the oocyte. The follicular cells secrete a **meiotic inhibitory factor** responsible for maintaining the first arrest of meiosis in the diplotene stage. The inhibitory factor is transferred from the follicular cells to the oocyte via the gap junctions that connect them. Within the oocyte, activity of the GTP-binding protein, $G_s$, main-

| Cell types | Meiotic events | Chromosomal complement |
|---|---|---|
| Spermatogonium (type B) | DNA replication | **2n, 4c** |
| Primary spermatocyte | First meiotic division in progress | **2n, 4c** |
| *First meiotic division completed* | | |
| Two secondary spermatocytes | Second meiotic division in progress | **1n, 2c** |
| *Second meiotic division completed* | | |
| 4 Spermatids | Immature haploid gametes | **1n, 1c** |
| *Spermiogenesis* | | |
| 4 Spermatozoa | Haploid gametes | **1n, 1c** |

Blood-testis barrier

Sertoli cell

**FIGURE 1-6** Summary of the major events in human spermatogenesis.

tains the state of meiotic arrest. The release of meiotic inhibition shortly before ovulation is associated with the luteinizing hormone surge and the subsequent disruption of the gap junction connections. The oocyte also appears to influence the development of the surrounding follicular cells, especially in mature follicles. Follicular functions that depend on interactions between the oocyte and surrounding follicular cells are summarized in Box 1-1.

As the primary follicle takes shape, a prominent, translucent, noncellular membrane called the **zona pellucida** forms between the primary oocyte and its enveloping follicular cells (Figure 1-9). The microvillous connections between the oocyte and follicular cells are maintained through the zona pellucida. In rodents, the characterized components of the zona pellucida (three glycoproteins and glycosaminoglycans) are synthesized almost entirely by the egg, but in other mammals, follicular cells also contribute materials to the zona. The zona pellucida contains sperm receptors and other components that are important in fertilization and early postfertilization development. (The functions of these molecules are discussed more fully in Chapter 2.)

In the prepubertal years, many of the primary follicles enlarge, mainly because of an increase in the size of the oocyte and the number of follicular cells. A basement membrane called the **membrana granulosa** surrounds the epithelial **granulosa cells** of the primary follicle. The

---

**Box 1-1   Functional Processes in Ovarian Follicles that Depend on Factors Exchanged Between Oocytes and Follicular Cells**

OOCYTE FUNCTIONS DEPENDENT ON FACTORS FROM GRANULOSA CELLS

Metabolism                          Meiotic arrest
Growth                              Maturation

GRANULOSA CELL FUNCTIONS DEPENDENT ON FACTORS FROM OOCYTES

Proliferation                       Follicle organization
Differentiation                     Cumulus expansion

From Eppig JJ: *Bioessays* 13:569–574, 1991.

---

membrana granulosa forms a barrier to capillaries, and as a result, both the oocyte and the granulosa cells depend on the diffusion of oxygen and nutrients for their survival.

An additional set of cellular coverings, derived from the ovarian connective tissue (**stroma**), begins to form

**CLINICAL CORRELATION 1-1**

## Meiotic Disturbances Resulting in Chromosomal Aberrations

Chromosomes sometimes fail to separate during meiosis, a phenomenon known as **nondisjunction**. As a result, one haploid daughter gamete contains both members of a chromosomal pair for a total of 24 chromosomes, whereas the other haploid gamete contains only 22 chromosomes (Figure 1-7). When such gametes combine with normal gametes of the opposite sex (with 23 chromosomes), the resulting embryos contain 47 chromosomes (with a **trisomy** of one chromosome) or 45 chromosomes (**monosomy** of one chromosome). (Specific syndromes associ-

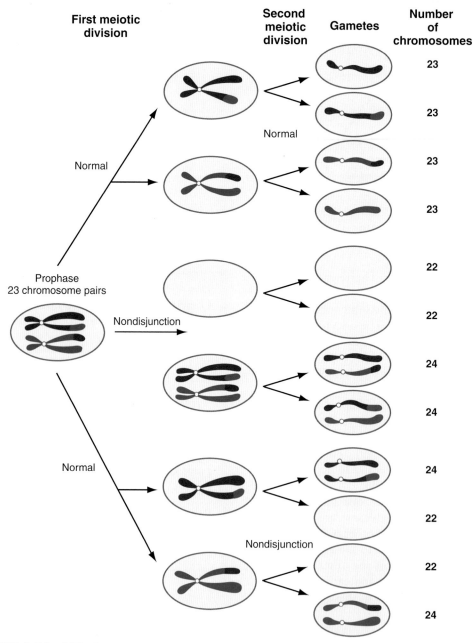

**FIGURE 1-7** Possibilities for nondisjunction. *Top arrow,* Normal meiotic divisions; *middle arrow,* nondisjunction during the first meiotic division; *bottom arrow,* nondisjunction during the second meiotic division.

ated with the nondisjunction of chromosomes are summarized in Chapter 8.) The generic term given to a condition characterized by an abnormal number of chromosomes is **aneuploidy**.

In other cases, part of a chromosome can be **translocated** to another chromosome during meiosis, or part of a chromosome can be **deleted**. Similarly, duplications or inversions of parts of chromosomes occasionally occur during meiosis. These conditions may result in syndromes similar to those seen after the nondisjunction of entire chromosomes. Under some circumstances (e.g., simultaneous fertilization by two spermatozoa, failure of the second polar body to separate from the oocyte during the second meiotic division), the cells of the embryo contain more than two multiples of the haploid number of chromosomes (**polyploidy**).

Chromosomal abnormalities are the underlying cause of a high percentage of spontaneous abortions during the early weeks of pregnancy. Over 75% of the spontaneous abortions occurring before the second week and over 60% of those occurring during the first half of pregnancy contain chromosomal abnormalities ranging from trisomies of individual chromosomes to overall polyploidy. Although the incidence of chromosomal anomalies declines with stillbirths occurring after the fifth month of pregnancy, it is close to 6%, a tenfold higher incidence over the 0.5% of living infants who are born with chromosomal anomalies. In counseling patients who have had a stillbirth or a spontaneous abortion, it can be useful to mention that this is often nature's way of handling an embryo destined to be highly abnormal.

around the developing follicle after it has become two to three cell layers thick. Known initially as the **theca folliculi**, this covering ultimately differentiates into two layers: a highly vascularized and glandular **theca interna** and a more connective tissue–like outer capsule called the **theca externa**. The early thecal cells secrete an **angiogenesis factor**, which stimulates the growth of blood vessels in the thecal layer. This nutritive support facilitates growth of the follicle.

Early development of the follicle occurs without the significant influence of hormones, but as puberty approaches, continued follicular maturation requires the action of the pituitary gonadotrophic hormone **follicle-stimulating hormone (FSH)** on the granulosa cells, which

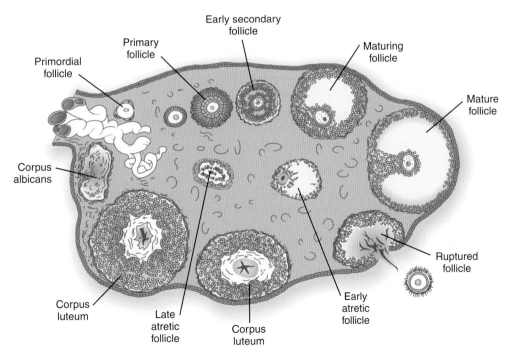

**FIGURE 1-8** The sequence of maturation of follicles within the ovary, starting with the primordial follicle and ending with the formation of a corpus albicans.

**FIGURE 1-9** Growth and maturation of a follicle along with major endocrine interactions in the theca cells and granulosa cells. *E,* Estrogen; *FSH,* follicle-stimulating hormone; *LH,* luteinizing hormone; *R,* receptor; *T,* testosterone.

have by this time developed FSH receptors on their surfaces (see Figure 1-9). After blood-borne FSH is bound to the FSH receptors, the stimulated granulosa cells produce small amounts of **estrogens**. The most obvious indication of the further development of some of the follicles is the formation of an **antrum**, a cavity filled with a fluid called **liquor folliculi**. Initially formed by secretions of the follicular cells, the antral fluid is later formed mostly as a transudate from the capillaries on the outer side of the membrana granulosa. With the appearance of the antrum, the follicle is called a **secondary follicle**.

Enlargement of the follicle results in large part from the proliferation of granulosa cells. The direct stimulus for granulosa cell proliferation is a locally produced signaling protein, **activin**, a member of the **transforming growth factor-β** family of signaling molecules (see Table 4-1). The local action of activin is enhanced by the actions of FSH.

Responding to the stimulus of pituitary hormones, secondary follicles produce significant amounts of steroid hormones. The cells of the theca interna possess receptors for **luteinizing hormone (LH)**, also secreted by the anterior pituitary (see Figure 1-14). The theca interna cells produce **androgens** (e.g., testosterone), which pass through the membrana granulosa to the granulosa cells. The influence of FSH induces the granulosa cells to synthesize the enzyme (**aromatase**) that converts the theca-derived androgens into estrogens (mainly 17β-estradiol). Not only does the estradiol leave the follicle to exert important effects on other parts of the body, but it also stimulates the formation of LH receptors on the granulosa cells. Through this mechanism, the follicular cells are able to respond to the large LH surge that immediately precedes ovulation (see Figure 1-15).

Under multiple hormonal influences, the follicle enlarges rapidly (Figures 1-9 and 1-10) and presses against the surface of the ovary. At this point, it is called a **tertiary (graafian) follicle**. About 10 to 12 hours before ovulation, meiosis resumes.

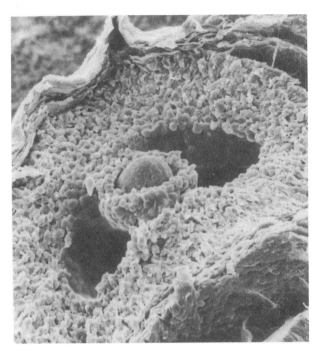

**FIGURE 1-10** Scanning electron micrograph of a mature follicle in the rat ovary. The spherical oocyte *(center)* is surrounded by smaller cells of the corona radiata, which projects into the antrum. (×840.) (Courtesy P. Bagavandoss, Ann Arbor, Michigan.)

The egg, now a secondary oocyte, is located in a small mound of cells known as the **cumulus oophorus**, which lies on one side of the greatly enlarged antrum. The oocyte appears to secrete a factor or factors that pass through the gap junctions into the surrounding cumulus cells. The factor enables the cumulus cells to respond to gonadotrophic hormones and to secrete hyaluronic acid, which results in an expansion of the cumulus oophorus. In keeping with the hormonally induced internal changes, the diameter of the follicle increases from about 6 mm early in the second week to almost 2 cm at ovulation.

The tertiary follicle protrudes from the surface of the ovary like a blister. The granulosa cells contain large numbers of both FSH and LH receptors, and LH receptors are abundant in the cells of the theca interna. The follicular cells secrete large amounts of estradiol (see Figure 1-15), which prepares many other components of the female reproductive tract for gamete transport. Within the antrum, the follicular fluid contains (1) a complement of proteins similar to that seen in serum but in a lower concentration; (2) as many as 20 enzymes; (3) dissolved hormones, including FSH, LH, and steroids; and (4) proteoglycans. The strong negative charge of the proteoglycans attracts water molecules, and with greater amounts of secreted proteoglycans, the volume of antral fluid increases correspondingly. The follicle is now poised for ovulation and awaits the stimulus of the preovulatory surge of FSH and LH released by the anterior pituitary gland.

The reason only one follicle normally matures to the point of ovulation is still not completely understood. Early in the cycle, as many as 50 follicles begin to develop, but only about 3 attain a diameter as great as 8 mm. Initial follicular growth is gonadotropin independent, but continued growth depends on a minimum "tonic" level of gonadotropins, principally FSH. During the phase of gonadotropin-induced growth, one dominant enlarging follicle becomes independent of FSH and secretes large amounts of **inhibin** (see p. 21). Inhibin suppresses the secretion of FSH by the pituitary, and when the FSH levels fall below the tonic threshold, the other developing follicles, which are still dependent on FSH for maintenance, become atretic. The dominant follicle acquires its status about 7 days before ovulation. It may also secrete an inhibiting substance that acts directly on the other growing follicles.

## Spermatogenesis

**Spermatogenesis** begins in the seminiferous tubules of the testes after the onset of puberty. In the broadest sense, the process begins with mitotic proliferation of the spermatogonia. At the base of the **seminiferous epithelium** are several populations of spermatogonia. **Type A spermatogonia** represent the stem cell population that mitotically maintains proper numbers of spermatogonia throughout life. Type A spermatogonia give rise to **type B spermatogonia**, which are destined to leave the mitotic cycle and enter meiosis. Many spermatogonia and their cellular descendants are connected by intercellular cytoplasmic bridges, which may be instrumental in maintaining the synchronous development of large clusters of sperm cells.

All spermatogonia are sequestered at the base of the seminiferous epithelium by interlocking processes of **Sertoli cells**, which are very complex cells that are regularly distributed throughout the periphery of the seminiferous epithelium and that occupy about 30% of its volume (see Figure 1-6). As the progeny of the type B spermatogonia (called *primary spermatocytes*) complete the leptotene stage of the first meiotic division, they pass through the Sertoli cell barrier to the interior of the seminiferous tubule. This translocation is accomplished by the formation of a new layer of Sertoli cell processes beneath these cells and slightly later, the dissolution of the original layer that was between them and the interior of the seminiferous tubule. The Sertoli cell processes are very tightly joined and form an immunological barrier (**blood-testis barrier** [see Figure 1-6]) between the forming sperm cells and the rest of the body, including the spermatogonia. Once they have begun meiosis, developing sperm cells are immunologically different from the rest of the body. Autoimmune infertility can arise if the blood-testis barrier is broken down.

The progeny of the type B spermatogonia, which have entered the first meiotic division, are the **primary**

**spermatocytes** (see Figure 1-6). Located in a characteristic position just inside the layer of spermatogonia and still deeply embedded in Sertoli cell cytoplasm, primary spermatocytes spend 24 days passing through the first meiotic division. During this time, the developing sperm cells use a strategy similar to that of the egg: namely, producing in advance molecules that are needed at later periods when changes occur very rapidly. Such preparation involves the production of mRNA molecules and their storage in an inactive form until they are needed to produce the necessary proteins.

A well-known example of preparatory mRNA synthesis involves the formation of **protamines**, which are small, arginine- and cysteine-rich proteins that displace the lysine-rich nuclear histones and allow the high degree of compaction of nuclear chromatin required during the final stages of sperm formation. Protamine mRNAs are first synthesized in primary spermatocytes but are not translated into proteins until the spermatid stage. In the meantime, the protamine mRNAs are complexed with proteins and are inaccessible to the translational machinery. If protamine mRNAs are translated before the

spermatid stage, the chromosomes condense prematurely and sterility results.

After completion of the first meiotic division, the primary spermatocyte gives rise to two **secondary spermatocytes**, which remain connected by a cytoplasmic bridge. The secondary spermatocytes enter the second meiotic division without delay. This phase of meiosis is very rapid, typically completed in approximately 8 hours. Each secondary spermatocyte produces two immature haploid gametes, the **spermatids**. The four spermatids produced from a primary spermatocyte progenitor are still connected to one another and typically to as many as 100 other spermatids as well. In mice, some genes are transcribed as late as the spermatid stage.

Spermatids do not divide further, but they undergo a series of profound changes that transform them from relatively ordinary looking cells to highly specialized **spermatozoa** (singular, **spermatozoon**). The process of transformation from spermatids to spermatozoa is called **spermiogenesis** or **spermatid metamorphosis**.

Several major categories of change occur during spermiogenesis (Figure 1-11). One is the progressive

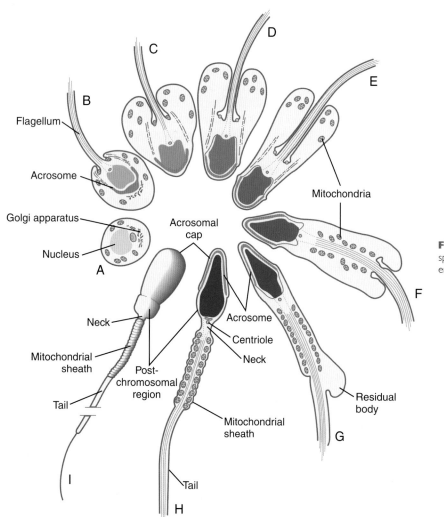

**FIGURE 1-11** Summary of the major stages in spermiogenesis, starting with a spermatid **(A)** and ending with a mature spermatozoon **(I)**.

reduction in the size of the nucleus and tremendous condensation of the chromosomal material, which is associated with the replacement of histones by protamines. Along with the changes in the nucleus, a profound reorganization of the cytoplasm occurs. Cytoplasm streams away from the nucleus, but a condensation of the Golgi apparatus at the apical end of the nucleus ultimately gives rise to the **acrosome**. The acrosome is an enzyme-filled structure that plays a very important role in the fertilization process. At the other end of the nucleus, a prominent **flagellum** grows out of the centriolar region. **Mitochondria** are arranged in a spiral around the proximal part of the flagellum. During spermiogenesis, the plasma membrane of the head of the sperm is partitioned into a number of antigenically distinct molecular domains. These domains undergo numerous changes as the sperm cells mature in the male and at a later point when the spermatozoa are traveling through the female reproductive tract. As spermiogenesis continues, the remainder of the cytoplasm (**residual body** [Figure 1-11, G]) moves away from the nucleus and is shed along the developing tail of the sperm cell. The residual bodies are phagocytized by Sertoli cells.

For many years, gene expression in postmeiotic (haploid) spermatids was considered to be impossible. However, molecular biological research on mice has shown that gene expression in postmeiotic spermatids is not only possible but common. Nearly 100 proteins that are produced only after the completion of the second meiotic division have been identified, and many additional proteins are synthesized both during and after meiosis (Figure 1-12).

After spermiogenesis (approximately 64 days after the start of spermatogenesis), the **spermatozoon** is a highly specialized cell well adapted for motion and the delivery of its packet of DNA to the egg. The sperm cell consists of a head (2 to 3 μm wide and 4 to 5 μm long) containing the nucleus and acrosome; a midpiece containing the centrioles, the proximal part of the flagellum, and the mitochondrial helix; and the tail (about 50 μm long), which consists of a highly specialized flagellum (see Figure 1-11). (Specific functional properties of these components of the sperm cell are discussed in Chapter 2.)

Although spermatozoa in the seminiferous tubules appear to be mature by morphological criteria, they are nonmotile and incapable of fertilizing an egg. From the

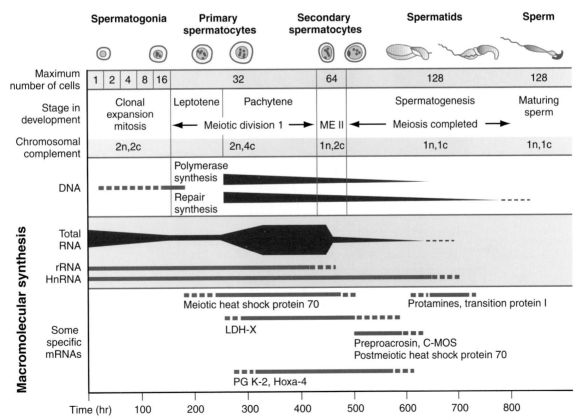

**FIGURE 1-12** Summary of the major events in spermatogenesis in the mouse, with specific examples of macromolecular synthesis superimposed. The solid lines represent qualitative periods of known synthesis. Broken segments in the lines represent uncertainty about the onset or duration of the activity. Bars with varying thicknesses represent relative amounts of the gene product that is represented. *LDH-X*, Lactic dehydrogenase; *ME II*, second meiotic division. (Modified from Erickson RP: *Trends Genet* 6:264–269, 1990.)

testis, they are carried to the **epididymis** via fluid currents that originate in the seminiferous tubules. While in transit through the epididymis, the spermatozoa undergo biochemical maturation, becoming covered with a glycoprotein coating and experiencing other surface modifications. The glycoprotein coating is removed in the female reproductive tract through the **capacitation** reaction, which renders the spermatozoa capable of fertilizing an egg. Further biochemical maturation and provision of the spermatozoa with an external energy source occur when the ejaculated sperm are mixed with secretions of the **prostate gland** and **seminal vesicles** during ejaculation. At this point, the spermatozoa are provided with an environment conducive to independent motion.

### Abnormal Spermatozoa

Substantial numbers (up to 10%) of mature spermatozoa are grossly abnormal. The spectrum of anomalies ranges from double heads or tails to defective flagella or variability in head size. Such defective sperm cells are highly unlikely to fertilize an egg. If the percentage of defective spermatozoa rises above 20% of the total, reduced fertility may result.

## PREPARATION OF THE FEMALE REPRODUCTIVE TRACT FOR PREGNANCY

### Structure

The structure and function of the female reproductive tract are well adapted for the transport of gametes and maintenance of the embryo. Many of the subtler features of this adaptation are under hormonal control and are cyclic. This section briefly reviews the aspects of female reproductive structure that are of greatest importance in understanding gamete transport and embryonic development.

### Ovaries and Uterine Tubes

The **ovaries** and **uterine** (or **fallopian**) **tubes** form a functional complex devoted to the production and transport of eggs. The almond-shaped ovaries, located on either side of the uterus, are positioned very near the open, funnel-shaped ends of the uterine tubes. Numerous small, fingerlike projections called **fimbriae** (Figure 1-13)

**FIGURE 1-13** Structure of the female reproductive tract.

project from the open **infundibulum** of the uterine tube toward the ovary and are involved in directing the ovulated egg into the tube. The uterine tube is characterized by a very complex internal lining with a high density of prominent longitudinal folds in the upper **ampulla** and a simpler lining nearer the uterus. The lining epithelium of the uterine tubes contains a mixture of ciliated cells that assist in gamete transport and secretory cells that produce a fluid supporting early development of the embryo. Layers of smooth muscle throughout the uterine tubes provide the basis for peristaltic contractions. The amount and function of many of these components are under cyclic hormonal control, and the overall effect of these changes is to facilitate the transport of gametes and the fertilized egg.

## Uterus

The principal functions of the uterus are to receive and maintain the embryo during pregnancy and to expel the fetus at the termination of pregnancy. The first function is carried out by the uterine mucosa (endometrium) and the second by the muscular wall (myometrium). Under the cyclic effect of hormones, the uterus undergoes a series of prominent changes throughout the course of each menstrual cycle.

The **uterus** is a pear-shaped organ with thick walls of smooth muscle (**myometrium**) and a complex mucosal lining (see Figure 1-13). The mucosal lining, called the **endometrium**, has a structure that changes daily throughout the menstrual cycle. The endometrium can be subdivided into two layers: a **functional layer** that is shed with each menstrual period or after parturition and a **basal layer** that remains intact. The general structure of the endometrium consists of (1) a columnar **surface epithelium**, (2) **uterine glands**, (3) a specialized connective tissue stroma, and (4) **spiral arteries** that coil from the basal layer toward the surface of the endometrium. All these structures participate in the implantation and nourishment of the embryo.

The lower outlet of the uterus is the **cervix**. The mucosal surface of the cervix is not typical uterine endometrium but is studded with a variety of irregular crypts. The cervical epithelium produces a glycoprotein-rich cervical mucus, the composition of which varies considerably throughout the menstrual cycle. The differing physical properties of cervical mucus make it easier or more difficult for spermatozoa to penetrate through the cervix and find their way into the uterus.

## Vagina

The **vagina** is a channel for sexual intercourse and also serves as the birth canal. It is lined with a stratified squamous epithelium, but the epithelial cells contain deposits of **glycogen**, which vary in amount throughout the menstrual cycle. Glycogen breakdown products contribute to the acidity (pH, 4.3) of the vaginal fluids. The low pH of the upper vagina serves a bacteriostatic function and prevents infectious agents from entering the upper genital tract through the cervix and ultimately spreading to the peritoneal cavity through the open ends of the uterine tubes.

## Hormonal Control of the Female Reproductive Cycle

Reproduction in the human female is governed by a complex series of interactions between hormones and the tissues that they influence. The hierarchy of cyclic control begins with input to the **hypothalamus** of the brain (Figure 1-14). The hypothalamus influences hormone production by the anterior lobe of the pituitary gland. The pituitary hormones are spread via the blood throughout the entire body and act on the ovaries, which are in turn stimulated to produce their own sex steroid hormones. During pregnancy, the placenta exerts a powerful effect on the mother by producing a number of hormones. The final level of hormonal control of female reproduction is that exerted by the ovarian or placental hormones on other reproductive target organs (e.g., uterus, uterine tubes, vagina, breasts).

## Hypothalamic Control

The first level of hormonal control of reproduction resides in the hypothalamus. Various inputs stimulate neurosecretory cells in the hypothalamus to produce **gonadotropin-releasing hormone (GnRH)**, along with releasing factors for other pituitary hormones. Releasing factors as well as an inhibiting factor are carried to the anterior lobe of the pituitary gland by blood vessels of the **hypothalamohypophyseal portal system**, where they stimulate the secretion of pituitary hormones (Table 1-1).

## Pituitary Gland (Hypophysis)

Producing its hormones in response to stimulation by the hypothalamus, the **pituitary gland** constitutes a second level of hormonal control of reproduction. The pituitary gland consists of two components: the **anterior pituitary (adenohypophysis)**, an epithelial glandular structure that produces various hormones in response to factors carried to it by the hypothalamohypophyseal portal system, and the **posterior pituitary (neurohypophysis)**, a neural structure that releases hormones by a neurosecretory mechanism.

Under the influence of GnRH and direct feedback by steroid hormone levels in the blood, the anterior pituitary secretes two polypeptide **gonadotrophic hormones**, FSH and LH, from the same cell type (see Table 1-1). In the

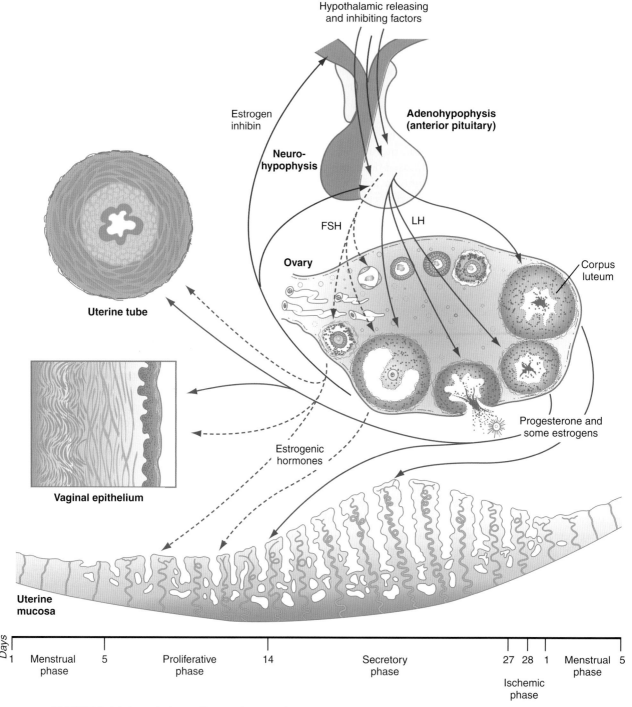

Hypothalamic releasing
and inhibiting factors

Estrogen
inhibin

**Adenohypophysis
(anterior pituitary)**

**Neuro-
hypophysis**

FSH          LH

**Ovary**

Corpus
luteum

Progesterone and
some estrogens

Estrogenic
hormones

**Uterine tube**

**Vaginal epithelium**

**Uterine
mucosa**

| *Days* | | | | | | | |
|---|---|---|---|---|---|---|---|
| 1 | 5 | | 14 | | 27 28 1 | | 5 |
| Menstrual phase | | Proliferative phase | | Secretory phase | | Menstrual phase | |
| | | | | | Ischemic phase | | |

**FIGURE 1-14** General scheme of hormonal control of reproduction in the female. Inhibitory factors are represented by purple arrows. Stimulatory factors are represented by red arrows. Hormones involved principally in the proliferative phase of the menstrual cycle are represented by dashed arrows; those involved principally in the secretory phase are solid.

absence of an inhibiting factor (**dopamine**) from the hypothalamus, the anterior pituitary also produces **prolactin**, which acts on the mammary glands.

The only hormone from the posterior pituitary that is directly involved in reproduction is **oxytocin**, an oligopeptide involved in childbirth and the stimulus for milk let-down from the mammary glands in lactating women.

## Ovaries and Placenta

The ovaries and, during pregnancy, the placenta constitute a third level of hormonal control. Responding to blood levels of the anterior pituitary hormones, the granulosa cells of the ovarian follicles convert androgens (**androstenedione** and **testosterone**) synthesized by the theca interna into estrogens (mainly **estrone** and the

| TABLE I-I *Major Hormones Involved in Mammalian Reproduction* | | |
|---|---|---|
| **Hormone** | **Chemical nature** | **Function** |
| **HYPOTHALAMUS** | | |
| Gonadotropin-releasing hormone (GnRH, LHRH) | Decapeptide | Stimulates release of LH and FSH by anterior pituitary |
| Prolactin-inhibiting factor | Dopamine | Inhibits release of prolactin by anterior pituitary |
| **ANTERIOR PITUITARY** | | |
| Follicle-stimulating hormone (FSH) | Glycoprotein ($\alpha$ and $\beta$ subunits) (MW, ~35,000) | Male: Stimulates Sertoli cells to produce androgen-binding protein<br>Female: Stimulates follicle cells to produce estrogen |
| Luteinizing hormone (LH) | Glycoprotein ($\alpha$ and $\beta$ subunits) (MW, ~28,000) | Male: Stimulates Leydig cells to secrete testosterone<br>Female: Stimulates follicle cells and corpus luteum to produce progesterone |
| Prolactin | Single-chain polypeptide (198 amino acids) | Promotes lactation |
| **POSTERIOR PITUITARY** | | |
| Oxytocin | Oligopeptide (MW, ~1100) | Stimulates ejection of milk by mammary gland |
| **OVARY** | | |
| Estrogens | Steroid | Has multiple effects on reproductive tract, breasts, body fat, and bone growth |
| Progesterone | Steroid | Has multiple effects on reproductive tract and breast development |
| Testosterone | Steroid | Is precursor for estrogen biosynthesis, induces follicular atresia |
| Inhibin | Protein (MW, ~32,000) | Inhibits FSH secretion, has local effects on ovaries |
| Activin | Protein (MW, ~28,000) | Stimulates granulosa cell proliferation |
| **TESTIS** | | |
| Testosterone | Steroid | Has multiple effects on male reproductive tract, hair growth, and other secondary sexual characteristics |
| Inhibin | Protein (MW, ~32,000) | Inhibits FSH secretion, has local effects on testis |
| **PLACENTA** | | |
| Estrogens | Steroid | Has same functions as ovarian estrogens |
| Progesterone | Steroid | Has same functions as ovarian progesterone |
| Human chorionic gonadotrophin (HCG) | Glycoprotein (MW, ~30,000) | Maintains activity of corpus luteum during pregnancy |
| Human placental lactogen (somatomammotropin) | Polypeptide (MW, ~20,000) | Promotes development of breasts during pregnancy |

*LHRH*, Luteinizing hormone–releasing hormone; *MW*, molecular weight.

tenfold more powerful **17β-estradiol**), which then pass into the bloodstream. After ovulation, **progesterone** is the principal secretory product of the follicle after its conversion into the corpus luteum (see Chapter 2). During later pregnancy, the placenta supplements the production of ovarian steroid hormone by synthesizing its own estrogens and progesterone. It also produces two polypeptide hormones (see Table 1-1). **Human chorionic gonadotropin (HCG)** acts on the ovary to maintain the activity of the corpus luteum during pregnancy. **Human placental lactogen (somatomammotropin)** acts on the corpus luteum; it also promotes breast development by enhancing the effects of estrogens and progesterone and stimulates the synthesis of milk constituents.

### Reproductive Target Tissues

The last level in the hierarchy of reproductive hormonal control constitutes the target tissues, which ready themselves both structurally and functionally for gamete transport or pregnancy in response to ovarian and placental hormones binding to specific cellular receptors. Changes in the number of ciliated cells and in smooth muscle activity in the uterine tubes, the profound changes in the endometrial lining of the uterus, and the cyclic changes in the glandular tissues of the breasts are some of the more prominent examples of hormonal effects on target tissues. These changes are described more fully later.

A general principle recognized some time ago is the efficacy of first priming reproductive target tissues with estrogen so that progesterone can exert its full effects. Estrogen induces the target cells to produce large quantities of progesterone receptors, which must be in place for progesterone to act on these same cells.

## Hormonal Interactions with Tissues During Female Reproductive Cycles

All tissues of the female reproductive tract are influenced by the reproductive hormones. In response to the hormonal environment of the body, they undergo cyclic modifications that improve the chances for successful reproduction.

Knowledge of the changes the ovaries undergo is necessary to understand hormonal interactions and tissue responses during the female reproductive cycle. Responding to both FSH and LH secreted by the pituitary just before and during a menstrual period, a set of secondary ovarian follicles begins to mature and secrete 17β-estradiol. By ovulation, all of these follicles except one have undergone atresia, their main contribution having been to produce part of the supply of estrogens needed to prepare the body for ovulation and gamete transport.

During the preovulatory, or **proliferative, phase** (days 5 to 14) of the menstrual cycle, estrogens produced by the ovary act on the female reproductive tissues (see Figure 1-14). The uterine lining becomes reepithelialized from the just-completed menstrual period. Then, under the influence of estrogens, the endometrial stroma progressively thickens, the uterine glands elongate, and the spiral arteries begin to grow toward the surface of the endometrium. The mucous glands of the cervix secrete a glycoprotein-rich but relatively watery mucus, which facilitates the passage of spermatozoa through the cervical canal. As the proliferative phase progresses, a higher percentage of the epithelial cells lining the uterine tubes becomes ciliated, and smooth muscle activity in the tubes

increases. In the days preceding ovulation, the fimbriated ends of the uterine tubes move closer to the ovaries.

Toward the end of the proliferative period, a pronounced increase in the levels of estradiol secreted by the developing ovarian follicle acts on the hypothalamohypophyseal system, causing increased responsiveness of the anterior pituitary to GnRH and a surge in the hypothalamic secretion of GnRH. Approximately 24 hours after the level of 17β-estradiol reaches its peak in the blood, a preovulatory surge of LH and FSH is sent into the bloodstream by the pituitary gland (Figure 1-15). The **LH surge** is not a steady increase in gonadotropin secretion; rather, it constitutes a series of sharp pulses of secretion that appear to be responding to a hypothalamic timing mechanism.

The LH surge leads to ovulation, and the graafian follicle becomes transformed into a **corpus luteum** (yellow body). The basal lamina surrounding the granulosa of the follicle breaks down and allows blood vessels to grow into

**FIGURE 1-15** Comparison of curves representing daily serum concentrations of gonadotropins and sex steroids and basal body temperature in relation to events in the human menstrual cycle. (Redrawn from Midgley AR and others. In Hafez ES, Evans TN, eds: *Human reproduction*, New York, 1973, Harper & Row.)

the layer of granulosa cells. Through proliferation and hypertrophy, the granulosa cells undergo major structural and biochemical changes and now produce progesterone as their primary secretory product. Some estrogen is still secreted by the corpus luteum. After ovulation, the menstrual cycle, which is now dominated by the secretion of progesterone, is said to be in the **secretory phase** (days 14 to 28 of the menstrual cycle).

After the LH surge and with the increasing concentration of progesterone in the blood, the basal body temperature rises (see Figure 1-15). Because of the link between a rise in basal body temperature and the time of ovulation, accurate temperature records are the basis of the **rhythm method** of birth control.

Around the time of ovulation, the combined presence of estrogen and progesterone in the blood causes the uterine tube to engage in a rhythmic series of muscular contractions designed to promote transport of the ovulated egg. Progesterone prompts epithelial cells of the uterine tube to secrete fluids that provide nutrition for the cleaving embryo. Later during the secretory phase, high levels of progesterone induce regression of some of the ciliated cells in the tubal epithelium.

In the uterus, progesterone prepares the estrogen-primed endometrium for implantation of the embryo. The endometrium, which has thickened under the influence of estrogen during the proliferative phase, undergoes further changes. The straight uterine glands begin to coil and accumulate glycogen and other secretory products in the epithelium. The spiral arteries grow farther toward the endometrial surface, but mitosis in the endometrial epithelial cells decreases. Through the action of progesterone, the cervical mucus becomes highly viscous and acts as a protective block, inhibiting the passage of materials into or out of the uterus. During the secretory period, the vaginal epithelium becomes thinner.

In the mammary glands, progesterone furthers the estrogen-primed development of the secretory components and causes water retention in the tissues. However, more extensive development of the lactational apparatus awaits its stimulation by placental hormones.

Midway through the secretory phase of the menstrual cycle, the epithelium of the uterine tubes has already undergone considerable regression from its midcycle peak, whereas the uterine endometrium is at full readiness to receive a cleaving embryo. If pregnancy does not occur, a series of hormonal interactions bring the menstrual cycle to a close. One of the early feedback mechanisms is the production of the protein **inhibin** by the granulosa cells. Inhibin is carried by the bloodstream to the anterior pituitary, where it directly inhibits the secretion of gonadotropins, especially FSH. Through mechanisms that are still unclear, the secretion of LH is also reduced. This inhibition results in regression of the corpus luteum and marked reduction in the secretion of progesterone by the ovary.

Some of the main consequences of the regression of the corpus luteum are the infiltration of the endometrial stroma with leukocytes, the loss of interstitial fluid, and the spasmodic constriction and breakdown of the spiral arteries, causing local ischemia. The ischemia results in local hemorrhage and the loss of integrity of areas of the endometrium. These changes initiate menstruation (by convention, constituting days 1 to 5 of the menstrual cycle). Over the next few days, the entire functional layer of the endometrium is shed in small bits, along with the attendant loss of about 30 ml of blood. By the time the menstrual period is over, only a raw endometrial base interspersed with the basal epithelium of the uterine glands remains as the basis for the healing and reconstitution of the endometrium during the next proliferative period.

## HORMONAL INTERACTIONS INVOLVED WITH REPRODUCTION IN MALES

Along with the homologies of certain structures between the testis and ovary, some strong parallels exist between the hormonal interactions involved in reproduction in males and females. The most important homologies are between granulosa cells in the ovarian follicle and Sertoli cells in the seminiferous tubule of the testis and between theca cells of the ovary and Leydig cells in the testis (Table 1-2).

The hypothalamic secretion of GnRH stimulates the anterior pituitary to secrete FSH and LH. The LH binds to the nearly 20,000 LH receptors on the surface of each Leydig (interstitial) cell, and through a cascade of second messengers, LH stimulates the synthesis of testosterone from cholesterol. Testosterone is released into the blood and is taken to the Sertoli cells and throughout the body, where it affects a variety of secondary sexual tissues, often after it has been locally converted to dihydrotestosterone.

### CLINICAL VIGNETTE

A 33-year-old woman has had both ovaries removed because of large bilateral ovarian cysts. The next year she is on an extended expedition in northern Canada, and her canoe tips, sending her replacement hormonal medication to the bottom of the lake. More than 6 weeks elapse before she is able to obtain a new supply of medication.

Which of the following would be least affected by the loss of the woman's medication?

A. Blood levels of FSH and LH
B. Ciliated cells of the uterine tube
C. Mass of the heart
D. Glandular tissue of the breasts
E. Thickness of the endometrium

Sertoli cells are stimulated by pituitary FSH via surface FSH receptors and by testosterone from the Leydig cells via cytoplasmic receptors. After FSH stimulation, the Sertoli cells convert some of the testosterone to estrogens (as the granulosa cells in the ovary do). Some of the estrogen diffuses back to the Leydig cells along with a **Leydig cell stimulatory factor**, which is produced by the Sertoli cells and reaches the Leydig cells by a **paracrine** (non–blood-borne) mode of secretion (Figure 1-16). The FSH-stimulated Sertoli cell produces **androgen-binding protein**, which binds testosterone and is carried into the fluid compartment of the seminiferous tubule, where it exerts a strong influence on the course of spermatogenesis. Like their granulosa cell counterparts in the ovary, the

| TABLE 1-2 *Homologies between Hormone-Producing Cells in Male and Female Gonads* | | | | |
|---|---|---|---|---|
| Parameter | Granulosa cells (female) | Sertoli cells (male) | Theca cells (female) | Leydig cells (male) |
| Origin | Rete ovarii | Rete testis | Stromal mesenchyme | Stromal mesenchyme |
| Major receptors | FSH | FSH | LH | LH |
| Major secretory products | Estrogens, progesterone, inhibin | Estrogen, inhibin, androgen-binding protein | Androgens | Testosterone |

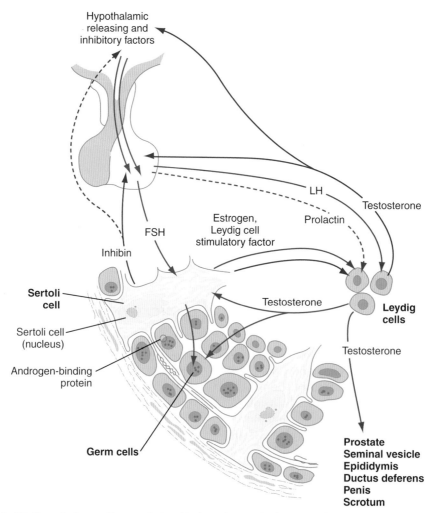

**FIGURE 1-16** General scheme of hormonal control in the male reproductive system. *Red arrows* represent stimulatory influences. *Purple arrows* represent inhibitory influences. Suspected interactions are represented by *dashed arrows.*

hormone-stimulated Sertoli cells produce inhibin, which is carried by the blood to the anterior pituitary and possibly the hypothalamus. There inhibin acts by negative feedback to inhibit the secretion of FSH. In addition to inhibin and androgen-binding protein, the Sertoli cells have a wide variety of other functions, the most important of which are summarized in Box 1-2.

## SUMMARY

○ Gametogenesis is divided into four phases:
  1. Extraembryonic origin of germ cells and their migration into the gonads
  2. An increase in the number of germ cells by mitosis
  3. A reduction in chromosomal material by meiosis
  4. Structural and functional maturation

○ Primordial germ cells are first readily recognizable in the yolk sac endoderm. They then migrate through the dorsal mesentery to the primordia of the gonads.

○ In the female, oogonia undergo intense mitotic activity in the embryo only. In the male, spermatogonia are capable of mitosis throughout life.

○ Meiosis involves a reduction in chromosome number from diploid to haploid, independent reassortment of paternal and maternal chromosomes, and further redistribution of genetic material through the process of crossing-over.

○ In the oocyte, there are two meiotic blocks—in diplotene of prophase I and in metaphase II. In the female, meiosis begins in the 5-month embryo; in the male, meiosis begins at puberty.

○ Failure of chromosomes to separate properly during meiosis results in nondisjunction, which is associated with

---

**Box 1-2  Major Functions of Sertoli Cells**

Maintenance of the blood-testis barrier
Secretion of tubular fluid (10 to 20 μL/gm of testis/hr)
Secretion of androgen-binding protein
Secretion of inhibin
Secretion of a wide variety of other proteins (e.g., growth factors, transferrin, retinal-binding protein, metal-binding proteins)
Maintenance and coordination of spermatogenesis
Phagocytosis of residual bodies of sperm cells

---

multiple anomalies depending on which chromosome is affected.

○ Developing oocytes are surrounded by layers of follicular cells and interact with them through gap junctions. When stimulated by pituitary hormones (e.g., FSH, LH), the follicular cells produce steroid hormones (estrogens and progesterone). The combination of oocyte and follicular (granulosa) cells is called a *follicle*. Under hormonal stimulation, certain follicles greatly increase in size, and each month, one of these follicles undergoes ovulation.

○ Spermatogenesis occurs in the testis and involves successive waves of mitosis of spermatogonia, meiosis of primary and secondary spermatocytes, and final maturation (spermiogenesis) of postmeiotic spermatids into spermatozoa. Functional maturation of spermatozoa occurs in the epididymis.

○ Female reproductive tissues undergo cyclic, hormonally induced preparatory changes for pregnancy. In the uterine tubes, this involves the degree of ciliation of the epithelium and smooth muscle activity of the wall. Under the influence of estrogens and then progesterone, the endometrium of the uterus builds up in preparation to receive the embryo. In the absence of fertilization and with the subsequent withdrawal of hormonal support, the endometrium breaks down and is shed (menstruation). Cyclic changes in the cervix involve thinning of the cervical mucus at the time of ovulation.

○ Hormonal control of the female reproductive cycle is hierarchical, with releasing or inhibiting factors from the hypothalamus acting on the adenohypophysis, causing the release of pituitary hormones (e.g., FSH, LH). The pituitary hormones sequentially stimulate the ovarian follicles to produce estrogens and progesterone, which act on the female reproductive tissues. In pregnancy, the remains of the follicle (corpus luteum) continue to produce progesterone, which maintains the early embryo until the placenta begins to produce sufficient hormones to maintain pregnancy.

○ In the male, LH stimulates the Leydig cells to produce testosterone, and FSH acts on the Sertoli cells, which support spermatogenesis. In both the male and the female, feedback inhibition decreases the production of pituitary hormones.

○ There are two systems for dating pregnancy:
  1. Fertilization age: dates the age of the embryo from the time of fertilization.
  2. Menstrual age: dates the age of the embryo from the start of the mother's last menstrual period. The menstrual age is 2 weeks greater than the fertilization age.

---

**CLINICAL CORRELATION 1-2**

## Dating of Pregnancy

Two different systems for dating pregnancies have evolved. One, used by embryologists, dates pregnancy from the time of fertilization (**fertilization age**), so that a 6-week-old embryo is 6 weeks (42 days) from the day of fertilization. The other system, used by obstetricians and many clinicians, dates pregnancy from the woman's last menstrual period (**menstrual age**) because this is a convenient reference point from the standpoint of a history taken from a patient. The menstrual age of a human embryo is 2 weeks greater than the fertilization age because usually 2 weeks elapse between the start of the last menstrual period and fertilization. Thus an embryo with a fertilization age of 6 weeks is assigned a menstrual age of 8 weeks, and the typical duration of pregnancy is 38 weeks' fertilization age and 40 weeks' menstrual age (Figure 1-17; see also Figure 18-16).

For valid clinical reasons, obstetricians subdivide pregnancy into three equal **trimesters**, whereas embryologists divide pregnancy into unequal periods corresponding to major developmental events.

0–3 weeks   Early development (cleavage, gastrulation)
4–8 weeks   Period of embryonic organogenesis
9–38 weeks  Fetal period

A recognition of the existence of different systems for dating pregnancy is essential. In a courtroom case involving a lawsuit about a birth defect, a 2-week misunderstanding about the date of a pregnancy could make the difference between winning or losing the case. In a case involving a cleft lip or cleft palate (see p. 336), the difference in development of the face between 6 and 8 weeks (see Figure 14-5) would make some scenarios impossible. For example, an insult at 6 weeks could potentially be the cause of a cleft lip, whereas by 8 weeks, the lips have formed, so a cleft would be most unlikely to form at that time.

**FIGURE 1-17** Comparison between dating events in pregnancy by the fertilization age and the menstrual age.

---

## Review Questions

1. During spermatogenesis, histone is replaced by what to allow better packing of the condensed chromatin in the head of the spermatozoon?
   A. Inhibin
   B. Prostaglandin E
   C. Testosterone
   D. Protamine
   E. Androgen-binding protein

2. Which cell type is located outside the blood-testis barrier?
   A. Spermatozoon
   B. Secondary spermatocyte
   C. Spermatid
   D. Primary spermatocyte
   E. Spermatogonium

3. Which of the following cells normally participates in mitotic divisions?
   A. Primary oocyte
   B. Oogonium
   C. Primary spermatocyte
   D. Spermatid
   E. Secondary spermatocyte

4. In a routine chest x-ray examination, the radiologist sees what appear to be teeth in a mediastinal mass. What is the likely diagnosis, and what is a probable embryological explanation for its appearance?

5. When does meiosis begin in the female and in the male?

6. At what stages of oogenesis is meiosis arrested in the female?

7. What is the underlying cause of most spontaneous abortions during the early weeks of pregnancy?

8. What is the difference between spermatogenesis and spermiogenesis?

9. The actions of what hormones are responsible for the changes in the endometrium during the menstrual cycle?

10. Sertoli cells in the testis are stimulated by what two major reproductive hormones?

## REFERENCES

Abou-Haila A, Tulsiani DRP: Mammalian sperm acrosome: formation, contents, and function, *Arch Biochem Biophys* 379:173–182, 2000.

Bellve AR, ed: The Male Germ Cell: Migration to Fertilization, *Seminars Cell Devel Biol* 9:379–489, 1998.

Browder LW, ed: *Developmental biology*, vol 1, *Oogenesis*, New York, 1985, Plenum.

Clermont Y: The cycle of the seminiferous epithelium in man, *Am J Anat* 112:35–51, 1963.

Dym M: Spermatogonial stem cells of the testis, *Proc Natl Acad Sci USA* 91:11287–11289, 1994.

Eddy EM and others: Origin and migration of primordial germ cells in mammals, *Gamete Res* 4:333–362, 1981.

Eppig JJ: Intercommunication between mammalian oocytes and companion somatic cells, *Bioessays* 13:569–574, 1991.

Erickson RP: Post-meiotic gene expression, *Trends Genet* 6(8):264–269, 1990.

Fawcett DW: *A textbook of histology*, Philadelphia, 1986, WB Saunders.

Filicori M: The role of luteinizing hormone in folliculogenesis and ovulation induction, *Fertil Steril* 71:405–414, 1999.

Gilbert EF, Opitz JM: Developmental and other pathological changes in syndromes caused by chromosome anomalies, *Perspect Pediatr Pathol* 7:1–63, 1982.

Grootegoed JA, Siep M, Baarends WM: Molecular and cellular mechanisms in spermatogenesis, *Baillere's Clin Endocrinol Metabol* 14:331–343, 2000.

Gougeon A: Regulation of ovarian follicular development in primates: facts and hypotheses, *Endocr Rev* 17:121–155, 1996.

Halvorson LM, DeCherney AH: Inhibin, activin, and follistatin in reproductive medicine, *Fertil Steril* 65:459–469, 1996.

Kerr JB: Functional cytology of the human testis, *Bailleres Clin Endocrinol Metab* 6(2):235–250, 1992.

Knobil E, Neill JD, eds: *The physiology of reproduction*, ed 2, New York, 1994, Raven.

Larson WJ and others: Expansion of the cumulus-oocyte complex during the preovulatory period: possible roles in oocyte maturation, ovulation, and fertilization. In Familiari G, Makabe S, Motta PM, eds: *Ultrastructure of the ovary*, Boston, 1991, Kluwer Academic, pp 45–61.

Mather JP, Moore A, Li R-H: Activins, inhibins, and follistatins: further thoughts on a growing family of regulators, *Proc Soc Exp Biol Med* 215:209–222, 1997.

Mehlmann LM, Jones TLZ, Jaffe LA: Meiotic arrest in the mouse follicle maintained by a $G_s$ protein in the oocyte, *Science* 297:1343–1345, 2002.

Moodbidri SB, Garde SV, Sheth AR: Inhibin: unity in diversity, *Arch Androl* 28:149–157, 1992.

Salustri A and others: Oocyte-granulosa cell interactions. In Adashi EY, Leung PCK, eds: *The ovary*, New York, 1993, Raven, pp 209–225.

Shoham Z and others: The luteinizing hormone surge: the final stage in ovulation induction: modern aspects of ovulation triggering, *Fertil Steril* 64:237–251, 1995.

Taieb F, Thibier C, Jessus C: On cyclins, oocytes and eggs, *Mol Reprod Devel* 48:397–411, 1997.

Verhoeven G: Local control systems within the testis, *Bailleres Clin Endocrinol Metab* 6(2):313–333, 1992.

Willard HF: Centromeres of mammalian chromosomes, *Trends Genet* 6(12):410–416, 1990.

Wynn RM: *Biology of the uterus*, New York, 1977, Plenum.

Zamboni L: Physiology and pathophysiology of the human spermatozoon: the role of electron microscopy, *J Electron Microsc Tech* 17:412–436, 1991.

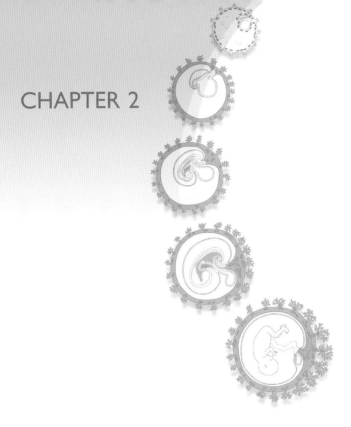

# CHAPTER 2

# Transport of Gametes and Fertilization

Chapter 1 describes the origins and maturation of male and female gametes and the hormonal conditions that make such maturation possible. It also describes the cyclic, hormonally controlled changes in the female reproductive tract that ready it for fertilization and the support of embryonic development. This chapter first explains the way the egg and sperm cells come together in the female reproductive tract so that fertilization can occur. It then outlines the complex set of interactions involved in fertilization of the egg by a sperm.

## OVULATION AND EGG AND SPERM TRANSPORT

### Ovulation

Toward the midpoint of the menstrual cycle, the mature graafian follicle, containing the egg that has been arrested in prophase of the first meiotic division, has moved to the surface of the ovary. Under the influence of follicle-stimulating hormone (FSH) and luteinizing hormone (LH), the follicle expands dramatically. The first meiotic division is completed, and the second meiotic division proceeds until the metaphase stage, at which the second meiotic arrest occurs. After the first meiotic division, the first polar body is expelled. By this point, the follicle bulges from the surface of the ovary. The apex of the protrusion is the **stigma**.

The stimulus for ovulation is the surge of LH secreted by the anterior pituitary at the midpoint of the menstrual cycle. Within minutes after the sharp rise in LH concentration in the blood, local blood flow increases in the outer layers of the follicular wall and throughout the ovary as well. Along with increased blood flow, plasma proteins leak into the tissues through the postcapillary venules, resulting in local edema. The edema and the release of a number of pharmacologically active compounds, such as prostaglandins, histamine, and vasopressin, provide the starting point for a series of reactions that result in the local production of **collagenase** (Figure 2-1). At the same time, the secretion of hyaluronic acid by the granulosa cells results in loosening of the granulosa layers. The collagen degradation, the ischemia, and the death of some of the overlying cells cause a weakness of the outer follicular wall. The weakened follicular wall, with possible contributions by the steady pressure of the antral fluid (about 15 to 20 mm Hg), and the contraction of local smooth muscle-like elements lead to rupture of the outer follicular wall about 28 to 36 hours after the LH surge.

Ovulation results in the expulsion of both antral fluid and the ovum from the ovary into the peritoneal cavity. The ovum, however, is not ovulated as a single naked cell but as a complex consisting of (1) the ovum, (2) the zona pellucida, (3) the two- to three-cell-thick corona radiata, and (4) a sticky matrix containing surrounding cells of the cumulus oophorus. By convention, the adhering cells are designated as **corona radiata** after ovulation has occurred.

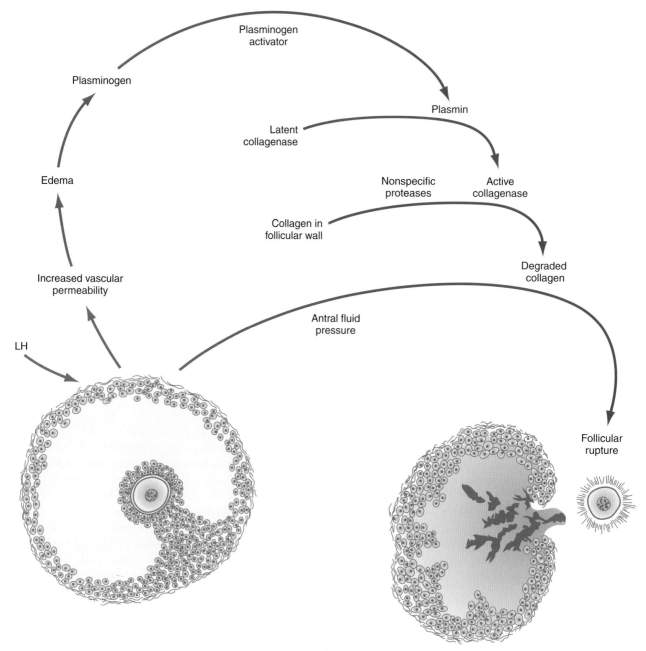

**FIGURE 2-1** Factors involved in mammalian ovulation. (Based on Lipner H. In Knobil E, Neill J, eds: *The physiology of reproduction*, vol 1, New York, 1988, Raven, pp 447–488.)

Normally, one egg is released at ovulation. The release and fertilization of two eggs can result in fraternal twinning.

Some women experience mild to pronounced pain at the time of ovulation. Often called **Mittelschmerz** (German for "middle pain"), such pain may accompany slight bleeding from the ruptured follicle. Another sign of ovulation is a slight rise in basal body temperature. This has often been used as a reference point in rhythm methods of contraception.

## Egg Transport

The first step in egg transport is capture of the ovulated egg by the uterine tube. Shortly before ovulation, the epithelial cells of the uterine tube become more highly ciliated, and smooth muscle activity in the tube and its suspensory ligament increases as the result of hormonal influences. By ovulation, the fimbriae of the uterine tube move closer to the ovary and seem to rhythmically sweep over its surface. This action, plus the currents set up by the cilia, efficiently captures the ovulated egg complex. Experimental studies on rabbits have shown that the bulk provided by the cellular coverings of the ovulated egg is important in facilitating the egg's capture and transport by the uterine tube. Denuded ova or inert objects of that size are not so readily transported. The human egg may rely less on its cellular coverings for transport than the egg of a rabbit. Capture of the egg complex by the uterine tube also appears to involve an adhesive interaction between the egg complex and the ciliary surface of the tube.

Even without these types of natural adaptations, the ability of the uterine tubes to capture eggs is remarkable. If the fimbriated end of the tube has been removed, egg capture occurs remarkably often, and pregnancies have even occurred in women who have had one ovary and the contralateral uterine tube removed. In such cases, the ovulated egg would have to travel free in the pelvic cavity for a considerable distance before entering the ostium of the uterine tube on the other side.

Once inside the uterine tube, the egg is transported toward the uterus, mainly as the result of contractions of the smooth musculature of the tubal wall. Although the cilia lining the tubal mucosa may also play a role in egg

transport, their action is not obligatory because women with **immotile cilia syndrome** are normally fertile.

While in the uterine tube, the egg is bathed in **tubal fluid**, which is a combination of secretion by the tubal epithelial cells and transudate from capillaries just below the epithelium. In some mammals, exposure to oviductal secretions is important to the survival of the ovum and for modifying the composition of the zona pellucida, but the role of tubal fluid in humans is less clear.

Tubal transport of the egg usually takes 3 to 4 days, regardless of whether fertilization occurs (Figure 2-2). Egg transport typically occurs in two phases: slow transport in the ampulla (approximately 72 hours) and a more rapid phase (8 hours) during which the egg or embryo passes through the isthmus and into the uterus (see p. 53). By a poorly understood mechanism, possibly local edema or reduced muscular activity, the egg is temporarily prevented from entering the isthmic portion of the tube, but under the influence of progesterone, the uterotubal junction relaxes and permits entry of the ovum.

By roughly 80 hours after ovulation, the ovulated egg or embryo has passed from the uterine tube into the uterus. If fertilization has not occurred, the egg

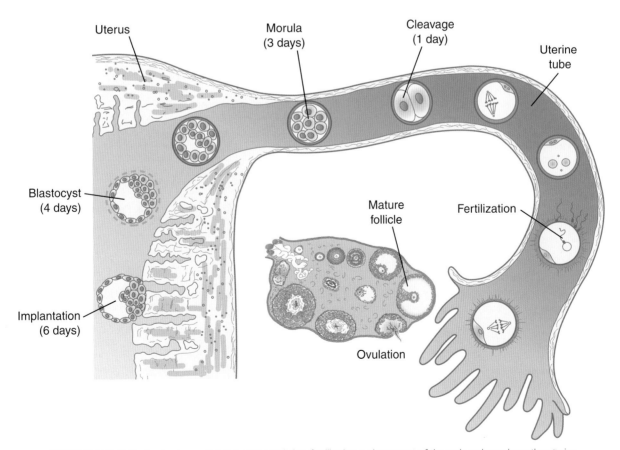

**FIGURE 2-2** Follicular development in the ovary, ovulation, fertilization, and transport of the early embryo down the uterine tube and into the uterus.

degenerates and is phagocytized. (Implantation of the embryo is discussed in Chapter 3.)

## Sperm Transport

Sperm transport occurs in both the male and the female. In the male, transport of spermatozoa is closely connected with their structural and functional maturation, whereas in the female reproductive tract, it is important for as many spermatozoa as possible to pass quickly to the upper uterine tube, where they can meet the ovulated egg.

After spermiogenesis in the seminiferous tubules, the spermatozoa are morphologically mature but are nonmotile and incapable of fertilizing an egg (Figure 2-3). Spermatozoa are passively transported via testicular fluid from the seminiferous tubules to the caput (head) of the epididymis through the rete testis and the efferent ductules. They are propelled by fluid pressure generated in the seminiferous tubules and are assisted by smooth muscle contractions and ciliary currents in the efferent ductules. Spermatozoa spend about 12 days in the highly convoluted duct of the epididymis, during which time they undergo biochemical maturation. This period of maturation is associated with changes in the glycoproteins in the plasma membrane of the sperm head. By the time the spermatozoa have reached the cauda

(tail) of the epididymis, they are capable of fertilizing an egg.

On ejaculation, the spermatozoa rapidly pass through the **ductus deferens** and become mixed with fluid secretions from the **seminal vesicles** and **prostate gland**. Prostatic fluid is rich in citric acid, acid phosphatase, zinc, and magnesium ions, whereas fluid of the seminal vesicle is rich in fructose (the principal energy source of spermatozoa) and prostaglandins. The 2 to 6 ml of ejaculate (**semen**, or **seminal fluid**) typically consists of 40 to 250 million spermatozoa mixed with alkaline fluid from the seminal vesicles (60% of the total) and acid secretion (pH, 6.5) from the prostate (30% of the total). The pH of normal semen is typically between 7.2 and 7.8. Despite the large number of spermatozoa normally present in an ejaculate, a number as small as 25 million per ejaculate may be compatible with fertility.

In the female, sperm transport begins in the upper vagina and ends in the ampulla of the uterine tube, where the spermatozoa make contact with the ovulated egg. During copulation, the seminal fluid is normally deposited in the upper vagina (see Figure 2-3), where its composition and buffering capacity immediately protect the spermatozoa from the acid fluid found in the upper vaginal area. The acidic vaginal fluid normally serves a bacteriocidal function in protecting the cervical canal from pathogenic organisms. Within about 10 seconds, the pH of the upper vagina is raised from 4.3 to as much

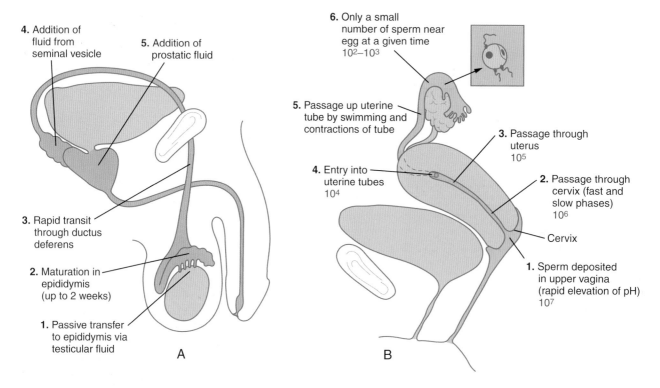

**FIGURE 2-3** Sperm transport in **(A)** the male and **(B)** the female reproductive tract. In **B,** numbers of spermatozoa typically found in various parts of the female reproductive tract are indicated in red.

as 7.2. The buffering effect lasts only a few minutes in humans but provides enough time for the spermatozoa to approach the cervix in an environment (pH, 6.0 to 6.5) optimal for sperm motility.

The next barrier that the sperm cells must overcome is the cervical canal and the cervical mucus that blocks it. Changes in intravaginal pressure may suck spermatozoa into the cervical os, but swimming movements also appear to be important for most spermatozoa in penetrating the cervical mucus.

The composition and viscosity of cervical mucus vary considerably throughout the menstrual cycle. Composed of **cervical mucin** (a glycoprotein with a high carbohydrate composition) and soluble components, cervical mucus is not readily penetrable. However, between days 9 and 16 of the cycle, its water content increases, which facilitates the passage of sperm through the cervix around the time of ovulation; such mucus is sometimes called **E mucus**. After ovulation, under the influence of progesterone, the production of watery cervical mucus ceases, and a new type of sticky mucus, which has a much decreased water content, is produced. This progestational mucus, sometimes called **G mucus**, is almost completely resistant to sperm penetration. A highly effective method of natural family planning makes use of the properties of cervical mucus.

There are two main modes of sperm transport through the cervix. One is a phase of initial rapid transport, by which some spermatozoa can reach the uterine tubes within 5 to 20 minutes of ejaculation. Such rapid transport relies more on muscular movements of the female reproductive tract than on the motility of the spermatozoa themselves. The second, slow phase of sperm transport involves the swimming of spermatozoa through the cervical mucus (traveling at a rate of 2 to 3 mm/hr), their storage in cervical crypts, and their final passage through the cervical canal as much as 2 to 4 days later.

Relatively little is known about the passage of spermatozoa through the uterine cavity, but the contraction of uterine smooth muscle, rather than sperm motility, seems to be the main intrauterine transport mechanism. At this point the spermatozoa enter one of the uterine tubes. According to some recent estimates, only several hundred spermatozoa enter the uterine tubes, with the majority entering the tube containing the ovulated egg.

Once inside the uterine tube, spermatozoa collect in the isthmus and temporarily bind to the tubal epithelium. During this time they are influenced by secretions of the tube to undergo the **capacitation** reaction, which consists of alterations of the plasma membrane, including the efflux of cholesterol. Capacitation is required for spermatozoa to be able to fertilize an egg (specifically, to undergo the acrosome reaction—see below). After the capacitation reaction, the spermatozoa undergo a period of hyperactivity and also detach from the tubal epithelium. There is evidence that capacitated spermatozoa are attracted to some type of chemotactic agent(s) present in follicular fluid or secreted by the cellular coverings of the egg.

Upon their release from the isthmus, the spermatozoa make their way up the tube through a combination of muscular movements of the tube and some swimming movements. The simultaneous transport of an egg down and spermatozoa up the tube is currently explained on the basis of peristaltic contractions of the uterine tube muscles. These contractions subdivide the tube into compartments. Within a given compartment, the gametes are caught up in churning movements that over 1 or 2 days bring the egg and spermatozoa together. Fertilization of the egg typically occurs in the ampullary portion (upper third) of the uterine tube. Estimates suggest that spermatozoa retain their function in the female reproductive tract for about 80 hours.

## Formation and Function of the Corpus Luteum of Ovulation and Pregnancy

While the ovulated egg is passing through the uterine tubes, the ruptured follicle from which it arose undergoes a series of striking changes that are essential for the progression of events leading to and supporting pregnancy (see Figure 1-8).

Soon after ovulation, the basement membrane that separates the granulosa cells from the theca interna breaks down, allowing thecal blood vessels to grow into the cavity of the ruptured follicle. The granulosa cells simultaneously undergo a series of major changes in form and function (**luteinization**). Within 30 to 40 hours of the LH surge, these cells, now called **granulosa lutein cells**, begin secreting increasing amounts of progesterone along with some estrogen. This pattern of secretion provides the hormonal basis for the changes in the female reproductive tissues during the last half of the menstrual cycle. During this period, the follicle continues to enlarge. Because of its yellow color, it is known as the **corpus luteum**. The granulosa lutein cells are terminally differentiated. They have stopped dividing, but they continue to secrete progesterone for 10 days.

In the absence of fertilization and a hormonal stimulus provided by the early embryo, the corpus luteum begins to deteriorate (**luteolysis**) late in the menstrual cycle. Luteolysis appears to involve both the preprogramming of the luteal cells to **apoptosis** (cell death) and **uterine luteolytic factors**, such as **prostaglandin F$_2$**. Regression of the corpus luteum and the accompanying reduction in progesterone production cause the hormonal withdrawal that results in the degenerative changes of the endometrial tissue during the last days of the menstrual cycle.

During the regression of the corpus luteum, the granulosa lutein cells degenerate and are replaced with collagenous scar tissue. Because of its white color, the former corpus luteum now becomes known as the **corpus albicans** ("white body").

If fertilization occurs, the production of the protein hormone **chorionic gonadotropin** by the future placental tissues maintains the corpus luteum in a functional condition and even causes an increase in its size and hormone production. Because the granulosa lutein cells are unable to divide and also cease producing progesterone after 10 days, the large **corpus luteum of pregnancy** is composed principally of theca lutein cells. The corpus luteum of pregnancy remains functional for the first few months of pregnancy. After the second month, the placenta produces enough estrogens and progesterone to maintain pregnancy on its own. At this point the ovaries can be removed, and pregnancy will continue.

## FERTILIZATION

Fertilization is a series of processes rather than a single event. Viewed in the broadest sense, these processes begin when spermatozoa start to penetrate the corona radiata that surrounds the egg and end with the intermingling of the maternal and paternal chromosomes after the spermatozoon has entered the egg.

### Penetration of the Corona Radiata

When the spermatozoa first encounter the ovulated egg in the ampullary part of the uterine tube, they are confronted by the corona radiata and possibly some remnants of the cumulus oophorus, which represents the outer layer of the egg complex (Figure 2-4). The corona radiata is a highly cellular layer with an intercellular matrix consisting of proteins and a high

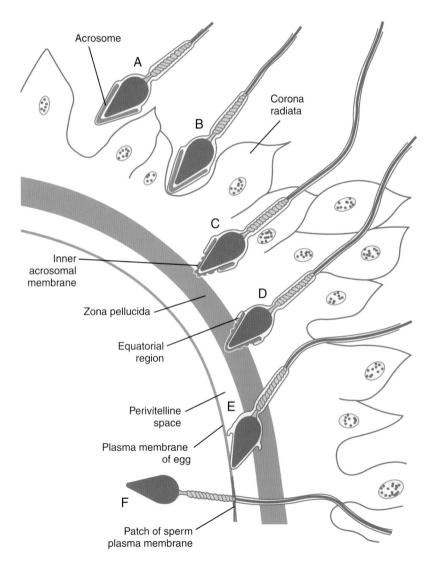

**FIGURE 2-4** The sequence of events in penetration of the coverings and plasma membrane of the egg. **A** and **B,** Penetration of the corona radiata. **C** and **D,** Attachment to the zona pellucida and acrosomal reaction. **E** and **F,** Binding to plasma membrane and entry into the egg.

concentration of carbohydrates, especially hyaluronic acid.

Although it has been widely believed that hyaluronidase emanating from the sperm head plays a major role in penetration of the corona radiata, the evidence is not unequivocal. The active swimming movements of the spermatozoa appear to play a significant role in penetration.

## Attachment to and Penetration of the Zona Pellucida

The **zona pellucida**, which is 13 μm thick in humans, consists principally of three glycoproteins—ZP1, ZP2, and ZP3—with molecular weights of 200,000, 120,000, and 83,000 daltons. ZP2 and ZP3 combine to form basic units that polymerize into long filaments. These filaments are periodically linked by cross-bridges of ZP1 molecules (Figure 2-5). The zona pellucida of the unfertilized mouse egg is estimated to contain over a billion copies of the ZP3 protein.

After they have penetrated the corona radiata, spermatozoa bind tightly to the zona pellucida by means of the plasma membrane of the sperm head (see Figure 2-4). The ZP3 molecule, specifically the O-linked oligosaccharides attached to the polypeptide core, acts as the sperm receptor in the zona in the mouse. Molecules on the surface of the sperm head are specific binding sites for the ZP3 sperm receptors on the zona pellucida. Over two dozen molecules have been proposed, but the identity of zona-binding molecule remains unknown. Interspecies molecular differences in the sperm-binding regions of the ZP3 molecule may serve as the basis for the inability of spermatozoa of one species to fertilize an egg of another species. In mammals, there is less species variation in the composition of ZP3; this may explain why penetration of the zona pellucida by spermatozoa of closely related mammalian species is sometimes possible, whereas it is rare among lower animals.

On binding to the zona pellucida, mammalian spermatozoa undergo the **acrosomal reaction**. The essence of the acrosomal reaction is the fusion of parts of the outer acrosomal membrane with the overlying plasma membrane and the pinching off of fused parts as small vesicles. This results in the liberation of the multitude of enzymes that are stored in the acrosome (Box 2-1).

### Box 2-1  Some Major Mammalian Acrosomal Enzymes

| | |
|---|---|
| Acid proteinase | β-Galactosidase |
| Acrosin | β-Glucuronidase |
| Arylaminidase | Hyaluronidase |
| Arylsulfatase | Neuraminidase |
| Collagenase | Phospholipase C |
| Esterase | Proacrosin |

**FIGURE 2-5 A,** Filamentous components of the mammalian (mouse) zona pellucida. **B,** Molecular organization of the filaments in the zona pellucida. *Far right,* Structure of the ZP3 glycoprotein. (**A** and **B** from Wassarman PM: *Sci Am* 259(6):82, 1988. Copyright Neil O. Hardy.)

The acrosomal reaction in mammals appears to be stimulated by the ZP3 molecule acting through G proteins in the plasma membrane on the sperm head (see Figure 2-5). In contrast to the sperm receptor function of ZP3, a large segment of the polypeptide chain of the ZP3 molecule must be present to induce the acrosomal reaction. One of the initiating events of the acrosomal reaction is a massive influx of $Ca^{++}$ through the plasma membrane of the sperm head. This process, accompanied by an influx of $Na^+$ and an efflux of $H^+$, raises the intracellular pH. Fusion of the outer acrosomal membrane with the overlying plasma membrane soon follows. As the vesicles of the fused membranes are shed, the enzymatic contents of the acrosome are freed and can assist the spermatozoa in making its way through the zona pellucida.

After the acrosomal reaction, the inner acrosomal membrane forms the outer surface covering of most of the sperm head (see Figure 2-4, *D*). Toward the base of the sperm head (in the equatorial region), the inner acrosomal membrane fuses with the remaining **postacrosomal plasma membrane** to maintain membrane continuity around the sperm head.

Only after completing the acrosomal reaction can the spermatozoon successfully begin to penetrate the zona pellucida. Penetration of the zona is accomplished by a combination of mechanical propulsion by movements of the sperm's tail and digestion of a pathway through the action of acrosomal enzymes. The most important enzyme is **acrosin**, a serine proteinase that is bound to the inner acrosomal membrane. Once the sperm has made its way through the zona and into the **perivitelline space** (the space between the egg's plasma membrane and the zona pellucida), it can make direct contact with the plasma membrane of the egg.

## Binding and Fusion of Spermatozoon and Egg

After a brief transit period through the perivitelline space, the spermatozoon makes contact with the egg. In two distinct steps, the spermatozoon first binds to and then fuses with the plasma membrane of the egg. Binding between the spermatozoon and egg occurs when the **equatorial region** of the sperm head contacts the microvilli surrounding the egg. Molecules on the plasma membrane of the sperm head, principally a sperm protein called **fertilin**, bind to **α6β1 integrin** molecules on the surface of the egg. The acrosomal reaction causes a change in the membrane properties of the spermatozoon because, if the acrosomal reaction has not occurred, the spermatozoon is unable to fuse with the egg. Actual fusion between spermatozoon and egg brings their plasma membranes into continuity. After initial fusion, the contents of the spermatozoon (the head, midpiece, and usually the tail) sink into the egg (Figure 2-6), whereas the sperm's plasma membrane, which is antigenically distinct from that of the egg, becomes incorporated into the egg's plasma membrane and remains recognizable at least until the start of cleavage. Although mitochondria located in the sperm neck enter the egg, they do not contribute to the functional mitochondrial complement of the zygote.

## Prevention of Polyspermy

Once a spermatozoon has fused with an egg, the entry of other spermatozoa into the egg (**polyspermy**) must be prevented or abnormal development will likely result. Two blocks to polyspermy, fast and slow, are typically present in vertebrate fertilization.

The **fast block to polyspermy**, which has been best studied in sea urchins, consists of a rapid electrical depolarization of the plasma membrane of the egg. The resting membrane potential of the egg changes from about −70 mV to +10 mV within 2 to 3 seconds after fusion of the spermatozoon with the egg. This change in membrane potential prevents other spermatozoa from adhering to the egg's plasma membrane. The fast block is short lived, usually lasting only about 5 minutes in mammals. This time is sufficient for the egg to mount the permanent slow block.

The **slow block to polyspermy** begins with the propagation of a wave of $Ca^{++}$ from the site of sperm-egg fusion. Within a couple of minutes, the $Ca^{++}$ wave has passed through the egg, sequentially acting on the cortical granules as it passes by them. Exposure to $Ca^{++}$ causes the cortical granules to fuse with the plasma membrane and to release their contents (hydrolytic enzymes and polysaccharides) into the perivitelline space. The polysaccharides released into the perivitelline space become hydrated and swell, causing the zona pellucida to elevate from the surface of the egg.

The secretory products of the cortical granules diffuse into the porous zona pellucida and hydrolyze the sperm receptor molecules (ZP3 in the mouse) in the zona. This reaction, called the **zona reaction**, essentially eliminates the ability of spermatozoa to adhere to and penetrate the zona. The zona reaction has been observed in human eggs that have undergone in vitro fertilization. In addition to changes in the zona pellucida, alterations in sperm receptor molecules on the plasma membrane of the human egg cause the egg itself to become refractory to penetration by other spermatozoa.

## Metabolic Activation of the Egg

One of the significant changes brought about by the penetration by a sperm is a rapid intensification of the egg's respiration and metabolism. The mechanisms underlying these changes are not fully understood even in the

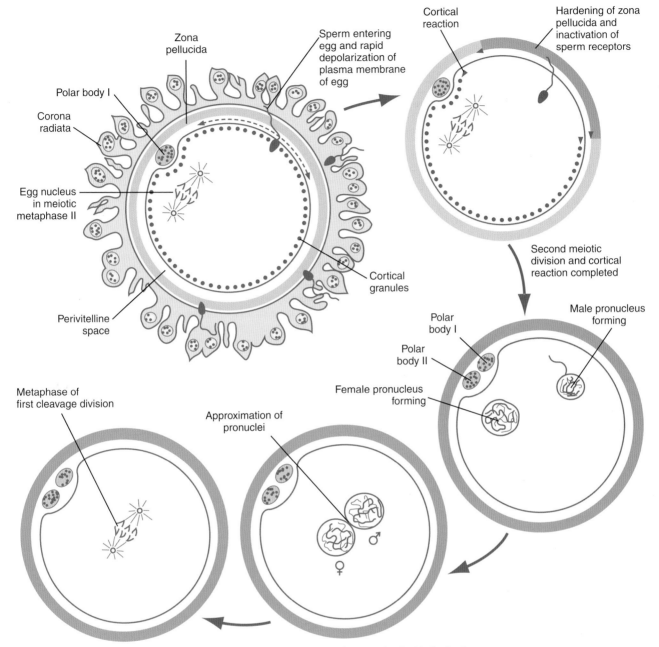

**FIGURE 2-6** Summary of the main events involved in fertilization.

best-studied systems, but the early release of Ca⁺⁺ from internal stores is believed to be the initiating event. In some species, Ca⁺⁺ release is shortly followed by an exchange of extracellular Na⁺ for intracellular H⁺ through the plasma membrane. This results in a rise in intracellular pH, which precedes an increase in oxidative metabolism.

## Decondensation of the Sperm Nucleus

In the mature spermatozoon, the nuclear chromatin is very tightly packed, due in large part to the —SS— (disulfide) cross-linking that occurs among the protamine molecules complexed with the DNA during spermatogenesis. Shortly after the head of the sperm enters the cytoplasm of the egg, the permeability of its nuclear membrane begins to increase, allowing cytoplasmic factors within the egg to affect the nuclear contents of the sperm. After reduction of the —SS— crosslinks of the protamines to sulfhydryl (—SH) groups by reduced glutathione in the ooplasm, the protamines are rapidly lost from the chromatin of the spermatozoon, and the chromatin begins to spread out within the nucleus (now called a **pronucleus**) as it moves closer to the nuclear material of the egg. After a short period during which the male chromosomes are naked, histones begin to associate with the chromosomes.

## Completion of Meiosis and the Development of Pronuclei in the Egg

After penetration of the egg by the spermatozoon, the nucleus of the egg, which had been arrested in metaphase of the second meiotic division, completes the last division, releasing a **second polar body** into the perivitelline space (see Figure 2-6). A pronuclear membrane, derived largely from the endoplasmic reticulum of the egg, forms around the female chromosomal material. Cytoplasmic factors appear to control the growth of both the female and the male pronuclei. DNA replication occurs in the developing haploid pronuclei, and each chromosome forms two chromatids as the pronuclei approach each other. When the male and female pronuclei come into contact, their membranes break down, and the chromosomes intermingle. The maternal and paternal chromosomes quickly become organized around a mitotic spindle in preparation for an ordinary mitotic division. At this point, the process of fertilization can be said to be complete and the fertilized egg is called a **zygote**.

## What Is Accomplished by Fertilization?

The process of fertilization ties together a number of biological loose ends:

1. It stimulates the egg to complete the second meiotic division.
2. It restores to the zygote the normal diploid number of chromosomes (46 in the human).
3. The sex of the future embryo is determined by the chromosomal complement of the spermatozoon. (If the sperm contains 22 autosomes and an X chromosome, the embryo will be a genetic female, and if it contains 22 autosomes and a Y chromosome, the embryo will be a male. See Chapter 16 for further details.)
4. Through the mingling of maternal and paternal chromosomes, the zygote is a genetically unique product of chromosomal reassortment, which is important for the viability of any species.
5. The process of fertilization causes metabolic activation of the egg, which is necessary for cleavage and subsequent embryonic development to occur.

---

**CLINICAL VIGNETTE**

A 33-year-old woman who has had her uterus surgically removed desperately wants her own child. She is capable of producing eggs because her ovaries remain functional. She and her husband want to attempt in vitro fertilization and embryo transfer. They find a woman who, for $10,000, is willing to allow the couple's embryo to be transferred to her uterus and will serve as a surrogate mother during the pregnancy. Induction of superovulation is very successful, and the physicians are able to fertilize eight eggs in vitro. Three embryos are implanted into the surrogate mother. The remaining embryos are frozen for possible future use. The embryo transfer is successful, and the surrogate mother becomes pregnant with twins. The twins are born, but the surrogate mother feels that she has bonded with them so much that she should have the right to raise them. The extremely wealthy genetic parents take the case to court, but before the case comes to trial they are both killed in an airplane accident. The surrogate mother now claims that she should get the large inheritance in the name of her twins, but the father's sister, equally aware of the financial implications, claims that she should care for the twins. The issue of what to do with the remaining five frozen embryos also comes up.

This case is fictitious, but all of its elements have occurred on an isolated basis. How would you deal with the following legal and ethical issues?

A. To whom should the twins be awarded?
B. What should be done with the remaining frozen embryos?

---

## SUMMARY

○ Ovulation is stimulated by a surge of LH and FSH in the blood. Expulsion of the ovum from the graafian follicle involves local edema, ischemia, and collagen breakdown, with a possible contribution by fluid pressure and smooth muscle activity in rupturing the follicular wall.

○ The ovulated egg is swept into the uterine tube and transported through it by ciliary action and smooth muscle contractions as it awaits fertilization by a sperm cell.

○ Sperm transport in the male involves a slow exit from the seminiferous tubules, maturation in the epididymis, and rapid expulsion at ejaculation, where the spermatozoa are joined by secretions from the prostate and seminal vesicles to form semen.

○ In the female, sperm transport involves entry into the cervical canal from the vagina, passage through the cervical mucus, and transport through the uterus into the uterine tubes, where capacitation occurs. The meeting of egg and sperm typically occurs in the upper third of the uterine tube.

Certain types of infertility caused by inadequate numbers or mobility of spermatozoa or by obstruction of the uterine tubes are now treatable by fertilizing an ovum in vitro and then transferring the cleaving embryo into the reproductive tract of the woman. Accomplishing this requires the sequential application of various techniques that were initially developed for the assisted reproduction of domestic animals, such as cows and sheep. The relevant techniques are (1) stimulating gamete production, (2) obtaining male and female gametes, (3) storing gametes, (4) fertilizing eggs, (5) culturing cleaving embryos in vitro, (6) preserving embryos, and (7) introducing embryos into the uterus (Figure 2-7).

## STIMULATION OF GAMETE PRODUCTION

Ovulation is stimulated by altering existing hormonal relationships. For women who are **anovulatory** (do not ovulate), these techniques alone may be sufficient to allow conception.

Three types of therapy have been commonly used to stimulate gamete production. The first consists of the administration of **clomiphene citrate**, a nonsteroidal antiestrogen that competes with estrogens for binding sites in the pituitary and possibly the hypothalamus and ovaries. Clomiphene acts to suppress the normal negative feedback by estrogens on the pituitary (see Figure 1-14),

resulting in an increase in the serum concentrations of LH and FSH. This typically results in multiple ovulation, a desired outcome for artificial fertilization because fertilizing more than one egg at a time is more efficient. Sometimes, however, a woman who has used clomiphene for the induction of ovulation produces multiple offspring, with a number of cases of quintuplet to septuplet births having been recorded.

Other methods of inducing ovulation are the application of **human menopausal gonadotropins (hMGs)** or the pulsatile administration of gonadotropin-releasing hormone (GnRH). These techniques are more expensive than the administration of clomiphene.

## OBTAINING GAMETES

For artificial insemination in vivo or artificial fertilization in vitro, spermatozoa are typically collected by masturbation. The collection of eggs, however, requires technological assistance. Ongoing monitoring of the course of induced ovulation is accomplished by the application of imaging techniques, especially diagnostic ultrasound.

The actual recovery of oocytes involves their aspiration from ripe follicles. Although originally accomplished by **laparoscopy** (direct observation by inserting a laparoscope through a small slit in the woman's abdominal wall), visualization is now done with the assistance of ultrasound. An aspiration needle is inserted into each

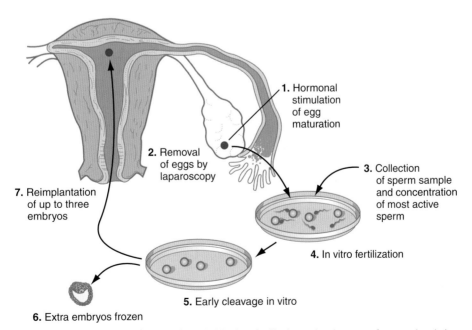

**FIGURE 2-7** Schematic representation of a typical in vitro fertilization and embryo transfer procedure in humans.

*Continued*

## Treatment of Infertility by In Vitro Fertilization and Embryo Transfer (Continued)

mature follicle, and the ovum is gently sucked into the needle and then placed into culture medium in preparation for fertilization in vitro.

### STORING GAMETES

Although eggs and sperm are usually placed together shortly after they are obtained, in some circumstances the gametes (especially spermatozoa) are stored for various periods of time before use. By bringing glycerinated preparations of spermatozoa down to the temperature of liquid nitrogen, spermatozoa can be kept for years without losing their normal fertilizing power. The freezing of eggs is possible, but much more problematic.

### IN VITRO FERTILIZATION AND EMBRYO CULTURE

Three ingredients for successful in vitro fertilization are (1) mature eggs; (2) normal, active spermatozoa; and (3) an appropriate culture environment.

One of the most important factors in obtaining successful in vitro fertilization is having oocytes that are properly mature. The eggs aspirated from a woman are sometimes at different stages of maturity. Immature eggs are cultured for a short time to become more fertilizable. The aspirated eggs are surrounded by the zona pellucida, the corona radiata, and a varying amount of cumulus oophorus tissue.

Spermatozoa, either fresh or frozen, are prepared by separating them as much as possible from the seminal fluid. Seminal fluid reduces their fertilizing capacity, in part because it contains decapacitating factors. After capacitation, which in the human can be accomplished by exposing spermatozoa to certain ionic solutions, a defined number of spermatozoa are added to the culture in concentrations from 10,000 to 500,000/ml. Rates of fertilization in vitro vary from one center to another, but 75% represents a realistic average.

In cases of infertility caused by **oligospermia** (too few spermatozoa) or excessively high percentages of abnormal sperm cells, multiple ejaculates may be obtained over an extended period. These are frozen and pooled to obtain adequate numbers of viable spermatozoa. In some cases, small numbers of spermatozoa are microinjected into the **perivitelline space** inside the zona pellucida. Although this procedure can compensate for very small numbers of viable spermatozoa, it introduces the risk of polyspermy because the normal gating function of the zona is bypassed. A recent variant on in vitro fertilization is direct injection of a spermatozoon into an oocyte (Figure 2-8). This technique has been used in cases of severe sperm impairment.

The initial success of in vitro fertilization is determined the next day by examination of the egg. If two pronuclei are evident (Figure 2-9), fertilization is assumed to have taken place.

Fortunately, the cleavage in vitro of human embryos is more successful than that of most other mammalian species. The embryos are usually allowed to develop to the two- to eight-cell stage before they are considered ready to implant into the uterus.

**FIGURE 2-8** Microinjection of a spermatozoon into a human oocyte. The micropipette containing the spermatozoon is entering the oocyte from the right side. (From Veeck LL: *Atlas of the human oocyte and early conceptus*, vol 2, Baltimore, 1991, Williams & Wilkins.)

Typically, all the eggs obtained from the multiple ovulations of the woman are fertilized in vitro during the same period. Very practical reasons exist for doing this. One is that because of the low success rate of embryo transfer, implanting more than one embryo (commonly up to three) into the uterus at a time is advisable. Another reason is financial and also relates to the low success rate of embryo transfer. Embryos other than those used during the initial procedure are stored for future use if the first embryo transfer proves unsuccessful. Such stockpiling saves a great deal of time and thousands of dollars for the patient.

## EMBRYO PRESERVATION

Embryos preserved for potential future use are treated with cryoprotectants (usually glycerol or dimethyl sulfoxide) to reduce ice crystal damage. They are slowly brought to very low temperatures (usually below −100°C) to halt all metabolic activity. The length of time frozen embryos should be kept and the procedure for handling them if the first implantation attempt is successful are questions with both technical and ethical aspects.

## EMBRYO TRANSFER INTO THE MOTHER

Transfer of the embryo into the mother is technically simple; yet this is the step in the entire operation that is subject to the greatest failure rate. Typically only 30% of the embryo transfer attempts result in a viable pregnancy.

Embryo transfer is commonly accomplished by introducing a catheter through the cervix into the uterine cavity and then expelling the embryo or embryos from the catheter. The patient remains quiet, preferably lying down for several hours after embryo transfer.

The reasons for the low success rate of embryo transfers are poorly understood, but the number of completed pregnancies after normal fertilization in vivo is also likely to be only about one third. If normal implantation does occur, the remainder of the pregnancy is typically uneventful and is followed by a normal childbirth.

## INTRAFALLOPIAN TRANSFER

Certain types of infertility are caused by factors such as hostile cervical mucus and pathological or anatomical abnormalities of the upper ends of the uterine tubes. A somewhat simpler method for dealing with these conditions is to introduce both male and female gametes directly into the lower end of a uterine tube (often at the junction of its isthmic and ampullary regions). Fertilization occurs within the tube, and the early events of embryogenesis occur naturally. The method of **gamete intrafallopian transfer** (**GIFT**) has resulted in slightly higher percentages of pregnancies than the standard in vitro fertilization and embryo transfer methods.

A variant on this technique is **zygote intrafallopian transfer** (**ZIFT**). In this case a cleaving embryo that has been produced by in vitro fertilization is implanted into the uterine tube.

## SURROGACY

In some circumstances a woman can produce fertile eggs but cannot become pregnant. An example would be the woman whose uterus has been removed but who still possesses functioning ovaries. One option in this case is in vitro fertilization and embryo transfer, but the embryo is transferred into the uterus of another woman (**surrogate mother**). From the biological perspective, this procedure differs little from embryo transfer into the uterus of the biological mother, but it introduces a host of social, ethical, and legal issues.

**FIGURE 2-9 A,** Photomicrograph of a mature human oocyte arrested at metaphase II. This oocyte will be fertilized in vitro. **B,** Photomicrograph of a human oocyte newly fertilized in vitro. Two pronuclei are visible. (From Veeck LL: *Atlas of the human oocyte and early conceptus,* vol 2, Baltimore, 1991, Williams & Wilkins.)

○ The fertilization process consists of several sequential events:

1. Penetration of the corona radiata
2. Attachment to the zona pellucida
3. Acrosomal reaction and penetration of the zona pellucida
4. Binding and fusion of sperm and egg
5. Prevention of polyspermy
6. Metabolic activation of the egg
7. Decondensation of the sperm nucleus
8. Completion of meiosis in the egg
9. Development and fusion of male and female pronuclei

○ Attachment of the spermatozoon to the zona pellucida is mediated by the ZP3 protein, which also stimulates the acrosomal reaction.

○ The acrosomal reaction involves fusion of the outer acrosomal membrane with the plasma membrane of the sperm call and the fragmentation of the fused membranes, leading to the release of the acrosomal enzymes. One of the acrosomal enzymes, acrosin, is a serine proteinase, which digests components of the zona pellucida and assists the penetration of the swimming spermatozoa through the zona.

○ After fusion of the spermatozoa to the egg membrane, a rapid electrical depolarization produces the first block to polyspermy in the egg. This is followed by a wave of $Ca^{++}$ that causes the cortical granules to release their contents into the perivitelline space and ultimately inactivate the sperm receptors in the zona pellucida.

○ Sperm penetration stimulates a rapid intensification of respiration and metabolism of the egg.

○ Within the egg, the nuclear material of the spermatozoon decondenses and forms the male pronucleus. At the same time, the egg completes the second meiotic division, and the remaining nuclear material becomes surrounded by a membrane, thereby forming the female pronucleus.

○ After DNA replication, the male and female pronuclei join, and their chromosomes become organized for a mitotic division. Fertilization is then complete, and the fertilized egg is properly called a *zygote*.

○ Treatment of infertility by in vitro fertilization and embryo transfer is a multistage process involving stimulating gamete production by drugs such as clomiphene citrate, obtaining eggs by laparoscopic techniques in the female, storing gametes by freezing, performing in vitro fertilization and culture of embryos, preserving the embryo, and transferring the embryo to the mother.

○ Other techniques used for the treatment of infertility are GIFT, the transfer of gametes directly into the uterine tube, and ZIFT, the transfer of zygotes into the uterine tube. These techniques can be used with both biological and surrogate mothers.

## Review Questions

1. Of the barriers to sperm survival and transport within the female reproductive tract, low pH is most important in the:
   A. Upper uterine tube
   B. Lower uterine tube
   C. Uterine cavity
   D. Cervix
   E. Vagina

2. The principal energy source for ejaculated spermatozoa is:
   A. Prostatic acid phosphatase
   B. Internal glucose
   C. Prostatic citric acid
   D. Fructose in seminal vesicle fluid
   E. Glycogen released from the vaginal epithelium

3. What is the principal hormonal stimulus for ovulation?

4. What is capacitation?

5. Where does fertilization take place?

6. Name two functions of the ZP3 protein of the zona pellucida.

7. What is polyspermy, and how is it prevented after a spermatozoon enters the egg?

8. A woman gives birth to septuplets. What is the likely reason for the multiple births?

9. When multiple oocytes obtained by laparoscopy are fertilized in vitro, why are up to three embryos implanted into the woman's uterus and why are the other embryos commonly frozen?

10. Why do some reproductive technology centers insert spermatozoa under the zona pellucida or even directly into the oocyte?

## REFERENCES

Austin CR: *Human embryos: the debate on assisted reproduction*, Oxford, England, 1989, Oxford University.

Braden TD, Belfiore CJ, Niswender GD: Hormonal control of luteal function. In Findlay JK, ed: *Molecular biology of the female reproductive system*, New York, 1994, Academic, pp 259–287.

Chang MC: Experimental studies of mammalian fertilization, *Zool Sci* 1:349–364, 1984.

Cho C and others: Fertilization defects in sperm from mice lacking fertilin β, *Science* 281:1857–1859, 1998.

Dietl J, ed: *The mammalian egg coat: structure and function*, Berlin, 1989, Springer-Verlag.

Eisenbach M, Ralt D: Precontact mammalian sperm-egg communication and role in fertilization, *Am J Physiol* 262(3):C1095–C1101, 1992.

Eisenbach M, Tur-Kaspa I: Do human eggs attract spermatozoa? *BioEssays* 21:203–210, 1999.

Espey LL, Lipner H: Ovulation. In Knobil E, Neill JD, eds: *The physiology of reproduction*, ed 2, New York, 1994, Raven, pp 725–780.

Familiari G, Makabe S, Motta PM: The ovary and ovulation: a three-dimensional study. In Van Blerkom J, Motta PM, eds: *Ultrastructure of human gametogenesis and early embryogenesis*, Boston, 1989, Kluwer Academic, pp 85–124.

Fukuda M and others: Right-sided ovulation favours pregnancy more than left-sided ovulation, *Human Reprod* 15:1921–1926, 2000.

Gaunt SJ: Spreading of the sperm surface antigen within the plasma membrane of the egg after fertilization in the rat, *J Embryol Exp Morph* 75:257–270, 1983.

Geerling JH: Natural family planning, *Am Fam Physician* 52:1749–1756, 1995.

Harper MJK: Gamete and zygote transport. In Knobil E, Neill JD, eds: *The physiology of reproduction*, vol 1, New York, 1988, Raven, pp 103–134.

Hoodbhoy T, Talbot P: Mammalian cortical granules: contents, fate, and function, *Mol Reprod Devel* 39:439–448, 1994.

Jones GS: Corpus luteum: composition and function, *Fertil Steril* 54:21–26, 1990.

Jones HW and others, eds: *In vitro fertilization*, Baltimore, 1986, Williams & Wilkins.

Klemm U, Muller-Esterl W, Engel W: Acrosin, the peculiar sperm-specific serine protease, *Hum Genet* 7:635–641, 1991.

Knoll M, Talbot P: Cigarette smoke inhibits oocyte cumulus complex pickup by the oviduct in vitro independent of ciliary beat frequency, *Reprod Toxicol* 12:57–68, 1998.

Kopf GS: Zona pellucida-mediated signal transduction in mammalian spermatozoa, *J Reprod Fertil* 42(suppl):33–49, 1990.

McLeskey SB and others: Molecules involved in mammalian sperm-egg interaction, *Int Rev Cytol* 177:57–113, 1998.

Metz CB, Monroy A, eds: *Biology of fertilization*, vols 1–3, New York, 1985, Academic.

Myles DG, Koppel DE, Primakoff P: Defining sperm surface domains. In Alexander NJ and others, eds: *Gamete interaction: prospects for immunocontraception*, New York, 1990, Wiley-Liss, pp 1–11.

Niswender GD, Nett TM: The corpus luteum and its control. In Knobil E, Neill JD, eds: *The physiology of reproduction*, vol 1, New York, 1988, Raven, pp 489–526.

Patrat C, Serres C, Jouannet P: The acrosome reaction in human spermatozoa, *Biol Cell* 92:255–266, 2000.

Phillips DM: Structure and function of the zona pellucida. In Familiari G, Makabe S, Motta PM, eds: *Ultrastructure of the ovary*, Boston, 1991, Kluwer Academic, pp 63–72.

Prasad SV and others: Structure and function of the proteins of the mammalian zona pellucida, *Cells Tiss Organs* 166:148–164, 2000.

Saling PM: How the egg regulates sperm function during gamete interaction: facts and fantasies, *Biol Reprod* 44:246–251, 1991.

Smith TT: The modulation of sperm function by the oviductal epithelium, *Biol Reprod* 58:1102–1104, 1998.

Snell WJ, White JM: The molecules of mammalian fertilization, *Cell* 85:629–637, 1996.

Suarez SS: The oviductal sperm reservoir in mammals: mechanisms of formation, *Biol Reprod* 58:1105–1107, 1998.

Talbot P and others: Oocyte pickup by the mammalian oviduct, *Mol Biol Cell* 10:5–8, 1999.

Tsafriri A, Reich R: Molecular aspects of mammalian ovulation, *Exp Clin Endocrinol Diabetes* 107:1–11, 1999.

Veeck LL: *Atlas of the human oocyte and early conceptus*, vols 1 and 2, Baltimore, 1986, 1991, Williams & Wilkins.

Visconti PE and others: The molecular basis of sperm capacitation, *J Androl* 19:242–248, 1998.

Wassarman PM: Mammalian fertilization: molecular aspects of gamete adhesion, exocytosis, and fusion, *Cell* 96:175–183, 1999.

Wassarman PM, Litscher ES: Towards the molecular basis of sperm and egg interaction during mammalian fertilization, *Cells Tiss Organs* 168:36–45, 2001.

Wood C, Trounson A, eds: *Clinical in vitro fertilization*, ed 2, London, 1989, Springer-Verlag.

Yanagimachi R: Mammalian fertilization. In Knobil E, Neill J, eds: *The physiology of reproduction*, ed 2, New York, 1994, Raven, pp 189–317.

# CHAPTER 3

# Cleavage and Implantation

The act of fertilization releases the ovulated egg from a depressed metabolism and prevents its ultimate disintegration within the female reproductive tract. Immediately after fertilization, the zygote undergoes a pronounced shift in metabolism and begins several days of **cleavage**. During this time, the embryo, still encased in its zona pellucida, is transported down the uterine tube and into the uterus. Roughly 6 days later, the embryo sheds its zona pellucida and attaches to the uterine lining.

With intrauterine development and a placental connection between the embryo and mother, higher mammals, including humans, have evolved greatly differing modes of early development from those found in most invertebrates and lower vertebrates. The eggs of lower animals, which are typically laid outside the body, must contain all the materials required for the embryo to attain the stage of independent feeding. Two main strategies have evolved. One is to complete early development as rapidly as possible, a strategy that has been adopted by *Drosophila*, the sea urchin, and many amphibians. This strategy involves storing a moderate amount of yolk in the oocyte and also preproducing much of the molecular machinery necessary for the embryo to move rapidly through cleavage to the start of gastrulation. The oocytes of such species typically produce and store huge amounts of ribosomes, mRNA and transfer RNA (tRNA). These represent maternal gene products, and it means that early development in these species is controlled predominantly by the maternal genome. The other strategy of independent development, adopted by birds and reptiles,

consists of producing a very large egg containing enough yolk that early development can proceed at a slower pace. This eliminates the need for the oocyte to synthesize and store large amounts of RNAs and ribosomes before fertilization.

Mammalian embryogenesis uses some fundamentally different strategies from those used by the lower vertebrates. Because the placental connection to the mother obviates the need for the developing oocyte to store large amounts of yolk, the eggs of mammals are very small. However, because mammalian development is internal and the embryo receives nourishment from the mother, cleavage is a prolonged process that typically coincides with the time required to transport the early embryo from the site of fertilization in the uterine tube to the place of implantation in the uterus. One of the prominent innovations in early mammalian embryogenesis is the formation of the **trophoblast**, the specialized tissue that forms the trophic interface between the embryo and the mother, during the cleavage period. The placenta represents the ultimate manifestation of the trophoblastic tissues.

## CLEAVAGE

### Morphology

In comparison with most other species, mammalian cleavage is a leisurely process measured in days rather than hours. Development proceeds at the rate of roughly one cleavage division per day for the first 2 days (Figures 3-1 and 3-2). After the two-cell stage, mammalian cleavage is asynchronous, with one of the two cells (**blastomeres**) dividing to form a three-cell embryo. When the embryo consists of approximately 16 cells, it is sometimes called a **morula** (derived from the Latin word meaning "mulberry").

After several cleavage divisions, the embryos of placental mammals enter into a phase called **compaction**, during which the individual outer blastomeres tightly adhere through gap and tight junctions and lose their individual identity when viewed from the surface. Compaction is mediated by the concentration of cell adhesion molecules, such as E-cadherin, in a ring around the apical surface of the blastomeres. Through the activity of an $Na^+$, $K^+$-ATPase-based $Na^+$ transport system, $Na^+$ and $H_2O$ move across the epithelium-like outer blastomeres and accumulate in spaces among the inner blastomeres. This process, which occurs about 4 days after fertilization, is called **cavitation**, and the fluid-filled space is known as the **blastocoele** (blastocyst cavity). At this stage, the embryo as a whole is known as a **blastocyst**.

At the blastocyst stage, the embryo consists of two types of cells: an outer epithelial layer (the **trophoblast**) that surrounds a small inner group of cells called the **inner cell mass** (see Figure 3-1). The end of the blastocyst that contains the inner cell mass is known as the **embryonic**

pole, and the opposite end is called the **abembryonic pole**. The appearance of these two cell types reflects major organizational changes that have occurred within the embryo and represents the specialization of the blastomeres into two distinct cell lineages. Cells of the inner cell mass give rise to the body of the embryo itself plus several extraembryonic structures, whereas cells of the trophoblast form only extraembryonic structures, including the outer layers of the placenta. There is increasing evidence that **fibroblast growth factor-4**, a growth factor secreted by cells of the inner cell mass, acts to maintain mitotic activity in the overlying trophoblast.

## Molecular Biology and Genetics

Most studies of the molecular biology and genetics of early mammalian development have been performed on the mouse. Until more information on early primate embryogenesis becomes available, results obtained from experimentation on mice must be used as a guide.

The consequence of the lack of massive advance storage of ribosomes and RNAs during mammalian oogenesis is that the zygote must rely on embryonic gene products very early during cleavage, typically by the two- or four-cell stage (four to eight cells in the human). There does not appear, however, to be a sharp transition between the cessation of reliance on purely maternal gene

**FIGURE 3-1** Drawings of early cleavage stages in human embryos. The drawings of the 58- and 107-cell stages represent sections made through the embryos.

**FIGURE 3-2** Photomicrographs of cleavage stages of human eggs fertilized in vitro. **A,** Two blastomeres 39 hours after fertilization. A polar body is seen to the right of the boundary between the blastomeres. **B,** Four blastomeres 42 hours after fertilization. **C,** Eight blastomeres 49 hours after fertilization. **D,** Hatching blastocyst 123 hours after fertilization. The empty zona pellucida is on the left. In **A** to **C,** numerous spermatozoa can be seen clinging to the zona pellucida. (From Veeck LL: *Atlas of the human oocyte and early conceptus,* vol 2, Baltimore, 1991, Williams & Wilkins.)

products and the initiation of transcription from the embryonic genome. For example, paternal gene products (e.g., isoforms of β-glucuronidase and β$_2$-microglobulin) appear in the embryo very early, while maternal actin and histone mRNAs are still being used for the production of corresponding proteins. As an indication of the extent to which the early embryo relies on its own gene products, development past the two-cell stage does not take place in the mouse if mRNA transcription is inhibited. In contrast, similar treatment of amphibian embryos does not disrupt development until late cleavage, at which time the embryos begin to synthesize the mRNAs required to control morphogenetic movements and gastrulation.

An important gene in early development is *oct-4* (formerly known as *oct-3*), a specific transcription factor that binds the octamer ATTTGCAT on DNA. There is a close relationship between the expression of the *oct-4* gene and the highly undifferentiated state of cells. In the mouse, maternally derived oct-4 protein is found in developing oocytes and is active in the zygote. After the experimentally induced loss of oct-4 protein, development is arrested at the one-cell stage. Such studies indicate that

maternally derived oct-4 protein is required to permit development to proceed to the two-cell stage, when the transcription of embryonic genes begins.

*Oct-4* is expressed in all blastomeres up to the morula stage. As various differentiated cell types begin to emerge in the embryo, the level of *oct-4* gene expression decreases until it is no longer detectable. Such a decrease is first noted in cells that become committed to forming extraembryonic structures and finally in cells of the specific germ layers as they emerge from the primitive streak (see Chapter 5). Even after virtually all cells of the embryo have ceased to express the *oct-4* gene, it is still detectable in the primordial germ cells as they migrate from the region of the allantois to the genital ridges. Because of its patterns of distribution, oct-4 protein is suspected of playing a regulatory role in maintenance of the undifferentiated state and in establishing the germ cells and maintaining their pluripotency.

Along with a small amount of preformed maternal mRNAs in mammalian embryos is a correspondingly low capacity for translation of mRNAs. Various injection experiments suggest that the factor limiting translational efficiency may be the small number of ribosomes stored in the egg.

Even at an early stage, the blastomeres of a cleaving embryo are not homogeneous. Simple staining methods reveal pronounced differences among cells in human embryos as early as the seven-cell stage (Figure 3-3). Autoradiographic studies have shown that all blastomeres of four-cell human embryos have low levels of extranucleolar and no nucleolar RNA synthesis. By the eight-cell stage, some blastomeres have very high levels of RNA synthesis, but other blastomeres still show the pattern seen in blastomeres of four-cell embryos. Morphological studies show corresponding differences between transcriptionally active and inactive blastomeres.

Once cleavage begins, transcription products from both maternally and paternally derived chromosomes are active in guiding development. Haploid embryos commonly die during cleavage or just after implantation. However, there is increasing evidence that the control of early development involves more than simply having a diploid set of chromosomes in each cell.

### Parental Imprinting

Experimentation, coupled with observations on some unusual developmental disturbances in mice and humans, has shown that the expression of certain genes derived from the egg differs from the expression of the same genes derived from the spermatozoon. Called **parental imprinting**, the effects are manifest in different ways. It is possible to remove a pronucleus from a newly inseminated mouse egg and replace it with a pronucleus taken from another inseminated egg at a similar stage of development (Figure 3-4). If a male or female pronucleus is removed and replaced with a corresponding male or

female pronucleus, development is normal. However, if a male pronucleus is removed and replaced with a female pronucleus (resulting in a zygote with two female pronuclei), the embryo itself develops fairly normally, but the placenta and yolk sac are poorly developed. Conversely, a zygote with two male pronuclei produces a severely stunted embryo, whereas the placenta and yolk sac are nearly normal.

Parental imprinting occurs during gametogenesis through the methylation of certain bases (especially cytosines in CpG sequences). This methylation results in the differential expression of paternal and maternal alleles of the imprinted genes during embryonic development. The imprinted genes operate during development and possibly into adulthood, but a given imprint is not passed on to that individual's progeny. Instead, the parental imprints on the genes in the gametes are erased and new imprints, corresponding to the sex of that individual, are established in the eggs or sperm during gametogenesis.

Not all genes are parentally imprinted. Present estimates suggest that 0.1 to 1.0% of all mammalian genes are imprinted (Table 3-1). Clinical Correlation 3-1 discusses some conditions and syndromes associated with parental imprinting.

### X-chromosome Inactivation

Another example of the inequality of genetic expression during early development is the pattern of X-chromosome inactivation in female embryos. It is well known from cytogenetic studies that one of the two X chromosomes in the cells of females is inactivated by extreme condensation. This is the basis for the **sex chromatin**, or **Barr body**, that can be demonstrated in cells of females but not those of normal males. The purpose of

**FIGURE 3-3** Seven-cell human embryo recovered from the uterine tube. Three small polar bodies are seen in the lower part of each photograph. The zona pellucida surrounds the blastomeres and polar bodies. **A,** Photograph of the intact embryo before fixation. **B,** Photomicrograph of a section through the embryo stained with toluidine blue. Two blastomeres stain differently (metachromatically) from the others. (Modified from Avendaño S and others: *Fertil Steril* 26:1167–1172, 1975.)

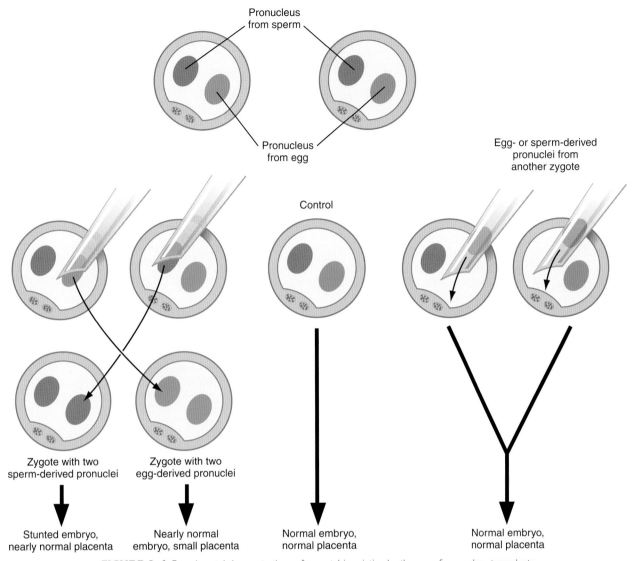

**FIGURE 3-4** Experimental demonstrations of parental imprinting by the use of pronuclear transplants.

| Function | Paternal imprinting | Maternal imprinting |
|---|---|---|
| **TABLE 3-1** *Differential Effects of Paternally and Maternally Expressed Genes* | | |
| Overall growth | Stimulated (IGF-2) | Reduced (H19) |
| Stem cell behavior | Proliferation | Differentiation |
| Enhanced differentiation | Muscle | Epidermis |
| Localization of activity in brain | Hypothalamus | Neocortex |
| Effect on behavior | Hyperkinetic | Hypokinetic |

Modified from Reik W: *Exp Physiol* 81:163, 1996.

X-chromosome inactivation is dosage compensation, or preserving the cells from an excess of X-chromosomal gene products.

Studies of levels of enzymes encoded in the DNA of the X chromosome in mice have shown that both X chromosomes are transcriptionally active during early cleavage of female embryos. After differentiation of the blastomeres into either trophoblast or inner cell mass, the pattern changes (Figure 3-5). Both X chromosomes continue to be active in cells of the inner cell mass, whereas in all cells of the trophoblast (**trophectoderm**), the paternally derived X chromosome is selectively inactivated. As the cells of the inner cell mass become subdivided into other lineages, differential X-chromosomal inactivation also occurs. X inactivation ultimately occurs in all cells, and only during oogenesis do both X chromosomes of the oocytes become active again. The selective inactivation of the paternal X chromosome in the trophoblast is

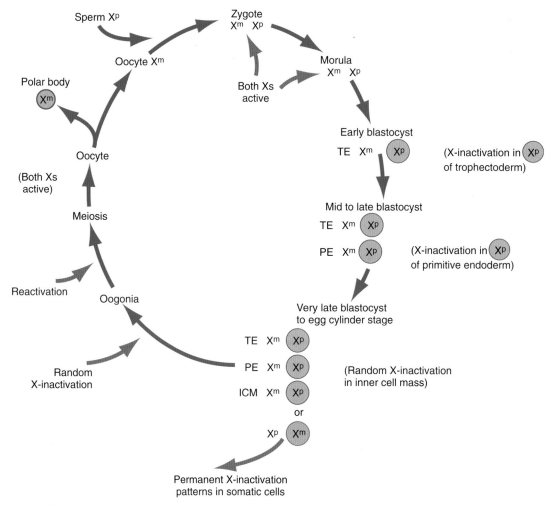

**FIGURE 3-5** X-chromosomal inactivation and reactivation during the mammalian life cycle. The red and green circles refer to inactivated paternally and maternally derived X chromosomes, respectively. *ICM,* Inner cell mass; *PE,* primitive (extraembryonic) endoderm; *TE,* trophectoderm; *X^m,* maternal X chromosome; *X^p,* paternal X chromosome. (Based on Gartler SM, Riggs HD: *Annu Rev Genet* 17:155–190, 1983.)

another example of parental genetic imprinting, although the mechanism of inactivation may be different.

X-chromosome inactivation is initiated at the **X-inactivation center** (XIC), a unique locus on the X chromosome. *XIST* (**X**-**i**nactive **s**pecific **t**ranscript), one of the genes in the XIC, produces a large RNA with no protein coding potential. XIST RNA remains in the nucleus and coats the entire inactive X chromosome, thus not allowing any further transcription from that chromosome. In the inactivated X-chromosome the *XIST* gene is unmethylated and expressed, whereas in the active X chromosome this gene is methylated and silent.

X-chromosomal inactivation occurs when cells undergo restriction and begin to differentiate, rather than remaining **totipotent** (capable of forming all types of progeny). Paternal imprinting on the *XIST* gene accounts for the selective inactivation of the paternal X chromosome in the extraembryonic trophectoderm and extraembryonic endoderm during cleavage (see Figure 3-5). Because they retain their totipotency longer, cells of the

inner cell mass do not undertake X-chromosomal inactivation until later, but why random inactivation of either a maternally or a paternally derived X chromosome occurs in these cells is not understood.

## Developmental Properties of Cleaving Embryos

Early mammalian embryogenesis is considered to be a highly regulative process. **Regulation** is the ability of an embryo or organ primordium to produce a normal structure if parts have been removed or added.* At the cellular

---

* Opposed to regulative development is **mosaic development**, which is characterized by the inability to compensate for defects or to integrate extra cells into a unified whole. In a mosaic system, the fates of cells are rigidly determined, and removal of cells results in an embryo or a structure missing the components that the removed cells were destined to form. Most regulative systems have an increasing tendency to exhibit mosaic properties as development progresses.

A striking example of paternal imprinting in the human is a **hydatidiform mole** (see Figure 7-18), which is characterized by the overdevelopment of trophoblastic tissues and the extreme underdevelopment of the embryo. This condition can result from the fertilization of an egg by two spermatozoa and the consequent failure of the maternal genome of the egg to participate in development or from the duplication of a sperm pronucleus in an "empty" egg. This form of highly abnormal development is consistent with the hypothesis that paternal imprinting favors the development of the trophoblast at the expense of the embryo.

Several other syndromes are also based on parental imprinting. The **Beckwith-Wiedemann syndrome**, characterized by fetal overgrowth and an increased incidence of childhood cancers, has been mapped to the imprinted region on chromosome 11, which contains the genes for insulin-like growth factor-2 (IGF-2, which promotes cell proliferation) and H19 (a growth suppressor). It occurs when both alleles of the *IGF-2* gene express a paternal imprinting pattern. Another instructive example involves deletion of the long arm of chromosome 15. Children of either sex who inherit the maternal deletion develop **Angelman's syndrome**, which includes severe mental retardation, seizures, and ataxia. A child who inherits a paternal deletion of the same region develops the **Prader-Willi syndrome**, characterized by obesity, short stature, hypogonadism, a bowed upper lip, and mild mental retardation.

level, it means that the fates of cells in a regulative system are not irretrievably fixed and that the cells can still respond to environmental cues. Because the assignment of blastomeres to different cell lineages is one of the principal features of mammalian development, identifying the environmental factors that are involved is important.

Of the experimental techniques used to demonstrate regulative properties of early embryos, the simplest is to separate the blastomeres of early cleavage–stage embryos and determine whether each one can give rise to an entire embryo. This method has been used to demonstrate that single blastomeres from two- and sometimes four-cell embryos can form normal embryos, although blastomeres from later stages cannot do so. In mammalian studies, a single cell is more commonly taken from an early cleavage–stage embryo and injected into the blastocoele of a genetically different host. Such injected cells become incorporated into the host embryo, forming cellular **chimeras** or **mosaics**. When genetically different donor blastomeres are injected into host embryos, the donor cells can be identified by histochemical or cytogenetic analysis, and their fate (the tissues that they form) can be determined. **Fate mapping** experiments are important in embryology because they allow one to follow the pathways along which a particular cell can differentiate. Fate mapping experiments, which involve different isozymes of the enzyme **glucose phosphate isomerase**, have shown that all blastomeres of an eight-cell mouse embryo remain **totipotent**; that is, they retain the ability to form any cell type in the body. Even at the 16-cell stage of cleavage, some blastomeres are capable of producing progeny that are found in both the inner cell mass and the trophoblastic lineage.

Another means of demonstrating the regulative properties of early mammalian embryos is to dissociate mouse embryos into separate blastomeres and then to combine the blastomeres of two or three embryos (Figure 3-6). The combined blastomeres soon aggregate and reorganize to become a single large embryo, which then goes on to become a normal-appearing **tetraparental** or **hexaparental mouse**. By various techniques of making chimeric embryos, it is even possible to combine blastomeres to produce interspecies chimeras (e.g., a sheep-goat).

One of the most important steps in early mammalian development is the decision that results in the appearance of two separate lines of cells—the trophoblast and the inner cell mass—from the early blastomeres. Up to the eight-cell stage in mice, all blastomeres are virtually identical in their developmental potential. Shortly thereafter, differences are noted between cells that have at least one surface situated on the outer border of the embryo and those that are completely enclosed by other blastomeres.

The relationship between the position of the blastomeres and their ultimate developmental fate was incorporated into the **inside-outside hypothesis**. The outer blastomeres ultimately differentiate into the trophoblast, whereas the inner blastomeres form the inner cell mass, from which the body of the embryo arises. Outer blastomeres apparently require contact with a nonadhesive surface, such as the inner surface of the zona pellucida, to differentiate into trophoblastic cells. If marked blastomeres from disaggregated embryos are placed on the outside of another early embryo, they typically contribute to the formation of the trophoblast. Conversely, if the same marked cells are introduced into the interior

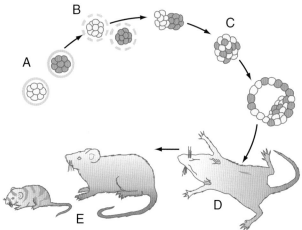

**FIGURE 3-6** Procedure for producing tetraparental embryos. **A,** Cleavage stages of two different strains of mice. **B,** Removal of the zona pellucida (dashed circles). **C,** Fusion of the two embryos. **D,** Implantation of embryos into a foster mother. **E,** Chimeric offspring obtained from the implanted embryos.

of the host embryo, they participate in the formation of the inner cell mass (Figure 3-7). Outer cells in the early mammalian embryo are linked by tight and gap junctions, but whether this morphological characteristic is a cause or an effect of their differentiation into trophoblast is not known. Expression of **E-cadherin** is associated with and may be required for the differentiation of blastomeres

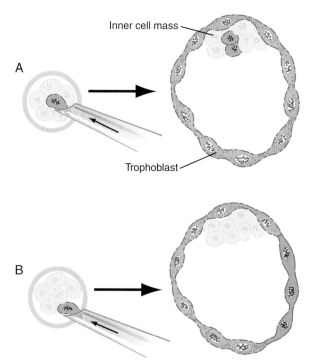

**FIGURE 3-7** Experiments illustrating the inside-outside hypothesis of cell determination in early mammalian embryos. **A,** If a marked blastomere is inserted into the interior of a morula, it and its progeny become part of the inner cell mass. **B,** If a marked blastomere is placed on the outside of a host morula, it and its descendants contribute to the trophoblast.

into trophoblastic cells. Experiments of this type demonstrate that the **developmental potential, or potency** (the types of cells that a precursor cell can form), of many cells is greater than their normal **developmental fate** (the types of cells that a precursor cell normally forms).

Although in many species the major body axes of the embryo are fixed very early in development (even before the first cleavage division), it has long been assumed that because of the high regulatory capacity of early mammalian embryos, their body axes do not become fixed until the end of cleavage or early gastrulation. Recent research, however, suggests that in mouse embryos, at least, the major body axes are recognizable as early as the two-cell stage. Marking experiments have shown that the second polar body, which in contrast to the first polar body may persist until the late blastocyst stage, marks the anterior end of the **anteroposterior axis** (Fig. 3-8). The **dorsoventral axis**, which corresponds to the embryonic/abembryonic axis of the blastocyst stage, can be identified in the very early cleaving embryo because of a slight obliquity in the cross-section. With two of the major body axes recognizable, the third (**mediolateral**) **axis** is automatically defined. Despite these axes being recognizable, how they are set up remains a mystery. Because of the highly regulative properties of early mammalian embryos, it would appear that after experimental manipulations, such as cellular dissociation, the major body axes can be reset.

## Experimental Manipulations of Cleaving Embryos

Much of the knowledge about the developmental properties of early mammalian embryos is the result of recently devised techniques for experimentally manipulating them. Typically, the use of these techniques must be combined with other techniques that have been designed for in vitro fertilization, embryo culture, and embryo transfer (see Chapter 2).

Classic strategies for investigating the developmental properties of embryos are (1) removing a part and determining the way that the remainder of the embryo compensates for the loss (such experiments are called **deletion** or **ablation experiments**) and (2) adding a part and determining the way that the embryo integrates the added material into its overall body plan (such experiments are called **addition experiments**). Although some deletion experiments have been done, the strategy of addition experiments has proved to be most fruitful in elucidating mechanisms controlling mammalian embryogenesis.

Blastomere deletion and addition experiments (Figure 3-9) have convincingly demonstrated the regulative nature (i.e., the strong tendency for the system to be restored to wholeness) of early mammalian embryos. Such knowledge is important in understanding why the exposure of early human embryos to unfavorable

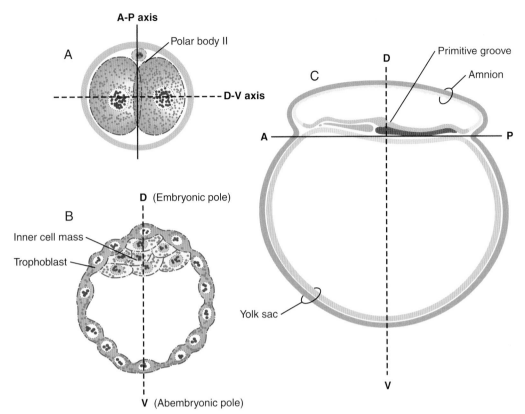

**FIGURE 3-8** The role of the polar body in establishing the main axes of the early mouse embryo. **A,** The future anteroposterior (A-P) axis runs in a plane between the first two blastomeres and bisects the second polar body. The dorsoventral (D-V) axis runs at right angles to the A-P axis through the first two blastomeres. **B,** By the blastocyst stage, the D-V axis runs from the embryonic to the abembryonic pole. **C,** During gastrulation, the A-P axis runs along the craniocaudal length of the flat three-layered embryo, whereas the D-V axis extends from the amnion, through the embryo and into the yolk sac below.

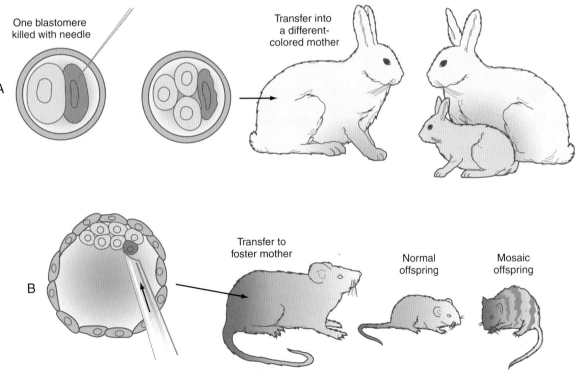

**FIGURE 3-9** Blastomere addition and deletion experiments. **A,** If one blastomere is killed with a needle and the embryo is transferred into a different-colored mother, a normal offspring of the color of the experimentally damaged embryo is produced. **B,** If a blastomere of a different strain is introduced into a blastocyst, a mosaic offspring with color markings characteristic of the strain of the introduced blastomere is produced.

environmental influences typically results in either death or a normal embryo.

One of the most powerful experimental techniques has been the injection of genetically or artificially labeled cells into the blastocyst cavity of a host embryo (see Figure 3-9, *B*). This technique has been used to show that the added cells become normally integrated into the body of the host embryo, providing additional evidence for embryonic regulation. An equally powerful use of this technique has been in the study of cell lineages in the early embryo. By identifying the progeny of the injected marked cells, investigators have been able to determine the developmental potency of the donor cells.

A technique that is providing great insight into the genetic control mechanisms of mammalian development is the production of **transgenic embryos**. Transgenic embryos (commonly mice) are produced by directly injecting foreign DNA into the pronuclei of zygotes (Figure 3-10, *A*). The DNA, typically recombinant DNA for a specific gene, can be fused with a different regulatory element that can be controlled by the investigator. For example, transgenic mice are created by injecting the rat growth hormone gene coupled with a metallothionein promoter region (*MT-I*) into the pronuclei of mouse zygotes. The injected zygotes are transplanted into the uteri of foster mothers, which give birth to normal-looking transgenic mice. Later in life, when these transgenic mice are fed a diet rich in zinc, which stimulates the MT-I promoter region, the rat growth hormone gene is activated, causing the liver to produce large amounts of the polypeptide growth hormone. The function of the transplanted gene is obvious; under the influence of the rat growth hormone that they were producing, the transgenic mice grow to a much larger size than their normal littermates (Figure 3-11). The technique of producing transgenic embryos is being increasingly used both to examine factors regulating the expression of specific genes in embryos and to disrupt genes in the host embryos. In addition, the efficacy of this technique to correct known genetic defects is being increasingly explored in mice.

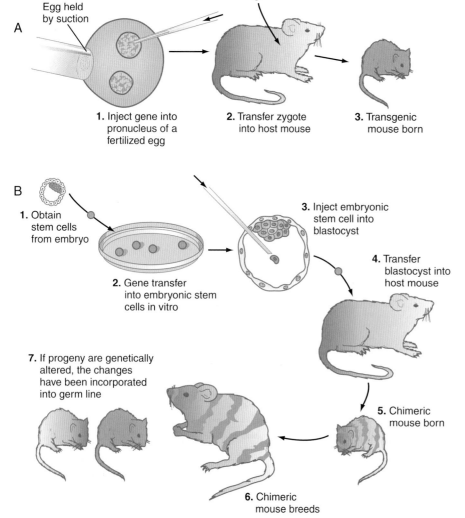

A

Egg held by suction

**1.** Inject gene into pronucleus of a fertilized egg

**2.** Transfer zygote into host mouse

**3.** Transgenic mouse born

B

**1.** Obtain stem cells from embryo

**2.** Gene transfer into embryonic stem cells in vitro

**3.** Inject embryonic stem cell into blastocyst

**4.** Transfer blastocyst into host mouse

**5.** Chimeric mouse born

**6.** Chimeric mouse breeds

**7.** If progeny are genetically altered, the changes have been incorporated into germ line

**FIGURE 3-10 A,** Procedure for creating transgenic mice by pronuclear injection. **B,** Procedure for inserting genes into mice by first introducing them into embryonic stem cells and then inserting the transfected stem cells into an otherwise normal blastocyst.

**FIGURE 3-11** Photograph of two 10-week-old mice. The one on the left (normal mouse) weighs 21.2 gm. The one on the right (a transgenic littermate of the normal mouse) carries a rat gene coding for growth hormone. It weighs 41.2 gm. (From Palmiter RD and others: Nature 300:611–615, 1982.)

An important technological advance is the creation of lines of embryo-derived stem cells (**ES cells**). ES cells are originally derived from inner cell masses and can be propagated in vitro as lines of pluripotential cells that can be either maintained in an undifferentiated condition or stimulated to undergo specific lines of differentiation.

### Stem Cells and Cloning

One of the major developments in biomedical research at the turn of this century was the realization that certain cells (**stem cells**) in both human embryos and adults have the capacity to develop into a variety of cell and tissue types in response to specific environments. In embryos, stem cells can be derived from the inner cell mass (**embryonic stem cells**) or primordial germ cells (**embryonic germ cells**). In adults, stem cells have been isolated from tissues as diverse as bone marrow, skeletal muscle, brain tissue, and fat. Regardless of their origin, stem cells are maintained and propagated in an undifferentiated state in culture. In response to specific combinations of exogenous agents, such as cocktails of growth factors, added to the culture medium, stem cells can be induced to differentiate into specific adult cell types, for example, red and white blood cells, neurons, skeletal and cardiac muscle, or cartilage. When introduced into living tissues, poorly defined local factors can direct the differentiation of adult or embryonic stem cells into specific adult cell types. These techniques have tremendous potential for the treatment of a variety of conditions, such as diabetes, Parkinsonism, blood diseases, or spinal cord injury, but many complicating factors such as immune rejection of

the implanted cells must be dealt with before they are practical and safe for human application.

**Cloning**, which is often confused with stem cell technology, consists of fusing or introducing an adult cell or nucleus into an enucleated oocyte and allowing the hybrid cell to develop into an embryo and ultimately mature into an adult. Although forms of cloning have been successfully accomplished for over 50 years, the creation of the sheep Dolly has had the greatest influence on the public imagination. Cloning is not easily accomplished and there appears to be a significant incidence of abnormal development in cloned individuals.

Both cloning and stem cell technology have brought to light significant ethical and societal issues. It will be fascinating to see how these issues, all sides of which have profound implications, are resolved.

It is now possible to genetically engineer specific genes in ES cells. When such genetically manipulated cells are introduced into blastocysts, they can become incorporated into the host embryo (see Figure 3-10, *B*). If the progeny of a genetically engineered ES cell become incorporated into the germ line, the genetic trait can be passed to succeeding generations.

Some types of twinning represent a natural experiment that demonstrates the highly regulative nature of early human embryos, as described in Clinical Correlation 3-2.

## EMBRYO TRANSPORT AND IMPLANTATION

### Transport Mechanisms by the Uterine Tube

The entire period of early cleavage takes place while the embryo is being transported from the place of fertilization to its implantation site in the uterus (see Figure 2-2). It is increasingly apparent that the early embryo and the female reproductive tract influence one another during this period of transport, but knowledge is still fragmentary.

At the beginning of cleavage, the zygote is still encased in the zona pellucida and the cells of the corona radiata. The corona radiata is lost within 2 days of the start of cleavage. The zona pellucida, however, remains intact until the embryo reaches the uterus.

The embryo remains in the ampullary portion of the uterine tube for approximately 3 days. It then traverses the isthmic portion of the tube in as little as 8 hours. Under the influence of progesterone, the uterotubal junction relaxes, allowing the embryo to enter the uterine cavity. A couple of days later (6 to 8 days after fertilization), the embryo implants into the midportion of the posterior wall of the uterus.

## Zona Pellucida

During the entire period from ovulation until its entry into the uterine cavity, the ovum and then the embryo are surrounded by the zona pellucida. During this time the composition of the zona changes, through contributions from the blastomeres and the maternal reproductive tissues. These changes facilitate the transport and differentiation of the embryo. After the embryo reaches the uterine cavity, it sheds the zona pellucida in preparation for implantation. The blastocyst "hatches" from the zona by digesting a hole through it by means of a trypsin-like enzyme that is secreted by a few trophoblastic cells. The blastocyst then extrudes itself through the hole. Very few specimens of human embryos have been taken in vivo from the period just preceding implantation, but in vitro studies on human embryos suggest a similar mechanism, which probably occurs 1 to 2 days before implantation (see Figure 3-2, *D*). Box 3-1 summarizes the functions of the zona pellucida.

---

### Box 3-1  Summary of Functions of the Zona Pellucida

1. The zona pellucida serves as a barrier that normally allows only sperm of the same species access to the egg.

2. It initiates the acrosomal reaction.

3. After fertilization, the modified zona prevents any additional spermatozoa from reaching the zygote.

4. During the early stages of cleavage, it acts as a porous filter through which certain substances secreted by the uterine tube can reach the embryo.

5. Because it lacks histocompatibility (human leukocyte) antigens, it serves as an immunological barrier between the mother and the antigenically different embryo.

6. It prevents the blastomeres of the early cleaving embryo from dissociating.

7. It facilitates the differentiation of trophoblastic cells.

8. It normally prevents premature implantation of the cleaving embryo into the wall of the uterine tube.

---

## Implantation into the Uterine Lining

Approximately 6 to 7 days after fertilization, the embryo begins to make a firm attachment to the epithelial lining of the endometrium. Soon thereafter, it sinks into the endometrial stroma, and its original site of penetration into the endometrium becomes closed over by the epithelium, much like a healing skin wound.

Successful implantation requires a high degree of preparation and coordination by both the embryo and the endometrium (Table 3-2). The complex hormonal preparations of the endometrium that began at the close of the previous menstrual period are all aimed at providing a suitable cellular and nutritional environment for the embryo. Dissolution of the zona pellucida signals the readiness of the embryo to begin implantation.

The first stage in implantation consists of attachment of the expanded blastocyst to the endometrial epithelium. The apical surfaces of the hormonally conditioned endometrial epithelial cells express a variety of adhesion molecules (such as integrins) that allow implantation to occur in the narrow window of 20 to 24 days in the ideal menstrual cycle. Correspondingly, the trophoblastic cells of the preimplantation blastocyst also express adhesion molecules on their surfaces. The blastocyst attaches to the endometrial epithelium through the mediation of bridging ligands. Both in vivo and in vitro studies have shown that attachment of the blastocyst occurs at the area above the inner cell mass (**embryonic pole**),

| TABLE 3-2 *Stages in Human Implantation* | |
|---|---|
| **Age (days)** | **Developmental event in embryos** |
| 5 | Maturation of blastocyst |
| 5 | Loss of zona pellucida from blastocyst |
| 6? | Attachment of blastocyst to uterine epithelium |
| 6–7 | Epithelial penetration |
| 7½–9 | Trophoblastic plate formation and invasion of uterine stroma by blastocyst |
| 9–11 | Lacuna formation along with erosion of spiral arteries in endometrium |
| 12–13 | Primary villus formation |
| 13–15 | Secondary placental villi, secondary yolk sac formation |
| 16–18 | Branching and anchoring villus formation |
| 18–22 | Tertiary villus formation |

Modified from Enders AC. In *Encyclopedia of human biology*, vol 4, New York, 1991, Academic.

## Twinning

Some types of twinning represent a natural experiment that demonstrates the highly regulative nature of early human embryos. In the United States, roughly one pregnancy in 90 results in twins, and one in 8000 results in triplets. Of the total number of twins born, approximately two thirds are **fraternal**, or **dizygotic**, twins and one third are **identical**, or **monozygotic**, twins. Dizygotic twins are the product of the fertilization of two ovulated eggs, and the mechanism of their formation involves the endocrine control of ovulation. Monozygotic twins and some triplets, on the other hand, are the product of one fertilized egg. They arise by the subdivision and splitting of a single embryo. Although monozygotic twins could theo-

retically arise by the splitting of a two-cell embryo, it is commonly accepted that most arise by the subdivision of the inner cell mass in a blastocyst, or possibly even splitting of the epithelial epiblast a few days later (Figure 3-12). Because the majority of monozygotic twins are normal, the early human embryo can obviously be subdivided and each component regulated to form a normal embryo. Inferences on the origin and relations of multiple births can be made from the arrangement of the extraembryonic membranes at the time of birth (see Chapter 7).

Quadruplets or higher orders of multiple births occur very rarely. In previous years, these could be combinations of multiple ovulations and splitting of single

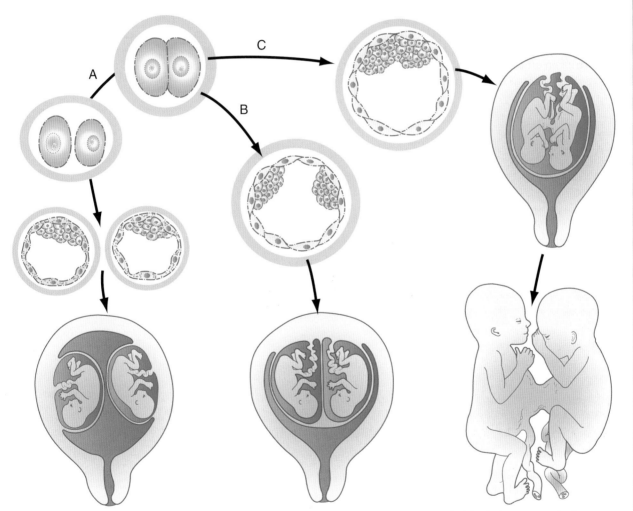

**FIGURE 3-12** Modes of monozygotic twinning. **A,** Cleavage of an early embryo, with each half developing as a completely separate embryo. **B,** Splitting of the inner cell mass of a blastocyst and the formation of two embryos enclosed in a common trophoblast. This is the most common mode of twinning. **C,** If the inner cell mass does not completely separate or if portions of the inner cell mass secondarily rejoin, conjoined twins may result.

*Continued*

embryos. In the modern era of reproductive technology, the majority of multiple births, sometimes up to septuplets, can be attributed to the side effects of fertility drugs taken by the mother.

The separation of portions of an embryo is sometimes incomplete, and although two embryos take shape, they are joined by a tissue bridge of varying proportions. When this occurs, the twins are called **conjoined twins** (sometimes colloquially called *Siamese twins*). The extent of bridging between the twins varies from a relatively thin connection in the chest or back to massive fusions along much of the body axis. Examples of the wide variety of types of conjoined twins are illustrated in Figures 3-13 and 3-14. With the increasing sophistication of surgical techniques, twins with more complex degrees of fusion can be separated. A much less common variety of conjoined twin is a **parasitic twin**, in which a much smaller but often remarkably complete portion of a body protrudes from the body of an otherwise normal host twin (Figure 3-15).

Common attachment sites of parasitic twins are the oral region, the mediastinum, and the pelvis. The mechanism of conjoined twinning has not been directly demonstrated experimentally, but possible theoretical explanations are the partial secondary fusion of originally separated portions of the inner cell mass or the formation of two primitive streaks in a single embryo (see Chapter 5).

One phenomenon often encountered in conjoined twins is a reversal of symmetry of the organs of one of the pair (see Figure 3-14, *B*). Such reversals of symmetry are common in duplicated organs or entire embryos. Over a century ago, this phenomenon was recorded in a large variety of biological situations and was incorporated into what is now called Bateson's rule, which states that when duplicated structures are joined during critical developmental stages, one structure is the mirror image of the other. Despite the long recognition of this phenomenon, only in recent years has there been any understanding of the mechanism behind the reversal of symmetry.

**FIGURE 3-13** Types of conjoined twins. **A,** Head-to-head fusion (cephalopagus). **B** and **C,** Rump-to-rump fusion (pygopagus). **D,** Massive fusion of head and trunk, resulting in a reduction in the number of appendages and a single umbilical cord. **E,** Fusion involving both head and thorax (cephalothoracopagus). **F,** Chest-to-chest fusion (thoracopagus).

**FIGURE 3-14 A,** Conjoined twins with broad truncal attachment (thoracopagus). **B,** Dissected intestinal tracts from the same twins showing partial fusion of the small intestine and mirror image symmetry of the stomachs. (Courtesy M. Barr, Ann Arbor, Michigan.)

**FIGURE 3-15** Parasitic twin arising from the pelvic region of the host twin. One well-defined leg and some hair can be seen on the parasitic twin. (Courtesy M. Barr, Ann Arbor, Michigan.)

suggesting that the surfaces of the trophoblast are not all the same.

The next stage of implantation is penetration of the uterine epithelium. In primates, the cellular trophoblast undergoes a further stage in its differentiation just before it contacts the endometrium. In the area around the inner cell mass, cells derived from the cellular trophoblast (**cytotrophoblast**) fuse to form a multinucleated **syncytiotrophoblast**. Although only a small area of syncytiotrophoblast is evident at the start of implantation, this structure (sometimes called the **syntrophoblast**) soon surrounds the entire embryo. Small projections of syncytiotrophoblast insert themselves between uterine epithelial cells. They then spread along the epithelial surface of the basal lamina that underlies the endometrial epithelium to form a somewhat flattened **trophoblastic plate**. Within a day or so, syncytiotrophoblastic projections from the small trophoblastic plate begin to penetrate the basal lamina. The early syncytiotrophoblast is a highly invasive tissue, and it quickly expands and erodes its way into the endometrial stroma (Figure 3-16, A and B). Although the invasion of the syncytiotrophoblast into the endometrium is obviously enzymatically mediated, the biochemical basis in humans is little understood. By 10 to 12 days after fertilization, the embryo is completely embedded in the endometrium. The site of initial penetration is first marked by a bare area or a noncellular plug and is later sealed by migrating uterine epithelial cells (Figure 3-16, C and D).

As early implantation continues, projections from the invading syncytiotrophoblast envelop portions of the maternal endometrial blood vessels. They erode into the vessel walls, and maternal blood begins to fill the isolated lacunae that have been forming in the trophoblast (see Figure 3-16, C and D). Trophoblastic processes enter the blood vessels and even share junctional complexes with the endothelial cells. By the time blood-filled lacunae have formed, the trophoblast changes character, and it is not as invasive as it was during the first few days of implantation. Leakage of blood from the uterus at this stage can produce "spotting," which is sometimes misinterpreted to be an abnormal menstrual period.

While the embryo burrows into the endometrium and some cytotrophoblastic cells fuse into syncytiotrophoblast, the fibroblast-like stromal cells of the somewhat edematous endometrium swell, with the accumulation of glycogen and lipid droplets (see Figure 7-6). These cells, called **decidual cells**, are tightly adherent and form a massive cellular matrix that first surrounds the implanting embryo and later occupies most of the endometrium. Concurrent with the **decidual reaction**, as this transformation is called, the leukocytes that have infiltrated the endometrial stroma during the late progestational phase of the endometrial cycle secrete **interleukin-2**, which prevents maternal recognition of the embryo as a foreign body during the early stages of implantation. An embryo

**CLINICAL VIGNETTE**

Within a week, two young women in their 20s come to the emergency room of a large city hospital, each complaining of acute pain in her lower right abdominal quadrant. On physical examination, both are exquisitely sensitive to mild pressure in that area.

Further questioning of the first woman reveals that she had a menstrual period 2 weeks previously. Emergency surgery was performed and found that the woman had a ruptured appendix.

The second young woman gives a history of gonorrhea and has been treated for pelvic inflammation. Her last menstrual period was 9 weeks previously. During emergency surgery, her right uterine tube is removed. What was the likely reason for doing so?

is antigenically different from the mother and consequently should be rejected by a cellular immune reaction similar to the type that rejects an incompatible heart or kidney transplant. It appears that a primary function of the decidual reaction is to provide an immunologically privileged site to protect the developing embryo from being rejected, but a real understanding of how this is accomplished has resisted years of intensive research.

Not infrequently, a blastocyst fails to attach to the endometrium, and implantation does not occur. Failure of implantation is a particularly vexing problem in in vitro fertilization and embryo transfer procedures, for which the success rate of implantation of transferred embryos remains at about 25% to 30% (see Clinical Correlation 2-1).

## Embryo Failure and Spontaneous Abortion

A high percentage of fertilized eggs (over 50%) do not develop to maturity and are spontaneously aborted. Most spontaneous abortions (**miscarriages**) occur during the first 3 weeks of pregnancy. Because of the small size of the embryo at that time, spontaneous abortions are often not recognized by the mother, who may equate the abortion and attendant hemorrhage with a late and unusually heavy menstrual period.

Examinations of early embryos obtained after spontaneous abortion or from uteri removed by hysterectomy during the early weeks of pregnancy have shown that many of the aborted embryos are highly abnormal. Chromosomal abnormalities represent the most common category of abnormality in abortuses (about 50% of the cases). When viewed in the light of the accompanying pathological conditions, spontaneous abortion can be viewed as a natural mechanism for reducing the incidence of severely malformed infants.

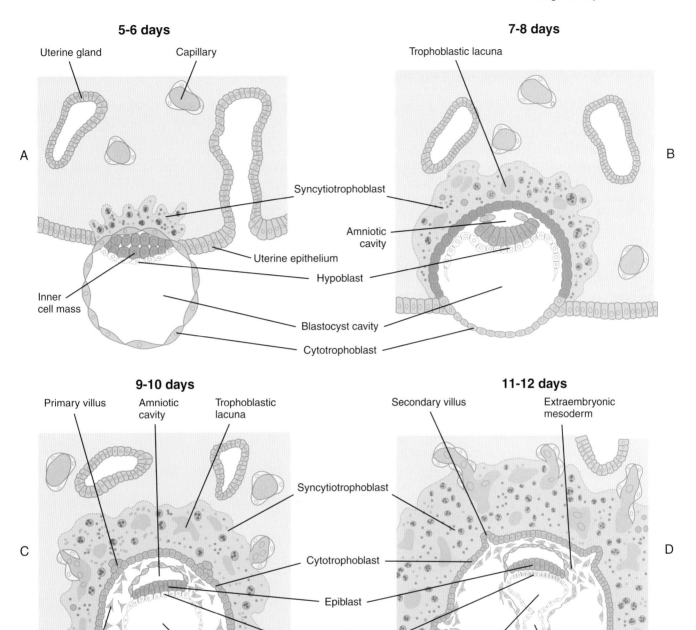

**5-6 days**

Uterine gland

Capillary

A

Syncytiotrophoblast

Uterine epithelium

Hypoblast

Inner
cell mass

Blastocyst cavity

Cytotrophoblast

**7-8 days**

Trophoblastic lacuna

B

Amniotic
cavity

**9-10 days**

Primary villus  Amniotic  Trophoblastic
cavity  lacuna

C

Extraembryonic
mesoderm

Primary yolk sac

Syncytiotrophoblast

Cytotrophoblast

Epiblast

Hypoblast

**11-12 days**

Secondary villus  Extraembryonic
mesoderm

D

Secondary  Extraembryonic  Remains of primary
yolk sac forming  coelom  yolk sac

**FIGURE 3-16** Major stages in implantation of a human embryo. **A,** The syncytiotrophoblast is just beginning to invade the endometrial stroma. **B,** Most of the embryo is embedded in the endometrium; there is early formation of the trophoblastic lacunae. The amniotic cavity and yolk sac are beginning to form. **C,** Implantation is almost complete, primary villi are forming, and the extraembryonic mesoderm is appearing. **D,** Implantation is complete; secondary villi are forming.

## SUMMARY

○ Early human cleavage is slow, with roughly one cleavage division occurring per day for the first 3 to 4 days. The cleaving embryo passes through the morula stage (16 cells) and enters a stage of compaction. By day 4, a fluid-filled blastocoele forms within the embryo, and the embryo becomes a blastocyst with an inner cell mass surrounded by a trophoblast.

○ The zygote relies on maternal mRNAs, but by the two-cell stage, the embryonic genome becomes activated. The

The blastocyst typically implants into the posterior wall of the uterine cavity, but in a low percentage (0.25% to 1.0%) of cases, implantation occurs in an abnormal site. Such a condition is known as an **ectopic pregnancy.**

**Tubal pregnancies** are by far the most common type of ectopic pregnancy. Although most tubal pregnancies are found in the ampullary portion of the tube, they can be located anywhere, from the fimbriated end to the uterotubal junction (Figure 3-17). Tubal pregnancies (Figure 3-18) are most commonly seen in women who have had **endometriosis** (a condition characterized by the presence of endometrium-like tissue in abnormal locations), prior surgery, or **pelvic inflammatory disease.** Scarring from inflammation or sometimes anatomical abnormalities result in blind pockets among the mucosal folds of the uterine tube; these can trap a blastocyst. Typically, the woman shows the normal signs of early

pregnancy, but at about 2 to 2½ months, the implanted embryo and its associated trophoblastic derivatives have grown to the point where the stretching of the tube causes acute abdominal pain. If untreated, a tubal pregnancy typically ends with rupture of the tube and hemorrhage, often severe enough to be life threatening to the mother.

Very rarely an embryo implants in the ovary (**ovarian pregnancy**) or in the abdominal cavity (**abdominal pregnancy**). Such instances can be the result of fertilization of an ovum before it enters the tube, the reflux of a fertilized egg from the tube, or very rarely, the penetration of a tubal pregnancy through the wall of the tube. The most common implantation site for an abdominal pregnancy is in the **rectouterine pouch (pouch of Douglas),** which is located behind the uterus. Implantation on the intestinal wall or mesentery is very dangerous because of

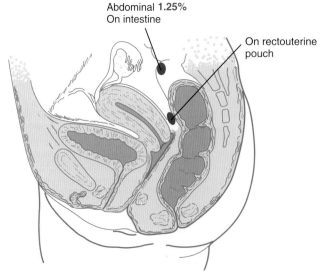

**FIGURE 3-17** Sites of ectopic pregnancy (indicated by red dots) and the frequency of their occurrence.

**FIGURE 3-18** Ruptured ectopic pregnancy in a 34-year-old woman. Because of the increasing size of the fetus and associated membranes, the uterine tube ruptured during the third month of pregnancy. (From Rosai J: *Ackerman's surgical pathology*, vol 2, ed 8, St Louis, 1996, Mosby.)

the likelihood of severe hemorrhage as the embryo grows. In some instances, an embryo has developed to full term in an abdominal location. If not delivered, such an embryo can calcify, forming a **lithopedion.**

Within the uterus, an embryo can implant close to the cervix. Although embryonic development is likely to be normal, the placenta typically forms a partial covering over the cervical canal. This condition, called **placenta previa,** can result in hemorrhage during late pregnancy and if untreated, would likely cause the death of the fetus, the mother, or both persons because of premature placental detachment with accompanying hemorrhage. Implantation directly within the cervical canal is extremely rare.

*oct-4* gene is important in very early development, and its expression is associated with the undifferentiated state of cells.

◯ Through parental imprinting, specific homologous chromosomes derived from the mother and father exert different effects on embryonic development. In female embryos, one X chromosome per cell becomes inactivated through the action of the *XIST* gene, forming the sex chromatin body. The early embryo has distinct patterns of X-chromosomal inactivation.

◯ The early mammalian embryo is highly regulative. It can compensate for the loss or addition of cells to the inner cell mass and still form a normal embryo. According to the inside-outside hypothesis, the position of a blastomere determines its developmental fate (i.e.,

whether it will become part of the inner cell mass or the trophoblast).

◯ Transgenic embryos are produced by injecting rDNA into the pronuclei of zygotes. Such embryos are used to study the effects of specific genes on development.

◯ Monozygotic twinning, usually caused by the complete separation of the inner cell mass, is possible because of the regulative properties of the early embryo. Incomplete splitting of the inner cell mass can lead to the formation of conjoined twins.

◯ After fertilization, the embryo spends several days in the uterine tube before entering the uterus. During this time, it is still surrounded by the zona pellucida, which prevents premature implantation.

◯ Implantation of the embryo into the uterine lining involves several stages: apposition of the expanded (hatched) blastocyst to the endometrial epithelium, penetration of the uterine epithelium, invasion into the tissues underlying the epithelium, and erosion of the maternal vascular supply. Connective tissue cells of the endometrium undergo the decidual reaction in response to the presence of the implanting embryo. Implantation is accomplished through the invasive activities of the syncytiotrophoblast, which is derived from the cytotrophoblast.

◯ Implantation of the embryo into a site other than the upper uterine cavity results in an ectopic pregnancy. Ectopic pregnancy is most often encountered in the uterine tube.

◯ A high percentage of fertilized eggs and early embryos do not develop and are spontaneously aborted. Many of these embryos contain major chromosomal abnormalities.

 *Review Questions*

1. **What is the most common condition associated with spontaneously aborted embryos?**
   A. Maternal imprinting
   B. Paternal imprinting
   C. Ectopic pregnancy
   D. Chromosomal abnormalities
   E. Lack of X-chromosomal inactivation

2. **What tissue from the implanting embryo directly interfaces with the endometrial connective tissue?**
   A. Corona radiata
   B. Inner cell mass
   C. Extraembryonic mesoderm
   D. Epiblast
   E. Syncytiotrophoblast

3. **Identical twinning is made possible by what process or property of the early embryo?**
   A. Regulation
   B. Aneuploidy
   C. Paternal imprinting
   D. Maternal imprinting
   E. X-chromosomal inactivation

4. **The zona pellucida:**
   A. Aids in penetration of the endometrial epithelium
   B. Serves as a source of nutrients for the embryo
   C. Prevents premature implantation of the cleaving embryo
   D. All of the above
   E. None of the above

5. **What is the importance of the inner cell mass of the cleaving embryo?**

6. **Parental imprinting is a phenomenon demonstrating that certain homologous maternal and paternal chromosomes have somewhat different influences on the development of the embryo. Excess paternal influences result in the abnormal development of what type of tissue at the expense of development of the embryo itself?**

7. **What is the function of integrins in implantation?**

8. **What is the cellular origin of the syncytiotrophoblast of the implanting embryo?**

9. **A woman who is 2 to 3 months pregnant suddenly develops severe lower abdominal pain. In the differential diagnosis, the physician must include the possibility of what condition?**

## REFERENCES

Aplin JD: The cell biology of human implantation, *Placenta* 17:269–275, 1996.
Baltz JM: Intracellular pH regulation in the early embryo, *BioEssays* 15:523–530, 1993.
Barlow DP: Genetic imprinting in mammals, *Science* 270:1610–1613, 1995.
Bateson W: *Materials for the study of variation*, London, 1894, Macmillan.
Carlson BM: Stem cells and cloning: what's the difference and why the fuss? *Anat Rec (New Anat)* 257:1–2, 1999.
Cassidy SB, Schwartz S: Prader-Willi and Angelman syndromes: disorders of genomic imprinting, *Medicine* 77:140–151, 1998.
Coucouuvanis E, Martin GR: Signals for death and survival: a two-step mechanism for cavitation in the vertebrate embryo, *Cell* 83:279–287, 1995.
Cruz YP: Role of ultrastructural studies in the analysis of cell lineage in the mammalian pre-implantation embryo, *Microsc Res Tech* 22:103–125, 1992.
Denker HW: Trophoblast-endometrial interactions at embryo implantation: a cell biological paradox. In Denker HW, Aplin JD, eds: *Trophoblast research*, vol 4, New York, 1990, Plenum, pp 3–29.
Denker H-W: Structural dynamics and functions of early embryonic coats, *Cells Tiss Organs* 166:180–207, 2000.
Enders AC: Trophoblast differentiation during the transition from trophoblastic plate to lacunar stage of implantation in the rhesus monkey and human, *Am J Anat* 186:85–98, 1989.
Enders AC: Implantation, embryology. In *Encyclopedia of human biology*, 2nd ed, vol 4, New York, 1997, Academic, pp 799–807.
Enders AC: Formation of monozygotic twins: when does it occur? *Placenta* 23:236–238, 2002.
Flemming TP and others: Assembly of tight junctions during early vertebrate development, *Seminars Cell Devel Biol* 11:291–299, 2000.
Gardner RL: Clonal analysis of early mammalian development, *Philos Trans R Soc Lond [Biol]* 312:163–178, 1985.
Gardner RL: The initial phase of embryonic patterning in mammals, *Internat Rev Cytol* 203:233–290, 2001.
Gualtieri R, Santella L, Dale B: Tight junctions and cavitation in the human pre-embryo, *Mol Reprod Dev* 32:81–87, 1992.
Heard E, Clerc P, Avner P: X-chromosome inactivation in mammals, *Annu Rev Genet* 31:571–610, 1997.
Kidder GM, Watson AJ: Gene expression required for blastocoele formation in the mouse. In Heyner S, Wiley LM, eds: *Early embryo development and paracrine relationships*, New York, 1990, Liss, pp 97–107.
King T, Brown NA: The embryo's one-sided genes, *Curr Biol* 5:1364–1366, 1995.
Kuroda MI, Meller VH: Transient XIST-ence, *Cell* 91:9–11, 1997.
Latham KE: X chromosome imprinting and inactivation in the early mammalian embryo, *Trends Genet* 12:134–138, 1996.
Latham KE, McGrath J, Solter D: Mechanistic and developmental aspects of genetic imprinting in mammals, *Int Rev Cytol* 160:53–98, 1995.
Leese HJ: The energy metabolism of the preimplantation embryo. In Heyner S, Wiley LM, eds: *Early embryo development and paracrine relationships*, New York, 1990, Liss, pp 67–78.

Lessey BA: Endometrial receptivity and the window of implantation, *Baillere's Clin Obstet Gyn* 15:775–788, 2000.

Levin M and others: A molecular pathway determining left-right asymmetry in chick embryogenesis, *Cell* 82:803–814, 1995.

Monk M, Surani A, eds: Genomic imprinting, *Development* 1990(suppl): 1–155, 1990.

Ovitt CE, Schoeler HR: The molecular biology of Oct-4 in the early mouse embryo, *Mol Human Reprod* 4:1021–1031, 1998.

Palmiter RD and others: Dramatic growth of mice that develop from eggs microinjected with metallothionein-growth hormone fusion genes, *Nature* 300:611–615, 1982.

Pederson RA, Burdsal CA: Mammalian embryogenesis. In Knobil E, Neill J, eds: *The physiology of reproduction*, ed 2, New York, 1988, Raven, pp 319–390.

Pfeifer K: Mechanisms of genomic imprinting, *Am J Human Genet* 67:777–787, 2000.

Reik W: Genetic imprinting: the battle of the sexes rages on, *Exp Physiol* 81:161–172, 1996.

Reik W, Walter J: Imprinting mechanisms in animals, *Curr Opin Genet Devel* 8:154–164, 1998.

Rosner MH and others: Oct-3 and the beginning of mammalian development, *Science* 253:144–145, 1991.

Sheardown SA and others: Stabilization of XIST RNA mediates initiation of X chromosome inactivation, *Cell* 91:99–107, 1997.

Spencer R: Rachipagus conjoined twins: they really do occur, *Teratology* 52:346–356, 1995.

Spencer R: Theoretical and analytical embryology of conjoined twins: part 1: embryogenesis, *Clin Anat* 13:36–53, 2000.

Surani MA: Imprinting and the initiation of gene silencing in the germ line, *Cell* 93:309–312, 1998.

Tanaka S and others: Promotion of trophoblast stem cell proliferation by FGF4, *Science* 282:2072–2075, 1998.

Tarkowski AJK, Ozdzendki W, Czolowska R: How many blastomeres of the 4-cell embryo contribute cells to the mouse body? *Int J Dev Biol* 45:811–816, 2001.

Tarkowski AK, Wroblewska J: Development of blastomeres of mouse eggs isolated at the 4- and 8-cell stage, *J Embryol Exp Morphol* 18:155–180, 1967.

Tesarik J and others: Early morphological signs of embryonic genome expression in human preimplantation development as revealed by quantitative electron microscopy, *Dev Biol* 128:15–20, 1988.

Thie M, Fuchs P, Denker H-W: Epithelial cell polarity and embryo implantation in mammals, *Int J Devel Biol* 40:389–393, 1996.

Uchida IA: Twinning in spontaneous abortions and developmental abnormalities, *Issues Rev Teratol* 5:155–180, 1990.

Wang S, Gearhart JD: Human pluripotential stem cells, *NeoReviews* 1:132–136, 2000.

Weitlauf HM: Biology of implantation. In Knobil E, Neill J, eds: *The physiology of reproduction*, New York, 1988, Raven, pp 231–262.

# CHAPTER 4

# Molecular Basis for Embryonic Development

Since 1990 the application of new techniques in molecular biology has revolutionized the understanding of the mechanisms underlying both normal and abnormal embryonic development. It is not possible to have a contemporary understanding of embryonic development without integrating fundamental molecular and morphological aspects of embryology. This chapter is a general introduction to the most important families of molecules known to direct embryonic development. Because new developmentally active molecules are reported almost weekly, the approach used in this text is to introduce important examples illustrating molecular correlates or control of developing systems rather than to attempt completeness in any way.

One of the most important realizations has been the conservatism of the genes that guide development. Sequencing studies have shown remarkably few changes in the nucleotide bases of many developmentally regulated genes that are represented in species ranging from worms to *Drosophila* to humans. Because of this phylogenetic conservatism, it has been possible to identify mammalian counterparts of genes that are known from genetic studies to have important developmental functions in other species (Box 4-1). It is also clear that the same gene may function at different periods of development and in different organs. Such reutilization greatly reduces the total number of molecules that are needed to control development. Both before and after birth, specific genes may be expressed in both normal and abnormal processes. One of the principal themes in contemporary cancer research is the role of mutant forms of developmentally important genes (e.g., protooncogenes) in converting normal cells to tumor cells.

## FUNDAMENTAL MOLECULAR PROCESSES IN DEVELOPMENT

From a functional standpoint, many of the important molecules that guide embryonic development can be grouped into a relatively small number of categories. Some of them remain in the cells that produced them and act as **transcription factors** (Figure 4-2). Transcription factors are proteins possessing domains that bind to the DNA of promoter or enhancer regions of specific genes. They also possess a domain that interacts with RNA polymerase II or other transcription factors and consequently regulates the amount of mRNA that the gene produces.

Other molecules act as intercellular **signaling molecules.** Such molecules leave the cells that produce them and exert their effects on other cells, which may be neighboring cells or cells located at greater distances from those that produce the signaling molecules. Many signaling molecules are members of large families of related proteins, called **growth factors.** To exert their effect, signaling molecules typically bind as **ligands** to **receptor molecules** that are often transmembrane proteins protruding through the plasma membrane of the cells that they affect. When these receptor molecules form complexes with signaling molecules, they set off a

Box 4-1    **Early Developmental Genetics in *Drosophila***

Despite the discovery and characterization of many developmentally important genes in mammals, the basic framework for understanding the molecular basis of embryonic development still rests largely on studies of developmental genetics in *Drosophila*. Although the very earliest stages of human development occur under less rigid genetic control than those of *Drosophila*, an exposure to the fundamental aspects of early *Drosophila* development nevertheless sets the stage for a deeper understanding of molecular embryogenesis in mammals.

Embryonic development of *Drosophila* is under tight genetic control. In the earliest stages the dorsoventral and

anteroposterior axes of the embryo are established by the actions of batteries of **maternal-effect genes** (Figure 4-1). Once these broad parameters have been established, the oval-shaped embryo undergoes a series of three sequential steps that result in the segmentation of the entire embryo along its anteroposterior axis. The first step in segmentation, under the control of what are called **gap genes**, subdivides the embryo into broad regional domains. Loss-of-function gap mutants result in loss of structure, or gaps, in the body pattern several segments in width. In the second step, a group of **pair-rule genes** is involved in the formation of seven pairs of stripes along

| Genetic hierarchy | Functions | Representative genes | Effects of mutation |
|---|---|---|---|
| **Maternal-effect genes** | Establish gradients from anterior and posterior poles of the egg | Bicoid Swallow Oskar Caudal Torso Trunk | Major disturbances in anteroposterior organization |
| **Segmentation genes** *Gap genes* | Define broad regions in the egg | Empty spiracles Hunchback Krüppel Knirps Orthodenticle Tailless | Adjacent segments missing in a major region of the body |
| *Pair-rule genes* | Define 7 segments | Hairy Even skipped Runt Fushi tarazu Odd paired Odd skipped Paired | Part of pattern deleted in every other segment |
| *Segment-polarity genes* | Define 14 segments | Engrailed Gooseberry Hedgehog Patched Smoothened Wingless | Segments replaced by their mirror images |
| **Homeotic genes** | Determine regional characteristics | Antennapedia complex Bithorax complex | Inappropriate structures form for a given segmental level |

**FIGURE 4-1** Sequence of genetic control of early development in *Drosophila*. Within each level of genetic control are listed representative genes.

the craniocaudal axis of the embryo. The third level in the segmentation process is controlled by the **segment-polarity genes**, which work at the level of individual segments and are involved in their anteroposterior organization.*

The segmentation process results in a regular set of subdivisions along the anteroposterior axis of the early *Drosophila* embryo, but none of the previously mentioned developmental controls imparts specific or regional characteristics to the newly formed segments. This function is relegated to two large clusters of **homeotic genes** found in the **antennapedia** complex and the **bithorax** complex. The specific genes in these two complexes determine the

morphogenetic character of the body segments, such as segments bearing antennae, wings, or legs. Mutations of homeotic genes have long been known to produce bizarre malformations in insects, such as extra sets of wings or legs instead of antennae (hence the term *antennapedia*).

---

\* In *Drosophila*, each stripe (segment) is subdivided into anterior and posterior halves. The posterior half of one segment and the anterior half of the next are collectively known as a **parasegment**. The genetics and developmental aspects of insect parasegments are beyond the scope of this text, but in chapter 6, when formation of the vertebral column is discussed, a similar set of divisions of the basic body segments in vertebrate embryos is introduced.

cascade of events in a **signal transduction pathway** that transmits the molecular signal to the nucleus of the responding cell. This signal influences the nature of the gene products produced by that cell and often the cell's future course of development. In the past decade, many new developmentally important molecules have been identified and their expression patterns during development described. Much effort is being expended toward understanding the molecular cascades or networks that control developmental processes.

## Transcription Factors

Many families of molecules act as **transcription factors**. Some transcription factors are general ones that are found in virtually all cells of an organism. Other transcription factors are specific for certain types of cells and stages of development. Specific transcription factors are often very important in initiating patterns of gene expression that result in major developmental changes. They typically do so by acting on promoters or enhancers of specific genes.

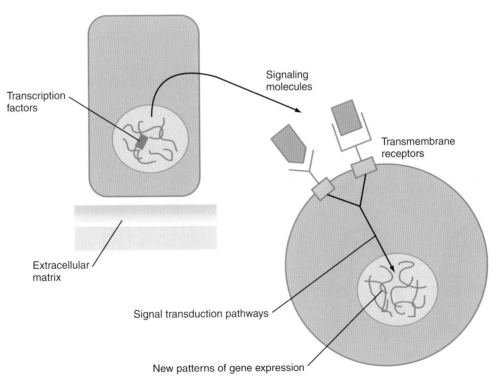

**FIGURE 4-2** Schematic representation of types of developmentally important molecules and their sites of action.

One class of transcription factors is the **basic helix-loop-helix protein**, which contains a short stretch of amino acids in which two α-helices are separated by an amino acid loop. This region, with an adjacent basic region, allows the regulatory protein to bind to specific DNA sequences. The basic regions of these proteins bind DNA, and the helix-loop-helix domain is involved in homodimerization or heterodimerization. This configuration is common in a number of the transcription factors that regulate myogenesis (see Figure 9-27).

Another family of transcription factors is the **zinc finger proteins**. In these proteins, regularly placed cystine and histidine units are bound by zinc ions to cause the polypeptide chain to pucker into fingerlike structures (Figure 4-3). These "fingers" can be inserted into specific regions in the DNA helix.

### Homeodomain Proteins and the Homeobox

One of the most important types of transcription factors is represented by the **homeodomain proteins**. These proteins contain a highly conserved **homeodomain** of 60 amino acids, which is a type of helix-loop-helix region (Figure 4-4). The 180 nucleotides that encode the homeodomain are collectively called a homeobox. Homeobox regions were first discovered in the homeotic genes of the *antennapedia* and *bithorax* complex in *Drosophila* (see Figure 4-1), hence their name. This designation sometimes confuses students, because homeoboxes have been found in a number of more distantly related genes outside the homeotic gene cluster since their initial description.

#### Hox Genes

The *Drosophila* **antennapedia-bithorax** complex consists of eight homeobox-containing genes located in two clusters on one chromosome. Mice and humans possess at

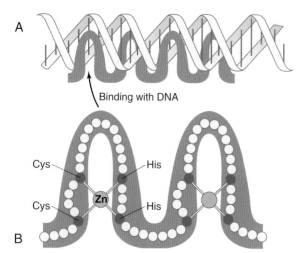

**FIGURE 4-3 A,** Binding to DNA of a zinc finger. **B,** Structure of a zinc finger DNA-binding sequence.

**FIGURE 4-4** Structure of a typical homeodomain protein.

least 39 homologous homeobox genes (called **Hox** genes in vertebrates [**HOX** in humans]), which are found in four clusters on four different chromosomes (Figure 4-5). The *Hox* genes on the four mammalian chromosomes are arranged in 13 **paralogous groups**.

Vertebrate *Hox* genes are strongly implicated in the craniocaudal segmentation of the body, and their spatiotemporal expression proceeds according to some remarkably regular rules. The genes are both activated and expressed according to a strict sequence in the 3' to 5' direction, corresponding to their positions on the chromosomes. Consequently, in *Drosophila* and mammals, 3' genes are expressed earlier and more anteriorly than the 5' genes (Figure 4-6). Mutations of *Hox* genes result in morphological transformations of the segmental structures in which a specific gene is normally expressed. In general, **loss-of-function mutations** result in posterior-to-anterior transformations (e.g., cells of a given segment form the structural equivalent of the next most anterior segment), and **gain-of-function mutations** result in anterior-to-posterior structural transformations. Figure 4-7 illustrates an experiment in which injection of an antibody to a homeodomain protein into an early frog embryo resulted in the transformation of the anterior spinal cord into an expanded hindbrain. Although *Hox* genes were originally described to operate along the main body axis, sequential arrays of expression are found in developing organs or regions as diverse as the gut, the limbs, blood cells, and the internal and external genitalia. The expression of isolated *Hox* genes also occurs in locations as diverse as hair follicles, blood cells, and developing sperm cells. It appears that, although the principal function of the *Hox* genes is involved in setting up structures along the main body axis, individual *Hox* genes are later reutilized in guiding the formation of several specific nonaxial structures.

A number of other gene families contain not only a homeobox but other conserved sequences (Figure 4-8). Some, such as **Engrailed** and **Lim** genes, consist of only a few members per group, but others, such as the **POU** and **Paired** (**Pax**) genes, constitute large families, members of which are expressed in many developing structures.

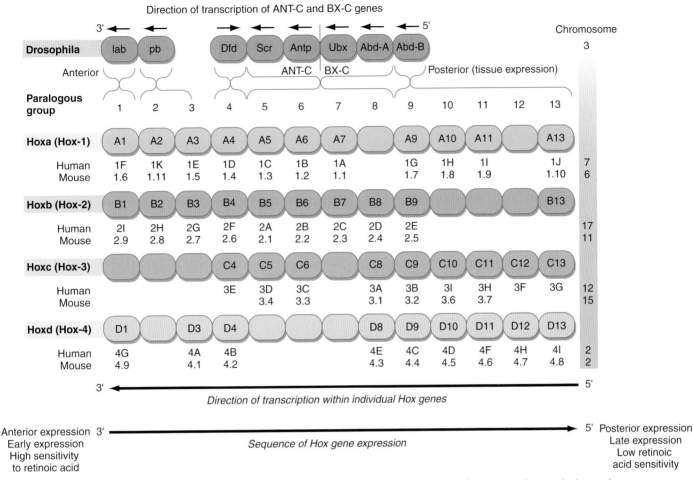

**FIGURE 4-5** Comparison of mouse and human *Hox* complexes. The old terminology for human and mouse is given under the colored ovals. Genes on the 3′ ends of the complexes are expressed earlier and more anteriorly than those on the 5′ end (*right*). (Based on review by Scott MP: *Cell* 71:551–553, 1992.)

## Pax Genes

The **Pax gene family**, consisting of nine known members, is an important group of genes that are involved in many aspects of mammalian development (Figure 4-9). The *Pax* genes are homologous to the *Drosophila* pair-rule segmentation genes (see Figure 4-1). All Pax proteins contain a paired domain of 128 amino acids, which binds to DNA. Various members of this group also contain entire or partial homeobox domains and a conserved octapeptide sequence. *Pax* genes play a variety of important roles in the sense organs and developing nervous system, and outside the nervous system they are involved in cellular differentiative processes when epithelial-mesenchymal transitions take place.

## Sox Genes

The **Sox genes** comprise a large family (over 20 members) that have in common an **HMG (high-mobility group) domain** on the protein. This domain is unusual for a transcription factor in that it binds to seven nucleotides on the minor instead of the major groove on the DNA helix and causes a pronounced conformational change in the DNA. Sox proteins were first recognized in 1990, when the *SRY* gene was demonstrated to be the male-determining factor in sex differentiation (see p. 408), and the name of this group, Sox, was derived from **S**ry HMG b**ox**. One characteristic of Sox proteins is that they work in concert with other transcription factors to influence expression of their target genes (Figure 4-10). As may be expected from their large number, Sox proteins are expressed by most structures at some stage in their development.

## Other Transcription Factors

The **POU gene family** is named for the acronym of the first genes identified, namely, **P**it-1, a gene uniquely expressed in the pituitary, **O**ct-1 and Oct-2, and **U**nc-86, a gene expressed in a nematode. Genes of the *POU* family contain, in addition to a homeobox, a region encoding 75 amino acids, which also bind to DNA through a helix-loop-helix structure. As was seen on p. 45, Oct-4 plays an important role during early cleavage.

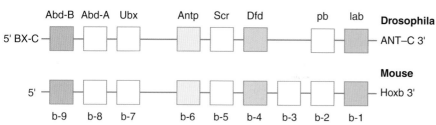

Abd-B  Abd-A  Ubx      Antp   Scr   Dfd        pb    lab   **Drosophila**

5' BX-C                                                    ANT–C 3'

**Mouse**

5'                                                         Hoxb 3'

b-9    b-8    b-7      b-6    b-5   b-4   b-3   b-2   b-1

**FIGURE 4-6** Organization of certain homeobox-containing genes of *Drosophila* and the mouse and their segmental expression in the body. (Based on review by DeRobertis EM, Oliver G, Wright CVE: *Sci Am* 263[1]:46–52, 1990. Copyright Patricia J. Wynne.)

Midbrain — Hindbrain

Forebrain

A

Band of XlHBox 1 expression

Inject with antibody to XlHBox 1 protein

Abnormal dorsal fin

B

Expanded hindbrain

**FIGURE 4-7** Effect of interference of *XlHbox 1* (~Hoxc-6) function on development in *Xenopus*. **A,** Normal larva, showing a discrete band (*green*) of *XlHbox 1* expression. **B,** Caudal expansion of the hindbrain after antibodies to *XlHbox 1* protein are injected into the early embryo. (Based on studies by Wright CV and others: *Cell* 59:81–93, 1989.)

**FIGURE 4-8** Schematic representation of classes of homeobox-containing genes also possessing conserved motifs outside the homeodomain. Names of the different classes of genes are listed on the left. The red boxes represent the homeodomain within each gene class. The other boxes represent conserved motifs specific to each class of genes. (Modified from Duboule D, ed: *Guidebook to the homeobox genes*, Oxford, 1994, Oxford University Press.)

| | Chromosomal localization | | | | | | Sites of expression | Mutants | |
|---|---|---|---|---|---|---|---|---|---|
| Gene | Human | N | PD | Oct | HD | C | | Mouse | Human |
| Pax-1 | 20p11 | | | | | | Sclerotome, perivertebral mesenchyme, thymus | *Undulated* (un) | |
| Pax-9 | 14q12 -q13 | | | | | | Sclerotome, perivertebral mesenchyme | | |
| Pax-2 | 10p25 | | | | | | Urogenital, CNS, eye, inner ear | KO: no kidneys | Ocular-renal syndromes |
| Pax-5 | 9p13 | | | | | | Pro-B cells, CNS | KO: no B cells | |
| Pax-8 | 2q12 -q14 | | | | | | Thyroid, kidney, CNS | KO: no follicular cells in thyroid | |
| Pax-3 | 2q35 | | | | | | Dermomyotome, neural crest, muscle, CNS | *Splotch* (Sp) | Waardenburg syndrome |
| Pax-7 | 1p36 | | | | | | Dermomyotome, neural crest, muscle, CNS | KO: cranial neural crest defects | Rhabdomyo- sarcoma |
| Pax-4 | 7q32 | | | | | | Pancreas | KO: no insulin | |
| Pax-6 | 11p13 | | | | | | Eye, pancreas, CNS | *Small eye* (Sey) | Aniridia |

**FIGURE 4-9** Summary diagram of the members of the *Pax* gene family, showing their location on human chromosomes, sites of expression, and known effects of mutants in both human and mouse. The structures of conserved elements of these genes are schematically represented. *CNS*, Central nervous system; *KO*, knockout. (Modified from Wehr R, Gruss P: *Int J Dev Biol* 40:369–377, 1996; and Epstein JC: *Trends Card Med* 6:255–260, 1996.)

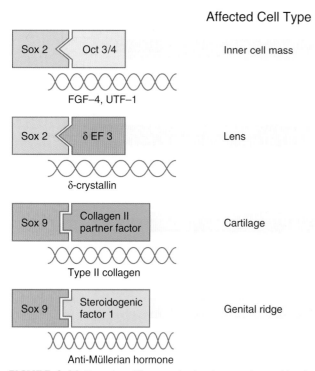

Affected Cell Type

FGF–4, UTF–1 — Inner cell mass

δ-crystallin — Lens

Type II collagen — Cartilage

Anti-Müllerian hormone — Genital ridge

**FIGURE 4-10** Examples of Sox proteins forming complexes with other transcription factors as they influence the expression of specific genes (labels below the helix representing DNA). (Right) Tissues influenced by the Sox-based gene regulation.

The **Lim proteins** constitute a large family of homeodomain proteins, some of which bind to the DNA in the nucleus and others of which are localized in the cytoplasm. Lim proteins are involved at some stage in the formation of virtually all parts of the body. As will be seen on page 94, the absence of certain Lim proteins results in the development of headless mammalian embryos.

The **T-box** genes get their names from the **brachyury (T) locus**, which was recognized as early as 1927 to cause short tails in heterozygotic mice. In 1990 the gene was cloned and found to contain a conserved region, the T-box, which acts as a transcription factor. Initially thought to be a single gene, an entire family of T-box genes has been identified. Genes in this family play important roles in development, such as the induction of the mesodermal germ layer and the specification of fore vs. hind limbs (see p. 216).

The **Dlx** gene family, like the Hox gene family, is a group of genes that have been phylogenetically conserved. The six members of this group in mammals are related to the single distalless gene in Drosophila, and they play important roles in patterning, especially of outgrowing structures, in early embryos. The mammalian Dlx genes operate in pairs, which are closely associated with Hox genes. Dlx-5 and Dlx-6 are located 5′ to Hoxa-13; Dlx-3, to Dlx-7 are 5′ to Hoxb-13; and Dlx-1, and Dlx-2 are 5′ to Hoxd-13. In addition to being involved in appendage

development, Dlx gene products are involved in morphogenesis of the jaws and inner ear.

## Signaling Molecules

Signaling molecules, sometimes called **cytokines**, are glycoproteins or polypeptide **growth factors** that mediate most interactions between groups of cells in embryos. **Nerve growth factor**, which stimulates the growth of sensory and sympathetic neurons, was the first growth factor to be intensively investigated, with research starting in the 1950s. Many of the signaling molecules that are most important in embryonic development are members of two large families with more than 20 members each—the **transforming growth factor-β (TGF-β)** and **fibroblast growth factor (FGF)** families. Other polypeptide signaling molecules, such as the **epidermal growth factor** and the **IGFs (insulin-like growth factors)**, belong to much smaller families. Members of another more recently discovered family of signaling molecules, the **hedgehog proteins**, mediate some of the most potent inductive interactions discovered to date.

### TGF-β Family

The TGF-β superfamily consists of a large number of molecules (up to 30) that play a wide variety of roles during embryogenesis and postnatal life. The TGF family was named because its first-discovered member (TGF-$\beta_1$) was isolated from virally transformed cells. Only later was it realized that many signaling molecules with greatly different functions during both embryological and postnatal life bear structural similarity to this molecule. Table 4-1 summarizes some of these molecules and their functions.

The formation, structure, and modifications of TGF-$\beta_1$ are representative of many types of signaling molecules and will be used as an example (Figure 4-11). TGF-$\beta_1$ is a disulfide-linked dimer, which is synthesized as a pair of inactive 390 amino acid precursors. The glycosylated precursor consists of a small N-terminal signal sequence, a much larger pro-region, and a 112–amino acid C-terminal bioactive domain. The pro-region is enzymatically cleaved off the bioactive domain at a site of four basic amino acids adjoining the bioactive domain. After secretion from the cell, the pro-region of the molecule remains associated with the bioactive region, causing the molecule to remain in a latent form. Only after dissociation of the pro-region from the bioactive region does the bioactive dimer acquire its biological activity.

### FGF Family

FGF was initially described in 1974 as a substance that stimulates the growth of fibroblasts in culture. Since then the originally described FGF has expanded into a family

| Member | Representative functions | Chapters |
|---|---|---|
| TABLE 4-1 *Members of the TGF-β Superfamily Mentioned in This Text* | | |
| TGF-β$_1$ to TGF-β$_5$ | Mesodermal induction | 5 |
| | Myoblast proliferation | 9 |
| | Invasion of cardiac jelly by atrioventricular endothelial cells | 17 |
| Activin | Granulosa cell proliferation | 1 |
| | Mesodermal induction | 5 |
| Inhibin | Inhibition of gonadotropin secretion by hypophysis | 1 |
| Müllerian inhibiting substance | Regression of paramesonephric ducts | 16 |
| Decapentaplegic | Signaling in limb development | 10 |
| Vg1 | Mesodermal and primitive streak induction | 5 |
| BMP-1 to -9 | Induction of neural plate, skeletal differentiation, and other inductions | 5, 9, 10 |
| Nodal | Formation of mesoderm and primitive streak, left-right axial fixation | 5 |
| Glial cell line–derived neurotrophic factor | Induction of outgrowth of ureteric bud, neural colonization of gut | 16, 12 |
| Lefty | Determination of body asymmetry | 5 |

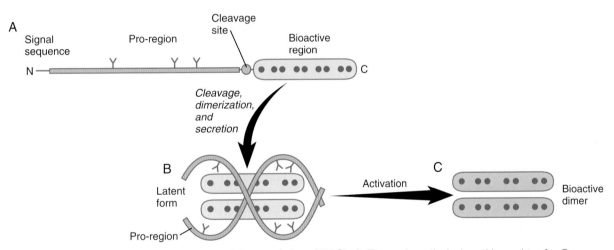

**FIGURE 4-11** Steps in the activation of the growth factor, TGF-β1. **A,** The newly synthesized peptide consists of a C-terminal bioactive region, to which is attached a long glycosylated pro-region and an N-terminal signal sequence. The pro-region is cleaved off from the bioactive region, and two secreted bioactive regions form a dimer **(B)** that is maintained in a latent form by being complexed with the separated pro-regions. Through an activation step **(C)** the bioactive dimer is released from the pro-regions and can then function as a signaling molecule.

of more than 10 members, each of which has distinctive functions. Many members of the FGF family play important roles in a variety of phases of embryonic development, as well as fulfilling functions, such as the stimulation of capillary growth, in the postnatal body. Some of the functions of the FGFs in embryonic development are listed in Table 4-2. Secreted fibroblast growth factors are closely associated with the extracellular matrix and must bind to heparan sulfate to activate their receptors.

## Other Signaling Molecules

Numerous families of signaling molecules have been identified. One of the most potent for embryological development is the **hedgehog family**. One member of this family, sonic hedgehog, is extremely important in many aspects of development, and it is treated as a model signaling molecule in Box 4-2. Members of the large **Wnt family** are related to the segment-polarity gene *Wingless* in *Drosophila* (see Figure 4-1), and like most signaling molecules they play a variety of roles in the development of many structures in the embryo. Many other individual signaling molecules from other families are mentioned in this text.

One of the important recent realizations in molecular embryology is how often signaling molecules act by inhibiting the actions of other signaling molecules. For example, the signaling molecules **chordin**, **noggin**, and **gremlin** all inhibit the activity of bone morphogenetic protein (BMP), which itself often acts as an inhibitor.

There is also evidence from several developing organ systems that some signaling molecules (e.g., sonic hedgehog and members of the FGF family) are positive regulators of growth and that others (e.g., some members of the BMP family) serve as negative regulators of growth. Normal development of a variety of organs requires a balance between the activities of these positive and negative regulators. Such interactions are described later in the text for developing organ systems as diverse as limbs, hair (or feathers), teeth, and the branching of ducts in the lungs, kidneys, and prostate gland.

## Receptor Molecules

For intercellular signaling molecules to exert an effect on target cells, they must normally interact with receptors in these cells. Most receptors are located on the cell surface, but some, especially those for lipid-soluble molecules, such as steroids, retinoids, and thyroid hormone, are intracellular.

**Cell surface receptors** are typically transmembrane proteins with extracellular, transmembrane, and cytoplasmic domains (see Figure 4-2). The extracellular domain contains a binding site for the **ligand**, which is typically a hormone, cytokine, or growth factor. When the ligand binds to a receptor, it effects a conformational change in the cytoplasmic domain of the receptor molecule. Cell surface receptors are two main types—(1) those with intrinsic protein kinase activity and (2) those that use a second messenger system to activate cytoplasmic protein kinases. An example of the first type is the family of receptors for FGFs, in which the cytoplasmic domain possesses **tyrosine kinase** activity. Receptors for growth factors of the TGF-β superfamily are also of this type, but in them the cytoplasmic domain contains **serine/threonine kinase** activity. In cell surface receptors of the second type, the protein kinase activity is separate from the receptor molecule itself. This type of receptor is also activated by binding with a ligand (e.g., neurotransmitter, peptide hormone, growth factor), but a series of intermediate steps is required to activate cytoplasmic protein kinases. A surface receptor, **Notch**, is introduced in greater detail in Box 4-3 as a specific example of a receptor that plays a number of important roles in embryonic development.

## Box 4-2   Sonic Hedgehog—A Busy Molecule in Development

The signaling molecule **sonic hedgehog (shh)** burst upon the vertebrate embryological scene in 1994, and since then it has proved to be one of the most important molecules in development (Table 4-3). It is related to the segment-polarity molecule hedgehog. In *Drosophila* shh is a member of an increasingly large family with whimsical names, such as desert hedgehog, Indian hedgehog, and tiggy-winkle hedgehog. The name hedgehog arose because mutant larvae in *Drosophila* contain batches of spikey outgrowths on their bellies.

Sonic hedgehog is a protein with a highly conserved N-terminal region and a more divergent C-terminal region. After its synthesis and release of the propeptide from the rough endoplasmic reticulum, the signal peptide is cleaved off and glycosylation occurs on the remaining peptide (Figure 4-12). Still within the cell, the shh peptide undergoes autocleavage through the catalytic activity of its C-terminal portion. During cleavage, the N-terminal segment becomes covalently bound with cholesterol. The 19kDa N-terminal peptide is then secreted from the cell, but remains bound to the surface of the cell

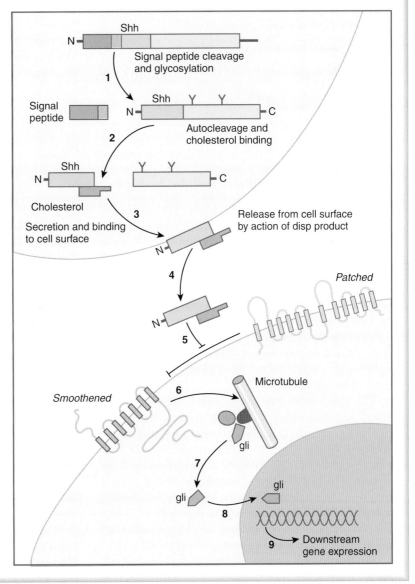

**FIGURE 4-12** The sonic hedgehog (shh) signaling pathway. (1) The signal peptide is cleaved off the newly synthesized polypeptide, and the remainder undergoes glycosylation. (2) The remaining peptide undergoes autocleavage under the influence of the C-terminal portion, and cholesterol binds to the N-terminal part, which is the active part of the molecule. (3) The N-terminal part is secreted and bound to the cell surface. (4) The bound shh molecule is released from the cell surface through the action of a product of *dispersed (disp)*. (5) The released shh inhibits the inhibitory effect of Patched upon smoothened. (6) Upon release from the inhibitory influence of Patched, smoothened emits a signal that (7) releases the transcription factor Gli from a complex of molecules bound to microtubules. (8) Gli enters the nucleus and binds to the DNA, (9) influencing the expression of a number of genes.

*Continued*

## Box 4-2   Sonic Hedgehog—A Busy Molecule in Development (Continued)

**TABLE 4-3** *Sites in the Embryo Where Sonic Hedgehog Serves as a Signaling Molecule*

| Signaling center | Chapter |
|---|---|
| Primitive node | 5 |
| Notochord | 6, 11 |
| Floor plate (nervous system) | 11 |
| Intestinal portals | 6 |
| Zone of polarizing activity (limb) | 10 |
| Hair and feather buds | 9 |
| Ectodermal tips of facial processes | 14 |
| Apical ectoderm of second pharyngeal arch | 14 |
| Tips of epithelial buds in outgrowing lung | 15 |
| Patterning of retina | 13 |
| Outgrowth of genital tubercle | 16 |

that produced it. All of the signaling activity of shh resides in the N-terminal segment. Through the activity of another gene product (*disp* in *Drosophila*), the N-terminal segment of shh, still bound with cholesterol, is released from the cell. The C-terminal peptide plays no role in signaling.

At the surface of a target cell, shh, still complexed with cholesterol, binds to a receptor, **Patched (Ptc)**. The cholesterol appears to facilitate binding. Ptc is closely associated with another transmembrane protein, **smoothened (smo)**. Ptc normally inhibits the signalling activity of smo, and shh inhibits the inhibitory activity of Ptc, thus allowing smo to give off an intracellular signal. Through the mediation of several other molecules, which are normally bound to microtubules, smo ultimately activates the 5-zinc finger transcription factor, Gli, which moves to the nucleus and binds to specific sites on the DNA of the target cell, thus affecting gene expression of the target cell.

## Box 4-3   Lateral Inhibition and the Notch Receptor

The normal development of many tissues begins with a population of developmentally equivalent cells. At some point, one of these cells begins to differentiate into a dominant mature cell type, such as a neuron, and in doing so, it transmits to its neighboring cells a signal that prevents them from differentiating into that same cell type. As a consequence, these neighboring cells are forced to differentiate into a secondary cell type, such as a glial cell in the central nervous system (Figure 4-13). This type of signaling of a dominant cell to its subservient neighbors is called **lateral inhibition.**

The common mechanism of lateral inhibition is the **Notch** signaling pathway, which is so basic that it has been preserved largely unchanged throughout the animal kingdom. Notch is a 300 kD cell surface receptor with a large extracellular domain and a smaller intracellular domain. The Notch receptor becomes activated when it combines with ligands (**Delta** or **Jagged** in vertebrates) that extend from the surface of the dominant cell. This sets off a pathway that inhibits the neighboring cell from differentiating into the dominant phenotype.

An abbreviated version of this pathway is as follows (Figure 4-14): The complexing of Notch with its ligand (e.g., Delta) stimulates an intracellular protease reaction that cleaves off the intracellular domain of the Notch molecule. The liberated intracellular domain of Notch becomes translocated to the nucleus, but on its way it may become associated with regulatory proteins, such as **Deltex**. Within the nucleus, the intracellular domain of Notch combines with several helix-loop-helix transcription factors, and this complex binds to the DNA of a gene called **enhancer of split**. The product of this gene, in turn, is another transcription factor that regulates other genes. For example, it represses certain genes of the **Achaete-Scute** complex, whose function is to promote neuronal development. By this complex pathway, the subservient cells are denied the opportunity to differentiate into neurons and they, instead, follow a secondary pathway, which leads to their becoming glial cells.

As complex as this appears, the above is a greatly abbreviated version of this inhibitory pathway and its controlling elements. When more is learned about all of the elements involved in this pathway, it will likely look like a component of an immense network of regulatory pathways that interact in very complex ways to integrate both internal and external environmental influences that determine the ultimate developmental fate of a cell.

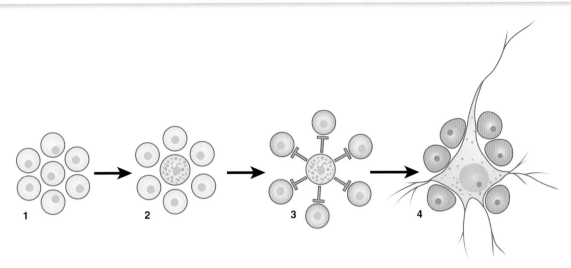

**FIGURE 4-13** An example of lateral inhibition. (1) A population of developmentally equivalent cells. (2) One cell, whether by its position or through stochastic (random) factors, begins to develop along a dominant pathway before its neighbors. (3) The selected cell then gives off inhibitory signals (lateral inhibition) that prevent its neighbors from differentiating into the dominant cell type. (4) The selected cell then differentiates into a mature cell type (e.g., a neuron), whereas its neighbors differentiate into secondary phenotypes (e.g., glial cells).

**FIGURE 4-14** The Delta-Notch pathway. When Delta from a dominant cell binds to Notch on the surface of the neighboring cell, proteolytic cleavage releases the intracellular domain of Notch, which complexes with Deltex and then enters the nucleus. There it becomes linked to Suppressor of hairless and serves as a transcription factor, which binds to *enhancer of split*. This sends off an inhibitory influence that represses the expression of genes, such as the *Achaete-Scute* complex, which would otherwise promote differentiation.

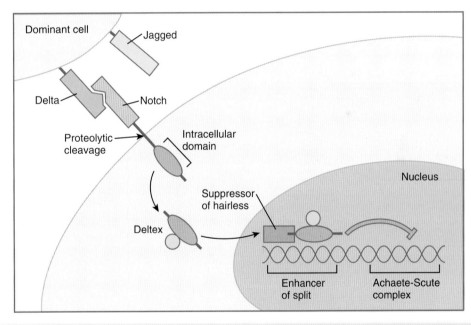

## Signal Transduction

**Signal transduction** is the process by which the signal provided by the **first messenger** (i.e., the growth factor or other signaling molecule) is translated into an intracellular response. Signal transduction begins when the first messenger, or ligand, binds to a receptor and changes its conformation. In the case of receptors that do not possess intrinsic protein kinase activity, binding of the ligand to the receptor stimulates a chain reaction, or **cascade**, leading to the production of a **second messenger**, which activates cytoplasmic protein kinases.

A typical cascade (see Figure 4-2) consists of a series of steps by which the activated receptor, acting through **G proteins** (proteins that bind guanosine triphosphate and guanosine diphosphate), stimulates an effector enzyme (e.g., adenyl cyclase) to convert precursor molecules into second messengers. (Two important second messengers are cyclic adenosine monophosphate and inosine triphosphate plus diacylglycerol.) The second messenger then activates cytoplasmic protein kinases, which phosphorylate (add phosphate groups to) target proteins, either activating or inactivating them. After additional steps typically involving other kinases and the translocation of activated molecules to the nucleus, DNA transcription is affected. In this way the transduction cascade leads to a cellular response, which in embryonic development could be the transformation of cell type during differentiation or the production of a specific product by the target cell.

## Retinoic Acid

For years, **vitamin A (retinol)** and its metabolite, **retinoic acid**, have been known to play a very important but equally enigmatic role in embryonic development. Over a half century ago it was found that either a severe deficiency or an excess of vitamin A results in a broad spectrum of severe congenital anomalies that can involve the face, eye, hindbrain, limbs, or urogenital system. It was only in the 1990s, when the binding proteins and receptors for the retinoids were characterized and the development of various knockouts was investigated, that specific clues to the function of vitamin A in embryogenesis began to emerge.

Vitamin A enters the body of the embryo as retinol and binds to a retinol binding protein, which attaches to specific cell surface receptors (Figure 4-15). Retinol is released from this complex and enters the cytoplasm, where it is bound to **cellular retinol-binding protein (CRBP I)**. In the cytoplasm the all-trans retinol is enzymatically converted first to all-trans retinaldehyde and then to all-trans retinoic acid, the retinoid with the most potent biological activity

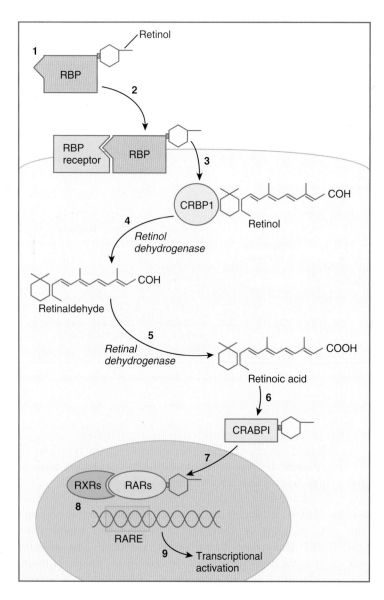

**FIGURE 4-15** The pathway of vitamin A in a cell. (1) Retinol becomes bound to a retinol-binding protein (RBP) outside the cell. (2) This complex is bound to an RBP receptor on the cell surface. (3) The retinol is then released into the cytoplasm and is bound to a cytoplasmic retinol-binding protein (CRBP I). (4) Through the action of retinol dehydrogenase, retinol is converted to retinaldehyde, which, in turn, (5) is converted to retinoic acid by retinal dehydrogenase. (6) Retinoic acid is bound to a cytoplasmic receptor (CRABP I) and taken into the nucleus. (7) Within the nucleus, retinoic acid is bound to a dimer of two nuclear retinoic acid receptors (RXR and RAR). (8) This complex binds to a retinoic acid response element (RARE) on the DNA and (9) activates transcription of target genes.

(see Figure 4-15). Both CRBP and **CRABP I (cellular retinoic acid–binding protein)** may function to control the amount of retinoids that enters the nucleus. Once released from CRABP, retinoic acid enters the nucleus, where it typically binds to a heterodimer consisting of a member of the **retinoic acid receptor (RAR)** α, β, or γ family and a member of the **retinoid X receptor (RXR)** α, β, or γ family. This complex of retinoic acid plus receptor heterodimer binds to a **retinoic acid response element (RARE)** on DNA, usually on the enhancer region of a gene, and it acts as a transcription factor, controlling the production of a gene product.

Retinoic acid appears to be produced and utilized in specific local regions at various times during prenatal and postnatal life. One of its well-defined targets early in development is certain of the *Hox* genes (e.g., *Hoxb-1*), where misexpression caused by either too little or too much retinoic acid can result in serious disturbances in the organization of the hindbrain and pharyngeal neural crest. One of the most spectacular examples of the power of retinoic acid is its ability to cause extra pairs of limbs to form alongside the regenerating tails of amphibians (Figure 4-16). This is a true example of a homeotic shift in a vertebrate, similar to the formation of double-winged flies or legs instead of antennae in *Drosophila*.

## Developmental Genes and Cancer

Many cancers are caused by mutated genes, and a number of these are genes that play a role in normal embryological development. Two main classes of genes are involved in tumor formation, and each class uses a different mechanism in stimulating tumor formation.

**FIGURE 4-16** A skeletal preparation showing a cluster of four supernumerary legs (*right*) growing out of the regenerating tail of a tadpole that had been placed in a solution of vitamin A following amputation of the tail. This is an example of a homeotic transformation. (Courtesy M. Maden, London, England.)

**Protooncogenes**, a class involving a variety of different types of molecules, induce tumor formation through dominant gain-of-function alleles that result in deregulated growth. Through several types of mechanisms, such as single-point mutations, selective amplification, or chromosomal rearrangements, protooncogenes can become converted to **oncogenes**, which are the actual effectors of poorly controlled cellular proliferation. Protooncogenes direct the normal formation of molecules as diverse as certain growth factors, growth-factor receptors, membrane-bound and cytoplasmic signal proteins, and transcription factors.

The other class of genes involved in tumor formation consists of the **tumor suppressor genes**, which normally function to limit the frequency of cell divisions. Recessive loss-of-function alleles of these genes fail to suppress cell division, resulting in uncontrolled divisions in defined populations of cells. A good example of a tumor suppressor gene is *Patched*, which has already been discussed as the transmembrane receptor for the signaling molecule, sonic hedgehog (see Box 4-2). Recall that *Patched* normally inhibits the activity of smoothened. Mutations of *Patched* eliminate the inhibition of smoothened, allowing uncontrolled downstream activity from smoothened, which stimulates the genome of the affected cell. Such a *Patched* mutation is the basis for the most common type of cancer, **basal cell carcinoma** of the skin.

## SUMMARY

○ Evidence is increasing that the basic body plan of mammalian embryos is under the control of many of the same genes that have been identified as controlling morphogenesis in *Drosophila*. In this species the basic axes are fixed through the actions of maternal-effect genes. Batteries of segmentation genes (gap, pair-rule, and segment-polarity genes) are then activated. Two clusters of homeotic genes next confer a specific morphogenetic character to each body segment. Because of their regulative nature, mammalian embryos are not as rigidly controlled by genetic instructions as *Drosophila* embryos.

○ The homeobox, a highly conserved region of 180 base pairs, is found in multiple different genes in almost all animals. The homeobox protein is a transcription factor. Homeobox-containing genes are arranged along the chromosome in a specific order and are expressed along the craniocaudal axis of the embryo in the same order. Activation of homeobox genes may involve interactions with other morphogenetically active agents, such as retinoic acid and TGF-β.

○ Many of the molecules that control development can be assigned to several broad groups. One group is the transcription factors, of which the products of homeobox-containing genes are just one of many types.

A second category is signaling molecules, many of which are effectors of inductive interactions. Some of these are members of large families, such as the TGF-β and FGF families. A very important class of signaling molecules is the hedgehog proteins, which mediate the activities of many important organizing centers in the early embryo. Signaling molecules interact with responding cells by binding to specific surface or cytoplasmic receptors. These receptors represent the initial elements of complex signal transduction pathways, which translate the signal to an intracellular event that results in new patterns of gene expression in the responding cells. Retinoic acid (vitamin A) is a powerful, but poorly understood developmental molecule. Misexpression of retinoic acid causes level shifts in axial structures through interactions with *Hox* genes.

○ Many cancers are caused by mutations of genes involved in normal development. Two major classes of cancer-causing genes are protooncogenes, which induce tumor formation through gain-of-function mechanisms, and tumor suppressor genes, which cause cancers through loss-of-function mutations.

## Review Questions

1. What is a homeobox?

2. Which of the following is a transcription factor?
   A. Fibroblast growth factor
   B. Pax
   C. Transforming growth factor
   D. Notch
   E. Wnt

3. Where in the cell is the retinoic acid receptor located?

4. A mutation of what receptor is the basis for basal carcinomas of the skin?
   A. Patched
   B. Retinoic acid
   C. Notch
   D. FGF receptor
   E. None of the above

5. Zinc fingers or helix-loop-helix arrangements are characteristic of members of what class of molecules?
   A. Protooncogenes
   B. Signaling molecules
   C. Receptors
   D. Transcription factors
   E. None of the above

6. Based on your knowledge of paralogous groups, which gene would be expressed most anteriorly in the embryo?
   A. *Hoxa-13*
   B. *Hoxc-9*
   C. *Hoxd-13*
   D. *Hoxb-1*
   E. *Hoxb-6*

7. Sonic hedgehog is produced in which signaling center?
   A. Notochord
   B. Intestinal portals
   C. Floor plate of neural tube
   D. Zone of polarizing activity in the limb bud
   E. All of the above

## REFERENCES

Bach I: The LIM domain: regulation by association, *Mech Devel* 91:5–17, 2000.

Cillo C and others: Homeobox genes and cancer, *Exp Cell Res* 248:1–9, 1999.

Cutforth T, Harrison CJ: Ephs and ephrins close ranks, *Trends Neurosci* 25:332–334, 2002.

DeRobertis EM, Oliver G, Wright CVE: Homeobox genes and the vertebrate body plan, *Sci Am* 263(1):46–52, 1990.

Duboule D, ed: *Guidebook to the homeobox genes*, Oxford, 1994, Oxford University Press.

Duboule D, Morata G: Colinearity and functional hierarchy among genes of the homeotic complexes, *Trends Genet* 10:358–364, 1994.

Gehring WJ: Homeobox genes, the homeobox, and the spatial organization of the embryo, *Harvey Lect* 81:153–172, 1987.

Goodman FR and others: Human *HOX* gene mutations, *Clin Genet* 59:1–11, 2001.

Graham A, Papalopulu N, Krumlauf R: The murine and *Drosophila* homeobox gene complexes have common features of organization and expression, *Cell* 57:367–378, 1989.

Hammerschmidt M, Brook A, McMahon AP: The world according to hedgehog, *Trends Genet* 13:14–21, 1997.

Hofmann C, Eichele G: Retinoids in development. In Sporn MB and others, eds: *The retinoids: biology, chemistry, and medicine*, 2nd ed., New York, 1994, Raven Press, pp. 387–441.

Ingham PW, McMahon AP: Hedgehog signaling in animal development: paradigms and principles, *Genes Dev* 15:3059–3087, 2001.

Johnson RL, Scott MP: New players and puzzles in the hedgehog signaling pathway, *Curr Opin Genet Devel* 8:450–456, 1998.

Kamachi Y, Uchikawa M, Kondoh H: Pairing Sox off with partners in the regulation of embryonic development, *Trends Genet* 16:182–187, 2000.

Kingsley DM: The TGF-β superfamily: new members, new receptors, and new genetic tests of function in different organisms, *Genes Dev* 8:133–146, 1994.

Kolodziejczyk SM, Hall BK: Signal transduction and TGF-β superfamily receptors, *Biochem Cell Biol* 74:299–314, 1996.

Kraus P, Lufkin T: Mammalian *Dlx* homeobox gene control of craniofacial and inner ear morphogenesis, *J Cell Biochem* (Suppl) 32/33:133–140, 1999.

Maden M: The role of retinoic acid in embryonic and post-embryonic development, *Proc Nutrition Soc* 59:65–73, 2000.

Mark M, Rijli FM, Chambon P: Homeobox genes in embryogenesis and pathogenesis, *Pediatr Res* 42:421–429, 1997.

Mansouri A, Goudreau G, Gruss P: *Pax* genes and their role in organogenesis, *Cancer Res* (Suppl) 59:1707s–1710s, 1999.

Mavillio F: Regulation of vertebrate homeobox-containing genes by morphogens, *Eur J Biochem* 212:273–288, 1993.

McGinnis W, Krumlauf R: Homeobox genes and axial patterning, *Cell* 68:283–302, 1992.

McMahon AP: The *Wnt* family of developmental regulators, *Trends Genet* 8:236–242, 1992.

Morriss-Kay GM, Ward SJ: Retinoids and mammalian development, *Internat Rev Cytol* 188:73–131, 1999.

Nusse R, Varmus HE: *Wnt* genes, *Cell* 69:1073–1087, 1992.

O'Rourke MP, Tam PPL: *Twist* functions in mouse development, *Int J Dev Biol* 46:401–413, 2002.

Papaioannou VE, Silver LM: The T-box gene family, *BioEssays* 20:9–19, 1998.

Patient RK, McGhee JD: The GATA family (vertebrates and invertebrates), *Curr Opin Genet Devel* 12:416–422, 2002.

Prior HM, Walter MA: *Sox* genes: architects of development, *Mol Med* 2:405–412, 1996.

Ross SA and others: Retinoids in embryonal development, *Physiol Revs* 80:1021–1054, 2000.

Saldanha G: The hedgehog signalling pathway and cancer, *J Pathol* 193:427–432, 2001.

Scott MP: Vertebrate homeobox nomenclature, *Cell* 71:551–553, 1992.

Simeone A, Puelles E, Acampora D: The Otx family, *Curr Opin Genet Devel* 12:409–415, 2002.

Stein S and others: Checklist: vertebrate homeobox genes, *Mech Devel* 55:91–108, 1996.

Tada M, Smith JC: T-targets: clues to understanding the functions of T-box proteins, *Devel Growth Differ* 43:1–11, 2001.

Von Bubnoff A, Cho KWY: Intracellular BMP signaling regulation in vertebrates: pathway or network? *Devel Biol* 239:1–14, 2001.

Walterhouse DO, Yoon JW, Iannaccone PM: Developmental pathways: sonic hedgehog-patched-GLI, *Environ Health Perspect* 107:169–171, 1999.

Wegner M: From head to toes: the multiple facets of Sox proteins, *Nucleic Acids Res* 27:1409–1420, 1999.

Wehr R, Gruss P: Pax and vertebrate development, *Int J Dev Biol* 40:369–377, 1996.

Wilkie AOM and others: Functions of FGFs and their receptors, *Curr Biol* 5:500–507, 1995.

Wilson M, Koopman P: Matching SOX: partner proteins and co-factors of the SOX family of transcriptional regulators, *Curr Opin Genet Devel* 12:441–446, 2002.

Wright CV and others: Interference with function of a homeobox gene in *Xenopus* embryos produces malformations of the anterior spinal cord, *Cell* 59:81–93, 1989.

# CHAPTER 5

# Formation of Germ Layers and Early Derivatives

As it is implanting into the uterine wall, the embryo undergoes profound changes in its organization. Up to the time of implantation, the blastocyst consists of the inner cell mass, from which the body of the embryo proper arises, and the outer trophoblast, which represents the future tissue interface between the embryo and mother. Both components of the blastocyst serve as the precursors of other tissues that appear in subsequent stages of development. Chapter 3 discusses the way that the cytotrophoblast gives rise to an outer syncytial layer, the syncytiotrophoblast, shortly before attaching to uterine tissue (see Figure 3-16). Not long thereafter, the inner cell mass begins to give rise to other tissue derivatives as well. The subdivision of the inner cell mass ultimately results in an embryonic body that contains the three primary embryonic germ layers: the **ectoderm** (outer layer), **mesoderm** (middle layer), and **endoderm** (inner layer). The process by which the germ layers are formed through cell movements is called **gastrulation**.

After the germ layers have been laid down, the continued progression of embryonic development depends on a series of signals called **embryonic inductions** that are exchanged between the germ layers or other tissue precursors. In an inductive interaction, one tissue (the **inductor**) acts on another (**responding tissue**) so that the developmental course of the latter is different from what it would have been in the absence of the inductor. The developments that can be seen with a microscope during this period are tangible reflections of profound changes in gene expression and cellular properties of implanting embryos.

## TWO-GERM-LAYER STAGE

Just before the embryo implants into the endometrium early in the second week, significant changes begin to occur in the inner cell mass as well as in the trophoblast. As the cells of the inner cell mass become rearranged into an epithelial configuration, sometimes referred to as the **embryonic shield**, a thin layer of cells appears ventral to the main cellular mass (see Figure 3-16). The main upper layer of cells is known as the **epiblast**, and the lower layer is called the **hypoblast**, or **primitive endoderm** (Figure 5-1).

How the hypoblast forms in human embryos is not understood, but comparative embryological data suggest that cells of this layer arise by **delamination** (a separation or dropping down) from the inner cell mass. The hypoblast is considered an **extraembryonic endoderm**, and it ultimately gives rise to the endodermal lining of the **yolk sac** (see Figure 3-16). Quite recently a localized region of the anterior hypoblast in mammalian embryos has been shown to possess the remarkable power of inducing much of the head and forebrain. Further details are given in Box 5-2. After the hypoblast has become a well-defined layer and the epiblast has taken on an epithelial configuration, the former inner cell mass is transformed into a **bilaminar disk**, with the epiblast on

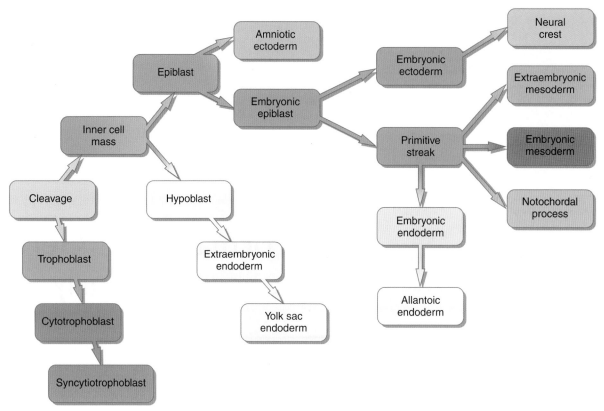

**FIGURE 5-1** Cell and tissue lineages in the mammalian embryo. (The colors in the boxes are found in all illustrations involving the embryonic and extraembryonic germ layers.)

the dorsal surface and the hypoblast on the ventral surface.

The epiblast contains the cells that will make up the embryo itself, but extraembryonic tissues also arise from this layer. The next layer to appear after the hypoblast is the **amnion**, a layer of extraembryonic ectoderm that ultimately encloses the entire embryo in a fluid-filled chamber called the **amniotic cavity** (see Chapter 7). Because of the paucity of specimens, the earliest stages in the formation of the human amnion and amniotic cavity are not completely understood. Studies on primate embryos indicate that a primordial amniotic cavity first arises by **cavitation** (formation of an internal space) within the preepithelial epiblast; it is covered by cells derived from the inner cell mass (Figure 5-2). According to some investigators, the roof of the amnion then opens, exposing the primordial amniotic cavity to the overlying cytotrophoblast. Soon thereafter (by about 8 days after fertilization), the original amniotic epithelium re-forms a solid roof over the amniotic cavity.

While the early embryo is still sinking into the endometrium (about 9 days after fertilization), cells of the hypoblast begin to spread, lining the inner surface of the cytotrophoblast with a continuous layer of extraembryonic endoderm called **parietal endoderm** (see Figure

5-2). When the endodermal spreading is completed, a vesicle called the **primary yolk sac** has taken shape (see Figure 3-16, C). At this point (roughly 10 days after fertilization), the embryo complex constitutes the bilaminar germ disk, which is located between the primary yolk sac on its ventral surface and the amniotic cavity on its dorsal surface. Shortly after it forms, the primary yolk sac becomes constricted, forming a secondary yolk sac and leaving behind a remnant of the primary yolk sac (see Figures 3-16, D, and 5-2, E).

Starting at about 12 days after fertilization, another extraembryonic tissue, the **extraembryonic mesoderm**, begins to appear (see Figure 5-2). The first extraembryonic mesodermal cells seem to arise from a transformation of parietal endodermal cells. These cells are later joined by extraembryonic mesodermal cells that have originated from the primitive streak. The extraembryonic mesoderm becomes the tissue that supports the epithelium of the amnion and yolk sac as well as the **chorionic villi**, which arise from the trophoblastic tissues (see Chapter 7). The support supplied by the extraembryonic mesoderm is not only mechanical but also trophic, since the mesoderm serves as the substrate through which the blood vessels supply oxygen and nutrients to the various epithelia.

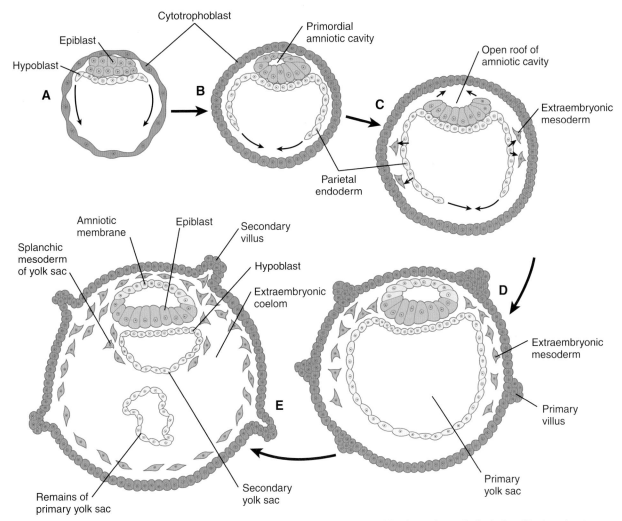

**FIGURE 5-2** Origins of the major extraembryonic tissues. The syncytiotrophoblast is not shown. **A,** Beginning of implantation at **6 days. B,** Implanted blastocyst at **7½ days. C,** Implanted blastocyst at **8 days. D,** Embryo at **9 days. E, Late second week.**

## GASTRULATION AND THE THREE EMBRYONIC GERM LAYERS

At the end of the second week the embryo consists of two flat layers of cells, the epiblast and the hypoblast. As the third week of pregnancy begins, the embryo enters the period of gastrulation, during which the three embryonic germ layers form from the epiblast (see Figure 5-1). The morphology of human gastrulation follows the pattern seen in birds. Because of the large amount of yolk in birds' eggs, the avian embryo forms the primary germ layers as three overlapping flat disks that rest on the yolk, much like a stack of pancakes. Only later do the germ layers fold to form a cylindrical body. Although the mammalian egg is essentially devoid of yolk, the morphological conservatism of early development still constrains the human embryo to follow a pattern of gastrulation similar to that seen in reptiles and birds. Because of the scarcity

of material, even the morphology of gastrulation in human embryos is not known in detail. Nevertheless, extrapolation from avian and mammalian gastrulation can provide a reasonable working model of human gastrulation.

Gastrulation begins with the formation of the **primitive streak**, a linear midline condensation of cells derived from the epiblast in the posterior region of the embryo, possibly through an induction by cells at the edge of the embryonic disk in that region (Figure 5-3). Initially triangular in shape, the primitive streak soon becomes linear and elongates, largely through internal cellular rearrangements, called **convergent-extension movements**. With the appearance of the primitive streak, the anteroposterior (craniocaudal) and right-left axes of the embryo can be readily identified (see Figure 5-3), but it is likely that the axes were set much earlier in development (Box 5-1).

The primitive streak is a region where cells of the epiblast converge in a well-defined sequence (Figure 5-4, *A*).

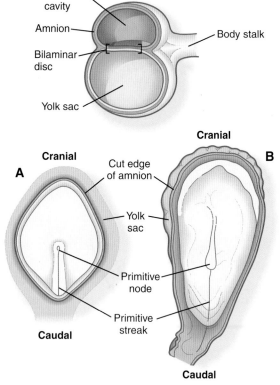

FIGURE 5-3 Dorsal views of **16-day (A)** and **18-day (B)** human embryos. *Top,* Sagittal section through an embryo and its extraembryonic membranes during early gastrulation.

As cells of the epiblast reach the primitive streak, they change shape and pass through it on their way to forming new cell layers beneath (ventral to) the epiblast (Figure 5-4, C). Marking studies have shown that cells in specific regions of the epiblast form specific structures in the mesoderm and endoderm. The composite results of such experiments are organized into **fate maps,** such as that illustrated in Figure 5-4, A. The movement of cells through the primitive streak results in the formation of a groove (**primitive groove**) along the midline of the primitive streak. At the anterior end of the primitive streak is a small but well-defined accumulation of cells, called **primitive node,** or **Hensen's node.*** This structure is of great developmental significance because it is the area through which migrating cells are channeled into a rodlike mass of mesenchymal cells called the **notochord** and a group of cells anterior to that called the **prechordal plate** (see Figure 4, A, C). (The important functions of the notochord and prechordal plate are discussed on p. 88.)

The movements of the cells passing through the primitive streak are accompanied by major changes in their structure and organization (Figure 5-6). While in the epiblast, the cells have the properties of typical epithelial cells, with well-defined apical and basal surfaces, and they

---

* Hensen's node is the commonly used designation for the primitive node in avian embryos, but this term is sometimes used in the mammalian embryological literature as well. This structure is the structural and functional equivalent of the dorsal lip of the blastopore in amphibians.

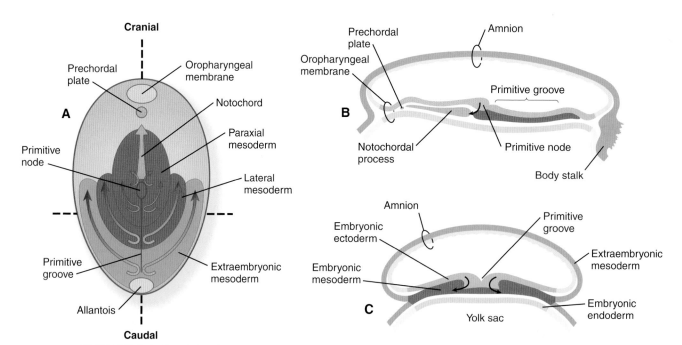

FIGURE 5-4 **A,** Dorsal view through a human embryo during gastrulation. The arrows show the directions of cellular movements across the epiblast toward, through, and away from the primitive streak as newly formed mesoderm. The illustrated fates of the cells that have passed through the primitive streak are based on studies of mouse embryos. **B,** Sagittal section through the craniocaudal axis of the same embryo. The curved arrow indicates cells passing through the primitive node into the notochord. **C,** Cross section through the level of the primitive streak in **A** (*dashed lines*).

## Box 5-1    Establishment of the Embryonic Axes

Both the early embryo and the adult body are organized along three axes—anteroposterior (craniocaudal), dorsoventral, and right-left. Although they are readily apparent at the time of gastrulation, these axes appear to be set considerably earlier in development. Research on the mouse suggests that the second polar body defines the anterior end of the anteroposterior axis (Figure 5-5, *A*). The embryonic-abembryonic axis in essence defines the dorsoventral axis. The portion of the blastocyst containing the inner cell mass is defined as the **embryonic pole**, and the region of trophoblast directly opposite is called the **abembryonic pole** (Figure 5-5, *B*). Because the side of the inner cell mass that abuts the blastocoele gives rise to the hypoblast, this is the ventral side of the inner cell mass. At what point in development the dorsoventral axis is specified remains uncertain. Once the dorsoventral and anteroposterior axes are set, the third (right-left) axis is automatically defined (Figure 5-5,*C*).

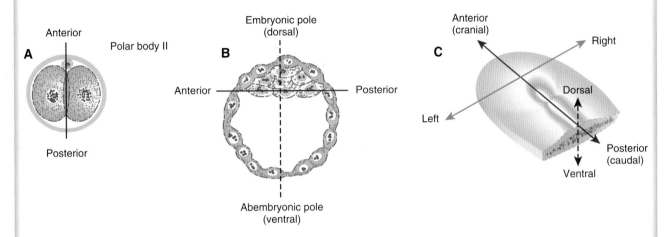

**FIGURE 5-5** Establishment of the embryonic axes. **A,** The anteroposterior (craniocaudal) axis is established by the location of the polar body during early cleavage. **B,** The dorsoventral axis is established in relation to the embryonic and abembryonic poles during the blastocyst stage. **C,** All three primary axes are apparent in the gastrulating embryo.

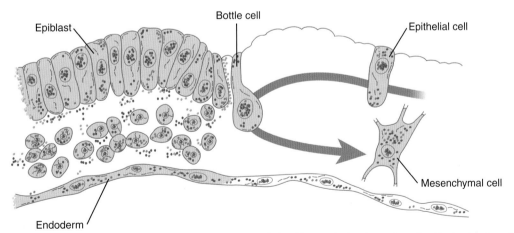

**FIGURE 5-6** Cross-sectional view of an embryo during gastrulation. Changes in the shape of a cell as it migrates along the epiblast (epithelium), through the primitive streak (bottle cell), and away from the groove as a mesenchymal cell that will become part of the mesodermal germ layer. The same cell can later assume an epithelial configuration as part of a somite.

are associated with a basal lamina that underlies the epiblast. As they enter the primitive streak, these cells elongate, lose their basal lamina, and take on a characteristic morphology that has led to their being called **bottle cells**. When they become free of the epiblastic layer in the primitive groove, the bottle cells assume the morphology and characteristics of **mesenchymal cells**, which are able to migrate as individual cells if provided with the proper extracellular environment (see Figure 5-6). Included in this transformation is the loss of specific cell adhesion molecules (see p. 99) as the cells convert from an epithelial to a mesenchymal configuration.

In birds, the first cells to leave the primitive streak enter the hypoblast layer, displacing some of the extraembryonic endodermal cells to form the definitive **embryonic endoderm**. This process has not been confirmed in the human embryo, but the morphology of human gastrulation is comparable to that seen in birds.

The most prominent feature of human gastrulation is the formation of mesoderm. Some cells that migrate through the primitive streak form extraembryonic mesoderm (see Figure 5-4, A). Much of the extraembryonic mesoderm forms the **body stalk**, which connects the caudal part of the embryo to the extraembryonic tissues that surround it (see Figures 5-4, B and 7-1). The body stalk later becomes the umbilical cord.

After the primitive streak is well established, the majority of cells passing through it spread out between the epiblast and the hypoblast to form the **embryonic mesoderm** (see Figure 5-4). Tracing studies have shown that cells leaving the node and primitive streak at given craniocaudal levels are destined to form specific types of mesoderm. For example, cells passing through the primitive node become either notochord or paraxial mesoderm, whereas cells leaving the primitive streak form paraxial mesoderm (see p. 108), lateral plate mesoderm (see p. 113), or extraembryonic mesoderm, depending on the craniocaudal level at which they exit the primitive streak (see Figure 5-4). The transformations of morphology and the behavior of the cells passing through the primitive streak are associated with profound changes not only in their adhesive properties and internal organization but also in the way that they relate to their external environment.

Starting in early gastrulation, cells of the epiblast produce **hyaluronic acid**, which enters the space between the epiblast and hypoblast. Hyaluronic acid, a polymer consisting of repeating subunits of D-glucuronic acid and N-acetylglucosamine, is frequently associated with cell migration in developing systems. The molecule has a tremendous capacity to bind water (up to 1000 times its own volume), and it functions to keep mesenchymal cells from aggregating during cell migrations. Although after leaving the primitive streak the mesenchymal cells of the embryonic mesoderm find themselves in a hyaluronic acid–rich environment, hyaluronic acid

alone is not enough to support their migration from the primitive streak. In all vertebrate embryos that have been investigated to date, the spread of mesodermal cells away from the primitive streak or the equivalent structure is found to depend on the presence of **fibronectin** associated with the basal lamina beneath the epiblast. The embryonic mesoderm ultimately spreads laterally as a thin sheet of mesenchymal cells between the epiblast and hypoblast layers (see Figure 5-4, C). By the time the mesoderm has formed a discrete layer in the human embryo, the upper germ layer (remains of the former epiblast) is called the **ectoderm**, and the lower germ layer, which has displaced the original hypoblast, is called the **endoderm**. This terminology is used for the remainder of this text.

## Regression of the Primitive Streak

After its initial appearance at the extreme caudal end of the embryo, the primitive streak expands cranially until about 18 days after fertilization (see Figure 5-3). Thereafter, it regresses caudally (see Figure 5-14), stringing out the notochord in its wake. Vestiges remain into the fourth week. During that time, the formation of mesoderm continues by means of cells migrating from the epiblast through the primitive groove.

The primitive streak normally disappears without a trace, but in rare instances, large tumors called teratomas appear in the sacrococcygeal region (see Figure 1-2, A). Teratomas often contain bizarre mixtures of many different types of tissue, such as cartilage, muscle, fat, hair, and glandular tissue. Because of this, sacrococcygeal teratomas are thought to arise from remains of the primitive streak (which can form all germ layers). Teratomas are also found in the gonads and the mediastinum. These tumors are thought to originate from germ cells.

## Notochord and Prechordal Plate

The notochord, the structure that is the basis for giving the name *Chordata* to the phylum to which all vertebrates belong, is a cellular rod running along the longitudinal axis of the embryo just ventral to the central nervous system. Although both phylogenetically and ontogenetically it serves as the original longitudinal support for the body, the notochord also plays an extremely important role as a prime mover in a series of signaling episodes (inductions) that transform unspecialized embryonic cells into definitive tissues and organs. In particular, inductive signals from the notochord (1) stimulate the conversion of overlying surface ectoderm into neural tissue, (2) specify the identity of certain cells (floor plate) within the early nervous system, (3) transform certain mesodermal cells of the somites into vertebral bodies, and (4) stimulate the earliest steps in the development of the dorsal pancreas.

Cranial to the notochord is a small region where embryonic ectoderm and endoderm abut without any intervening mesoderm. Called the **oropharyngeal membrane** (see Figure 5-4), this structure marks the site of the future oral cavity. Between the cranial tip of the notochordal process and the oropharyngeal membrane is a small aggregation of mesodermal cells closely apposed to endoderm, called the **prechordal plate** (see Figure 5-4). The prechordal plate emits molecular signals that are instrumental in stimulating the formation of the forebrain (see p. 93).

Both the prechordal plate and the notochord arise from the ingression of a population of epiblastic cells, which join other cells of primitive streak origin, within the primitive node. As the primitive streak regresses, the cellular precursors of first the prechordal plate and then the notochord migrate rostrally from the node, but are then left behind as a rodlike aggregation of cells (**notochordal process**, see Figure 5-4, *A, B*) in the wake of the regressing primitive streak. In mammals, shortly after ingression, the cells of the notochordal process temporarily spread out and fuse with the embryonic endoderm (Figure 5-7, *B*), resulting in the formation of a transitory **neurenteric canal** that connects the emerging amniotic cavity with the yolk sac. Later, the cells of the notochord separate from the endodermal roof of the yolk sac and form the definitive notochord, a solid rod of cells in the midline between the embryonic ectoderm and endoderm (Figure 5-7, *C*).

## INDUCTION OF NERVOUS SYSTEM

### Neural Induction

The inductive relationship between the notochord (**chordamesoderm**) and the overlying ectoderm in the genesis of the nervous system was recognized in the early 1900s. Although the original experiments were done on amphibians, similar experiments in higher vertebrates have shown that the essential elements of **neural** (or **primary**) **induction** are the same in all vertebrates.

Deletion and transplantation experiments in amphibians set the stage for the present understanding of neural induction. (See Chapters 6 and 11 for further details on the formation of the nervous system.) In the absence of chordamesoderm moving from the dorsal lip of the blastopore (the amphibian equivalent of the primitive node), the nervous system, which is first represented by a thickened plate of transformed ectodermal cells situated along the dorsal midline of the embryo, does not form from the dorsal ectoderm. On the other hand, if the dorsal lip of the blastopore is grafted beneath the belly ectoderm of another host, a secondary nervous system and body axis form in the area of the graft (Figure 5-8). The dorsal lip has been called the **organizer** because of its ability to stimulate the formation of a secondary body axis. Subsequent research has shown that the interactions occurring in the region of the dorsal lip in amphibians are far more complex than a single induction between chordamesoderm and ectoderm. Deletion and transplantation experiments have also been conducted on embryos of

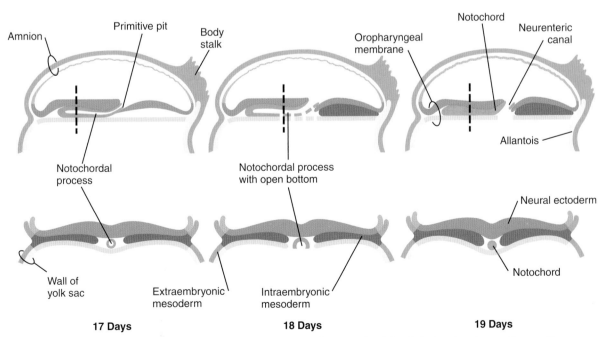

**FIGURE 5-7** From left to right, sequential stages in formation of the notochord. *Top,* Sagittal sections. *Bottom,* Cross sections at the level of the vertical line in the upper figure. In the upper row, the cranial end is on the left. The function of the neurenteric canal remains obscure.

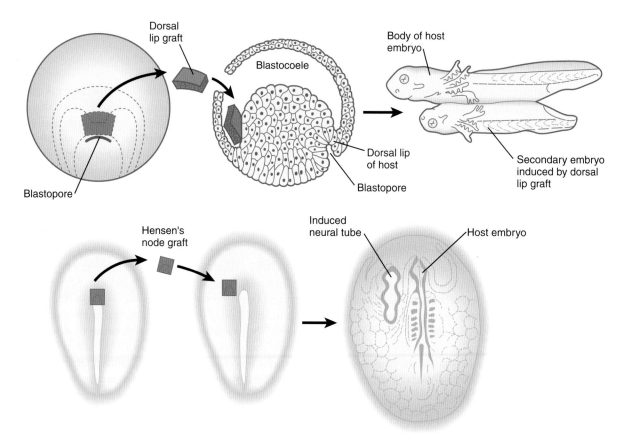

**FIGURE 5-8** Early experiments demonstrating neural induction. *Top*, Graft of the dorsal lip of the blastopore in a salamander embryo induces a secondary embryo to form. *Bottom*, Graft of Hensen's node from one avian embryo to another induces the formation of a secondary neural tube. (*Top* based on studies by Spemann H: *Embryonic development and induction*, New York, 1938, Hafner; *bottom* based on studies by Waddington C: *J Exp Biol* 10:38–46, 1933.)

birds and mammals (see Figure 5-8); clearly the primitive node and the notochordal process in birds and mammals are homologous in function to the dorsal lip and chordamesoderm in amphibians. This means that in higher vertebrates the primitive node and the notochordal process act as the neural inductor and the overlying ectoderm is the responding tissue. This fundamental relationship was established more than a half century ago. Since that time, embryologists have devoted an enormous amount of research to identifying the nature of the inductive signal that passes from the chordamesoderm to the ectoderm.

Early attempts to uncover the nature of the inductive stimulus were marked by a great deal of optimism. As early as the 1930s, various laboratories had proposed that molecules as diverse as proteins and steroids were the inductive stimulus. Soon thereafter came the discovery that an even wider variety of stimuli, such as inorganic ions or killed tissues, could elicit neural induction. With such a plethora of possible inductors, attention turned to the properties of the responding tissue (the dorsal ectoderm) and ways that it might react, through a final common pathway, to the inductive stimulus. The quest

for the neural inductive molecules and their mode of action has been arduous and frustrating, with many blind alleys and wrong turns along the way.

A number of laboratories found that isolated ectoderm could respond in vitro to inductive stimuli and become transformed into neural tissue. A very useful technique for studying induction in vitro involved separating the responding tissue from the inducing tissue by a filter with pores that permitted the passage of molecules but not cells. This technique has been used in the analysis of a variety of mammalian inductive systems.

Various experimental manipulations have clearly shown that neural induction is not a simple all-or-nothing process. Rather, considerable regional specificity exists. (For example, certain artificial inductors stimulate the formation of more anterior neural structures, and others stimulate the formation of more posterior ones.) In amphibian embryos, anterior chordamesoderm has different inducing properties from posterior chordamesoderm.

Recent research has identified specific molecules that bring about neural induction. In amphibians, three signaling molecules, **noggin**, **follistatin**, and **chordin**, given off by the notochord, are the inductive agents. It was first thought that these molecules directly stimulate uncommitted cells of the dorsal ectoderm to form neural tissue, but subsequent research on amphibians has shown that these inductors act by blocking the action of an inhibitor, **bone morphogenetic protein-4 (BMP-4)**, in the dorsal ectoderm (see Figure 5-10). In the absence of BMP-4 activity, dorsal ectoderm forms neural tissue as a default state. In birds and mammals, the inactivation of BMP-4 is also likely the immediate mechanism of neural induction, but the role of noggin and chordin as inactivators of BMP-4 is less clear. This set of molecular interactions commits ectodermal cells over the notochord to becoming neural tissue, but it is only the first step in the formation of the nervous system. An important second step is regionalization of the central nervous system.

**Regionalization** refers to the subdivision of the central nervous system into broad craniocaudal regions. Experimentation has shown that explants of the early primitive node can induce a nervous system with both anterior (head) and posterior (trunk) components, whereas explants of older node tissue only induce trunk components. Earlier experiments also showed that certain inductors cause the formation of more cranial, and others more caudal, neural structures. From studies on birds, it is known that the early cells that pass through the primitive node become incorporated into the prechordal plate, which is the head inducer in birds (see Box 5-2), and that the cells that leave the node later form the notochord, which induces trunk structures. Some evidence suggests that the prechordal plate alone cannot induce dorsal ectoderm to become neural tissue, but once neural induction has occurred, the prechordal plate plays an important role

in the forebrain regionalization of the central nervous system. However, in the presence of either **retinoic acid** or **fibroblast growth factor**, the induced neural structures are posteriorized, and more caudal structures (hindbrain) form.

## Mesodermal Induction

When initially described, neural induction was considered the first inductive process that takes place in the embryo, and it was often called **primary induction**. Subsequent experimentation conducted principally on amphibians has shown that other important inductions occur before neural induction. The best understood of these is the induction of mesoderm in the amphibian blastula. The mesoderm normally arises from a ring of cells around the equatorial region of the blastula (Figure 5-9). If the ectoderm located at the roof of the blastocoele is isolated, it remains general ectoderm and produces normal levels of **keratin** proteins, which are ectoderm-specific molecules. If the same piece of ectoderm is apposed to endoderm, it differentiates into mesoderm, as indicated by its producing α-actin, a molecule characteristic of muscle. In recent years, understanding of the nature of mesodermal induction has been greatly enhanced by the demonstration that certain specific proteins—**activin, noggin**, and **Vg1**—are effectors of mesodermal induction.

Although most current research on induction in early embryos is being conducted on amphibians, many principles learned from amphibians can be transferred to the embryos of higher vertebrates. If an early avian epiblast is isolated and grown in culture, a notochord and axial

**FIGURE 5-9** Experiments illustrating the induction of mesoderm in the amphibian blastula. The animal pole is the region of yolk-poor cells corresponding to the future rostral end of the amphibian embryo. The vegetal pole is the region of yolk-rich cells corresponding to the future caudal region of the amphibian embryo.

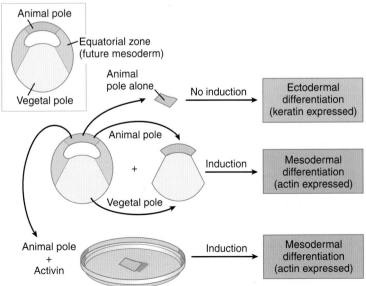

## Box 5-2  Molecular Aspects of Gastrulation

Many decades of research on birds and amphibians have resulted in a reasonable understanding of the cellular and molecular aspects of gastrulation in these species. Recent research suggests that despite some species differences, the basic aspects of gastrulation in mammals are fundamentally similar to those in birds.

The events of gastrulation are guided by a series of molecular inductions emanating from a succession of signaling centers in the caudalmost part of the embryo, but the evidence for a mammalian counterpart, sometimes called the **early gastrula organizer**, is less certain. Once the primitive streak is established, the primitive node takes over as the center that organizes the fundamental structure of the body axis. As the prechordal plate and the notochord take shape from cells that flow through the node, they, in turn, become important signaling centers, with the prechordal plate involved in the organization of

the head (anterior to rhombomere 3, see. p. 106 and the notochord organizing the development of the axial structures of the trunk. A recently discovered variant in mammals is that a region of anterior hypoblast is likely the initial head signaling region and functions even before the prechordal plate and notochord have taken shape (see below). Gene expression in the major signaling centers is not confined to the production of signaling molecules. Important transcription factors are also expressed.

### INDUCTION OF THE PRIMITIVE STREAK (THE EARLY GASTRULA ORGANIZER)

The basis for primitive streak formation is still poorly understood in any species, but four major signaling molecules, **chordin**, **nodal**, **cripto**, and **Vg1**, are active in the caudalmost area where the primitive streak first takes shape (Figure 5-10). In the chick embryo, ectopically

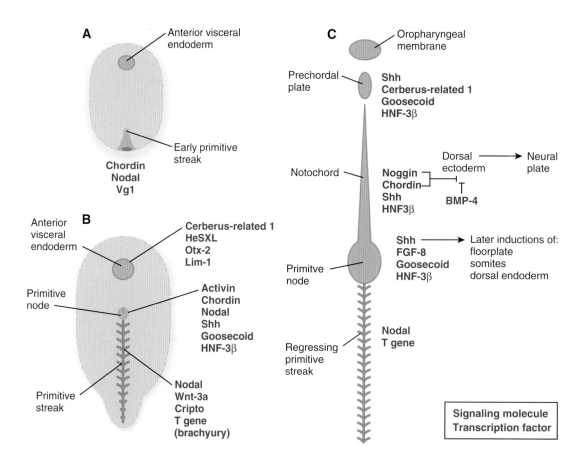

**FIGURE 5-10** Summary of major genes involved in various stages of early embryonic development. **A,** Early formation of the primitive streak. **B,** Gastrulation (period of germ layer formation). **C,** Late gastrulation and neural induction. The molecules in red are signaling molecules and those in blue are transcription factors. Names of specific molecules (bold) are placed by the structures in which they are expressed.

administered **chordin** and **Vg1** both induce the formation of an ectopic primitive streak.

## THE PRIMITIVE NODE (ORGANIZER)

As the primitive streak elongates, migrating cells of the epiblast join the tip of the streak, and a dynamic mass of cells, called the **primitive node**, becomes evident at the tip of the primitive streak. Cells of the node express many genes, including three classical molecular markers of the organizer region in many vertebrates—**chordin**, **goosecoid**, and **hepatic nuclear factor**-3β (HNF-3β). Not only is the winged helix transcription factor, HNF-3β, important for the formation of the node itself, but it is vital for the establishment of midline structures cranial to the node. HNF-3β is required for the initiation of notochord function. In its absence, not only the notochord, but also the floor plate of the neural tube (see Chapter 11) fail to form. On the other hand, endoderm, the primitive streak, and intermediate mesoderm do develop. The exact molecular action of **goosecoid**, a homeodomain transcription factor, is still not well understood, but this gene is prominently expressed in the organizer region of all vertebrates studied. Goosecoid activates *chordin*, *noggin*, and other genes of the organizer region. If ectopically expressed, it stimulates the formation of a secondary body axis. **Chordin**, **noggin**, and signaling molecules associated with the node (such as sonic hedgehog (shh), nodal, and activin) are involved in the setting of left-right asymmetry (see Box 5-3).

Two genes, *T* and *nodal*, play prominent roles in the function of the primitive streak and posterior mesoderm formation. Expression of the *T* **gene** appears to be activated by products of the *HNF-3β* and *goosecoid* genes. In *T* mutants (**brachyury**) the notochord begins to form through the activity of HNF-3β, but it fails to complete development. Studies on *T* mutants have shown that activity of the *T* gene is necessary for normal movements of future mesodermal cells through the primitive streak during gastrulation. In brachyury (short tail) mutant mice, mesodermal cells pile up at a poorly formed primitive streak, and the embryos show defective elongation of the body axis (including a short tail) posterior to the forelimbs. *T* gene mutants may be responsible for certain gross caudal body defects in humans. ***Nodal***, a member of the TGF-β family of growth factor genes (see Table 4-1), is expressed throughout the epiblast before gastrulation, but its activity is concentrated at the primitive node during gastrulation. Like the *T* gene, the

effects of *nodal* are strongly seen in the caudal region of the embryo. In the null mutant of *nodal*, the primitive streak fails to form, and the embryo is deficient in mesoderm. Similarly, mutants of *cripto*, an early acting member of the epidermal growth factor family and an essential cofactor in the *nodal* signaling pathway, produce a trunkless phenotype.

## THE PRECHORDAL PLATE AND NOTOCHORD

The first cells passing through the primitive node form a discrete midline mass of cells, the **prechordal plate**, which is closely associated with endoderm in the region just caudal to the oropharyngeal membrane. The next generation of cells passing through the node forms the notochord.

The **notochord** is a major axial signaling center of the trunk in the early embryo (see page 88), and it is important in the formation of many axial structures. Under the influence of HNF-3β, cells of the forming notochord produce **noggin** and **chordin**, molecules known to be potent neural inducers in many species. The notochord also produces sonic hedgehog, the effector molecule for many notochordal inductions of axial structures after the neural plate is induced. Despite inducing the neural plate within the overlying ectoderm, however, the notochord does not stimulate the formation of anterior parts of the brain or head structures. This function is reserved for the prechordal plate and the anterior visceral endoderm.

The **prechordal plate**, sometimes called the **head organizer**, consists of early mesodermal cells passing through the primitive node. These cells are structurally and functionally closely associated with cells of the underlying anterior endoderm.

## ANTERIOR VISCERAL ENDODERM (HYPOBLAST)

In mammals, even before mesodermal cells begin migrating through the primitive node, the anterior hypoblast (called the **anterior visceral endoderm** by mouse embryologists) expresses genes characteristic of the prechordal plate and probably initiates head formation. The anterior visceral endoderm itself is subdivided into an anterior part, which will serve as a signaling center for early heart formation (see page 115), and a more posterior part, which becomes part of the prechordal plate complex and induces formation of the head. According

*Continued*

## Box 5-2 Molecular Aspects of Gastrulation (Continued)

to one recent model, induction of the head and forebrain in mammals is a two-step process, in which an early induction by the anterior visceral endoderm confers a labile anterior character to the head and brain and a later induction by the prechordal plate mesoderm reinforces and maintains this induction. In avian embryos, in which much experimental work has been done, the prechordal plate alone seems to serve as the head signaling center.

To produce a head, it is necessary to block the BMP-4 signal and also a signal from the **Wnt** signaling pathway. Both signaling molecules and transcription factors are produced in the head signaling centers. In mice bearing mutants of **Lim-1**, a homeobox-containing transcription factor, and **cereberus-related 1**, a signaling molecule, headless mice are born (see Figure 5-11). The headless mice are born without neural structures anterior to rhombomere 3 (see Figure 6-3). Otx-2, another transcription factor present in the head signaling center, is also a general marker of the induced anterior region of the central nervous system. Many other molecules are also expressed in the head signaling center. How these orchestrate the formation of the head remains to be determined.

**FIGURE 5-11** Newborn headless mice and a normal mouse. The headless mice have a null mutant of the *Lim-1* gene. (From Shawlot W, Behringer RR: *Nature* 374:425–430, 1994.)

## Box 5-3 Molecular Basis for Left-Right Asymmetry

Up to the time of gastrulation the embryo is bilaterally symmetrical, but at that time mechanisms are set in place that ultimately result in the right-sided looping of the heart, followed by asymmetrical looping of the gut and the asymmetrical positioning of the liver, spleen, and lobation of the lungs. In mammalian embryos, the currently earliest known manifestation of asymmetry involves the beating of cilia around the primitive node (Figure 5-12). Their beat results in a directional current that appears to displace symmetry-breaking molecules (possibly **fibroblast growth factor [FGF]-8**) to the left. This, in turn, causes the appearance of two signaling

molecules in the TGF-β family, **nodal** in the lateral plate mesoderm to the left of the primitive node and **lefty-1** along the left side of the primitive streak. Lefty-1 may function to prevent the diffusion of left-determining molecules to the right side of the embryo. A sequence of molecular interactions downstream of nodal results in the activation of the *Pitx2* gene, a transcription factor, also on the left side. The Pitx2 protein is responsible for later asymmetrical development, such as rotation of the gut and stomach, position of the spleen, and the asymmetrical lobation of the lungs. Although the left-sided expression of nodal in the lateral mesoderm seems to be a point

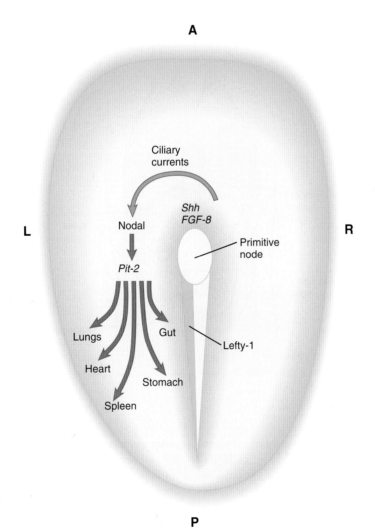

**FIGURE 5-12** Summary of the molecular basis for body asymmetry. Ciliary currents at the primitive node sweep the highest concentrations of sonic hedgehog (shh) and fibroblast growth factor-8 (FGF-8) toward the left side of the embryo, where they stimulate an asymmetric cascade of gene expression, starting with nodal. Lefty-1, expressed in the left side of the primitive streak, appears to prevent diffusion of molecules to the right side of the embryo. Only the most important molecules in a complex cascade are shown.

*Continued*

## Box 5-3   Molecular Basis for Left-Right Asymmetry (Continued)

of commonality in the determination of left-right asymmetry in all vertebrates, earlier (upstream) molecular events differ from those that operate in mammals.

In roughly one in 10,000 persons the left-right asymmetry of the body is totally reversed, a condition called **situs inversus** (Figure 5-13). This condition is often not recognized until the individual is examined relatively late in life by an astute diagnostician. Several mutations and syndromes are associated with this condition, but one of the most instructive is **Kartagener's syndrome**, in which situs inversus is associated with respiratory symptoms (sinusitis and bronchiectasis) due to abnor-

malities of the dynein arms in cilia (immotile cilia). In a similar mouse mutant, the cilia around the primitive node do not function properly, and the lack of directionality of the resulting fluid currents around the node is suspected to result in the random localization of nodal and other asymmetry-producing molecules to the right side of the embryo. Partial situs inversus, such as an isolated right-sided heart (**dextrocardia**), can also occur. With over 24 genes presently known to be involved in left-right asymmetry it is likely that such isolated occurrences of organ asymmetry are due to mutations of genes farther downstream in the asymmetry cascade.

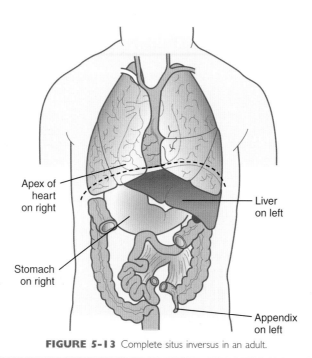

**FIGURE 5-13** Complete situs inversus in an adult.

mesoderm do not form. If an intact hypoblast or even dissociated and then reaggregated hypoblastic cells are juxtaposed to the cultured epiblast, axial structures form. Another experiment has shown that adding tissue culture medium exposed to a mesodermal inductor (XTC cells) to an isolated avian epiblast results in the induction of the epiblast to form axial mesodermal structures. Activin alone can induce axial structures in the avian epiblast. In mammals, other members of the TGF-β family of signaling molecules, **BMPs**, and **nodal** are also important in stimulating the formation of mesoderm, but despite the demonstration that these and many

other genes are involved in the induction of mesoderm, the sequence of molecular interactions leading to the formation of mesoderm in mammals remains poorly understood.

## Early Formation of the Neural Plate

The first obvious morphological response of the embryo to neural induction is the transformation of the dorsal ectoderm overlying the notochordal process into an

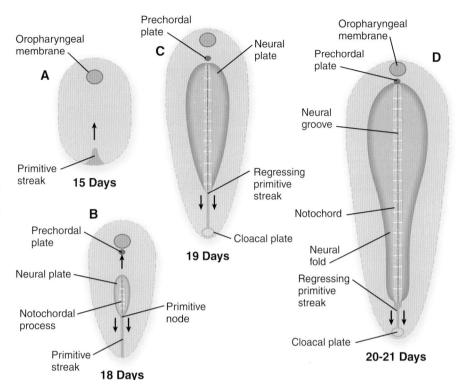

**FIGURE 5-14** Relationships between the neural plate and primitive streak. **A, Day 15. B, Day 18. C, Day 19. D, Days 20 to 21.**

elongated patch of thickened epithelial cells called the **neural plate** (Figure 5-14).

With the formation of the neural plate, the ectodermal germ layer becomes subdivided into two developmental lineages: neural and nonneural. This example illustrates several fundamental developmental concepts: **restriction, determination,** and **differentiation.** The zygote and blastomeres resulting from the first couple of cleavage divisions are **totipotent** (i.e., capable of forming any cell in the body). As development progresses, certain decisions are made that narrow the developmental options of cells (Figure 5-15). For example, at an early stage in cleavage, some cells become committed to the extraembryonic trophoblastic line and are no longer capable of participating in the formation of the embryo itself. At the point where cells become committed to becoming trophoblast, a restriction event has occurred. When a group of cells has gone through its last restriction event (e.g., the transition from cytotrophoblast to syncytiotrophoblast), their fate is fixed, and they are said to be determined. These terms, which were coined in the early days of experimental embryology, are now understood to reflect limitations in gene expression as cell lineages follow their normal developmental course. The rare instances in which cells or tissues strongly deviate from their normal developmental course, a phenomenon called **metaplasia,** are of considerable interest to pathologists and those who study the control of gene expression.

Restriction and determination signify the progressive limitation of the developmental capacities in the embryo.

Differentiation describes the actual morphological or functional expression of the portion of the genome that remains available to a particular cell or group of cells. Differentiation commonly connotes the course of phenotypic specialization of cells. One example of differentiation occurs in spermatogenesis, when spermatogonia, relatively ordinary-looking cells, become transformed into highly specialized spermatozoa.

## CELL ADHESION MOLECULES

In the early 1900s, researchers determined that suspended cells of a similar type have a strong tendency to aggregate. If different types of embryonic cells are mixed together, they typically sort according to tissue type. Their patterns of sorting even give clues to their properties and behavior in the mature organism. For example, if embryonic ectodermal and mesodermal cells are mixed, they come together into an aggregate with a superficial layer of ectodermal cells surroundings a central aggregate of mesodermal cells.

Contemporary research has begun to provide a molecular basis for many of the cell aggregation and sorting phenomena described by earlier embryologists. Several families of **cell adhesion molecules (CAMs)** have been characterized. CAMs have been extensively studied in relation to early developmental events. In pregastrulation avian embryos, cells of both epiblast and hypoblast contain two CAMs (neuronal CAM [N-CAM] and L-

**Potential of Cells**

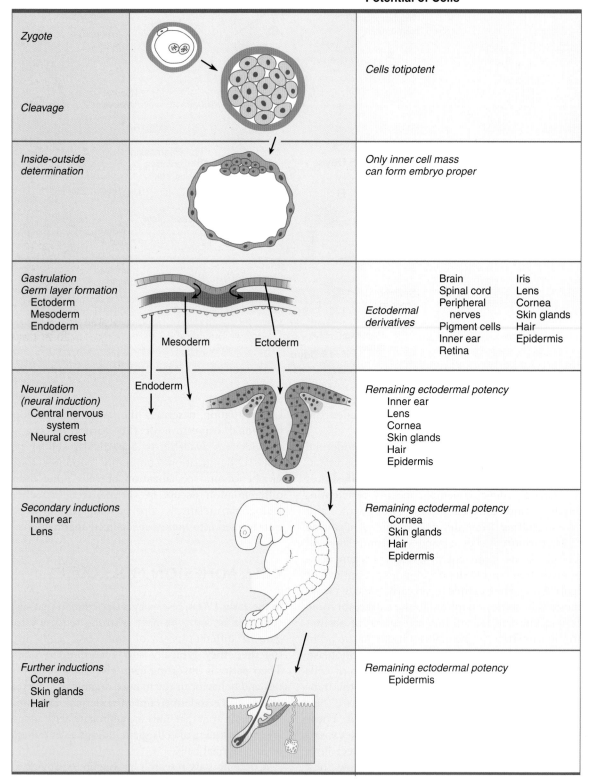

*Zygote*

*Cleavage*

*Cells totipotent*

*Inside-outside determination*

*Only inner cell mass can form embryo proper*

*Gastrulation*
*Germ layer formation*
  Ectoderm
  Mesoderm
  Endoderm

Mesoderm    Ectoderm

*Ectodermal derivatives*

| | |
|---|---|
| Brain | Iris |
| Spinal cord | Lens |
| Peripheral | Cornea |
| nerves | Skin glands |
| Pigment cells | Hair |
| Inner ear | Epidermis |
| Retina | |

*Neurulation*
*(neural induction)*
  Central nervous
    system
  Neural crest

Endoderm

*Remaining ectodermal potency*
  Inner ear
  Lens
  Cornea
  Skin glands
  Hair
  Epidermis

*Secondary inductions*
  Inner ear
  Lens

*Remaining ectodermal potency*
  Cornea
  Skin glands
  Hair
  Epidermis

*Further inductions*
  Cornea
  Skin glands
  Hair

*Remaining ectodermal potency*
  Epidermis

**FIGURE 5-15** Restriction during embryonic development. The labels on the right illustrate the progressive restriction of the developmental potential of cells that are in the line leading to the formation of the epidermis. On the left are developmental events that remove groups of cells from the epidermal track.

CAM) on their surfaces. A significant change occurs when cells of the epiblast migrate through the primitive streak. They lose the expression of both CAMs during the migratory phase and while they are beginning to form an organized mesoderm. Later, certain mesodermal cell derivatives reexpress CAMs. In general, when an epithelial cell type becomes transformed into a mesenchymal cell, its surface CAMs are lost.

The expression of CAMs is a sensitive indicator of primary induction in the early embryo. Before induction, the epiblast expresses both **N-CAM** and L-CAM (also called **E-cadherin**). After primary induction of the nervous system, the cells of the neural plate retain N-CAM but lose the expression of E-cadherin. Conversely, in nonneural ectoderm, N-CAM expression is lost, but E-cadherin expression is retained.

Some CAMs require the presence of $Ca^{++}$ to function, whereas others are independent of $Ca^{++}$. N-CAM, a $Ca^{++}$-independent CAM, binds directly to other N-CAM molecules on neighboring cells of the same type (Figure 5-16). N-CAM is unusual in having a high concentration of negatively charged sialic acid groups in the carbohydrate component of the molecule, and embryonic forms of N-CAM have three times as much sialic acid as the adult form of the molecule.

## SUMMARY

○ Just before implantation, the inner cell mass becomes reorganized as an epithelium (epiblast), and a second layer (hypoblast) begins to form beneath it. Within the epiblast, the amniotic cavity forms by cavitation; outgrowing cells of the hypoblast give rise to the endodermal lining of the yolk sac. Extraembryonic mesoderm appears to form by an early transformation of parietal endodermal cells and cells migrating through the primitive streak.

○ During gastrulation, a primitive streak forms in the epiblast at the caudal end of the bilaminar embryo. Cells migrating through the primitive streak form the mesoderm and endoderm, and the remaining epiblast becomes ectoderm.

○ The primitive node, located at the cranial end of the primitive streak, is the source of the cells that become the notochord. It also functions as the organizer or primary inductor of the future nervous system.

### CLINICAL VIGNETTE

A 35-year-old married man with a history of chronic respiratory infections is found on a routine x-ray examination to have dextrocardia. Further physical examination and imaging studies reveal that he has complete situs inversus. He has also been going to another clinic for a completely different problem, which is related to the same underlying defects.

Which is the most likely clinic?
A. Urology
B. Dermatology
C. Infertility
D. Orthopedic
E. Oncology

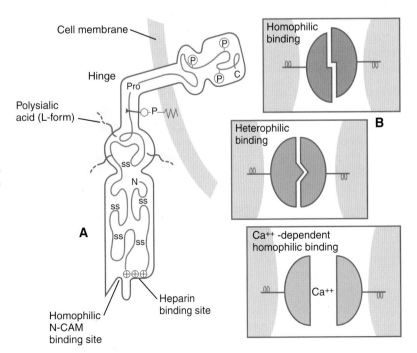

**FIGURE 5-16** *A,* Structure of the neuronal cell adhesion molecule (N-CAM). *B,* Types of intercellular adhesion. *P,* Phosphate; *Pro,* proline; *ss,* disulfide.

◌ As they pass through the primitive streak, future mesodermal cells in the epiblast change in morphology from epithelial epiblastic cells to bottle cells and then to mesenchymal cells. Extraembryonic mesodermal cells form the body stalk. The migration of mesenchymal cells during gastrulation is facilitated by extracellular matrix molecules such as hyaluronic acid and fibronectin.

◌ Late in the third week after fertilization, the primitive streak begins to regress caudally. Normally the primitive streak disappears, but sacrococcygeal teratomas occasionally form in the area of regression.

◌ The essential elements of neural induction are the same in all vertebrates. In mammals, the primitive node and the notochordal process act as the primary inductor of the nervous system. Mesodermal induction occurs even earlier than neural induction. Growth factors such as Vg1 and activin are the effective agents in mesodermal induction.

◌ A number of signaling centers control the organization of many important embryonic structures during early development. Each is associated with a constellation of important developmental genes. The early gastrula organizer is involved in initiation of the primitive streak. The primitive node organizes the formation of the notochord and nervous system, as well as many aspects of cellular behavior associated with the primitive streak. The notochord is important in the induction of many axial structures, such as the nervous system and somites. Formation of the head is coordinated by the anterior visceral endoderm (hypoblast) and the prechordal plate.

◌ Early blastomeres are totipotent. As development progresses, cells pass through restriction points that limit their differentiation. When the fate of a cell is fixed, the cell is said to be determined. Differentiation refers to the actual expression of the portion of the genome that remains available to a determined cell, and the term connotes the course of phenotypic specialization of a cell.

◌ Embryonic cells of the same type adhere to one another and will reaggregate if separated. The molecular basis for cell aggregation and adherence is the presence of CAMs on their surfaces. Among the several families of adhesion molecules, some are $Ca^{++}$ dependent and some are $Ca^{++}$ independent.

## ▌ Review Questions

1. The principal inductor in primary neural induction is the:
   A. Hypoblast
   B. Primitive streak
   C. Extraembryonic mesoderm
   D. Notochordal process
   E. Embryonic ectoderm

2. Which of the following tissues arises from cells passing through the primitive streak?
   A. Embryonic endoderm
   B. Hypoblast
   C. Cytotrophoblast
   D. Primary yolk sac
   E. Amnion

3. Cells of which germ layer are not present in the oropharyngeal membrane?
   A. Ectoderm
   B. Mesoderm
   C. Endoderm
   D. All are present

4. The prechordal plate plays an important role in regionalization of the:
   A. Notochord
   B. Forebrain
   C. Embryonic mesoderm
   D. Primitive node
   E. Hindbrain

5. Brachyury, a deficiency in caudal tissues in the body, is caused by a mutation in what gene?
   A. *Lim-1*
   B. *Noggin*
   C. *T*
   D. *Sonic hedgehog*
   E. *Activin*

6. Which layer of the bilaminar (two-layered) embryo gives rise to all of the embryonic tissue proper?

7. Of what importance is the primitive node in embryonic development?

8. The migration of mesodermal cells from the primitive streak is facilitated by the presence of what molecules of the extracellular matrix?

9. What molecules can bring about mesodermal induction in an early embryo?

10. At what stage in the life history of many cells are cell adhesion molecules lost?

## REFERENCES

Beddington RSP, Robertson EJ: Anterior patterning in the mouse, *Trends Genet* 14:277–284, 1998.

Boettger T and others: The avian organizer, *Int J Devel Biol* 45:281–2887, 2001.

Boncinelli E, Mallamaci A: Homeobox genes in vertebrate gastrulation, *Curr Opin Genet Devel* 5:619–627, 1995.

Campione M and others: The homeobox gene Pitx2: mediator of asymmetric left-right signaling in vertebrate heart and gut looping, *Development* 126:1225–1234, 1999.

Capdevila J and others: Mechanisms of left-right determination in vertebrates, *Cell* 101:9–21, 2000.

Casey B, Hackett BP: Left-right axis malformations in man and mouse, *Curr Opin Genet Devel* 10:257–261, 2000.

De Souza FSJ, Niehrs C: Anterior endoderm and head induction in early vertebrate embryos, *Cell Tiss Res* 300:207–217, 2000.

Edelman GM: Cell adhesion molecules in the regulation of animal form and tissue pattern, *Annu Rev Cell Biol* 2:81–116, 1986.

Enders AC: Trophoblastic differentiation during the transition from trophoblastic plate to lacunar stage of implantation in the rhesus monkey and human, *Am J Anat* 186:85–98, 1989.

Enders AC, King BF: Formation and differentiation of extraembryonic mesoderm in the rhesus monkey, *Am J Anat* 181:327–340, 1988.

Foley AC, Storey KG, Stern CD: The prechordal region lacks neural inducing ability, but can confer anterior character to more posterior neuroepithelium, *Development* 124:2983–2996, 1997.

Fujinaga M: Development of sidedness of asymmetric body structures in vertebrates, *Int J Devel Biol* 41:153–186, 1997.

Gardner RL: The initial phase of embryonic patterning in mammals, *Internat Rev Cytol* 203:233–290, 2001.

Gilbert SF: Continuity and change: paradigm shifts in neural induction, *Int J Devel Biol* 45:155–164, 2001.

Hemmati-Brivanlou A, Melton D: Vertebrate embryonic cells will become nerve cells unless told otherwise, *Cell* 88:13–17, 1997.

Herrmann BG, ed: The brachyury gene, *Semin Devel Biol* 6:381–435, 1995.

Kavka AI, Green JBA: Tales of tails: brachyury and the T-box genes, *Biochem Biophys Acta* 1333:F73–F84, 1997.

Lemaire L, Kessel M: Gastrulation and homeobox genes in chick embryos, *Mech Devel* 67:3–16, 1997.

Luckett WP: The development of primordial and definitive amniotic cavities in early rhesus monkey and human embryos, *Am J Anat* 144:149–168, 1975.

Luckett WP: Origin and differentiation of the yolk sac and extraembryonic mesoderm in presomite human and rhesus monkey embryos, *Am J Anat* 152:59–98, 1978.

Matsuo I and others: Otx and Emx functions in patterning of the vertebrate rostral head, *Cold Spring Harbor Symp Quant Biol* LXII:545–553, 1997.

Melloy PG and others: No turning, a mouse mutation causing left-right and axial patterning defects, *Devel Biol* 193:77–89, 1998.

Meyers EN, Martin GR: Differences in left-right axis pathways in mouse and chick: Functions of FGF8 and SHH, *Science* 285:403–406, 1999.

Mitrani E and others: Activin can induce the formation of axial structures and is expressed in the hypoblast of the chick, *Cell* 63:495–501, 1990.

Pera EM, Kessel M: Patterning of the chick forebrain anlage by the prechordal plate, *Development* 124:4153–4162, 1997.

Schneider H, Brueckner M: Of mice and men: Dissecting the genetic pathway that controls left-right asymmetry in mice and humans, *Am J Med Genet* 97:258–270, 2000.

Shawlot W, Behringer RR: Requirement for Lim1 in head organizer function, *Nature* 374:425–430, 1994.

Smith JL, Schoenwolf GC: Getting organized: new insights into the organizer of higher vertebrates, *Curr Top Devel Biol* 40:79–110, 1998.

Spemann H: Embryonic development and induction, New York, 1938, Hafner.

Spemann H, Mangold H: Ueber Induktion von Embryonenanlagen durch Implantation ortfremder Organisatoren, *Arch Microskop Anat Entw-Mech* 100:599–638, 1924.

Sulik K and others: Morphogenesis of the murine node and notochordal plate, *Devel Dynam* 201:260–278, 1994.

Supp DM and others: Mutation of an axonemal dynein affects left-right asymmetry in inversus viscerum mice, *Nature* 389:963–966, 1997.

Supp DM and others: Molecular motors: the driving force behind mammalian left-right development, *Trends Cell Biol* 10:41–45, 2000.

Takeichi M: The cadherins: cell-cell adhesion molecules controlling animal morphogenesis, *Development* 102:639–655, 1988.

Tam PPL, Behringer RR: Mouse gastrulation: the formation of a mammalian body plan, *Mech Devel* 68:3–25, 1997.

Townes PL, Holtfreter J: Directed movements and selective adhesion of embryonic amphibian cells, *J Exp Zool* 128:53–120, 1955.

Watson CM, Tam PPL: Cell lineage determination in the mouse, *Cell Struct Funct* 26:123–129, 2001.

Zernicka-Goetz M: Patterning of the embryo: the first spatial decisions in the life of a mouse, *Development* 129:815–892, 2002.

# CHAPTER 6

# Establishment of the Basic Embryonic Body Plan

After gastrulation is complete, the embryo proper consists of a flat, three-layered disk containing the ectodermal, mesodermal, and endodermal germ layers. Its cephalocaudal axis is defined by the location of the primitive streak. Because of the pattern of cellular migration through the primitive streak and the regression of the streak toward the caudal end of the embryo, a strong **cephalocaudal gradient** of maturity is established. This gradient is marked initially by the formation of the notochord and later by the appearance of the neural plate, which results from the primary induction of the dorsal ectoderm by the notochord.

As was seen in Chapter 5, despite the relatively featureless appearance of the gastrulating embryo, complex patterns of gene expression set up the basic body plan of the embryo. One of the earliest morphological manifestations of this pattern is the regular segmentation that becomes evident along the craniocaudal axis of the embryo. Such a segmental plan, which is a dominant characteristic of all early embryos, becomes less obvious as development progresses. Nonetheless, even in the adult the regular arrangement of the vertebrae, ribs, and spinal nerves persists as a reminder of humans' highly segmented phylogenetic and ontogenetic past. Only recently have embryologists begun to understand the molecular and cellular controls that underlie the process of segmentation.

Another major change critical in understanding the fundamental organization of the body plan is the lateral folding of the early embryo from three essentially flat, stacked, pancakelike disks of cells (the primary embryonic germ layers) to a cylinder, with the ectoderm on the outside, the endoderm on the inside, and the mesoderm between them. The cellular basis for lateral folding still remains better described than understood.

This chapter concentrates on the establishment of the basic overall body plan. In addition, it charts the appearance of the primordia of the major organ systems of the body from the undifferentiated primary germ layers (see Figure 6-25).

## DEVELOPMENT OF THE ECTODERMAL GERM LAYER

### Neurulation: Formation of the Neural Tube

The principal early morphological response of the embryonic ectoderm to neural induction is an increase in the height of the cells that are destined to become components of the nervous system. These transformed cells are evident as a thickened **neural plate** visible on the dorsal surface of the early embryo (Figures 6-1, *A*, and 6-2, *A*). Unseen but also important is the restricted expression of cell adhesion molecules (CAMs), from N-CAM and L-CAM/E-cadherin in the preinduced ectoderm to N-CAM and N-cadherin in the neural plate.

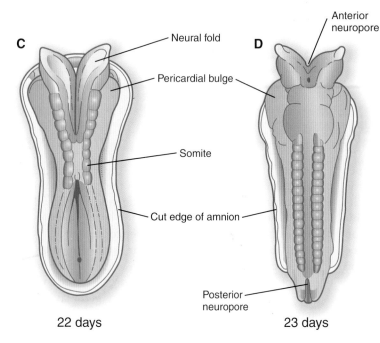

A
Cut edge of amnion
Neural fold
Neural plate

B

Neural groove
Somite

Primitive node
Primitive streak

18 days

20 days

C
Neural fold

Pericardial bulge

Somite

Cut edge of amnion

D
Anterior neuropore

Posterior neuropore

22 days

23 days

**FIGURE 6-1** Early stages in the formation of the human central nervous system. **A,** At **18 days. B,** At **20 days. C,** At **22 days. D,** At **23 days.**

The first of four major stages in the formation of the neural tube is transformation of the general embryonic ectoderm into a thickened neural plate. The principal activity of the second stage is further shaping of the overall contours of the neural plate so that it becomes narrower and longer. Shaping of the neural plate is accomplished to a great extent by region-specific changes in the shape of the neuroepithelial cells (e.g., an increase in height at the expense of basal surface area) and by rearrangements of these cells relative to one another.

The third major stage in the process of **neurulation** is the lateral folding of the neural plate, resulting in the elevation of each side of the neural plate along a midline **neural groove** (see Figures 6-1, *B,* and 6-2, *B*). Many explanations have been proposed for lateral folding of the neural plate and ultimate closure of the neural tube. Most have invoked a single or dominant mechanism, but it is

now becoming apparent that lateral folding is the result of a number of region-specific mechanisms, both intrinsic and extrinsic to the neural plate.

The ventral midline of the neural plate, sometimes called the **median hinge point,** appears to act like an anchoring point about which the two sides become elevated at a sharp angle from the horizontal. At the median angle, bending can be largely accounted for by notochord-induced changes in the shape of the neuroepithelial cells of the neural plate. These cells become narrower at their apex and broader at their base (see Figure 6-2, *C*) through a combination of a basal position of the nuclei (causing a lateral expansion of the cell in that area) and a purse string–like contraction of a ring of actin-containing microfilaments in the apical cytoplasm. Throughout the lateral folding of the neural plate in the region of the spinal cord, much of the wall area of the

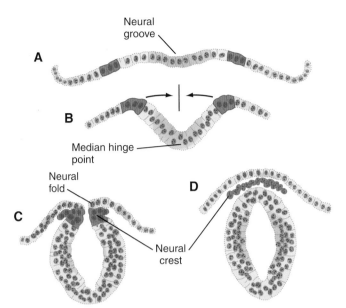

A

Neural
groove

B

Median hinge
point

Neural
fold

C

D

Neural
crest

**FIGURE 6-2** Cross sections through the forming neural tube. **A,** Neural plate. **B,** Neural fold. **C,** Neural folds apposed. **D,** Neural tube complete. (Neural crest before and after its exit from the neural epithelium is shown in green.)

neural plate remains flat (see Figure 6-2, *B*). Elevation of the **neural folds** appears to be accomplished largely by factors extrinsic to the neural epithelium, in particular, pushing forces generated by the expanding surface epithelium lateral to the neural plate.

The fourth stage in the formation of the neural tube consists of apposition of the two most lateral apical surfaces of the neural folds, their fusion (mediated by cell surface glycoconjugates), and the separation of the completed segment of the neural tube from the overlying ectodermal sheet (see Figure 6-2, *C* and *D*). At the same time, cells of the **neural crest** begin to separate from the neural tube.

Closure of the neural tube begins almost midway along the craniocaudal extent of the nervous system of the 21- to 22-day-old embryo (see Figure 6-1, *C*). Over the next couple of days, closure extends caudally in a zipperlike fashion, but cranially there are commonly two additional discontinuous sites of closure. The unclosed cephalic and caudal parts of the neural tube are called the **anterior** (cranial) and **posterior** (caudal) **neuropores.** The neuropores also ultimately close off so that the entire future central nervous system resembles an irregular cylinder sealed at both ends. Occasionally, one or both neuropores remain open, resulting in serious birth defects (see p. 268).

Caudal to the posterior neuropore, the remaining neural tube (more prominent in animals with large tails) is formed by the process of **secondary neurulation.** Secondary neurulation in mammals appears to begin with the formation of a rodlike condensation of mesenchymal cells beneath the dorsal ectoderm of the **tail bud.** Within the mesenchymal rod, a central canal forms directly by **cav-**

**itation** (the formation of a space within a mass of cells). This central canal becomes continuous with the one formed during primary neurulation by the lateral folding of the neural plate and closure of the posterior neuropore. Because of the poor development of the tail bud, secondary neurulation in humans is not a prominent process.

## Segmentation in the Neural Tube

### Morphological Manifestations of Segmentation

Soon after the neural tube has taken shape, the region of the future brain can be distinguished from the spinal cord. The brain-forming region undergoes a series of subdivisions that constitute the basis for the fundamental gross organization of the adult brain. Segmentation by subdivision of an existing structure (in the case of the neural tube) contrasts to segmentation by adding terminal segments, as is the case in the formation of somites (see p. 110). An early set of subdivisions results in a three-part brain, consisting of a forebrain (**prosencephalon**), midbrain (**mesencephalon**), and hindbrain (**rhombencephalon**). Later the prosencephalon subdivides into a **telencephalon** and **diencephalon,** and the rhombencephalon subdivides into a **metencephalon** and **myelencephalon** (see Figure 11-2).

Superimposed on the traditional gross morphological organization of the developing brain is another, more subtle, level of segmentation, which subdivides certain regions of the brain into transiently visible series of regular segments called **neuromeres** (Figure 6-3). In the hindbrain, the neuromeres, often called **rhombomeres,** are visible from early in the fourth to late in the fifth week. The midbrain does not appear to be segmented, but there is evidence for a more subtle segmentation of the prosencephalon into a less regular series of **prosomeres.**

Rhombomeres are arranged as odd and even pairs, and once established, they act like isolated compartments in insect embryos. Because of specific surface properties, cells from adjacent rhombomeres do not intermingle across boundaries between even and odd segments; however, marked cells from two even or two odd rhombomeres placed side by side do intermingle. During their brief existence, rhombomeres provide the basis for the fundamental organization of the hindbrain. In the adult, the segmental organization of the rhombomeres is manifest in the rhombomere-specific origin of many cranial nerves and parts of the reticular formation within the brainstem (see Figure 11-12).

### Mechanisms of Early Segmentation of the Neural Tube

Even while gastrulation is still taking place, the newly induced neural tube is subjected to yet undefined vertical

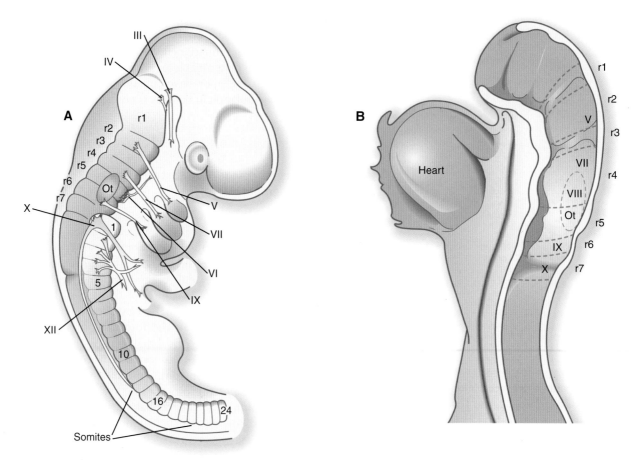

**FIGURE 6-3** Neuromeres in 3-day-old chick brain **(A)** and **24-day-old** human **(B)** brain. *Ot,* Otic vesicle; *r,* rhombomeres (neuromeres in rhombencephalon); Roman numerals, cranial nerves; numbers, somites.

inductions from the notochord and head organizing regions (anterior visceral endoderm and prechordal plate), which effectively subdivide it into forebrain/midbrain and hindbrain/spinal cord segments. This subdivision is marked by the expression of two transcription factors, **Otx-2** (orthodenticle homologue 2) in the forebrain/midbrain region and in the hindbrain, **Gbx-2** (gastrulation brain homeobox 2), whose boundaries sharply define the midbrain-hindbrain border (Figure 6-4, *A*). Fibroblast growth factors (FGF), produced in the early primitive streak, are known to exert a posteriorizing effect on the newly forming neural plate.

The midbrain-hindbrain border becomes a powerful local signaling center, called the **isthmic organizer**. The signaling molecule **Wnt-1** (a gene homologous with *Wingless,* a segment-polarity gene in *Drosophila* [see Figure 4-1]) is synthesized in the neural ectoderm anterior, and **FGF-8** is formed posterior to the isthmic organizer (Figure 6-4, *B*). The transcription factors, **Pax-2** and **Pax-5** and **engrailed** (**En-1** and **En-2**), are expressed on both sides of the isthmic organizer as gradients that are critical in organizing the development of both the midbrain and the cerebellum, a hindbrain derivative.

Another putative secondary organizer in the forebrain region is located in the **anterior pole (anterior neural ridge)** of the brain (Fig. 6-4, *B*). It is a site of sonic hedgehog and FGF-8 activity, but its functions are less well defined than those of the isthmic organizer. Additional information on the organization and segmentation of the forebrain is presented in Chapter 11.

### Segmentation in the Hindbrain Region

Segmentation of the hindbrain into 7 rhombomeres in the human, and 8 in some other animals, is the result of the expression of several categories of genes, which operate in a manner remarkably reminiscent of the way in which the early *Drosophila* embryo becomes subdivided into segments (see Figure 4-1). Individual rhombomeres are initially specified through the ordered expression of unique combinations of transcription factors; this patterning is then translated into cellular behavior by the patterned expression of cell surface molecules.

After the *Gbx-2*-expressing area defines the rough limits of the hindbrain, several **segmentation genes** are involved in setting up the basic pattern of segmentation

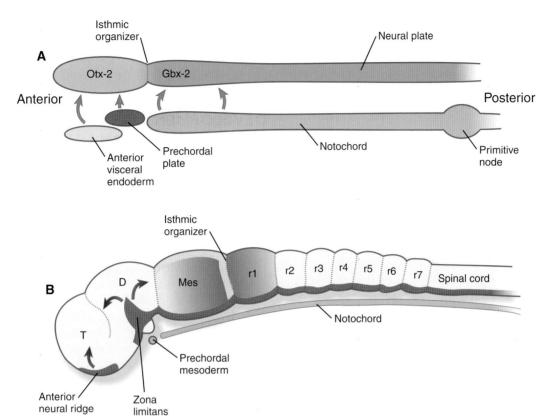

**FIGURE 6-4** Schematic representation of signaling centers acting on and within the early embryonic brain. **A,** In response to signals *(green arrows)* from the anterior visceral endoderm, the prechordal plate, and the notochord, the neural tube expresses Otx-2 in the future forebrain and midbrain regions and Gbx-2 in the hindbrain and spinal cord. **B,** Later in development, signals (FGF-8 *[green]* and Wnt-1 *[yellow]*) from the isthmic organizer induce decreasing gradients of En-1 and En-2 *(blue)* on either side. Sonic hedgehog *(red)* is secreted from two other organizers, the anterior neural ridge and the zona limitans, as well as the ventral part (floor plate) of the neural tube. D, Diencephalon; *Mes,* Mesencephalon; *r,* rhombomere; *T,* Telencephalon. (Part B after Lumsden A, Krumlauf R: *Science* 274:1109–1115, 1996.)

that leads to rhombomere formation. **Krox 20,** a zinc finger transcription factor, is expressed in and guides the formation of rhombomeres 3 and 5 (r3 and r5; see Figure 11-11), whereas **kreisler,** another transcription factor, and **Hoxa-1** are also involved in the formation of r5. **Retinoids,** produced by the anterior somites, play an important, but less well-defined role in the formation of the posterior rhombomeres (r4 to r7), but they do not play a role in the specification of r1 to r3, which is regulated by Gbx-2.

The *Hox* genes are principally involved in specifying segmental identity. Under the influence of segmentation genes, various *Hox* paralogues are expressed in a highly specific sequence along the hindbrain and spinal cord. As will be seen in Chapters 11 and 14, the pattern of *Hox* gene expression determines the morphological identity of the cranial nerves and other pharyngeal arch derivatives that arise from specific rhombomeres. The orderly expression of *Hox* gene paralogues extends anteriorly through rhombomere 2; Hox proteins are not found in r1. This is largely due to the antagonistic action of FGF-8, which is produced in response to signals from the isthmic organizer at the anterior end of r1. In the absence

of FGF-8, Hox proteins are expressed in r1. Another rhombencephalic protein, **sprouty 2,** acts as an antagonist of FGF-8, and this, plus the presence of Hoxa-2 in r2, confines FGF-8 mostly to r1 and contains the primordium of the cerebellum to the anterior part of r1.

Another family of genes, the **ephrins** and their receptors, determines the behavioral properties of the cells in the rhombomeres. The action of *ephrins,* which are expressed in even-numbered rhombomeres (2, 4, and 6), and ephrin receptors, which are expressed in odd-numbered rhombomeres (3 and 5), appears to account for the lack of mixing behavior of cells from adjacent rhombomeres, as well as maintaining the separation of the various streams of neural crest cells that emigrate from the rhombomeres (see Figure 12-9).

### Segmentation of the Spinal Cord

Although neuromeres are not seen in the region of the neural tube that gives rise to the spinal cord, the regular arrangement of the exiting motor and sensory nerve roots is evidence of a fundamental segmental organization in this region of the body, as well. In contrast to the brain, however, segmentation of the spinal cord is to a great extent imposed by signals emanating from the paraxial mesoderm rather than from molecular signals intrinsic to the neural tube. (see Figure 6-10 for the relationship between the spinal nerves and the mesodermal segments of the body [somites and their derivatives]).

## Neural Crest

When the neural tube has just closed and is separating from the general cutaneous ectoderm, a population of cells called the **neural crest** leaves the dorsal part of the neural tube and begins to spread throughout the body of the embryo (see Figure 6-2). The neural crest produces an astonishing array of structures in the embryo (see Table 12-1), and its importance is such that the neural crest is sometimes called the *fourth germ layer of the body*. (Further consideration of the neural crest is presented in Chapter 12.)

## Sensory Placodes and Secondary Inductions in the Cranial Region

As the cranial region begins to take shape, several series of **ectodermal placodes** (thickenings) appear lateral to the neural tube and neural crest (Figure 6-5). These placodes arise as the result of a variety of secondary inductive processes between neural or mesenchymal tissues and the overlying ectoderm. In several cases, cells from the placodes and neural crest interact closely to form the sensory ganglia of cranial nerves (V, VII, IX, and X). Defi-

ciencies of one of these two components can often be made up by an increased contribution by the other component. Further details of placodes and their developmental fate are given in the introduction to Chapter 13.

# DEVELOPMENT OF THE MESODERMAL GERM LAYER

## Basic Plan of the Mesodermal Layer

After passing through the primitive streak, the mesodermal cells spread laterally between the ectoderm and endoderm as a continuous layer of mesenchymal cells (see Figure 5-6). Subsequently, three regions can be recognized in the mesoderm of cross-sectioned embryos (Figure 6-6, *B*). Nearest the neural tube is a thickened column of mesenchymal cells known as the **paraxial mesoderm**, or **segmental plate**. This tissue is soon organized into somites. Lateral to the paraxial mesoderm is a compact region of **intermediate mesoderm**, which ultimately gives rise to the urogenital system. Beyond that, the **lateral mesoderm** ultimately splits into two layers and forms the bulk of the tissues of the body wall, the wall of the digestive tract, and the limbs (see Figure 6-25).

## Paraxial Mesoderm

As the primitive node and the primitive streak regress toward the caudal end of the embryo, they leave behind the notochord and the induced neural plate. Lateral to the neural plate, the paraxial mesoderm appears to be a

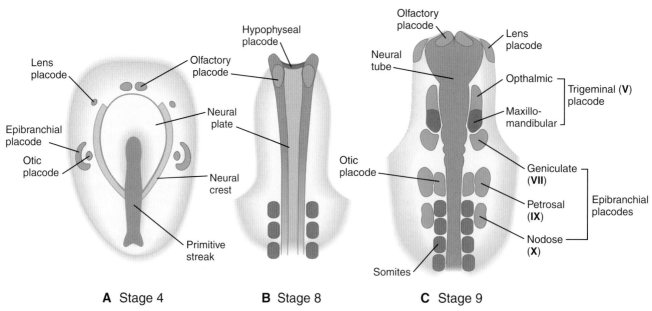

**FIGURE 6-5** Early stages in the formation of cranial ectodermal placodes in the chick embryo, as viewed from the dorsal aspect. The placodes are shown in blue.

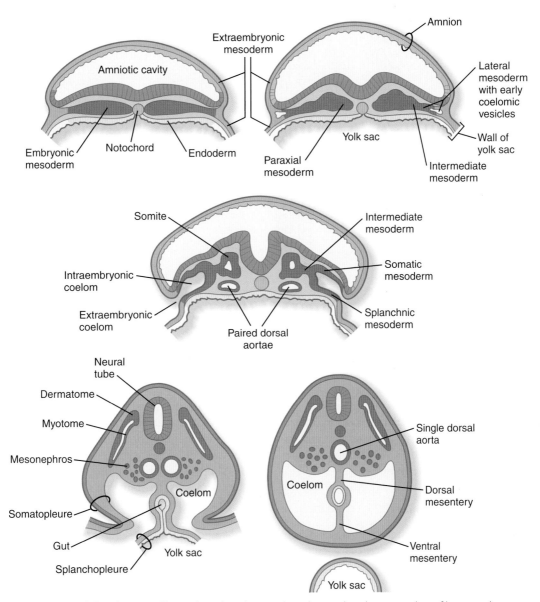

**FIGURE 6-6** Development of intraembryonic and extraembryonic mesoderm in cross sections of human embryos.

homogeneous strip of closely packed mesenchymal cells. However, if scanning electron micrographs of this mesoderm are examined with stereoscopic techniques, a series of regular pairs of segments can be discerned. These segments, called **somitomeres,** have been most studied in avian embryos, but they are also found in mammals. New pairs of somitomeres form along the primitive node as it regresses toward the caudal end of the embryo (Figure 6-7). Not until almost 20 pairs of somitomeres have formed and the primitive node has regressed quite far caudally does the first pair of **somites** (brick-shaped masses of paraxial mesoderm) form behind the seventh pair of somitomeres.

After the first pair of somites has been established (approximately 20 days after fertilization), a regular relationship develops between the regression of the primitive streak and the formation of additional somites and somitomeres. The first seven pairs of somitomeres in the cranial region do not undergo further separation or segmentation; the first pair of somites forms at the expense of the eighth pair of somitomeres. In the types of embryos studied to date, there is a constant relationship between the most caudal pair of definitive somites and the number of somitomeres (usually 10 to 11) that can be demonstrated behind them. Every few hours the pair of somitomeres located caudal to the last-formed somites becomes transformed into a new pair of somites, and a new pair of somitomeres is laid down at the caudal end of the paraxial mesoderm near the primitive node (see Figure 6-7). As regression of the primitive streak comes to a close, the formation of paraxial mesoderm continues through the contribution of cells contributed by the tail

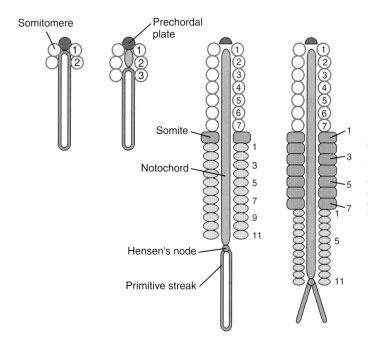

**FIGURE 6-7** Relationship between somitomeres and somites in the early chick embryo. Cranial somitomeres *(open circles)* take shape along Hensen's node until seven pairs have formed. Caudal to the seventh somitomere, somites *(rectangles)* form from caudal somitomeres *(ovals)*. As the most anterior of the caudal somitomeres transform into somites, additional caudal somitomeres take shape posteriorly. For a while, the equilibrium between transformation into somites anteriorly and new formation posteriorly keeps the number of caudal somitomeres at 11.

bud. The cervical and thoracic vertebrae and associated structures are derived from cells migrating through the primitive streak, whereas the cellular precursors of the sacrum and coccyx come from the tail bud. The mechanism that terminates somite formation in the most posterior end of the embryo remains obscure.

### Formation of Individual Somites

The formation of individual somites from a seemingly homogeneous strip of paraxial mesoderm is a complex process that involves a variety of levels of molecular control and changes in cellular behavior within the paraxial mesoderm. Our basic understanding of **somitogenesis** (somite formation) comes from studies on the chick. The first significant step in somitogenesis is **segmentation** of the paraxial mesoderm. In contrast to segmentation in the hindbrain (see page 106), somite formation occurs by the sequential addition of new segments in a craniocaudal sequence. This is initiated with the aid of a molecular clock that stimulates a regular cycle of expression of mRNA of *c-hairy*, a homologue of the pair-rule segmentation gene, *hairy*, which is involved in segmentation of the *Drosophila* embryo (see Figure 4-1). At the start of the 90-minute somite-producing cycle in the chick embryo, *c-hairy* is expressed throughout the nonsegmented preaxial mesoderm, but by the end of the cycle its expression is narrowed to a thin band corresponding to the posterior edge of a new somite. Then the cycle repeats itself. Molecules in the Notch signaling pathway, such as **lunatic fringe**, which are important in setting boundaries in a variety of developmental situations (see also p. 217), are expressed in a 90-minute cyclical pattern similar to

that of *c-hairy*, but in the chick lunatic fringe becomes localized in the anterior part of the forming somite. During this very early stage in segmentation, the specific segmental identity of future somites is fixed by the expression of a unique sequence of *Hox* genes (see Figure 9-16). In the unsegmented presomitic mesoderm, an environment rich in the signaling molecule **FGF-8** keeps the cells in a developmentally labile state. More anteriorly, in areas where levels of FGF-8 are reduced, the mesodermal cells respond to the segmentation clock and become determined to form somites.

The formation of boundaries between somites involves interactions between cells on one side of the boundary expressing the Notch receptor and those on the other expressing the Delta ligand. Mutants affecting the Notch pathway result in abnormal somitogenesis. Through a poorly understood mechanism, lunatic fringe and the Notch pathway also interact in setting up the boundaries between adjacent somites. The mesodermal precursor cells of the somites express the CAM **N-cadherin**, on their surfaces. This assists in their condensation to form the somite.

While in the earliest stages of its formation, a somite also undergoes an internal subdivision into anterior and posterior halves. Differences in cellular properties stemming from this subdivision are of great significance in the formation of vertebrae and in guiding the migration of neural crest cells and outgrowing axons. As is the case in the rhombomeres, ephrins are involved in the internal subdivision of the somite. The ephrin receptor is expressed by cells in the anterior half of a somite, whereas the ephrin ligand is expressed in cells of the posterior half.

The continued development of a somite involves the transformation of segmented blocks of cells with a mesenchymal morphology into a sphere of epithelial cells within the paraxial mesoderm (Figure 6-8, A). Although the segmentation of the paraxial mesoderm is intrinsically controlled, epithelialization of the early somites depends on a yet unknown inductive signal from the overlying ectoderm. This signal stimulates the expression of a gene called *paraxis*, a basic helix-loop-helix transcription factor. Through the mediation of *paraxis*, the transformation from mesenchyme to epithelium is preceded by an increase in the intercellular adhesive properties of the presomitic cells. The cells of the epithelial somite are arranged so that their apical surfaces surround a small central lumen, the **somitocoel** (which contains a small number of core cells), and their outer basal surfaces are surrounded by a basal lamina (containing laminin, fibronectin, and other components of the extracellular matrix).

Shortly after the formation of the epithelial somite, the cells of its ventromedial wall are subjected to an inductive stimulus in the form of the signaling molecule **sonic hedgehog**, originating from the notochord and the ventral wall of the neural tube. The response is the expression of *Pax-1* and *Pax-9* in the ventral half of the

somite, which is now called the **sclerotome** (Figure 6-9). This leads to a burst of mitosis, the loss of intercellular adhesion molecules (**N-cadherin**), the dissolution of the basal lamina in that region, and the transformation of the epithelial cells (and somitocoel core cells [see Figure 6-8, A]) in that region back to a mesenchymal morphology (these cells are called **secondary mesenchyme**). These secondary mesenchymal cells migrate or are otherwise displaced medially from the remainder of the somite (Figure 6-8, B) and begin to produce **chondroitin sulfate proteoglycans** and other molecules characteristic of cartilage matrix as they aggregate around the notochord.

Under the influence of secreted products of *Wnt* genes produced by the dorsal neural tube, which function in concert with sonic hedgehog, the dorsal half of the epithelial somite becomes transformed into the **dermomyotome** (see Figure 6-8, B) and expresses its own characteristic genes (*Pax-3, Pax-7, paraxis*). Mesenchymal cells arising from the dorsomedial border of the dermomyotome form a separate layer, the **myotome**, beneath the remaining somitic epithelium, which is now called the **dermatome** (Figure 6-8, C). As their names imply, cells of the myotome produce muscle, and cells of the dermatome contribute to the dermis.

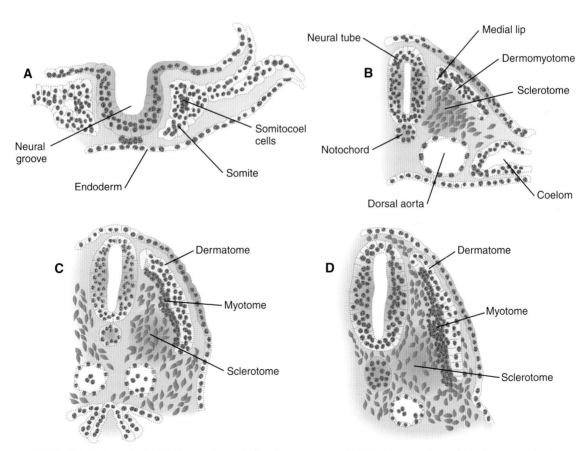

**FIGURE 6-8** Stages in the life history of a somite in a human embryo. **A,** Epithelial stage of a somite in the preneural tube stage. **B,** Epitheliomesenchymal transformation of the ventromedial portion into the sclerotome. **C,** Appearance of a separate myotome from the original dermomyotome. **D,** Early stage of breakup of the epithelial dermatome into dermal fibroblasts.

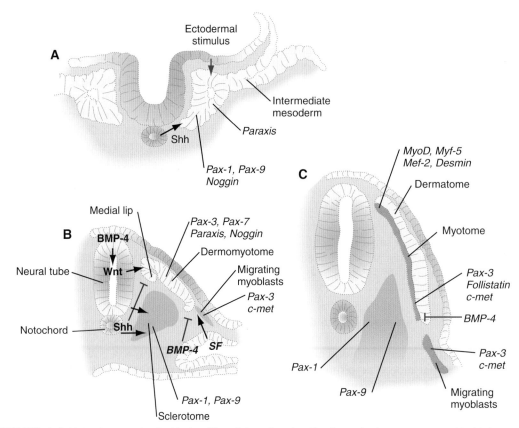

**FIGURE 6-9** Molecular events involved in the differentiation of somites. Signaling molecules are represented by black arrows. Inhibitory signals are represented by red arrows. Genes expressed in responding tissues are indicated in italics. *SF,* Scatter factor. (Modified from Brand-Saberi B and others: *Int J Dev Biol* 40:411–420, 1996.)

## Organization of the Somite and the Basic Segmental Body Plan

The epithelial somite can be subdivided into four cross-sectional quadrants, each of which gives rise to a different set of derivatives (Table 6-1). As described in the previous section, under the influence of sonic hedgehog secreted by the notochord, the ventral half of the somite becomes transformed into the sclerotome and goes on to form the vertebral body. Two mouse mutants illustrate the importance of the interacting components in differentiation of the somite. In the **Danforth short tail** mutant, degeneration of the notochord (inducer of the sclerotome) is followed by poor formation of the vertebral bodies and intervertebral disks. A disruption of *Pax-1* expression in the sclerotome in the **undulated** mutant also leads to vertebral defects.

After the *Wnt*-mediated induction of the dorsal half of the somite to form the dermomyotome, a medial lip of cells forms from the dermomyotome (see Figure 6-8, *B*). The medial lip spreads out beneath the dermomyotome to form a separate muscle-forming layer, the **myotome** (see Figure 6-8, *C*). The medial portion of the myotome goes on to express several **myogenic regulatory factors**

(see p. 197) as the cells prepare to form the intrinsic back muscles (see Table 6-1). **Bone morphogenetic protein-4 (BMP-4),** which is produced by the dorsal ectoderm, can suppress myogenesis, but the presence of **noggin** in the region of the medial myotomal lip counteracts this effect of BMP-4 in a manner similar to the way in which noggin induces the neural plate by inhibiting BMP-4 during gastrulation (see page 91). Under the influence of BMP-4, also produced by the lateral mesoderm, the expression of myogenic regulatory factors in cells of the lateral dermomyotome is suppressed, and they continue to express *Pax-3* and also a receptor molecule, **c-met.** A growth factor, **scatter factor** (also called **hepatic growth factor**), secreted in the region of the limb buds, binds to the c-met receptor of lateral dermomyotome cells. This stimulates these cells (30 to 100 cells per somite) to migrate out of the somite and into the limb bud even before the myotome forms, while they continue to express their dermomyotomal marker, *Pax-3*, as well as the cell adhesion molecule, N-cadherin.

As the cells of the sclerotome disperse around the notochord, cells of the anterior half of one somite aggregate with cells of the posterior half of the more cranial somite. Ultimately, this aggregate forms a single vertebra.

| TABLE 6-1 *Subdivisions of the Epithelial Somite* | | | |
|---|---|---|---|
| **Dorsal** | | | |
| **DERMATOME** | | **DERMATOME** | |
| Dermis | | Dermis | |
| Myotome | | Myotome | |
| Intrinsic back muscles (epaxial) | | Limb muscles | |
| | | Muscles of ventrolateral body wall | |
| **MEDIAL** | **SOMITOCOEL CELLS** | | **LATERAL** |
| | Intervertebral joint surfaces | | |
| **SCLEROTOME** | | **SCLEROTOME** | |
| Vertebral body | | Vertebral arch | |
| Intervertebral disk | | Pedicle of vertebra | |
| Proximal part of rib | | Distal part of rib | |
| Connective tissue | | Connective tissue around dorsal root ganglion | |
| **Ventral** | | | |

Such an arrangement places the bony vertebrae out of phase with the myotomally derived segmental muscles of the trunk (Figure 6-10, C). This allows the contracting segmental muscles to move the vertebral column laterally. The relationship between the anterior half of one somite and the adjoining posterior half of its neighboring somite is reminiscent of the parasegments of *Drosophila* (similarly arranged subdivisions of the segments into two parts), but whether they are functionally similar in terms of genetic control is undetermined.

## Intermediate Mesoderm

Connecting the paraxial mesoderm and the lateral mesoderm in the early embryo is a small cord of cells called the **intermediate mesoderm** that runs along the entire length of the trunk (see Figure 6-6, C). Possibly through a lack of receptors, the intermediate mesoderm does not appear to be influenced by the BMP-4 that is secreted by the lateral mesoderm, whereas somitic mesoderm exposed to high concentrations of BMP-4 assumes the characteristics of the lateral mesoderm. The intermediate mesoderm is the precursor of the urogenital system. The earliest signs of differentiation of the intermediate mesoderm are in the most cranial regions, where vestiges of the earliest form of the kidney, the **pronephros**, briefly appear. In the lateral region of the intermediate mesoderm, a longitudi-

nal **pronephric duct** appears on each side of the embryo. The pronephric duct is important in organizing the development of much of the adult urogenital system, which forms largely from cells of the caudal portions of the intermediate mesoderm (see Chapter 16).

## Lateral Mesoderm

Shortly after gastrulation, the ectoderm overlying the most lateral mesoderm produces BMP-4. Soon thereafter, the lateral mesoderm itself begins to produce BMP-4. Experimental studies have shown that this molecule has the ability to cause mesoderm, whether paraxial or lateral, to assume the molecular and cellular properties of lateral mesoderm. Whether early mesoderm develops the properties of paraxial or lateral mesoderm appears to depend on a balance between medializing influences emanating from the axial structures (neural tube and notochord) and lateralizing influences initially produced by lateral ectoderm.

The **lateral mesoderm** soon divides into two layers as the result of the formation and coalescence of coelomic (body cavity) spaces within it (see Figure 6-6, B and C). The dorsal layer, which is closely associated with the ectoderm, is called **somatic mesoderm**, and the combination of somatic mesoderm and ectoderm is called the **somatopleure** (see Figure 6-6, D). The ventral layer,

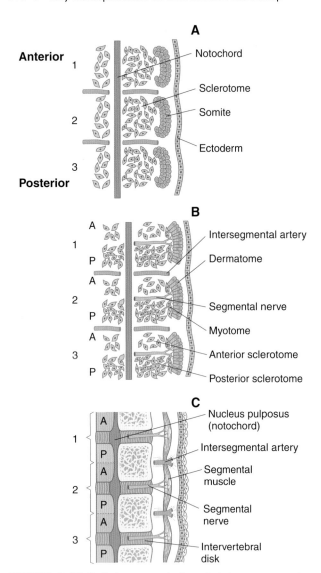

**FIGURE 6-10 A,** Early movement of seemingly homogeneous sclerotome from the somite. **B,** Breakup of the sclerotomal portions of the somites into anterior **(A)** and posterior **(P)** halves and the coalescence of the posterior portion of one somite with the anterior portion of the one caudal to it to form the body of a vertebra. **C,** With this rearrangement, the segmental muscles (derived from the myotomes) extend across intervertebral joints and are supplied by spinal nerves that grow out between the anterior and posterior halves of the somites.

called **splanchnic mesoderm,** is closely associated with the endoderm, and the combined endoderm and splanchnic mesoderm is called the **splanchnopleure.** The intraembryonic somatic and splanchnic mesodermal layers are continuous with the layers of extraembryonic mesoderm that line the amnion and yolk sac.

While the layers of somatic and splanchnic mesoderm are taking shape, the entire body of the embryo undergoes a lateral folding process that effectively transforms its shape from three flat germ layers to a cylinder, with a tube of endoderm (gut) in the center, an outer tubular covering of ectoderm (epidermis), and an intermediate layer of mesoderm. This transformation occurs before the appearance of the limbs.

## Formation of the Coelom

As the embryo undergoes lateral folding, the small coelomic vesicles that formed within the lateral mesoderm coalesce into the coelomic cavity (see Figure 6-6). Initially, the **intraembryonic coelom** is continuous with the **extraembryonic coelom,** but as folding is completed in a given segment of the embryo, the two coelomic spaces are separated. The last region of the embryo to undergo complete lateral folding is the area occupied by the yolk sac. In this area, small channels connecting the intraembryonic and extraembryonic coeloms persist until the ventral body wall is completely sealed.

In the cylindrical embryo, the somatic mesoderm constitutes the lateral and ventral body wall, and the splanchnic mesoderm forms the mesentery and the wall of the digestive tract. The somatic mesoderm of the lateral plate also forms the mesenchyme of the limb buds, which begin to appear late in the fourth week of pregnancy (see Figure 10-1).

## Extraembryonic Mesoderm and the Body Stalk

The thin layers of extraembryonic mesoderm that line the ectodermal lining of the amnion and the endodermal lining of the yolk sac are continuous with the intraembryonic somatic and splanchnic mesoderm, respectively (see Figure 6-6, A and B). The posterior end of the embryo is connected with the trophoblastic tissues (future placenta) by the mesodermal **body stalk** (see Figure 7-1). As the embryo grows and a circulatory system becomes functional, blood vessels from the embryo grow through the body stalk to supply the placenta, and the body stalk itself becomes better defined as the **umbilical cord.** The extraembryonic mesoderm that lines the inner surface of the cytotrophoblast ultimately becomes the mesenchymal component of the placenta.

## Early Stages in the Formation of the Circulatory System

As the embryo grows during the third week, it attains a size that does not permit simple diffusion to distribute oxygen and nutrients to all of its cells or efficiently remove waste products. The early development of the heart and circulatory system is an embryonic adaptation that permits the rapid growth of the embryo by providing an efficient means for the distribution of nutrients. The circulatory system faces the daunting task of having to grow and become continuously remodeled to keep pace with the embryo's overall growth while remaining fully functional in supplying the needs of the embryo's cells.

## Heart and Great Vessels

The earliest development of the circulatory system consists of the migration of heart-forming cells arising in the epiblast through the primitive streak in a well-defined anteroposterior order. Those cells passing through the streak closest to the primitive node will form the outflow tract, those passing through the midstreak will form the ventricles, and the cells that will form the atria enter the streak most posteriorly (Figure 6-11, *A*). After leaving the primitive streak, the precardiac cells, which are associated with endodermal cells as a splanchnic mesoderm, become arranged in the same anteroposterior order in a U-shaped region of **cardiogenic mesoderm** (Figure 6-11, *B*). Following an inductive influence (involving members of the BMP and FGF families) by the endoderm (likely the anterior visceral endoderm, which also serves as the head organizer in mammals), the cells in this field are committed to the heart-forming pathway. In response,

these cells express genes for several sets of transcription factors (*Nkx2-5*, *MEF2*, and *GATA-4*) that are important in early heart development. From the cardiogenic mesoderm, the heart and great vessels form from bilaterally paired tubes that fuse in the midline beneath the foregut to produce a single tube (Figures 6-11, *C*, 6-12, and 6-13).

In human embryos the earliest recognizable precardiac mesoderm is a crescent-shaped zone of thickened mesoderm rostral to the embryonic disk of the gastrulating embryo early in the third week (Figure 6-11, *B*). As the mesoderm begins to split into the splanchnic and somatic layers, a **cardiogenic plate** is recognizable in the splanchnic mesoderm rostral to the oropharyngeal membrane (see Figure 6-14, *A*). In this area the space between the two layers of mesoderm is the forerunner of the **pericardial cavity**. The main layer of splanchnic mesoderm in the precardiac region thickens to become the **myocardial primordium**. Between this structure and the endoderm of

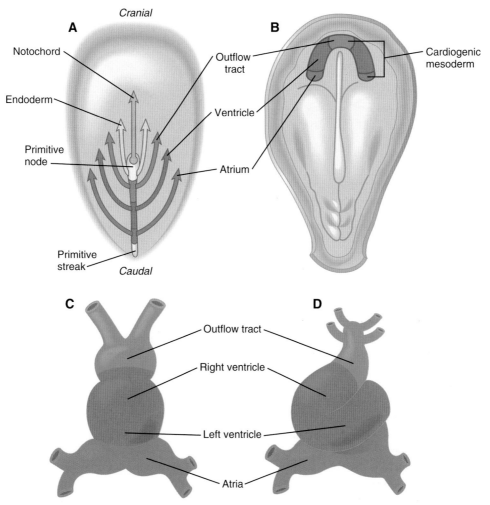

**FIGURE 6-11** Early stages in heart formation. **A,** Topographically precise movements of cardiogenic cells through the primitive streak. **B,** Horseshoe-shaped distribution of cardiogenic cells after their migration through the primitive streak. At this stage the cardiogenic area is anterior to the rostralmost extent of the neural plate. **C,** The straight tubular heart. **D,** Ventral view of the S-shaped heart.

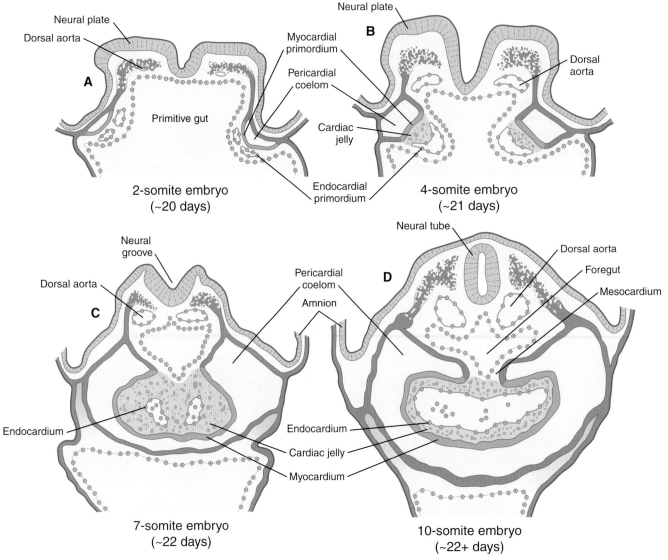

**FIGURE 6-12** Cross sections through the level of the developing heart from **20 to 22 days. A,** Two-somite embryo. **B,** Four-somite embryo. **C,** Seven-somite embryo. **D,** Ten-somite embryo.

the primitive gut, isolated mesodermal vesicles appear, which soon fuse to form the tubular **endocardial primordia** (see Figure 6-12, *A* and *B*). The endocardial primordia ultimately fuse and become the inner lining of the heart.

As the head of the embryo takes shape by both lateral and ventral folding, the bilateral cardiac primordia come together in the midline ventral to the gut and fuse to form a primitive single tubular heart. This structure consists of an inner **endocardial lining** surrounded by a loose layer of specialized extracellular matrix that has historically been called **cardiac jelly** (see Figure 6-12, *C*). Outside the cardiac jelly is the **myocardium,** which ultimately forms the muscular part of the heart. The outer lining of the heart, called the **epicardium,** is derived from the proepicardial primordium, which is located near the dorsal

mesocardium (see Figure 6-16, *B*). Cells migrating from the proepicardium cover the surface of the tubular heart. The entire tubular heart is located in the space known as the **pericardial coelom.** Shortly after the single tubular heart is formed, it begins to form a characteristic S-shaped loop that presages its eventual organization into the configuration of the adult heart (Figure 6-15). (Additional cellular and molecular aspects of early cardiogenesis are covered in Chapter 17.)

The heart is formed from a variety of cell lineages. Within the cardiogenic mesoderm are cells that express N-cadherin and those that do not (Figure 6-16, *A*). Depending upon their location within the cardiogenic mesoderm, N-cadherin–positive cells will go on to form either atrial or ventricular myocytes, whereas N-cadherin–negative cells will form the endocardial lining

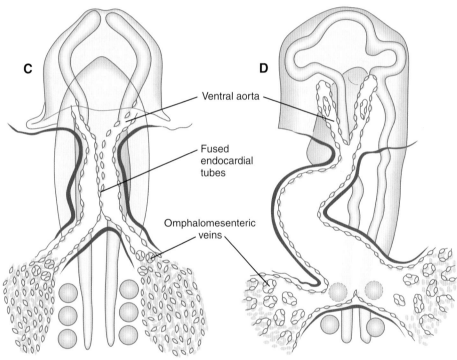

**FIGURE 6-13** Formation of the tubular heart in the chick embryo from paired primordia. The embryo is viewed from the ventral side. **A,** Stage 8. **B,** Stage 9. **C,** Stage 10. **D,** Stage 11.

and, later, cells of the endocardial cushions (see page 447). Cells of the cardiac conduction system are derived from modified atrial and ventricular cardiac myocytes.

The early heart does not form in isolation. At its caudal end, the endocardial tubes do not fuse but rather extend toward the posterior part of the body as the venous inflow tract of the heart (see Figure 6-15, *A*). Similarly, the endothelial tube leading out from the heart at its cranial end produces vascular arches that loop around the pharynx. Migrating neural crest cells form much of the walls of these vessels. By 21 or 22 days after fertilization, differentiation of cardiac muscle cells in the myocardium

is sufficiently advanced to allow the heart to begin beating.

## Blood and Blood Vessels

The formation of blood and blood vessels begins in the mesodermal wall of the yolk sac as well as in the wall of the chorion outside the embryo proper. Stimulated by an inductive interaction with the endoderm of the yolk sac, many small **blood islands**, consisting of stem cells called **hemangioblasts**, appear in the extraembryonic splanchnic mesoderm of the yolk sac (Figure 6-17). Recent

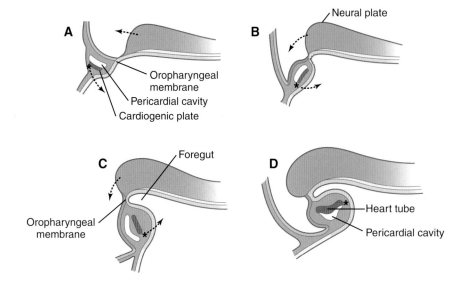

**FIGURE 6-14 A** to **D,** Sagittal sections through the cranial ends of **18- to 22-day-old** embryos showing the roughly 180-degree rotation of the primitive heart tube and pericardium with the expansion of the cranial end of the embryo.

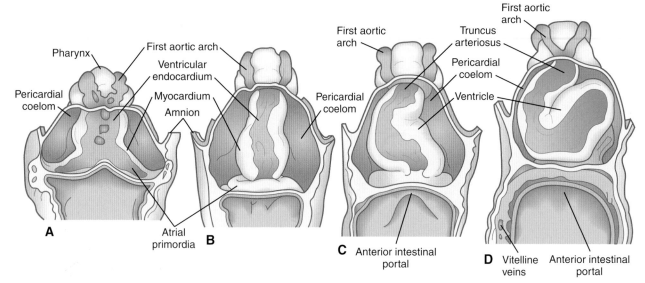

**FIGURE 6-15** Formation of the S-shaped heart from fused cardiac tubes in the human embryo at about **21 to 23 days. A,** Four-somite embryo. **B,** Eight-somite embryo. **C,** Ten- to eleven-somite embryo. **D,** Twelve-somite embryo.

experimental evidence suggests that the inductive signal from the yolk sac endoderm is the signaling molecule **Indian hedgehog.** The yolk sac mesoderm responds to this signal by producing **BMP-4,** which feeds back onto itself. In a yet undefined manner, this interaction triggers the formation of blood islands within the mesoderm of the yolk sac. Once the blood islands form, the central cells become blood-forming cells (**hemocytoblasts**), whereas those on the outside acquire the characteristics of **endothelial lining cells,** which form the inner walls of blood vessels. As the vesicular blood islands in the wall of the yolk sac fuse, they form primitive vascular channels that extend toward the body of the embryo. Connections are made with the endothelial tubes associated with the tubular heart and major vessels, and the primitive plan of the circulatory system begins to take shape.

## DEVELOPMENT OF THE ENDODERMAL GERM LAYER

As soon as it forms during gastrulation, the endoderm receives information that determines anterior or posterior characteristics of the appropriate regions. There is evidence that **FGF-4,** secreted by primitive streak mesoderm, imparts a posterior character to the endoderm. Further signals from surrounding tissues prepare the endoderm for more region-specific inductions of the gut tube.

Development of the endodermal germ layer continues with the transformation of the flat intraembryonic endodermal sheet into a tubular gut as a result of the lateral folding of the embryonic body and the ventral bending of the cranial and caudal ends of the embryo into a

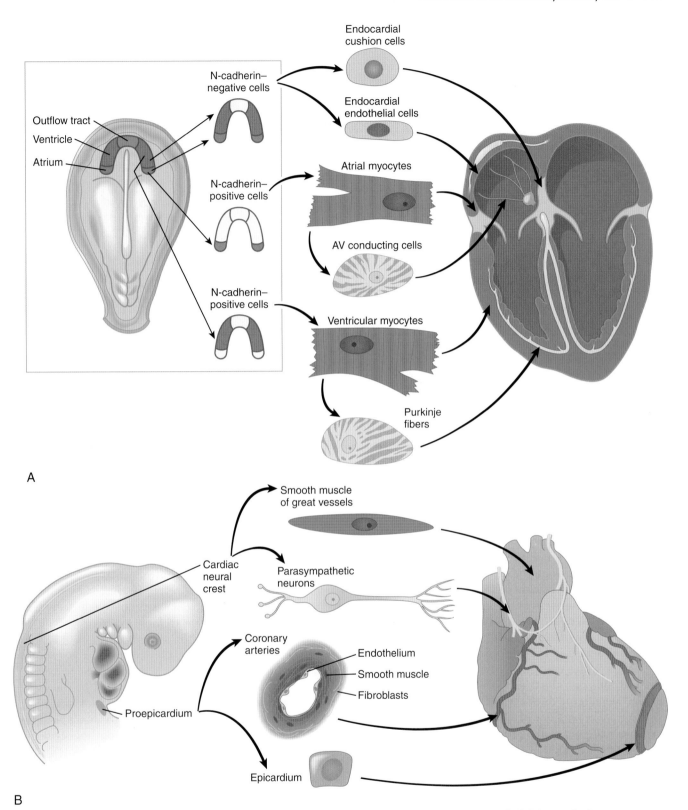

**FIGURE 6-16** Cell lineages in the developing heart. **A,** Derivatives of cardiogenic mesodermal cells. **B,** Cellular contributions of the cardiac neural crest and proepicardium to the heart.

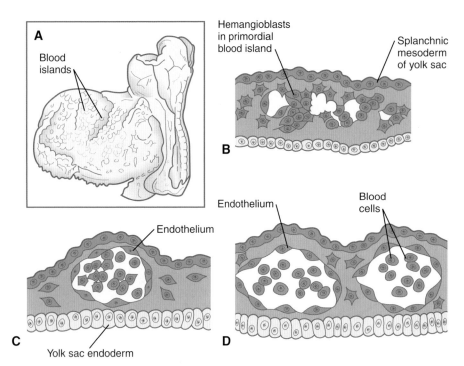

**FIGURE 6-17** Development of blood islands in the yolk sac of human embryos. **A,** Gross view of a 10-somite human embryo showing the location of blood islands on the yolk sac. **B** to **D,** Successive stages in the formation of blood islands. (From Corner G: *Carnegie Contr* Embryol 20:81–102, 1929.)

roughly **C**-shaped structure (Figures 6-6 and 6-18). A major morphological consequence of these folding processes is the sharp delineation of the **yolk sac** from the digestive tube.

Early in the third week, when the three embryonic germ layers are first laid down, the intraembryonic endoderm constitutes the roof of the roughly spherical yolk sac (see Figure 6-18). Expansion of either end of the neural plate, particularly the tremendous growth of the future brain region, results in the formation of the **head fold** and **tail fold** along the sagittal plane of the embryo. This process, along with concomitant lateral folding, results in the formation of the beginnings of the tubular **foregut** and **hindgut**. This process also begins to delineate the yolk sac from the gut proper. The sequence of steps in the formation of the tubular gut can be likened to a purse string constricting the ventral region of the embryo, although the actual mechanism is more related to the overall growth of the embryo than to a real constriction. The region of the imaginary purse string becomes the **yolk stalk** (also called the **omphalomesenteric** or **vitelline duct**), with the embryonic gut above and the yolk sac below (see Figures 6-6, *D*, and 6-18, *D*). The portion of the gut that still opens into the yolk sac is called the **midgut,** and the points of transition between the open-floored midgut and the tubular anterior and posterior regions of the gut are called the **anterior** and **posterior intestinal portals** (see Figure 6-18, *B*).

The endodermal edges of the anterior and posterior intestinal portals are also sites of expression of the signaling molecule **sonic hedgehog.** In the posterior intestinal portal, the appearance of sonic hedgehog in the

endoderm is followed shortly by the expression of another signaling molecule, BMP-4. This in turn is followed by the appearance of a gradient of mesodermal expression of paralogous groups 9–13 of the *Hox* genes (see Figure 4-5 for an illustration of paralogous groups), with *Hoxa-d-9* being expressed most cranially and *Hoxa-d-13* being expressed most caudally, near the cloaca. This distribution of *Hox* gene expression associated with hindgut formation is reminiscent of that already described for the early hindbrain region (see p. 107). It is likely that this gradient is instrumental in guiding the regional differentiation of the gut because later in development the gut-associated mesoderm is able to induce undifferentiated endoderm to form structures specific to the craniocaudal level of the mesoderm.

In some cases, normal development of the gut and its related structures can only proceed when sonic hedgehog signaling is repressed. For example, as will be discussed further on page 372, the dorsal pancreatic bud (see Figure 6-18, *D*) is induced by the notochord. A direct result of this induction is repression of sonic hedgehog signaling within the gut endoderm in the area of the dorsal pancreas. This allows the expression of the genes associated with the formation of the pancreas. At roughly the same anteroposterior level, but on the ventral side of the gut where the liver will form, hepatic endoderm expresses **albumin** in response to signals from the adjacent precardiac mesoderm.

The anterior end of the foregut remains temporarily sealed off by an ectodermal-endodermal bilayer called the **oropharyngeal membrane** (see Figure 6-18, *B*). This membrane separates the future mouth (**stomodeum**),

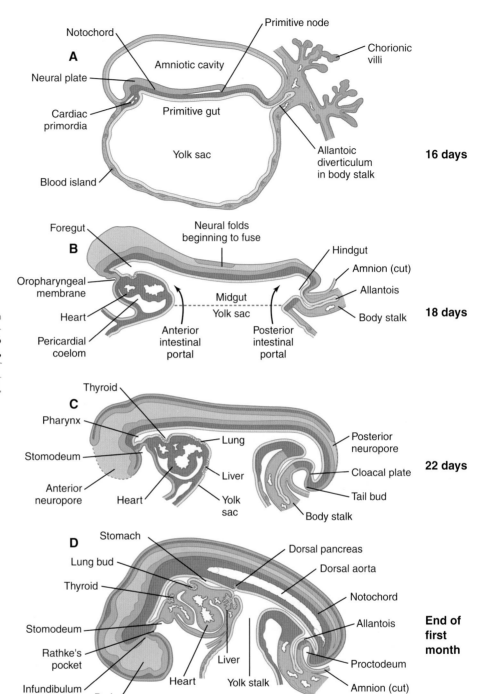

A

Notochord

Neural plate

Cardiac primordia

Blood island

Amniotic cavity

Primitive node

Chorionic villi

Primitive gut

Yolk sac

Allantoic diverticulum in body stalk

**16 days**

FIGURE 6-18 Sagittal sections through human embryos showing the early establishment of the digestive system. **A,** At **16 days. B,** At **18 days. C,** At **22 days. D,** At the **end of the first month.** (After Patten. From Carlson BM: *Patten's foundations of embryology,* ed 6, New York, 1996, McGraw-Hill.)

B

Foregut

Oropharyngeal membrane

Heart

Pericardial coelom

Neural folds beginning to fuse

Midgut
Yolk sac

Anterior intestinal portal

Posterior intestinal portal

Hindgut

Amnion (cut)

Allantois

Body stalk

**18 days**

C

Thyroid

Pharynx

Stomodeum

Anterior neuropore

Heart

Lung

Liver

Yolk sac

Posterior neuropore

Cloacal plate

Tail bud

Body stalk

**22 days**

D

Stomach

Lung bud

Thyroid

Stomodeum

Rathke's pocket

Infundibulum

Brain

Heart

Liver

Yolk stalk

Dorsal pancreas

Dorsal aorta

Notochord

Allantois

Proctodeum

Amnion (cut)

**End of first month**

which is lined by ectoderm, from the **pharynx,** the endodermally lined anterior part of the foregut. Without an intervening layer of mesoderm, this bilayer of two epithelial sheets is inherently unstable and eventually breaks down.

The rapid bulging of the cephalic region, in conjunction with the constriction of the ventral region, has a major topographic effect on the rapidly developing cardiac region. In the early embryo the cardiac primordia are located cephalic to the primitive gut. The forces that

shape the tubular foregut, however, cause the bilateral cardiac primordia to turn 180 degrees in the craniocaudal direction while the paired cardiac tubes are moving toward one another in the ventral midline (see Figure 6-14).

In the region of the hindgut the expansion of the embryo's body is not as prominent as it is in the cranial end, but nevertheless a less exaggerated ventral folding also occurs in that region. Even as the earliest signs of the tail fold are taking shape, a tubular evagination of the hindgut extends into the mesoderm of the body stalk. This evagination is called the **allantois** (Figure 6-18, *B*). In most mammals and birds the allantois represents a major structural adaptation for the exchange of gases and the removal of urinary wastes. Because of the efficiency of the placenta, however, the allantois never becomes a prominent structure in the human embryo. Nevertheless, because of the blood vessels that become associated with it, the allantois remains a vital part of the link between the embryo and the mother (see Chapter 7).

Caudal to the allantois is another ectodermal-endodermal bilayer called the **cloacal plate,** or **proctodeal membrane** (see Figure 6-18, *C*). This membrane, which ultimately breaks down, covers the cloaca, which in the early embryo represents a common outlet for both the digestive and the urogenital systems. The shallow depression outside the proctodeal membrane is called the **proctodeum.**

As the gut becomes increasingly tubular, a series of local inductive interactions between the epithelium of the digestive tract and the surrounding mesenchyme initiate the formation of most of the major digestive and endocrine glands (e.g., thyroid gland, salivary glands, pancreas), the respiratory system, and the liver. In the region of the stomodeum, an induction between forebrain and stomodeal ectoderm initiates the formation of the anterior pituitary gland. (Further development of these organs is discussed in Chapters 14 and 15.)

## BASIC STRUCTURE OF 4-WEEK-OLD EMBRYO

### Gross Appearance

By the end of the fourth week of pregnancy the embryo, which is still only about 4 mm long, has established the rudiments of most of the major organ systems except for the limbs (which are still absent) and the urogenital system (which has developed only the earliest traces of the embryonic kidneys). Externally, the embryo is **C**-shaped, with a prominent row of somites situated along either side of the neural tube (Figures 6-19 and 6-20). Except for the rudiments of the eyes and ears and the oropharyngeal membrane, which is beginning to break down (Figure 6-21), the head is relatively featureless. In the cervical region, **pharyngeal arches** are prominent (Figures 6-19, *B* and *C*, and 6-22). The body stalk still occupies a significant part of the ventral body wall, and cephalic to the body stalk, the heart and liver make prominent bulges in the contours of the ventral body wall. Posterior to the body stalk, the body tapers to a somewhat spiraled tail, which is prominent in embryos of this age.

Another prominent but little understood feature of embryos of this age is a ring of thickened ectoderm, called the **wolffian ridge,** that encircles the lateral aspect of the body (Figure 6-23). Its function is not well

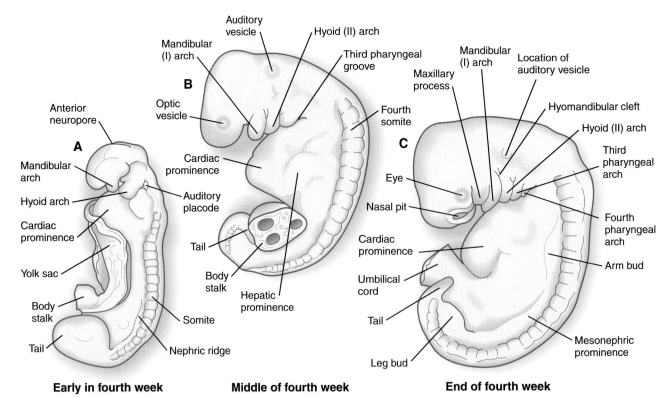

**Early in fourth week**       **Middle of fourth week**       **End of fourth week**

**FIGURE 6-19** Gross development of human embryos during the period of early organogenesis. **A, Early in the fourth week. B, Middle of the fourth week. C, End of the fourth week.**

**FIGURE 6-20** Scanning electron micrograph of a 3-mm human embryo approximately **26 days** old. *S*, Somite. (From Jirásek JE: *Atlas of human prenatal morphogenesis*, Amsterdam, 1983, Martinus Nijhoff.)

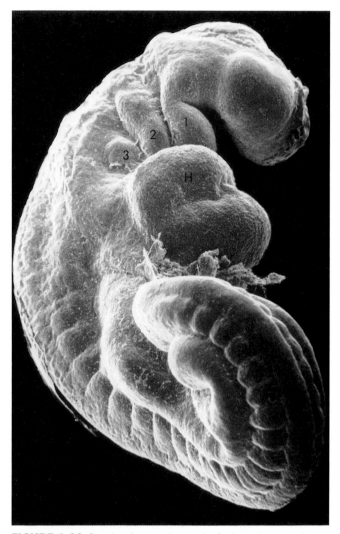

**FIGURE 6-22** Scanning electron micrograph of a 4-mm human embryo **30 days** old. *1* to *3*, Pharyngeal arches; *H*, heart. (From Jirásek JE: *Atlas of human prenatal morphogenesis*, Amsterdam, 1983, Martinus Nijhoff.)

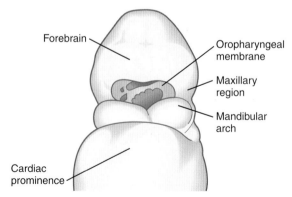

**FIGURE 6-21** Face of a human embryo during the **fourth week** showing the breakdown of the oropharyngeal membrane.

understood, but it spans the primordia of many structures (e.g., nose, eye, inner ear, pharyngeal arches, limbs) that require tissue interactions for their early development. What role the thickened ectoderm plays in early organogenesis remains to be determined.

## Circulatory System

At 4 weeks of age, the embryo has a functioning two-chamber heart and a blood vascular system that consists of three separate circulatory arcs (Figure 6-24). The first, the **intraembryonic circulatory arc**, is organized in a manner similar to that of a fish. A ventral aortic outflow tract from the heart splits into a series of aortic arches passing around the pharynx through the pharyngeal arches and then collecting into a cephalically paired dorsal aorta that distributes blood throughout the body. A system of cardinal veins collects the blood and returns it to the heart via a common inflow tract.

The second arc, commonly called the **vitelline** or **omphalomesenteric arc**, is principally an extraembryonic circulatory loop that supplies the yolk sac (see Figure 6-24). The third circulatory arc, also extraembryonic, consists of the vessels associated with the allantois. In the human, this third arc consists of the **umbilical vessels**,

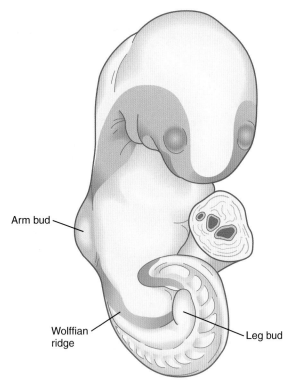

**FIGURE 6-23** Ventrolateral view of a 30-somite (4.2 mm) human embryo showing the thickened ectodermal ring *(blue)*. The portion of the ring between the upper and lower limb buds is the wolffian ridge. (Based on studies by O'Rahilly R, Gardner E: *Anat Embryol* 148:1–23, 1975.)

which course through the body stalk and spread in an elaborate network in the placenta and chorionic tissues. This set of vessels represents the real lifeline between the embryo and mother. Although the two extraembryonic circulatory loops do not persist as such after birth, the intraembryonic portions of these arcs are retained as vessels or ligaments in the adult body.

## Derivatives of the Embryonic Germ Layers

By the end of the fourth week of development, primordia of most of the major structures and organs in the body have been laid down, many of them the result of local inductive interactions. Each of the embryonic germ layers contributes to the formation of many of these structures. Figure 6-25 summarizes the germ layer origins of most of the major structures in the embryonic body. This figure is designed to be a guide that will allow specific structures that are being studied to be viewed in the context of the whole body rather than something that should be memorized at this stage. Students have found that a table like this is useful for review at the end of an embryology course.

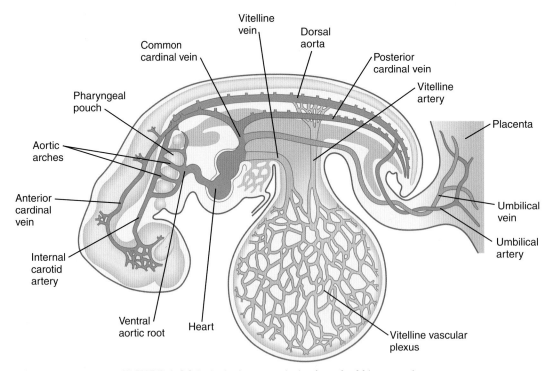

**FIGURE 6-24** Basic circulatory arcs in the **4-week-old** human embryo.

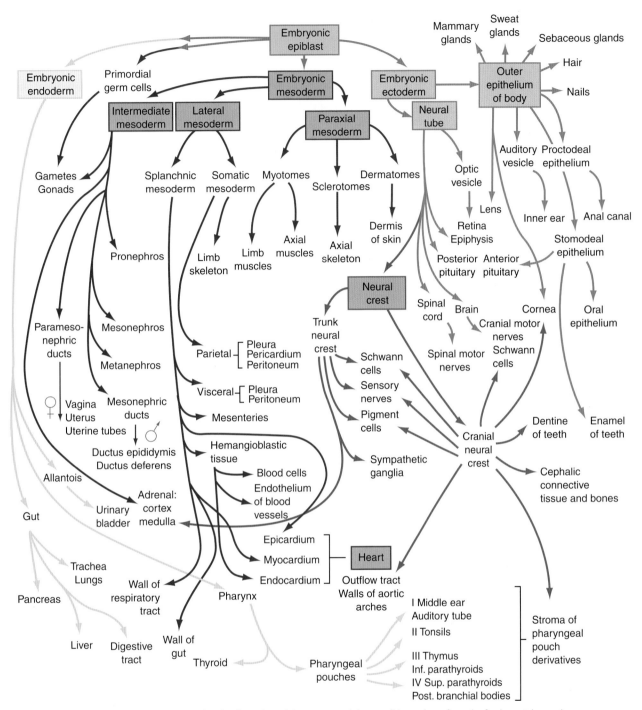

**FIGURE 6-25** Flow chart showing the formation of the organs and tissues of the embryo from the fundamental germ layers. The arrows are color-coded according to the germ layer of origin of the structure (see Figure 4-1 for color code).

## SUMMARY

○ The response of dorsal ectodermal cells to primary induction is to thicken, forming a neural plate. Neurulation consists of lateral folding of the neural plate at hinge points to form a neural groove. Opposing sides of the thickened epithelium of the neural groove join to form a neural tube. The temporarily unclosed cranial and caudal ends of the neural tube are the anterior and posterior neuropores.

○ Cranially, the neural tube subdivides into a primitive three-part brain consisting of the prosencephalon, mesencephalon, and rhombencephalon. The caudal part of the early brain also becomes subdivided into segments called *neuromeres*, of which the rhombomeres are most prominent. Specific homeobox genes are expressed in a regular order in the rhombomeres. A signaling center, the isthmic organizer, located at the midbrain and hindbrain junction acts via the production of Wnt-1 anteriorly and FGF-8 posteriorly.

◯ As the neural tube closes, neural crest cells emigrate from the neural epithelium and spread through the body along welldefined paths. Secondary inductions acting on ectoderm in the cranial region result in the formation of several series of ectodermal placodes, which are the precursors of sense organs and sensory ganglia of cranial nerves.

◯ The embryonic mesoderm is subdivided into three craniocaudal columns: the paraxial, intermediate, and lateral plate mesoderm. Paraxial mesoderm is the precursor tissue to the paired somites and somitomeres. Segmentation of the paraxial mesoderm into somites occurs through the action of a clock mechanism that leads to the periodic expression of *c-hairy* and a variety of downstream molecules. As the result of a complex series of inductive interactions involving a variety of signaling molecules, the epithelial somites become subdivided into sclerotomes (precursors of vertebral bodies) and dermomyotomes, which in turn form dermatomes (dermal precursors) and myotomes (precursors of axial muscles). In further subdivisions, precursor cells of limb muscles are found in the lateral halves of the somites, and precursor cells of axial muscles are found in the medial halves. The posterior half of one sclerotome joins with the anterior half of the next caudal somite to form a single vertebral body.

◯ Intermediate mesoderm forms the organs of the urogenital system. The lateral mesoderm splits to form somatic mesoderm (associated with ectoderm) and splanchnic mesoderm (associated with endoderm). The space between becomes the coelom. The limb bud arises from lateral mesoderm, and extraembryonic mesoderm forms the body stalk.

◯ Blood cells and blood vessels form initially from blood islands located in the mesodermal wall of the yolk sac. The heart, originating from a horseshoe-shaped region of splanchnic mesoderm anterior to the oropharyngeal membrane, forms two tubes on either side of the foregut. As the foregut takes shape, the two cardiac tubes come together to form a single tubular heart, which begins to beat around 22 days after fertilization.

◯ The embryonic endoderm initially consists of the roof of the yolk sac. As the embryo undergoes lateral folding, the endodermal gut forms cranial and caudal tubes (foregut and hindgut), but the middle region (midgut) remains open to the yolk sac ventrally. Regional specification of the gut begins with sonic hedgehog signals from the endoderm of the intestinal portals, which are trans-

lated to gradients of *Hox* gene expression in the neighboring mesoderm. As the tubular gut continues to take shape, the connection to the yolk sac becomes attenuated to form the yolk stalk. The future mouth (stomodeum) is separated from the foregut by an oropharyngeal membrane, and the hindgut is separated from the proctodeum by the cloacal plate. A ventral evagination from the hindgut is the allantois, which in many animals is an adaptation for removing urinary and respiratory wastes.

◯ In the 4-week-old embryo, the circulatory system includes a functioning two-chamber heart and a blood vascular system that consists of three circulatory arcs. In addition to the intraembryonic circulation, the extraembryonic vitelline circulatory arc, which supplies the yolk sac, and the umbilical circulation, which is associated with the allantois and supplies the placenta, are present.

 # Review Questions

1. **The sclerotome arises from cells that were located in the:**
   A. Notochord
   B. Paraxial mesoderm
   C. Intermediate mesoderm
   D. Lateral mesoderm
   E. None of the above

2. **The cardiogenic plate arises from:**
   A. Embryonic endoderm
   B. Somatic mesoderm
   C. Splanchnic mesoderm
   D. Intermediate mesoderm
   E. Neural crest

3. **An inductive stimulus from which structure stimulates the transformation of the epithelial sclerotome into secondary mesenchyme?**
   A. Neural crest
   B. Somite
   C. Ectodermal placodes
   D. Embryonic endoderm
   E. Notochord

4. **Which of these structures in the embryo is unsegmented?**
   A. Somitomeres
   B. Neuromeres
   C. Notochord
   D. Somites

5. **The intermediate mesoderm is the precursor of the:**
   A. Urogenital system
   B. Heart
   C. Somites
   D. Body wall
   E. Vertebral bodies

6. What forces are involved in the folding of the neural plate to form the neural tube?

7. What role do neuromeres play in the formation of the central nervous system?

8. From what structures do the cells that form skeletal muscles arise?

9. Where do the first blood cells of the embryo form?

# REFERENCES

Alvarez IS, Schoenwolf GC: Expansion of surface epithelium provides the major extrinsic force for bending of the neural plate, *J Exp Zool* 261:340–348, 1992.

Amthor H and others: The expression and regulation of *follistatin* and a *follistatin-like* gene during avian somite compartmentalization and myogenesis, *Dev Biol* 178:343–362, 1996.

Baker CVH, Bronner-Fraser M: Vertebrate cranial placodes I. Embryonic induction, *Devel Biol* 232:1–61, 2001.

Begemann G, Meyer A: Hindbrain patterning revisited: timing and effects of retinoic acid signalling, *BioEssays* 23:981–986, 2001.

Bergquist H: Studies on the cerebral tube in vertebrates: the neuromeres, *Acta Zool* 33:117–187, 1952.

Brand-Saberi B and others: The formation of somite compartments in the avian embryo, *Int J Dev Biol* 40:411–420, 1996.

Brent AE, Tabin CJ: Developmental regulation of somite derivatives: muscle, cartilage and tendon, *Curr Opin Genet Devel* 12:548–557, 2002.

Christ B and others: Segmentation of the vertebrate body, *Anat Embryol* 197:1–8, 1998.

Cleaver O, Krieg PA: Notochord patterning of the endoderm, *Devel Biol* 234:1–12, 2001.

Colas J-F, Schoenwolf GC: Towards a cellular and molecular understanding of neurulation, *Devel Dyn* 221:117–145, 2001.

Dietrich S, Schubert FR, Lumsden A: Control of dorsoventral pattern in the chick paraxial mesoderm, *Development* 124:3895–3908, 1997.

Dubrulle J, Pourquié O: From head to tail: links between the segmentation clock and antero-posterior patterning of the embryo, *Curr Opin Genet Devel* 12:519–523, 2002.

Fishman MC, Chien KR: Fashioning the vertebrate heart: earliest embryonic decisions, *Development* 124:2099–2117, 1997.

Gavalas A, Krumlauf R: Retinoid signaling and hindbrain patterning, *Curr Opin Genet Devel* 10:380–386, 2000.

Harvey RP, Rosenthal N, eds: *Heart Development*, San Diego, 1999, Academic Press.

Jacobson AG: Somitomeres: mesodermal segments of the head and trunk. In Hanken J, Hall BK, eds: *The skull*, vol 1, *Development*, Chicago, 1993, University of Chicago Press.

Jacobson AG, Sater AK: Features of embryonic induction, *Development* 104:341–359, 1988.

Lassar AB, Munsterberg AE: The role of positive and negative signals in somite patterning, *Curr Opin Neurobiol* 6:57–63, 1996.

Lobe CG: Transcription factors and mammalian development, *Curr Topics Dev Biol* 27:351–382, 1992.

Lough J, Sugi Y: Endoderm and heart development, *Devel Dyn* 217:327–342, 2000.

Lumsden A, Krumlauf R: Patterning the vertebrate neuraxis, *Science* 274:1109–1115, 1996.

Marcelle C, Stark MR, Bronner-Fraser M: Coordinate actions of BMPs, Wnts, Shh and Noggin mediate patterning of the dorsal somite, *Development* 124:3955–3963, 1997.

Martinez S: The isthmic organizer and brain regionalization, *Int J Devel Biol* 45:367–371, 2001.

Meier S: Development of the chick embryo mesoblast: formation of the embryonic axis and establishment of the embryonic pattern, *Dev Biol* 73:24–45, 1979.

Müller F, O'Rahilly R: The timing and sequence of appearance of neuromeres and their derivatives in staged human embryos, *Acta Anat* 158:83–99, 1997.

Nakatsu T, Uwabe C, Shiota K: Neural tube closure in humans initiates at multiple sites: evidence from human embryos and implications for the pathogenesis of neural tube defects, *Anat Embryol* 201:455–466, 2000.

O'Rahilly R, Müller F: The origin of the ectodermal ring in staged human embryos of the first 5 weeks, *Acta Anat* 122:145–157, 1985.

Ordahl CP, ed: *Somitogenesis*, Parts 1 and 2, *Curr Topics Dev Biol*, vols 47 and 48, 2000.

Pourquie O: The vertebrate segmentation clock, *J Anat* 199:169–175, 2001.

Pourquie O and others: Lateral and axial signals involved in avian somite patterning: a role for BMP4, *Cell* 84:461–471, 1996.

Rhinn M, Brand M: The midbrain-hindbrain boundary organizer, *Curr Opin Neurobiol* 11:34–42, 2001.

Rossant JU, Tam PPL, eds: *Mouse Development: Patterning, Morphogenesis, and Organogenesis*, San Diego, 2002, Academic Press.

Roberts DJ and others: Sonic hedgehog is an endodermal signal inducing *Bmp-4* and *Hox* genes during induction and regionalization of the chick hindgut, *Development* 121:3163–3174, 1995.

Rubenstein JLR and others: The embryonic vertebrate forebrain: the prosomeric model, *Science* 266:578–580, 1994.

Sasai Y, De Robertis EM: Ectodermal patterning in vertebrate embryos, *Dev Biol* 182:5–20, 1997.

Schoenwolf GC: Histological and ultrastructural studies of secondary neurulation in mouse embryos, *Am J Anat* 169:361–376, 1984.

Schoenwolf GC: Mechanisms of neurulation: traditional viewpoint and recent advances, *Development* 109:243–270, 1990.

Smith JL, Schoenwolf GC: Neurulation: coming to closure, *Trends Neurol Sci* 20:510–517, 1997.

Sosic D and others: Regulation of *paraxis* expression and somite formation by ectoderm- and neural tube-derived signals, *Dev Biol* 185:229–243, 1997.

Stockdale FE, Nikivits W, Christ B: Molecular and cellular biology of avian somite development, *Devel Dyn* 219:304–321, 2000.

Tajbakhsh S, Sporie R: Somite development: Constructing the vertebrate body, *Cell* 92:9–16, 1998.

Tam PPL, Meier S, Jacobson AG: Differentiation of the metameric pattern in the embryonic axis of the mouse. II. Somitomeric organization of the presomitic mesoderm, *Differentiation* 21:109–122, 1982.

Tam PPL, Quinlan GA, Trainor PA: The patterning of progenitor tissues for the cranial region of the mouse embryo during gastrulation and early organogenesis, *Adv Devel Biol* 5:137–200, 1997.

Tonegawa A and others: Mesodermal subdivision along the mediolateral axis in chicken controlled by different concentrations of BMP-4, *Development* 124:1975–1984, 1997.

Trainor PA, Krumlauf R: Patterning the cranial neural crest: Hindbrain segmentation and *Hox* gene plasticity, *Nature Revs Neurosci* 1:116–124, 2000.

Vaage S: The segmentation of the primitive neural tube in chick embryos (*Gallus domesticus*), *Adv Anat Embryol Cell Biol* 41(3):1–88, 1969.

Williams BA, Ordahl CP: Emergence of determined myotome precursor cells in the somite, *Development* 124:4983–4997, 1997.

Wurst W, Bally-Cuif L: Neural plate patterning: upstream and downstream of the isthmic organizer, *Nature Revs Neurosci* 2:99–108, 2001.

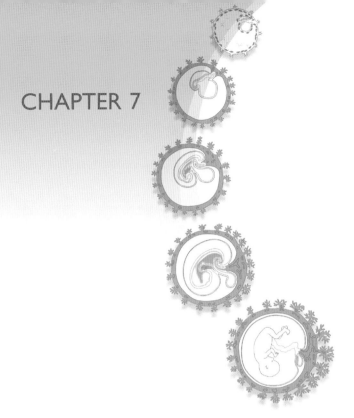

# CHAPTER 7

# Placenta and Extraembryonic Membranes

One of the most characteristic features of human embryonic development is the intimate relationship between the embryo and mother. The fertilized egg brings little with it except genetic material. To survive and grow during intrauterine life, the embryo must maintain an essentially parasitic relationship with the body of the mother for acquiring oxygen and nutrients and eliminating wastes. It must also avoid being rejected like a foreign body by the immune system of its maternal host. These exacting requirements are met by the placenta and extraembryonic membranes that surround the embryo and serve as the interface between the embryo and mother.

The tissues that make up the fetal-maternal interface (**placenta** and **chorion**) are derivatives of the **trophoblast**, which separates from the inner cell mass and surrounds the cellular precursors of the embryo proper even as the cleaving zygote travels down the uterine tube on its way to implanting into the uterine wall (see Figure 3-16). Other extraembryonic tissues are derived from the inner cell mass. These include the **amnion** (an ectodermal derivative), which forms a protective fluid-filled capsule around the embryo; the **yolk sac** (an endodermal derivative), which in mammalian embryos no longer serves a primary nutritive function; the **allantois** (an endodermal derivative), which is associated with the removal of embryonic wastes; and much of the **extraembryonic mesoderm**, which forms the bulk of the umbilical cord, the connective tissue backing of the extraembryonic membranes, and the blood vessels that supply them.

## EXTRAEMBRYONIC TISSUES

### Amnion

The origin of the amniotic cavity within the ectoderm of the inner cell mass in the implanting embryo was described in Chapter 5 (see Figures 3-16 and 5-2). As the early embryo undergoes cephalocaudal and lateral folding, the amniotic membrane surrounds the body of the embryo like a fluid-filled balloon (Figure 7-1), allowing the embryo to be suspended in a liquid environment for the duration of pregnancy. The amniotic fluid serves as a buffer against mechanical injury to the fetus; in addition, it accommodates growth, allows normal fetal movements, and protects the fetus from adhesions.

The thin amniotic membrane consists of a single layer of extraembryonic ectodermal cells lined by a nonvascularized layer of extraembryonic mesoderm. Keeping pace with fetal growth, the amniotic cavity steadily expands until its fluid content reaches a maximum of nearly 1 L by weeks 33 to 34 of pregnancy (Figure 7-2).

In many respects, amniotic fluid can be viewed as a dilute transudate of maternal plasma, but the origins and exchange dynamics of amniotic fluid are complex and not completely understood. There are two phases in amniotic fluid production. The first phase encompasses the first 20 weeks of pregnancy, during which the composition of amniotic fluid is quite similar to that of fetal fluids. During this period, the fetal skin is unkeratinized, and there is evidence that fluid and electrolytes are able to diffuse

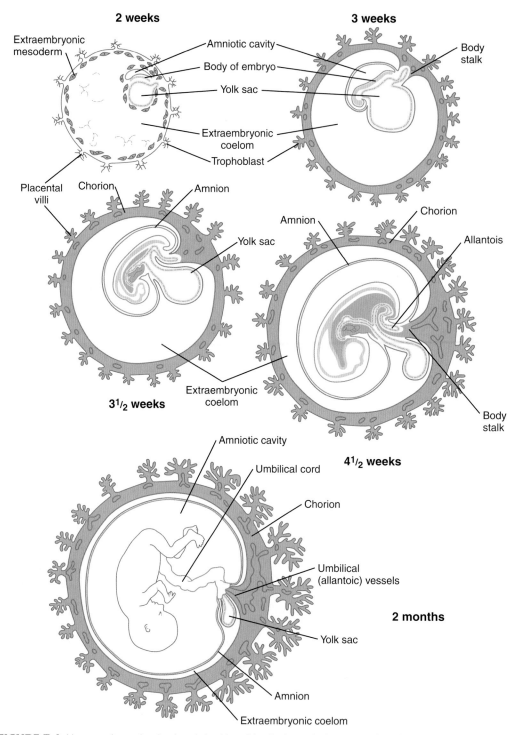

**FIGURE 7-1** Human embryos showing the relationships of the chorion and other extraembryonic membranes. (Modified from Carlson BM: *Patten's foundations of embryology*, ed 6, New York, 1996, McGraw-Hill.)

freely through the embryonic ectoderm of the skin. In addition, the amniotic membrane itself secretes fluid, and components of maternal serum pass through the amniotic membrane.

As pregnancy advances (especially after week 20, when the fetal epidermis begins to keratinize), changes occur in the source of amniotic fluid. There is not com-

plete agreement on the sources (and their relative contributions) of amniotic fluid in the second half of pregnancy. Nonetheless, there are increasing contributions from fetal urine, filtration from maternal blood vessels near the chorion laeve (which is closely apposed to the amniotic membrane at this stage), and possibly filtration from fetal vessels in the umbilical cord and chorionic plate.

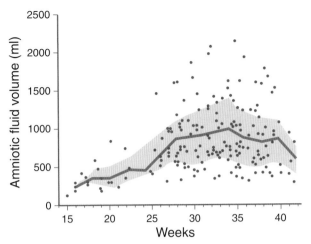

**FIGURE 7-2** Volumes of amniotic fluid in women at various weeks of pregnancy. The lined and colored area represents the mean plus or minus standard deviation. Dots represent outlying values. (Data from Queenan JT and others: *Am J Obstet Gynecol* 114:34–38, 1972.)

In the third trimester of pregnancy, the amniotic fluid turns over completely every 3 hours, and at term, the fluid-exchange rate may approach 500 ml/hr. Although much of the amniotic fluid is exchanged across the amniotic membrane, fetal swallowing is an important mechanism in late pregnancy, with about 20 ml/hr of fluid being swallowed by the fetus. Swallowed amniotic fluid ultimately enters the fetal bloodstream after absorption through the gut wall. The ingested water can leave the fetal circulation through the placenta.

Clinical Correlation 7-1 discusses conditions related to the amount of amniotic fluid or substance concentrations in the fluid.

## Yolk Sac

The yolk sac, which is lined by extraembryonic endoderm, is formed ventral to the bilayered embryo when the amnion appears dorsal to the embryonic disk (see Figure 5-2). In contrast to birds and reptiles, the yolk sac of mammals is small and devoid of yolk. Although vestigial in terms of its original function as a source of nutrition, the yolk sac remains vital to the embryo because of other functions that have become associated with it.

When it first appears, the yolk sac is in the form of a hemisphere bounded at the equatorial region by the dorsal wall of the primitive gut (see Figure 7-1). As the embryo grows and undergoes lateral folding and curvature along the craniocaudal axis, the connection between the yolk sac and forming gut becomes attenuated in the shape of a progressively narrowing stalk attached to a more spherical yolk sac proper at its distal end. In succeeding weeks the yolk stalk becomes very long and attenuated as it is incorporated into the body of the

umbilical cord. The yolk sac itself moves nearer the chorionic plate of the placenta (Figure 7-3).

The endoderm of the yolk sac is lined on the outside by well-vascularized extraembryonic mesoderm. Cells found in each of these layers contribute vital components to the body of the embryo. During the third week, **primordial germ cells**, which arise in the extraembryonic mesoderm near the base of the allantois, become recognizable in the lining of the yolk sac (see Figure 1-1). Soon these cells migrate into the wall of the gut and the dorsal mesentery as they make their way to the gonads, where they differentiate into oogonia or spermatogonia.

In the meantime, groups of extraembryonic mesodermal cells in the wall of the yolk sac become organized into **blood islands** (see Figure 6-17), and many of the cells differentiate into primitive blood cells. **Extraembryonic hematopoiesis** continues in the yolk sac until about the sixth week, when blood-forming activity transfers to intraembryonic sites, especially the liver.

As the tubular gut forms, the attachment site of the yolk stalk becomes progressively less prominent, until by 6 weeks it has effectively lost contact with the gut. In a small percentage of adults, traces of the yolk duct persist as a fibrous cord or an outpouching of the small intestine known as a **Meckel's diverticulum** (see Figure 15-12, A). The yolk sac itself may persist throughout much of pregnancy, but it is not known to have a specific function in the fetal period. The proximal portions of the blood

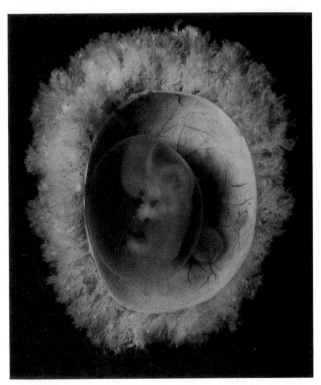

**FIGURE 7-3** A 7-week-old human embryo surrounded by its amnion. The embryo was exposed by cutting open the chorion. The small sphere to the right of the embryo is the yolk sac. (Carnegie embryo No. 8537A, Chester Reather, Baltimore.)

vessels of the yolk sac (the vitelline circulatory arc) persist as vessels that supply the midgut region.

## Allantois

The allantois arises as an endodermally lined ventral out-pocketing of the hindgut (see Figure 7-1). In the human embryo, it is just a vestige of the large, saclike structure that is used by the embryos of many mammals, birds, and reptiles as a major respiratory organ and repository for urinary wastes. Like the yolk sac, the allantois in the human retains only a secondary function, in this case respiration. However, in the human, this function is served by the blood vessels that differentiate from the mesodermal wall of the allantois. These vessels form the umbilical circulatory arc, consisting of the arteries and veins that supply the placenta (see Figure 6-24). (The postnatal fate of these vessels is discussed in Chapter 18.)

The allantois proper, which consists of little more than a cord of endodermal cells, is embedded in the umbilical cord. Later in development, the proximal part of the allantois (called the urachus) is continuous with the forming urinary bladder (see Figure 16-2). After birth, it becomes transformed into a dense fibrous cord (median umbilical ligament), which runs from the urinary bladder to the umbilical region (see Figure 18-18).

## CHORION AND PLACENTA

Formation of the placental complex represents a cooperative effort between the extraembryonic tissues of the embryo and the endometrial tissues of the mother. (Early stages of implantation of the embryo and the decidual reaction of the uterine lining are described in Chapter 3.) After implantation is complete, the original trophoblast surrounding the embryo has undergone differentiation into two layers: the inner cytotrophoblast and the outer syncytiotrophoblast (see Figure 3-16, D). Lacunae in the rapidly expanding trophoblast have filled with maternal blood, and the connective tissue cells of the endometrium have undergone the decidual reaction (containing increased amounts of glycogen and lipids) in response to the trophoblastic invasion.

### Formation of Chorionic Villi

In the early implanting embryo the trophoblastic tissues have no consistent gross morphological features;

---

### CLINICAL CORRELATION 7-1

#### Conditions Related to Amniotic Fluid

The normal amount of amniotic fluid at term is typically between 500 and 1000 ml. An excessive amount (over 2000 ml) is **hydramnios**. This condition is frequently associated with multiple pregnancies and **esophageal atresia** or **anencephaly** (a congenital anomaly characterized by gross defects of the head and often the inability to swallow [see Figure 8-4]). Such circumstantial evidence supports the important role of fetal swallowing in the overall balance of amniotic fluid exchange. Too little amniotic fluid (less than 500 ml) is **oligohydramnios**. This condition is often associated with bilateral **renal agenesis** (absence of kidneys) and points to the role of fetal urinary excretion in amniotic fluid dynamics. Oligohydramnios can also be a consequence of preterm rupture of the amniotic membrane, which occurs in about 10% of pregnancies.

There are many components, both fetal and maternal, in amniotic fluid; for example, over 200 proteins of both maternal and fetal origin have been detected in amniotic fluid. With the analytical tools available, much can be learned about the condition of the fetus by examining the composition of amniotic fluid. **Amniocentesis** involves removing a small amount of amniotic fluid by inserting a needle through the mother's abdomen and into the amniotic cavity. Because of the small amount of amniotic fluid in early embryos, amniocentesis is usually not performed until the thirteenth or fourteenth week of pregnancy. Amniotic fluid has bacteriostatic properties, which may account for the low incidence of infections after amniocentesis is performed.

Fetal cells present in the fluid can be cultured and examined for various chromosomal and metabolic defects. Recent techniques now permit the examination of chromosomes in the cells immediately obtained instead of having to wait up to 2 to 3 weeks for cultured amniotic cells to proliferate to the point of being suitable for genetic analysis. In addition to the detection of chromosomal defects (e.g., trisomies), it is possible to determine the sex of the fetus by direct chromosomal analysis. A high concentration of $\alpha$-fetoprotein (a protein of the central nervous system) in amniotic fluid is a strong indicator of a neural tube defect. Fetal maturity can be assessed by determining the concentration of creatinine or the **lecithin/sphingomyelin ratio** (which is a reflection of the maturity of the lungs). The severity of **erythroblastosis fetalis** (Rh disease) can also be assessed by examination of amniotic fluid.

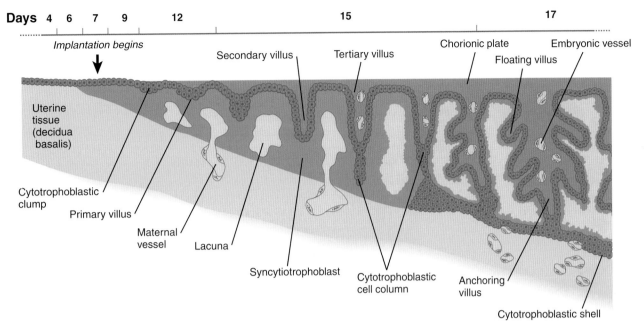

**FIGURE 7-4** Stages in the formation of a chorionic villus, starting with a cytotrophoblastic clump at the far left and progressing over time to an anchoring villus at right.

consequently, this is called the period of the **previllous embryo.** Late in the second week, defined cytotrophoblastic projections called **primary villi** begin to take shape (see Figure 5-2). Shortly thereafter, a mesenchymal core appears within an expanding villus, at which point it is properly called a **secondary villus** (Figure 7-4). Surrounding the mesenchymal core of the secondary villus is a complete layer of cytotrophoblastic cells, and outside of that is the syncytiotrophoblast. By definition, the secondary villus becomes a **tertiary villus** when blood vessels penetrate its mesenchymal core and newly formed branches. This occurs toward the end of the third week of pregnancy. Although individual villi undergo considerable branching, most of them retain the same basic structural plan throughout pregnancy. While the placental villi are becoming established, the homeobox-containing genes, *Msx-2* and *Dlx-4* (*distal-less-4*), are expressed near the interface between the trophoblast and underlying extraembryonic mesenchyme. These transcription factors are often seen at sites of epithelio-mesenchymal interactions.

The terminal portion of a villus remains trophoblastic, consisting of a solid mass of cytotrophoblast called a **cytotrophoblastic cell column** (see Figure 7-4) and a relatively thin covering of syncytiotrophoblast over that. The villus is bathed in maternal blood. A further development of the tip of the villus occurs when, under the influence of the local hypoxic environment, the cytotrophoblastic cell column expands distally, penetrating the syncytiotrophoblastic layer (Figure 7-5). These cytotrophoblastic cells abut directly on maternal decidual cells and spread over them to form a complete cellular layer

known as the **cytotrophoblastic shell,** which surrounds the embryo complex. The villi that give off the cytotrophoblastic extensions are known as **anchoring villi** (see Figure 7-4) because they represent the real attachment points between the embryo complex and the maternal tissues.

It is important to understand the overall relationships of the various embryonic and maternal tissues at this stage of development (see Figure 7-5). The embryo, attached by the **body stalk,** or **umbilical cord,** is effectively suspended in the **chorionic cavity.** The chorionic cavity is bounded by the **chorionic plate,** which consists of extraembryonic mesoderm overlain with trophoblast. The chorionic villi extend outward from the chorionic plate, and their trophoblastic covering is continuous with that of the chorionic plate. The villi and the outer surface of the chorionic plate are bathed in a sea of continually exchanging maternal blood. Because of this, the human placenta is designated as the **hemochorial type.***

Although chorionic villi are structurally very complex, it is convenient to liken the basic structure of a villus complex to the root system of a plant. The anchoring villus is equivalent to the central tap root; by means of the cytotrophoblastic cell columns, it attaches the villus complex to the outer cytotrophoblastic shell. The unattached branches of the **floating villi** (see Figure 7-12)

---

* Other mammals have various arrangements of tissue layers through which materials must pass to be exchanged between mother and fetus. For example, in an epitheliochorial placenta, which is found in pigs, the fetal component of the placenta (chorion) rests on the uterine epithelium instead of being directly bathed in maternal blood.

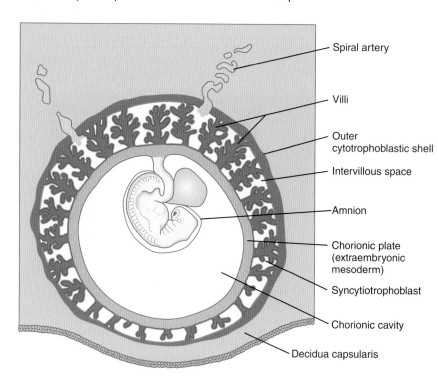

Spiral artery

Villi

Outer
cytotrophoblastic shell

Intervillous space

Amnion

Chorionic plate
(extraembryonic
mesoderm)

Syncytiotrophoblast

Chorionic cavity

Decidua capsularis

**FIGURE 7-5** Overall view of a **5-week-old** embryo plus membranes showing the relationships of the chorionic plate, villi, and outer cytotrophoblastic shell.

dangle freely in the maternal blood that fills the space between the chorionic plate and the outer cytotrophoblastic shell. All surfaces of the villi, chorionic plate, and cytotrophoblastic shell that are in contact with maternal blood are lined with a continuous layer of syncytiotrophoblast.

## Establishing the Uteroplacental Circulation

One of the critical features of the developing embryonic-maternal interface is the establishment of a **uteroplacental circulation** that serves as the medium for bringing food and oxygen to and removing wastes from the embryo. This is accomplished by erosion of the walls of the **spiral arteries** of the uterus and their modification so that, as the embryo grows, they can provide an increasing flow of blood at low pressure to bathe the syncytiotrophoblastic surface of the placenta (see Figure 7-10). Specialized **invasive cytotrophoblastic cells**, migrating out from the anchoring villi, invade the spiral arteries (but not the veins) and cause major modifications of their walls by secreting a specialized extracellular matrix and displacing many of the normal cellular elements of the spiral arteries. As a result, the arteries become wider, but the blood escaping from their open ends leaves at a much lower pressure than normal arterial pressure.

The first maternal fluid that bathes the embryonic trophoblast is not highly cellular, and the oxygen tension is low. During this period, the fetal erythrocytes contain embryonic hemoglobin, which is adapted to bind oxygen under low tension.

Interestingly, hypoxia stimulates cytotrophoblastic cells to undergo mitosis. This may be one of the environmental conditions that underlies the rapid growth of the cytotrophoblast during the early embryonic period. After 12 weeks, when the maternal blood in the placental space contains large numbers of erythrocytes and is more highly oxygenated, the fetal erythrocytes, through an isoform switch, begin to produce fetal hemoglobin, which requires higher oxygen tension to bind oxygen efficiently. The maternal blood that leaves the spiral arteries freely percolates throughout the intervillous spaces and bathes the surfaces of the villi. The maternal blood is then picked up by the open ends of the uterine veins, which also penetrate the cytotrophoblastic shell (see Figure 7-10).

## Gross Relations of Chorionic and Decidual Tissues

Within days after implantation of the embryo, the stromal cells of the endometrium undergo a striking transformation called the **decidual**† **reaction**. After the stromal cells swell as the result of the accumulation of glycogen and lipid in their cytoplasm, they are known as **decidual cells**

---

† The term *deciduum* refers to tissues that are shed at birth. These include the extraembryonic tissues plus the superficial layers of the endometrial connective tissue and epithelium.

(Figure 7-6). The decidual reaction spreads throughout stromal cells in the superficial layers of the endometrium. The maternal decidua are given topographic names based on where they are located in relation to the embryo.

The decidual tissue that overlies the embryo and its chorionic vesicle is the **decidua capsularis,** whereas the decidua that lies between the chorionic vesicle and the uterine wall is the **decidua basalis** (see Figure 7-7). With continued growth of the embryo, the decidua basalis becomes incorporated into the maternal component of the definitive placenta. The remaining decidua, which consists of the decidualized endometrial tissue on the sides of the uterus not occupied by the embryo, is the **decidua parietalis.**

In human embryology the **chorion** is defined as the layer consisting of the trophoblast plus the underlying extraembryonic mesoderm (see Figure 7-1). The chorion forms a complete covering (**chorionic vesicle**) that surrounds the embryo, amnion, yolk sac, and body stalk. During the early period after implantation, primary and secondary villi project almost uniformly from the entire outer surface of the chorionic vesicle. The formation of tertiary villi, however, is asymmetrical, and the invasion of the cytotrophoblastic core of the primary villi by mesenchyme and embryonic blood vessels occurs preferentially in the primary villi located nearest the decidua basalis. As these villi continue to grow and branch, those located on the opposite side (the abembryonic pole) of the chorionic vesicle fail to keep up and eventually atrophy as the growing embryo complex bulges into the uterine cavity (Figure 7-7). The region that contains the flourishing chorionic villi and that ultimately becomes the placenta is the **chorion frondosum.** The remainder of

the chorion, which ultimately becomes smooth, is the **chorion laeve** (Figure 7-8).

The overall growth of the chorionic vesicle (Figure 7-9), with its bulging into the uterine lumen, pushes the decidua capsularis progressively farther from the endometrial blood vessels. By the end of the first trimester, the decidua capsularis itself undergoes pronounced atrophy. Within the next month, portions of the atrophic decidua capsularis begin to disappear, leaving the chorion laeve in direct contact with the decidua parietalis on the opposite side of the uterus (see Figure 7-7). By mid-pregnancy, the decidua capsularis has fused with the tissues of the decidua parietalis, thus effectively obliterating the original uterine cavity.

While the chorion laeve and decidua capsularis are undergoing progressive atrophy, the placenta takes shape in its definitive form and acts as the main site of exchange between the mother and embryo.

## Formation and Structure of the Mature Placenta

As the distinction between the chorion frondosum and chorion laeve becomes more prominent, the limits of the placenta proper can be defined. The placenta consists of a fetal and a maternal component (Figure 7-10). The fetal component is that part of the chorionic vesicle represented by the chorion frondosum. It consists of the wall of the chorion, called the **chorionic plate,** and the chorionic villi that arise from that region. The maternal component is represented by the decidua basalis, but covering the decidua basalis is the fetally derived outer

**FIGURE 7-6 A,** Histological section through the endometrium during the late secretory stage of the endometrial cycle. A large uterine gland with an irregular epithelial border is on the left. On the right, note the stromal cells with compact nuclei and scanty cytoplasm. **B,** Endometrial stroma, showing the decidual reaction. Note the expanded cytoplasm and less compact nuclei of the decidual cells. (Hematoxylin and eosin stain.) (Courtesy D. MacCallum, Ann Arbor, Mich.)

A                    B

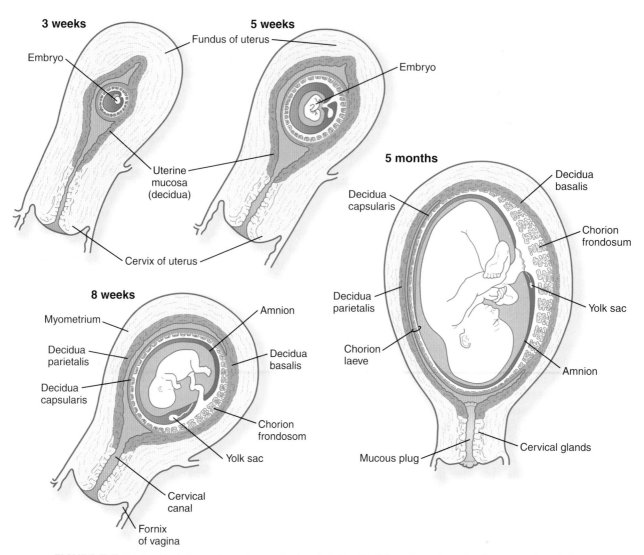

**FIGURE 7-7** Relationships between the embryo and maternal decidua *(pink)* from the early weeks of pregnancy through the fifth month. In the **5-month-old** fetus the placenta is represented by the white tissue to the right of the fetus. (Modified from Carlson BM: *Patten's foundations of embryology,* ed 6, New York, 1996, McGraw-Hill.)

**FIGURE 7-8** Early formation of the chorion laeve. The small bare area in this photograph of a human chorionic vesicle is a region where the chorionic villi have atrophied. This will enlarge in succeeding weeks. (From Gilbert-Barness E, ed: *Potter's pathology of the fetus and infant,* St Louis, 1997, Mosby.)

A                                                    B

**FIGURE 7-9  A,** Intact chorionic vesicle containing an embryo in the **fourth week** of development. The outline of the embryo can be seen through the thinned chorion laeve region. **B,** Opened chorionic vesicle, showing the disposition of the embryo inside. The yolk sac is indicated by the arrow. (From Gilbert-Barness E, ed: *Potter's pathology of the fetus and infant,* St Louis, 1997, Mosby.)

**FIGURE 7-10**  Structure and circulation of the mature human placenta. Blood enters the intervillous spaces from the open ends of the uterine spiral arteries. After bathing the villi, the blood *(blue)* is drained via endometrial veins. (From Bloom W, Fawcett DW: *Textbook of histology,* Philadelphia, 1986, WB Saunders.)

cytotrophoblastic shell. The intervillous space between the fetal and maternal components of the placenta is occupied by freely circulating maternal blood. In keeping with its principal function as an organ-mediating exchange between the fetal and maternal circulatory systems, the overall structure of the placenta is organized to provide a very large surface area (over 10 m²) for that exchange.

## Structure of the Mature Placenta

The mature placenta is disklike in shape, with a thickness of 3 cm and a diameter of about 20 cm (Table 7-1). A typical placenta weighs about 500 gm. The fetal side of the placenta is shiny because of the apposed amniotic membrane. From the fetal side, the attachment of the umbilical cord to the chorionic plate and the large placental branches of the umbilical arteries and vein radiating from it are evident.

The maternal side of the placenta is dull and subdivided into as many as 35 lobes. The grooves between lobes are occupied by placental septa, which arise from the decidua basalis and extend toward the basal plate. Within a placental lobe are several cotyledons, each of which consists of a main stem villus and all its branches. The intervillous space in each lobe represents a nearly isolated compartment of the maternal circulation to the placenta.

## Umbilical Cord

The originally broad-based body stalk elongates and becomes relatively narrower as pregnancy progresses.

The umbilical cord becomes the conduit for the umbilical vessels, which traverse its length between the fetus and the placenta (Figure 7-10). The umbilical vessels are embedded in a mucoid connective tissue that is often called **Wharton's jelly.**

The umbilical cord, which commonly attains a length of 50 to 60 cm by the end of pregnancy, is typically twisted many times. The twisting can be readily observed by gross examination of the umbilical blood vessels. In about 1% of full-term pregnancies, true knots occur in the umbilical cord. If they tighten as the result of fetal movements, they can cause anoxia and even death of the fetus.

Occasionally an umbilical cord contains two umbilical veins if the right umbilical vein does not undergo its normal degeneration (see Figure 17-13). Approximately 0.5% of mature umbilical cords contain only one umbilical artery. This condition is associated with a 15% to 20% incidence of associated cardiovascular defects in the fetus.

## Placental Circulation

Both the fetus and the mother contribute to the placental circulation (see Figure 7-10). The fetal circulation is contained in the system of umbilical and placental vessels. Fetal blood reaches the placenta through the two umbilical arteries, which ramify throughout the chorionic plate. Smaller branches from these arteries enter the chorionic villi and then break up into capillary networks in the terminal branches of the chorionic villi, where the exchange of materials with the maternal blood occurs

## TABLE 7-1 Developing Placenta

| Age of embryo (weeks after fertilization) | Placental diameter (mm) | Placental weight (gm) | Placental thickness (mm) | Length of umbilical cord (mm) | Embryo weight (gm)/ placental weight (gm) | Villous mass (gm) | Total villous surface area (cm²) | Diffusion distance from maternal to fetal circulation (μm) | Mean trophoblastic thickness on villi (μm) |
|---|---|---|---|---|---|---|---|---|---|
| 6 | — | 6 | — | — | 0.18 | 5 | 830 | 55.9 | 15.4 |
| 10 | — | 26 | — | — | 0.65 | 18 | 3020 | — | — |
| 14 | 70 | 65 | 12 | 180 | 0.92 | 28 | 5440 | 40.2 | 9.6 |
| 18 | 95 | 115 | 15 | 300 | 2.17 | 63 | 14,800 | 27.7 | 9.9 |
| 22 | 120 | 185 | 18 | 350 | 3.03 | 102 | 28,100 | 21.6 | 7.4 |
| 26 | 145 | 250 | 20 | 400 | 4.00 | 135 | 42,200 | — | — |
| 30 | 170 | 315 | 22 | 450 | 4.92 | 191 | 72,200 | 20.6 | 6.9 |
| 34 | 195 | 390 | 24 | 490 | 5.90 | 234 | 101,000 | 11.7 | 5.2 |
| 38 | 220 | 470 | 25 | 520 | 7.23 | 273 | 125,000 | 4.8 | 4.1 |

Modified from Kaufmann P, Scheffen I. In Polin R, Fox W, eds: *Fetal and neonatal physiology*, vol 1, Philadelphia, 1992, WB Saunders, p 48.

(see Figure 7-14). From the villous capillary beds, the blood vessels consolidate into successively larger venous branches. These retrace their way through the chorionic plate into the large single umbilical vein and to the fetus.

In contrast to the fetal circulation, which is totally contained within blood vessels, the maternal blood supply to the placenta is a free-flowing lake that is not bounded by vessel walls. As a result of the trophoblast's invasive activities, roughly 80 to 100 spiral arteries of the endometrium open directly into the intervillous spaces and bathe the villi in about 150 ml of maternal blood, which is exchanged 3 to 4 times each minute.

The maternal blood enters the intervillous space under reduced pressure because of the cytotrophoblastic plugs that partially occlude the lumens of the spiral arteries. Nevertheless, the maternal blood pressure is sufficient to force the oxygenated maternal arterial blood to the bases of the villous trees at the chorionic plate (see Figure 7-10). The overall pressure of the maternal placental blood is about 10 mm Hg in the relaxed uterus. From the chorionic plate, the blood percolates over the terminal villi as it returns to venous outflow pathways located in the decidual (maternal) plate of the placenta. An adequate flow of maternal blood to the placenta is vital to the growth and development of the fetus, and a reduced

maternal blood supply to the placenta leads to a small fetus.

In the terminal (floating) villi, the fetal capillaries are located next to the trophoblastic surface to facilitate exchange between the fetal and maternal blood (Figure 7-11). The placental barrier of the mature placenta consists of the syncytiotrophoblast, its basal lamina, the basal lamina of the fetal capillary, and the capillary endothelium. Often the two basal laminae seem to be consolidated. In younger embryos a layer of cytotrophoblast is present in the placental barrier, but by 4 months the cytotrophoblastic layer begins to break up, and by 5 months, it is essentially gone.

### Structure of a Mature Chorionic Villus

Mature chorionic villi constitute a very complex mass of seemingly interwoven branches (Figure 7-12). The core of a villus consists of blood vessels and mesenchyme that is similar in composition to the mesenchyme of the umbilical cord (see Figure 7-11). Scattered among the mesenchymal cells are large **Hofbauer cells,** which function like fetal macrophages.

The villus core is covered by a continuous layer of syncytiotrophoblast, with minimum numbers of

**FIGURE 7-11** Low-power transmission electron micrograph through a typical terminal villus of a human placenta. *C,* Capillary; *Ct,* cytotrophoblast; *S,* sinusoid (dilated capillary); *St,* syncytiotrophoblast. (From Benirschke K, Kaufmann P: *Pathology of the human placenta,* ed 2, New York, 1990, Springer-Verlag.)

FIGURE 7-12 Scanning electron micrograph of long, intermediate, knoblike terminal (floating) villi from a normal placenta near the termination of pregnancy. (From Benirschke K, Kaufmann P: *Pathology of the human placenta,* ed 2, New York, 1990, Springer-Verlag.)

cytotrophoblastic cells beneath it. The surface of the syncytiotrophoblast is covered by immense numbers of microvilli (over 1 billion/cm² at term), which greatly increase the total surface area of the placenta (Figure 7-13). The size and density of the microvilli are not constant but change with increasing age of the placenta and differing environmental conditions. For example, under conditions of poor maternal nutrition or oxygen transport, the microvilli increase in prominence. Poor adaptation of the microvilli to adverse conditions can lead to newborns with low birth weight.

The trophoblastic surface is not homogeneous but rather seems to be arranged into territories. Among the many functional components of the microvillous surface are (1) a wide variety of transport systems for substances ranging from ions to macromolecules, (2) hormone and growth factor receptors, (3) enzymes, and (4) numerous proteins with poorly understood functions. The placental surface is deficient or lacking in major histocompatibility antigens, the absence of which presumably plays a role in protecting against maternal immune rejection of the fetus and fetal membranes. In keeping with its active role in both synthesis and transport, the syncytiotrophoblast is well supplied with a high density and a wide variety of subcellular organelles.

## Placental Physiology

### Placental Transfer

The transport of substances both ways between the placenta and the maternal blood that bathes it is facilitated by the great surface area of the placenta, which expands from 5 m² at 28 weeks to almost 11 m² at term. Approximately 5% to 10% of the human placental surface consists of scattered areas where the barrier between fetal and maternal blood is extremely thin, measuring only a few microns. These areas, sometimes called **epithelial plates,** appear to be morphological adaptations designed to facilitate the diffusion of substances between the fetal and maternal circulations (Figure 7-14).

The transfer of substances occurs both ways across the placenta. The bulk of the substances transferred from mother to fetus consists of oxygen and nutrients.

FIGURE 7-13 Scanning electron micrograph of the surface of the syncytiotrophoblast of a human placenta in the twelfth week of pregnancy. The numerous microvilli increase the absorptive surface of the placenta. (×9000.) (Courtesy S. Bergström, Uppsala, Sweden.)

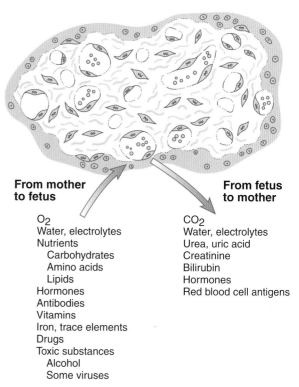

**From mother to fetus**

$O_2$
Water, electrolytes
Nutrients
    Carbohydrates
    Amino acids
    Lipids
Hormones
Antibodies
Vitamins
Iron, trace elements
Drugs
Toxic substances
    Alcohol
    Some viruses

**From fetus to mother**

$CO_2$
Water, electrolytes
Urea, uric acid
Creatinine
Bilirubin
Hormones
Red blood cell antigens

FIGURE 7-14 Exchange of substances across the placenta between the fetal and maternal circulation.

The placenta represents the means for the final elimination of carbon dioxide and other fetal waste materials into the maternal circulation. Under some circumstances, other substances, some of them harmful, can be transferred across the placenta. Clinical Correlation 7-2 describes abnormal placental transfer.

Gases, principally oxygen from the mother and carbon dioxide from the fetus, readily cross the placental barrier by diffusion. The amount of exchange is limited more by blood flow than by the efficiency of diffusion. The placenta is also permeable to carbon monoxide and many inhalational anesthetics. The latter can interfere with the transition of the newborn to independent function (e.g., breathing) if used during childbirth.

Like gases, water and electrolytes are readily transferred across the placenta. The rates of transfer are modified by colloid osmotic pressure in the case of water and the function of ion channels in the case of electrolytes. Fetal wastes (e.g., **urea, creatinine, bilirubin**) are rapidly transferred across the placenta from the fetal circulation to the maternal blood bathing the villi.

The placenta is highly permeable to certain nutrients such as **glucose**; on the other hand, it is considerably less permeable to **fructose** and several common disaccharides.

Amino acids are transported across the placenta through the action of specific receptors. A certain degree of transfer of maternal free **fatty acids** occurs, but more must be learned about the mechanism of transfer. Vitamins, especially water-soluble ones, are transferred from the maternal to the fetal circulation.

**Steroid hormones** cross the placental barrier from the maternal blood. Newborn males show evidence of the effects of exposure to maternal sex hormones. For example, the **prostatic utricle**, the vestigial rudiment of the uterine primordium (fused müllerian ducts [see Chapter 16]), is slightly enlarged in newborn males. Conversely, female fetuses exposed to testosterone or certain synthetic progestins (especially during the 1950s and 1960s before the effects were recognized) undergo masculinization of the external genitalia. Protein hormones are, in general, poorly transported across the placenta, although symptoms of maternal diabetes may be reduced during late pregnancy because of insulin produced by the fetus. Maternal thyroid hormone gains slow access to the fetus.

Some proteins are transferred very slowly through the placenta, mainly by means of pinocytosis (uptake by membrane-bound vesicles in the cells). Of considerable

## CLINICAL CORRELATION 7-2
### Abnormal Placental Transfer

Unfortunately, the placenta is permeable to substances that can be damaging to the embryo. Numerous maternally ingested drugs readily cross the placental barrier. Certain drugs can cause major birth defects if they reach the embryo during critical periods of morphogenesis. (Several classic examples of these are described in Chapter 8.) The placenta is highly permeable to alcohol, and excessive alcohol ingestion by the mother can produce **fetal alcohol syndrome** (see p. 162). The tragedy of newborns who are born addicted to heroin or crack cocaine is all too common in contemporary society.

In addition to drugs, certain infectious agents can penetrate the placental barrier and infect the fetus. Some (e.g., rubella virus) can cause birth defects if they infect the embryo at critical periods in development. Normally, bacteria cannot penetrate the placental barrier. Common viruses that can infect the fetus are rubella virus, cytomegalovirus, poliovirus, varicella virus, variola virus, human immunodeficiency virus, and coxsackieviruses. The spirochete *Treponema pallidum*, which causes syphilis, can cause devastating fetal infections. The protozoan parasite *Toxoplasma gondii* can cross the placental barrier and cause birth defects.

### CELLULAR TRANSFER AND Rh INCOMPATIBILITY

Small quantities of fetal blood cells often escape into the maternal circulation, either through small defects in the placental vasculature or through hemorrhage at birth. If the fetal erythrocytes are positive for the Rh antigen and the mother is Rh negative, the presence of fetal erythrocytes in the maternal circulation can stimulate the formation of anti-Rh antibody by the immune system of the mother. The fetus in the first pregnancy is usually spared the effects of the maternal antibody (often because it has not formed in sufficient quantities), but in subsequent pregnancies, Rh-positive fetuses are attacked by the maternal anti-Rh antibodies, which make their way into the fetal bloodstream. This antibody causes hemolysis of the Rh-positive fetal erythrocytes, and the fetus develops **erythroblastosis fetalis**, sometimes known as **hemolytic disease**. In severe cases the bilirubin released from the lysed red blood cells causes jaundice and brain damage in addition to anemia. When recognized, this condition is treated by exchange transfusions of Rh-negative donor blood into either the fetus or the newborn. An indication of the severity of this condition can be gained by examining the amniotic fluid.

importance is the transfer of maternal antibodies, mainly of the immunoglobulin G class. Because of its immature immune system, the fetus produces only small amounts of antibodies. The transfer of antibodies from the mother provides a passive immunity of the newborn to certain common childhood diseases such as smallpox, diphtheria, and measles until the infant's immune system begins to function more efficiently.

Another maternal protein, **transferrin**, is important because, as its name implies, it carries iron to the fetus. The placental surface contains specific receptors for this protein. It appears that the iron is dissociated from its transferrin carrier at the placental surface and then is actively transported into the fetal tissues.

## Placental Hormone Synthesis and Secretion

The placenta, specifically the syncytiotrophoblast, is an important endocrine organ during much of pregnancy. It produces both protein and steroid hormones.

The first protein hormone produced is **human chorionic gonadotropin (HCG)**, which is responsible for maintaining the corpus luteum and its production of progesterone and estrogens. With synthesis beginning even before implantation, the presence of this hormone in maternal urine is the basis for many of the common tests for pregnancy. The production of HCG peaks at approximately the eighth week of gestation and then gradually declines. By the end of the first trimester, the placenta produces enough progesterone and estrogens so that pregnancy can be maintained even if the corpus luteum is surgically removed. The placenta can independently synthesize progesterone from acetate or cholesterol precursors, but it does not contain the complete enzymatic apparatus for the synthesis of estrogens. For estrogen to be synthesized, the placenta must operate in concert with the fetal adrenal gland and possibly the liver; these structures possess the enzymes that the placenta lacks.

Another placental protein hormone is **chorionic somatomammotropin**, sometimes called **human placental lactogen**. Similar in structure to human growth hormone, it influences growth, lactation, and lipid and carbohydrate metabolism. The placenta also produces small amounts of **chorionic thyrotropin** and **chorionic corticotropin**. When they are secreted into the maternal bloodstream, some placental hormones stimulate changes in the metabolism and cardiovascular function of the mother. These changes ensure that appropriate types and amounts of fundamental nutrients and substrates reach the placenta for transport to the fetus.

A good example of a placental hormone that influences the mother is **human placental growth hormone**. This hormone, which differs by 13 amino acids from pituitary growth hormone, is produced by the syncytiotrophoblast. Placental growth hormone is not detectable in fetal serum, although it appears to influence growth of the placenta in a paracrine manner. This fetal hormone exerts a profound effect on the mother. During the first 15 to 20 weeks of pregnancy, maternal pituitary growth hormone is the main form present in the maternal circulation, but from 15 weeks to term, placental growth hormone gradually replaces maternal pituitary growth hormone to the extent that the maternally derived hormone becomes undetectable in the mother's serum. A major function of this hormone appears to be the regulation of maternal blood glucose levels so that the fetus is ensured of an adequate nutrient supply. Placental growth hormone secretion is stimulated by low maternal glucose levels. The increased hormone levels then stimulate gluconeogenesis in the maternal liver and other organs, thus increasing the supply of glucose available for fetal use.

In certain respects, the placenta duplicates the multilevel control system that regulates hormone production in the postnatal body. Cells of the cytotrophoblast produce a homologue of gonadotropin-releasing hormone (GnRH), as is normally done by the hypothalamus. GnRH then passes into the syncytiotrophoblast, where it, along with certain opiate peptides and their receptors (which have been identified in the syncytiotrophoblast), stimulates the release of HCG from the syncytiotrophoblast. The opiate peptides and their receptors are also involved in the release of chorionic somatomammotropin from the syncytiotrophoblast. Finally, HCG appears to be involved in regulating the synthesis and release of placental steroids from the syncytiotrophoblast.

In addition to hormones, the placenta produces a wide variety of other proteins that have principally been identified immunologically. The functions of the dozens of placental proteins that have been discovered are still very poorly understood.

## Placental Immunology

One of the major mysteries of pregnancy is why the fetus and placenta, which are immunologically distinct from the mother, are not recognized as foreign tissue and rejected by the mother's immune system. (Immune rejection of foreign tissues normally occurs by the activation of cytotoxic lymphocytes, but humoral immune responses are also possible.) Despite considerable research, the answer to this question is still unknown. Several broad explanations have been suggested to account for the unusual tolerance of the mother to the prolonged presence of the immunologically foreign embryo during pregnancy.

The first possibility is that the fetal tissues, especially those of the placenta, which constitute the direct interface between fetus and mother, do not present foreign antigens to the mother's immune system. To some extent this hypothesis is true, since neither the syncytiotrophoblast nor the nonvillous cytotrophoblast (**cytotrophoblastic shell**) expresses the two major classes of major histocompatibility antigens that trigger the immune response of the host in the rejection of typical foreign tissue grafts (e.g., a kidney transplant). However, these antigens are present on cells of the fetus and in stromal tissues of the placenta. The expression of minor histocompatibility antigens (e.g., the HY antigen in male fetuses [see Chapter 16]) follows a similar pattern. Nevertheless, other minor antigens are expressed on trophoblastic tissues. In addition, because of breaks in the placental barrier, fetal red and white blood cells are frequently found circulating in the maternal blood. These cells should be capable of sensitizing the mother's immune system.

A second major possibility is that the mother's immune system is somehow paralyzed during pregnancy so that it does not react to the fetal antigens to which it is exposed. Yet the mother is capable of mounting an immune response to infections or foreign tissue grafts. There still remains the possibility of a selective repression of the immune response to fetal antigens, although the Rh incompatibility response shows that this is not universally the case.

A third possibility is that local decidual barriers prevent either immune recognition of the fetus by the mother or the reaching of competent immune cells from the mother to the fetus. Again, there is evidence for a functioning decidual immune barrier, but in a significant number of cases that barrier is known to be breached through trauma or disease.

A fourth possibility is that molecules formed on the fetal placental surface are able to locally inactivate the T cells or other immune cells that could reject the embryo or that they paralyze the local cellular immune response. In mice, for example, inactivation of a complement regulator results in immune rejection of the fetus. It is currently not known if a similar system operates during human pregnancy.

Currently, studies are being directed toward conditions such as recurrent spontaneous abortion with the hope of finding further clues to the complex immunological interrelationships between the fetus and mother. What is abundantly clear is that this is not a simple relationship. Nevertheless, the solution to this problem may yield information that might be applied to the problem of reducing the host rejection of tissue and organ transplants.

## PLACENTA AFTER BIRTH

About 30 minutes after birth, the placenta, embryonic membranes, and remainder of the umbilical cord, along with much of the maternal decidua, are expelled from the uterus as the **afterbirth**. The fetal surface of the placenta is smooth, shiny, and grayish because of the amnion that covers the fetal side of the chorionic plate. The maternal surface, on the other hand, is a dull red and may be punctuated with blood clots. The maternal surface of the placenta must be examined carefully because if a cotyledon is missing and is retained in the uterine wall, it could cause serious postpartum bleeding. Recognition of certain types of placental pathology can provide valuable clues to intrauterine factors that could affect the well-being of the newborn (see Clinical Correlation 7-3).

## PLACENTA AND MEMBRANES IN MULTIPLE PREGNANCIES

Several different configurations of the placenta and extraembryonic membranes are possible in multiple pregnancies. Dizygotic twins or monozygotic twins resulting from complete separation of blastomeres very early in cleavage can have completely separate placentas and membranes if the two embryos implant in distant sites on the uterine wall (Figure 7-15, A). In contrast, if the implantation sites are closer together, the placentas and chorions (which were initially separate at implantation) can fuse, although the vascular systems of the two embryos remain separate (Figure 7-15, B).

When monozygotic twins form by splitting of the inner cell mass in the blastocyst, it is usual to have a common placenta and a common chorion, but inside the chorion the twin embryos each develop within separate amnions (Figure 7-15, C). In this case, there can be separate or fused vascular systems within the common placenta. When the vascular systems are fused, one twin may receive a greater proportion of the placental blood flow than the other. This may result in mild to severe stunting of growth of the embryo that receives the lesser amount of blood from the placenta. The twin from which the blood is siphoned is often highly misshapen and is commonly called an **acardiac monster** (Figure 7-16).

In conjoined twins and rarely in dizygotic twins with minimal separation of the inner cell mass, the embryos develop within a single amnion and chorion and have a common placenta with a common blood supply (Figure 7-15, D and E). This and the previously described conditions can be readily determined by examination of the membranes of the afterbirth. At one time it was thought that it could be determined whether twins were monozygotic or dizygotic by simple examination of the membranes. Although in most cases the correct inference can be made, this method is by no means foolproof. Other methods ranging from simple observation of gender, eye color, and fingerprint patterns to determination of blood

**FIGURE 7-15** Extraembryonic membranes in multiple pregnancies. **A,** Completely separate membranes in dizygotic or completely separated monozygotic twins. **B,** Common fused placenta, separate amnions, and partially fused chorions. **C,** Common placenta with separate or common fused vessels and separate amnions enclosed in a common chorion. **D** and **E,** Common placenta and amniotic cavity in separate or conjoined twins.

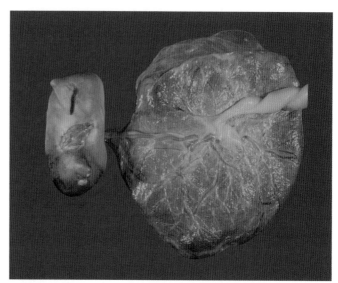

**FIGURE 7-16** Fused-twin placenta with an umbilical cord coming from its center and connecting to an anatomically normal fetus *(right)*. A shapeless acardiac monster *(left)*. This condition is related to the siphoning of blood through a common circulation from the acardiac embryo to the other member of the pair. (Photograph #7702 from the Arey-Depeña Pediatric Pathology Photographic Collection, Human Development Anatony Center, National Museum of Health and Medicine, Armed Forces Institute of Pathology.)

## CLINICAL VIGNETTE

A 32-year-old woman's obstetrician notes that her weight gain during late pregnancy is excessive. At least part of her weight gain appears to be the result of a greater-than-normal volume of amniotic fluid. She lives in a remote rural area far from an imaging center. Amniocentesis is performed, and the laboratory report indicates the presence of a high level of $\alpha$-fetoprotein in the amniotic fluid. The obstetrician is concerned that this pregnancy will not result in a normal single birth.

What condition does the doctor suspect and why?
A. Esophageal atresia
B. Renal agenesis
C. Triplets
D. Anencephaly
E. Placenta previa

types or even DNA fingerprinting should be used for a definitive determination. In the current age of organ and cell transplantation, it can be vital to know whether twins are monozygotic in the event that one develops a condition that can be treated by a transplant.

## SUMMARY

◯ The extraembryonic membranes consist of the chorion (the combination of trophoblast plus underlying extraembryonic mesoderm), amnion, yolk sac, and allantois.

◯ The amnion, a thin ectodermal membrane lined with mesoderm, grows to enclose the embryo like a balloon. It is filled with a clear fluid, which is generated from many sources such as the fetal skin, the amnion itself, the fetal kidneys, and possibly the fetal vessels. At term the volume of amniotic fluid approaches 1 L. Amniotic fluid is removed by exchange across the amniotic membrane and by fetal swallowing.

Placental pathological conditions cover a wide spectrum, ranging from the abnormalities of implantation site to neoplasia to frank bacterial infections. Much can be learned about the past history and future prospects of a newborn by examining the placenta. This box deals only with those aspects of placental pathology that are relevant to developmental mechanisms.

## ABNORMAL IMPLANTATION SITES

An abnormal implantation site within the uterine cavity is known as **placenta previa**. (Ectopic pregnancy is covered in Chapter 3.) When part of the placenta covers the cervical outlet of the uterine cavity, its presence is a mechanical obstacle in the birth canal. In addition,

**FIGURE 7-17** Variations in placental shape. **A,** Marginal insertion of the umbilical cord. **B,** Velamentous insertion of the umbilical cord. (From Naeye RL: *Disorders of the placenta, fetus, and neonate,* St Louis, 1992, Mosby.)

*Continued*

## Placental Pathological Conditions (Continued)

hemorrhage, which can be fatal to the fetus or even the mother, is a common consequence of placenta previa as a result of the premature separation of part of the placenta from the uterus.

### GROSS PLACENTAL ANOMALIES

Many variations in shape of the placenta have been described, but few appear to be of any functional significance. One involves marginal rather than central attachment of the umbilical cord (Figure 7-17, *A*). If the umbilical cord attaches to the smooth membranes outside the boundaries of the placenta itself, the condition is known as a **velamentous insertion** of the umbilical cord (Figure 7-17, *B*).

The placenta itself can be subdivided into **accessory lobes** (Figure 7-17, *C*). It can also be completely divided into two parts, with smooth membrane between (Figure 7-17, *D*).

### HYDATIDIFORM MOLE

A **hydatidiform mole** is a noninvasive condition in which many of the chorionic villi are characterized by nodular

**FIGURE 7-17, CONT. C,** Placenta with accessory (succenturiate) lobes. **D,** Completely bilobed placenta.

swellings, giving them an appearance almost like bunches of grapes. Commonly, much of the villous surface of the placenta takes on this appearance; in addition, the embryo is either absent or not viable (Figure 7-18). The villi show no evidence of vascularization.

Genetic analysis has determined that hydatidiform moles represent the results of paternal imprinting where the female pronucleus of the egg does not participate in development (see Chapter 3). Instead, the chromosomal material is derived from two sperm that had penetrated the egg or by duplication of a single sperm pronucleus within the egg. The chromosomes of hydatidiform moles are paternally derived 46,XX, since the number of lethal genes in 46,YY embryos is not compatible with tissue survival.

## CHORIOCARCINOMA

**Choriocarcinomas** are malignant tumors derived from embryonic cytotrophoblast and syncytiotrophoblast.

These tumors are highly invasive into the maternal decidual tissues and blood vessels. Like hydatidiform moles, most choriocarcinomas contain only paternally derived chromosomes and are thus products of paternal imprinting.

## BIOPSIES OF CHORIONIC VILLI

In recent years, biopsies of chorionic villi during the latter half of the second embryonic month have sometimes been performed instead of sampling of amniotic fluid. Performed with the assistance of ultrasonography, chorionic villus biopsies are obtained for the analysis of possible chromosomal disorders or the diagnosis of certain metabolic disorders.

**FIGURE 7-18 A,** Distended uterus containing a hydatidiform mole. The ovaries *(top* and *bottom)* contain bilateral theca lutein cysts. **B,** View at greater magnification showing swollen villi. (**A** from Benirschke K, Kaufmann P: *Pathology of the human placenta,* ed 2, New York, 1990, Springer-Verlag. **B** courtesy K. Benirschke, San Diego.)

○ The yolk sac is a ventral endodermally lined structure that does not serve a nutritive function in mammalian embryos. Mesodermal blood islands in the wall of the yolk sac form the first blood cells and vessels. Primordial germ cells are recognizable in the wall of the yolk sac, but they originate in extraembryonic mesoderm at the base of the allantois.

○ The allantois is a small, endodermally lined diverticulum off the ventral side of the hindgut. It does not serve a direct function of respiration or storage of wastes in humans. These functions are carried out through the placenta and the umbilical vessels that arise in conjunction with the allantois.

Chorionic villi form as outward projections from the trophoblast. Primary villi consist of projections of trophoblast alone. When a mesenchymal core forms within a villus, it is a secondary villus, and when the mesenchyme becomes vascularized, the villus is a tertiary villus. As villi mature, the cytotrophoblast in some villi grows through the syncytiotrophoblast as cytotrophoblastic cell columns and makes contact with the maternal endometrial tissue. Cytotrophoblast continues to grow around the blood-filled space surrounding the chorion to form a cytotrophoblastic shell, which is the direct interface between the fetal and maternal tissues. Villi that make direct contact with maternal tissues are anchoring villi; villi that do not make such contact are floating villi. Because chorionic villi float in a pool of maternal blood, the human placenta is designated as a hemochorial placenta.

Stimulated by the implanting embryo, endometrial stromal cells undergo the decidual reaction. Maternal tissues that are lost at childbirth are, collectively, the decidua. The decidua basalis underlies the placenta; the decidua capsularis encircles the remainder of the chorion like a capsule; portions of the uterine wall not occupied by the fetal chorion are the decidua parietalis. As the fetal chorion matures, it becomes subdivided into a chorion laeve, in which the villi regress, and the chorion frondosum, which is the region of chorion nearest the basal tissues of the endometrium. The chorion frondosum ultimately develops into the placenta.

The mature placenta consists of the wall of the chorion (the chorionic plate) and numerous villi protruding from it. The fetal surface of the placenta is smooth and shiny because of the apposed amniotic membrane. The maternal surface is dull and lobulated, with cotyledons of numerous placental villi and their branches. The umbilical cord (formerly the body stalk) enters the middle of the placenta. Blood from the fetus reaches the placenta via the umbilical arteries. These branch out into numerous small vessels, terminating into capillary loops in the ends of the placental villi. There, oxygen, nutrients, and wastes are exchanged between fetal and maternal blood, which bathes the villi. Fetal blood returns to the body of the mature fetus via a single umbilical vein. Maternal blood exiting open-ended spiral arteries of the endometrium bathes the placental villi.

The transfer of substances from fetal to maternal blood must occur across the endothelium of the fetal capillaries, a basal lamina, and trophoblastic tissues before reaching the maternal blood. The transfer of substances is accomplished by both passive and active mechanisms. In addition to normal substances, alcohol, certain drugs, and some infectious agents can pass from the maternal blood into the fetal circulation and interfere with normal development. If a fetus is Rh positive and the mother is Rh negative, maternal anti-Rh antibodies from a previous pregnancy can pass to the fetus to cause erythroblastosis fetalis.

The placenta produces a wide variety of hormones, many of which are normally synthesized in the hypothalamus and anterior pituitary gland. The first hormone released is HCG, which serves as the basis of many pregnancy tests. Other placental hormones are chorionic somatomammotropin (human placental lactogen), steroid hormones, human placental growth hormone, and chorionic thyrotropin and corticotropin.

The fetal and placental tissues are immunologically different from those of the mother, but the placenta and fetus are not immunologically rejected. The reason is still not clear, but some explanations involve reduced antigenicity of the trophoblastic tissues, paralysis of the mother's immune system during pregnancy, and local immunological barriers between the fetus and mother.

The placenta is delivered about 30 minutes after the fetus as the afterbirth. Inspection of the placenta can reveal placental pathological conditions, missing cotyledons, or the arrangement of membranes in multiple pregnancies. The last finding can help to determine whether a multiple birth is monozygotic in origin. Placental pathological findings include abnormal gross shape, benign hydatidiform moles, and malignant choriocarcinomas.

## Review Questions

1. **In the mature placenta, which fetal tissue directly interfaces with the maternal uterine connective tissue?**
   A. Cytotrophoblast
   B. Syncytiotrophoblast
   C. Extraembryonic mesoderm
   D. Decidual cells
   E. None of the above

2. **Which condition is related to paternal imprinting?**
   A. Accessory placental lobes
   B. Placenta previa
   C. Oligohydramnios
   D. Single umbilical artery
   E. Hydatidiform mole

3. **Blood vessels associated with which structure enter the fetal component of the placenta?**
   A. Decidua basalis
   B. Allantois
   C. Amnion
   D. Yolk sac
   E. Decidua parietalis

4. What type of cells invades the maternal spiral arteries and reduces the flow of blood from their open ends?
   A. Hofbauer cells
   B. Syncytiotrophoblast
   C. Fetal erythrocytes
   D. Cytotrophoblast
   E. Amniotic epithelium

5. Which condition of the extraembryonic membranes can be found in uteri containing identical twins?
   A. Common placenta and amniotic membrane
   B. Common placenta and chorion, separate amnions
   C. Separate placentas and extraembryonic membranes
   D. Common placenta, partially fused chorions
   E. All of the above

6. A 28-year-old Rh-negative woman's second son is born severely jaundiced. What statement most likely characterizes her first child?
   A. Male
   B. Female
   C. Rh positive
   D. Rh negative
   E. Hydramnios

7. Why is the human placenta designated a hemochorial type of placenta?

8. Through what layers of a placental villus must a molecule of oxygen pass to go from the maternal blood into the embryonic circulation?

9. What embryonic hormone has served as the basis for many standard pregnancy tests and why?

10. Why must a pregnant woman be very careful of what she eats and drinks?

## REFERENCES

Alsat E and others: Physiological role of human placental growth hormone, *Mol Cell Endocrinol* 140:121–127, 1998.

Alsat E and others: Le cytotrophoblaste humain, un casse-tête pour le biologiste, *Med Sci* 15:1236–1243, 1999.

Aplin JD: Implantation, trophoblast differentiation and haemochorial placentation: mechanistic evidence in vivo and in vitro, *J Cell Sci* 99:681–692, 1991.

Benirschke K, Kaufmann P: *Pathology of the human placenta*, ed 4, New York, 2000, Springer-Verlag.

Blankenship TN, Enders AC: Trophoblast cell-mediated modifications to uterine spiral arteries during early gestation in the macaque, *Acta Anat* 158:227–236, 1997.

Bohn H, Dati F, Lueben G: Human trophoblast specific products other than hormones. In Loke YW, Whyte A, eds: *Biology of trophoblast*, Amsterdam, 1983, Elsevier Science, pp 317–352.

Boyd JD, Hamilton WJ: *The human placenta*, Cambridge, England, 1970, Heffer & Sons.

Chamberlain GVP, Wilkinson AW, eds: *Placental transfer*, Tunbridge Wells, Kent, England, 1979, Pitman Medical.

Cullen TS: *Embryology, anatomy and diseases of the umbilicus, together with diseases of the urachus*, Philadelphia, 1916, WB Saunders.

Dallaire L, Potier M: Amniotic fluid. In Milunsky A, ed: *Genetic disorders and the fetus*, New York, 1986, Plenum, pp 53–97.

Dearden L, Ockleford CD: Structure of human trophoblast: correlation with function. In Loke YW, Whyte A, eds: *Biology of trophoblast*, Amsterdam, 1983, Elsevier Science, pp 69–110.

Demir R and others: Classification of human placental stem villi: review of structural and functional aspects, *Micros Res Techn* 38:29–41, 1997.

Enders AC: Trophoblast differentiation during the transition from trophoblastic plate to lacunar stage of implantation in the rhesus monkey and human, *Am J Anat* 186:85–98, 1989.

Faber JJ, Thornburg KL, eds: *Placental physiology*, New York, 1983, Raven.

Foidart J-M and others: The human placenta becomes haemochorial at the 13th week of pregnancy, *Int J Dev Biol* 36:451–453, 1992.

Garnica AD, Chan W-Y: The role of the placenta in fetal nutrition and growth, *J Am Coll Nutr* 15:206–222, 1996.

Genbacev O and others: Regulation of human placental development by oxygen tension, *Science* 277:1669–1672, 1997.

Johnson PM, Christmas SE, Vince GS: Immunological aspects of implantation and implantation failure, *Human Reprod* 14(supple 2):26–36, 1999.

Kaufmann P: Basic morphology of the fetal and maternal circuits in the human placenta, *Contrib Gynecol Obstet* 13:5–17, 1985.

Kaufmann P, Burton G: Anatomy and genesis of the placenta. In Knobil E, Neill JD, eds: *The physiology of reproduction*, ed 2, New York, 1994, Raven, pp 441–484.

Kliman HJ: Uteroplacental blood flow, *Am J Path* 157:1759–1768, 2000.

Knipp GT, Audus KL, Soares MJ: Nutrient transport across the placenta, *Adv Drug Deliv Revs* 38:41–58, 1999

Knoll BJ: Gene expression in the human placental trophoblast: a model for developmental gene regulation, *Placenta* 13:311–327, 1992.

Lavrey JP, ed: *The human placenta: clinical perspectives*, Rockville, Md, 1987, Aspen.

Loke YW, King A: *Human implantation*, Cambridge, England, 1995, Cambridge University Press.

Morriss FJ, Boyd RDH, Mahendran D: Placental transport. In Knobil E, Neill JD, eds: *The physiology of reproduction*, ed 2, New York, 1994, Raven, pp 813–861.

Naeye RL: *Disorders of the placenta, fetus, and neonate*, St Louis, 1992, Mosby.

Quinn LM, Latham SE, Kalionis B: The homeobox genes Msx2 and Mox2 are candidates for regulating epithelial-mesenchymal cell interactions in the human placenta, *Placenta* 21(suppl A 14):S50–S54, 2000.

Ramsey EM: *The placenta: human and animal*, New York, 1982, Praeger.

Schneider H: Placental transport function, *Reprod Fertil Dev* 3:345–353, 1991.

Schneider H: The role of the placenta in nutrition of the human fetus, *Am J Obstet Gynecol* 164:967–973, 1991.

Schroeder J: Review article: transplacental passage of blood cells, *J Med Genet* 12:230–242, 1975.

Sibley CP, Boyd RDH: Mechanisms of transfer across the human placenta. In Polin R, Fox W, eds: *Fetal and neonatal physiology*, vol 1, Philadelphia, 1992, WB Saunders, pp 62–74.

Truman P, Ford HC: The brush border of the human term placenta, *Biochem Biophys Acta* 779:139–160, 1984.

Xu C and others: A critical role for murine complement regulatory Crry in fetomaternal tolerance, *Science* 287:298–501, 2000.

# CHAPTER 8

# Developmental Disorders: Causes, Mechanisms, and Patterns

Congenital malformations have attracted attention since the dawn of human history. When seen in either humans or animals, malformations were often interpreted as omens of good or evil. Because of the great significance attached to congenital malformations, they were frequently represented in folk art, either as sculptures or paintings. As far back as the classical Greek period, people speculated that maternal impressions during pregnancy (e.g., being frightened by an animal) caused development to go awry. In other cultures, women who gave birth to malformed infants were assumed to have had dealings with the devil or other evil spirits.

Earlier representations of some malformed infants are remarkable in their anatomical accuracy, and it is often possible to diagnose specific conditions or syndromes from the ancient art (Figure 8-1, A). By the Middle Ages, however, representations of malformations were much more imaginative, with hybrids of humans and other animals often represented (Figure 8-1, B).

Among the first applications of scientific thought to the problem of congenital malformations were those of the sixteenth-century French surgeon Ambrose Paré, who suggested a role for hereditary factors and mechanical influences such as intrauterine compression in the genesis of birth defects. Less than a century later, William Harvey, who is also credited with first describing the circulation of blood, elaborated the concept of developmental arrest and further refined thinking on mechanical causes of birth defects.

In the early nineteenth century, Etienne Geoffroy de St. Hilaire coined the term **teratology**, which literally means "the study of monsters," as a descriptor for the newly emerging study of congenital malformations. Late in the nineteenth century, scientific study of teratology was put on a firm foundation with the publication of several encyclopedic treatises that exhaustively covered anatomical aspects of recognized congenital malformations.

After the flowering of experimental embryology and genetics in the early twentieth century, laboratory researchers began to produce specific recognizable congenital anomalies by means of defined experimental genetic or laboratory manipulations on laboratory animals. This led to the demystification of congenital anomalies and to a search for rational scientific explanations for birth defects. Nevertheless, old beliefs are very tenacious, and even today patients may adhere to traditional beliefs.

The first of two major milestones in human teratology occurred in 1941, when Gregg in Australia recognized that the **rubella** virus was a cause of a recognizable **syndrome** of abnormal development, consisting of defects in the eyes, ears, and heart. About 20 years later, the tragic story of **thalidomide** sensitized the medical community to the potential danger of certain drugs and other environmental **teratogens** (agents that produce birth defects) to the developing embryo.

Thalidomide is a very effective sedative that was widely used in West Germany, Australia, and other

**FIGURE 8-1 A,** Chalk carving from New Ireland in the South Pacific showing dicephalic, dibrachic conjoined twins *(left).* Note also the "collar" beneath the heads, which is a representation of the malformation cystic hygroma colli *(right).* **B,** The bird-boy of Paré (about 1520) *(left).* Stillborn fetus with sirenomelia (fused legs) *(right).* Compare with the lower part of the bird-boy. (**A** *[left]* from Brodsky I: *Med J Aust* 1:417–420, 1943. **A** *[right]* and **B** *[right]* courtesy M. Barr, Ann Arbor, Mich.)

countries during the late 1950s. Soon, physicians began to see infants born with extremely rare birth defects. One example is **phocomelia** (which means "seal limb"), a condition in which the hands and feet seem to arise almost directly from the shoulder and hip (Figure 8-2). Another is **amelia**, in which a limb is entirely missing. Only after some careful epidemiological detective work, involving the collection of individual case reports and sorting of the drugs taken by mothers during the early period of their pregnancies, was it possible to identify thalidomide as the certain cause. Thalidomide is still a drug of choice in the treatment of leprosy, and it is currently used in South America, where infants with thalidomide embryopathy continue to be born. With the intense investigations that followed the thalidomide disaster, modern teratology came of age. It is remarkable, however, that despite much

effort, the causes for most congenital malformations are still unknown.

## GENERAL PRINCIPLES

According to most studies, approximately 2% to 3% of all living newborns show at least one recognizable congenital malformation. This percentage is doubled when one considers anomalies diagnosed in children during the first few years after birth. With the decline in infant mortality caused by infectious diseases and nutritional problems, congenital malformations now rank high among the causes of infant mortality (currently over 20%), and an ever-increasing percentage (up to 30%) of infants admitted to neonatology or pediatric units

**FIGURE 8-2** Phocomelia in all four limbs. This fetus had not been exposed to thalidomide. (Courtesy M. Barr, Ann Arbor, Mich.)

come as a result of various forms of genetic diseases or congenital defects.

Congenital defects range from enzyme deficiencies caused by single nucleotide substitutions in the DNA molecule to very complex associations of gross anatomical abnormalities. Although medical embryology textbooks traditionally cover principally structural defects—congenital malformations—there is a continuum between purely biochemical abnormalities and those that are manifested as abnormal structures. This continuum includes defects that constitute abnormal structure, function, metabolism, and behavior.

The genesis of congenital defects can be viewed as an interaction between the genetic endowment of the embryo and the environment in which it develops. The basic information is encoded in the genes, but as the genetic instructions unfold, the developing structures or organs are subjected to microenvironmental or macroenvironmental influences that either are compatible with or interfere with normal development. In the case of genetically based malformations or anomalies based on chromosomal aberrations, the defect is intrinsic and commonly expressed even in a normal environment. Purely environmental causes interfere with embryological processes in the face of a normal genotype. However, in other cases, environment and genetics interact. Penetrance (the degree of manifestation) of an abnormal gene

or expression of one component of a genetically multifactorial cascade can sometimes be profoundly affected by environmental conditions.

One of the first clear-cut examples of the interactions between genetics and environment was provided in the 1950s by the experiments of Fraser on cleft palate formation in mice. In the presence of cortisone (the teratogen), 100% of the embryos of the A/J strain of mice developed cleft palate, whereas only about 20% of offspring of the C57BL strain were born with the anomaly. With crosses of the two strains, the incidence of cleft palate was approximately 40%. These results were ultimately shown to be related to strain-specific differences in the growth rate of the palatal shelves and to the width of the head at specific days of embryogenesis.

Several factors are associated with various types of congenital malformations. At present, they are understood more at the level of statistical associations than as points of interference with specific developmental controls, but they are important clues to why development can go wrong. Among the factors associated with increased incidences of congenital malformations are (1) parental age, (2) season of the year, (3) country of residence, (4) race, and (5) familial tendencies.

Well-known correlations exist between parental age and the incidence of certain malformations, a classic one being the increased incidence of **Down syndrome** (see Figure 8-9) in children born to women over 35 years of age. Other conditions are related to paternal age (Figure 8-3).

Some types of anomalies have a higher incidence among infants born at certain seasons of the year. For example, **anencephaly** (Figure 8-4) occurs more frequently in January. Recognizing that the primary factors leading to anencephaly occur during the first month of embryonic life, researchers must seek the potential environmental causes that are more prevalent in April. Anencephaly has been shown to be highly correlated with maternal **folic acid deficiency**. Its high incidence in pregnancies beginning in the early spring may relate to nutritional deficiencies of mothers during the late winter months. Folic acid supplementation in the diet of women of child-bearing age significantly reduces the incidence of neural tube defects, such as anencephaly.

The relationship between the country of residence and an increased incidence of specific malformations can be related to various factors, including racial tendencies, local environmental factors, and even governmental policies. A classic example of the last is the incidence of severely malformed infants as a result of exposure to thalidomide. These cases were concentrated in West Germany and Australia because the drug was commonly sold in these locations. Because thalidomide was not approved by the Food and Drug Administration (FDA), the United States was spared from this epidemic of birth defects. Another classic example of the influence of

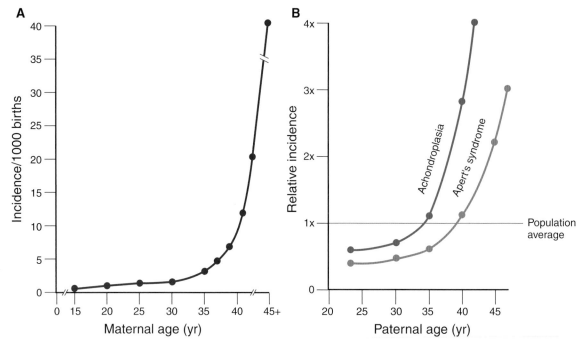

**FIGURE 8-3** The increased incidence of (**A**) Down syndrome with increasing maternal age and (**B**) achondroplasia and Apert's syndrome with increasing paternal age. Apert's syndrome (acrocephalosyndactyly) is characterized by a towering skull and laterally fused digits.

**FIGURE 8-4** Frontal *(left)* and lateral *(right)* views of anencephaly. (Courtesy M. Barr, Ann Arbor, Mich.)

country as a factor in the incidence of malformations is seen in neural tube defects (Table 8-1). The reason neural tube defects (especially anencephaly) are so common in Ireland has been the topic of much speculation. In light of the recognition of the importance of folic acid in the prevention of neural tube defects, it is possible that the high incidence of anencephaly in Ireland has resulted from poor nutrition in pregnant women during the winter.

Race is a factor in many congenital malformations and a variety of diseases. In humans as well as mice, there are racial differences in the incidence of cleft palate. The

| TABLE 8-1 | *Incidence of Neural Tube Defects* |
|---|---|
| **Site** | **Incidence*** |
| India | 0.6 |
| Ireland | 10 |
| United States | 1 |
| Worldwide | 2.6 |

*Per 1000 live births.

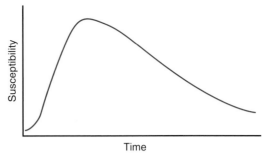

**FIGURE 8-5** Generalized susceptibility curve to teratogenic influences by a single organ.

incidence of cleft palate among Caucasians is twice as high as it is among African Americans and twice as high among Orientals as among Caucasians.

A number of malformations, particularly those with a genetic basis, are found more frequently with certain families, especially if there is any degree of consanguinity in the marriages over the generations. A good example is the increased occurrence of extra digits among some families within the American Amish community.

## Periods of Susceptibility to Abnormal Development

At certain critical periods during pregnancy, embryos are more susceptible to agents or factors causing abnormal development than at other times. The results of many investigations have allowed the following generalization: Insults to the embryo during the first 3 weeks of embryogenesis (the early period before organogenesis begins) are unlikely to result in defective development because they either kill the embryo or are compensated for by the powerful regulatory properties of the early embryo. The period of maximal susceptibility to abnormal development occurs between weeks 3 and 8, which is the period when most of the major organs and body regions are first being established. Major structural anomalies are unlikely to occur after the eighth week of pregnancy because by this point, most organs have become well established. Anomalies arising from the third to the ninth month of pregnancy tend to be functional (e.g., mental retardation) or involve disturbances in the growth of already-formed body parts. Such a simplified view of susceptible periods does not, however, take into account the possibility that a teratogen or some other harmful influence might be applied at an early stage of development but not be expressed as a developmental disturbance until later during embryogenesis. On the other hand, certain other influences (e.g., intrauterine diseases, toxins), may result in the destruction of all or parts of structures that have already been formed.

Typically, a developing organ has a curve of susceptibility to teratogenic influences similar to that illustrated in Figure 8-5. Before the critical period, exposure to a known teratogen has little influence on development. During the first days of the critical period, the susceptibility, measured as incidence or severity of malformation, increases sharply and then declines over a much longer period.

Different organs have different periods of susceptibility during embryogenesis (Figure 8-6). Organs that form the earliest (e.g., heart) tend to be sensitive to the effects of teratogens earlier than those that form later (e.g., external genitalia). Some very complex organs, especially the brain and major sense organs, show prolonged periods of high susceptibility to disruption of normal development.

Not all teratogenic influences act in the same developmental periods (Table 8-2). Some cause anomalies if the embryo is exposed to them early in development, but they are innocuous at later periods of pregnancy. Others affect only later developmental periods. A good example of the former is thalidomide, which has a very narrow and well-defined danger zone during the embryonic period (4 to 6 weeks). In contrast, tetracycline, which stains bony structures and teeth, exerts its effects after hard skeletal structures in the fetus have been formed.

## Patterns of Abnormal Development

Although isolated structural or biochemical defects are not rare, it is common to find multiple abnormalities in the same individual. This can result from a number of reasons. One possibility is that a single teratogen acted on the primordia of several organs during susceptible periods of development. Another is that a genetic or chromosomal defect spanned genes affecting a variety of structures or that a single metabolic defect affected different developing structures in different ways.

## CAUSES OF MALFORMATIONS

Despite considerable research over the past 50 years, the cause of at least 50% of human congenital malformations remains unknown (Figure 8-7). Roughly 18% of

|  | Cleavage | | Embryonic period (wk) | | | | | | Fetal period (mo) | | | | | |
|---|---|---|---|---|---|---|---|---|---|---|---|---|---|---|
|  | 1 | 2 | 3 | 4 | 5 | 6 | 7 | 8 | 4 | 5 | 6 | 7 | 8 | 9 |

Response to teratogens

Death or regulation

Heart

Central nervous system

Eyes

Ears

Lips and midface

Palate

Teeth

Upper limbs

Lower limbs

External genitalia

◼ Highly sensitive period (major structural anomalies)

◼ Less sensitive period (functional and/or minor structural anomalies)

**FIGURE 8-6** Periods and degrees of susceptibility of embryonic organs to teratogens. (Modified from Moore KL, Persaud TVN: *The developing human*, ed 5, Philadelphia, 1993, WB Saunders.)

**TABLE 8-2** *Developmental Times at Which Various Human Teratogens Exert Their Effects*

| Teratogens | Critical periods (gestational days) | Common malformations |
|---|---|---|
| Rubella virus | 0–60 | Cataract or heart malformations |
|  | 0–120+ | Deafness |
| Thalidomide | 21–40 | Reduction defects of limbs |
| Adrogenic steroids | Earlier than 90 | Clitoral hypertrophy and labial fusion |
|  | Later than 90 | Clitoral hypertrophy only |
| Coumadin anticoagulants | Earlier than 100 | Nasal hypoplasia |
|  | Later than 100 | Possible mental retardation |
| Radioiodine therapy | Later than 65–70 | Fetal thyroid deficiency |
| Tetracycline | Later than 120 | Staining of dental enamel in primary teeth |
|  | Later than 250 | Staining of crowns of permanent teeth |

Modified from Persaud TVN, Chudley AE, Skalko RG, eds: *Basic concepts in teratology*, New York, 1985, Liss.

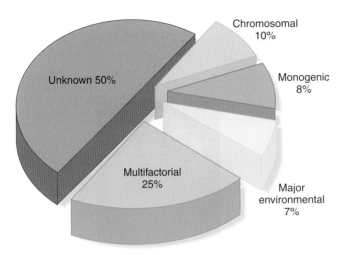

**FIGURE 8-7** Major causes of congenital malformations. (Data from Persaud TVN, Chudley AE, Skalko RG, eds: *Basic concepts in teratology*, New York, 1985, Liss.)

malformations can be attributed to genetic causes (chromosomal defects or mutations based on mendelian genetics), and 7% are caused by environmental factors, such as physical or chemical teratogens. Of all malformations, 25% are multifactorial, for example, caused by environmental factors acting on genetic susceptibility.

## Genetic Factors

Genetically based malformations can be caused by abnormalities of chromosomal division or mutations of genes. Chromosomal abnormalities are usually classified as structural or numerical errors. These arise during cell division, especially meiosis. Numerical errors of chromosomes result in **aneuploidy**, defined as a total number of chromosomes other than the normal 46.

### Abnormal Chromosome Numbers

#### Polyploidy

Polyploidy is the condition in which the chromosomal number is a higher multiple than 2 of the haploid number (23) of chromosomes. In the majority of cases, polyploid embryos abort spontaneously early in pregnancy. In fact, a high percentage of spontaneously aborted fetuses show major chromosomal abnormalities. Causes for polyploidy, especially triploidy, are likely to be either the fertilization of an egg by more than one sperm or the lack of separation of a polar body during meiosis.

#### Monosomy and Trisomy

Monosomy (the lack of one member of a chromosome pair) and **trisomy** (a triplet instead of the normal chromosome pair) are typically the result of nondisjunction

during meiosis (see Figure 1-7). When this happens, one gamete shows monosomy and the other shows trisomy of the same chromosome.

In most cases, embryos with monosomy of the autosomes or sex chromosomes are not viable. However, some individuals with monosomy of the sex chromosomes (45, XO genotype) can survive (Figure 8-8). Such individuals, who are said to have **Turner's syndrome**, exhibit a female phenotype, but the gonads are sterile.

Three autosomal trisomies produce infants with characteristic associations of anomalies. The best known is **trisomy 21**, also called **Down syndrome**. Individuals with Down syndrome are typically mentally retarded and have a characteristic broad face with a flat nasal bridge, wide-set eyes, and prominent epicanthic folds. The hands are also broad, and the palmar surface is marked by a characteristic transverse **simian crease** (Figure 8-9). Heart defects, especially atrial and ventricular septal defects, are common, with an incidence approaching 50%. Duodenal

**FIGURE 8-8** Woman with Turner's syndrome. Note the short stature, webbed neck, and infantile sexual characteristics. (From Connor J, Ferguson-Smith M: *Essential medical genetics*, ed 2, Oxford, England, 1987, Blackwell Scientific.)

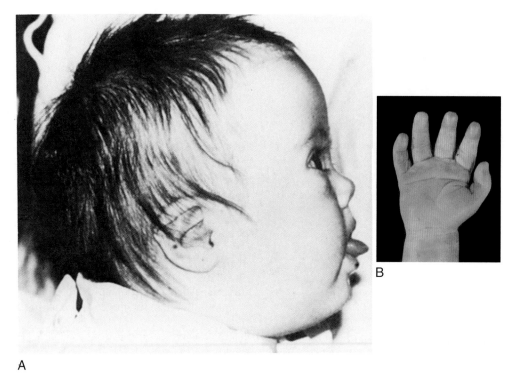

A

**FIGURE 8-9 A,** Profile of a child with Down syndrome. Note the flat profile, protruding tongue, saddle-shaped bridge of nose, and low-set ears. **B,** Hand of an infant with Down syndrome, showing the prominent simian crease that crosses the entire palm. (**A** from Garver K, Marchese S: *Genetic counseling for clinicians*, Chicago, 1986, Mosby. **B** courtesy M. Barr, Ann Arbor, Mich.)

atresia and other intestinal anomalies are also seen in patients with Down syndrome. Individuals with Down syndrome are prone to the early appearance of Alzheimer disease and typically have a shortened life span.

Other trisomies of chromosomes 13 and 18 result in severely malformed fetuses, many of which do not survive to birth. Both **trisomy 13** and **trisomy 18** infants show severe mental retardation and other defects of the central nervous system. Cleft lip and cleft palate are common. Polydactyly is often seen in trisomy 13, and infants with both syndromes exhibit other anomalies of the extremities such as "**rocker bottom feet,**" meaning a rounding under and protrusion of the heels (Figure 8-10). Most infants born with trisomy 13 or 18 die within the first 1 or 2 months after birth.

Abnormal numbers of the sex chromosomes are relatively common and can be detected by examination of the sex chromatin (X chromosome) or the fluorescence reactions of the Y chromosomes. Some of the various types of deletions and duplications of the sex chromosomes are summarized in Table 8-3.

### Abnormal Chromosome Structure

Various abnormalities of chromosome structure can give rise to malformations in development. Some chromosomal abnormalities result from chromosome breakage induced by environmental factors such as radiation and certain chemical teratogens. This type of structural error is usually unique to a given individual and is not transmitted to succeeding generations.

Other types of structural abnormalities of chromosomes are generated during meiosis and, if present in the germ cells, can be inherited. Common types of errors in chromosome structure are **reciprocal translocations, isochromosome formation,** and **deletions** and **duplications** (Figure 8-11). One well-defined congenital malformation resulting from a deletion in the short arm of chromosome 5 is the **cri du chat syndrome.** Infants with this syndrome are severely retarded, have microcephaly, and make a cry that sounds like the mewing of a cat.

### Genetic Mutations

Many genetic mutations are expressed as morphological abnormalities. These can be dominant or recessive genes of either the autosomes or the sex chromosomes. For some of these conditions (e.g., hemophilia, Lesch-Nyhan syndrome, muscular dystrophy, cystic fibrosis), the molecular or biochemical lesion has been identified, but the manner in which these defects are translated into abnormal development is unclear. Many of these conditions are extensively discussed in textbooks of human genetics, and only representative examples are listed here (Table 8-4).

**FIGURE 8-10 A,** Front and lateral views of the head of a 34-week-old fetus with trisomy 13. This fetus shows pronounced cebocephaly with a keel-shaped head, a flattened nose, abnormal ears, and a reduction of forebrain and upper facial structures. **B,** Rocker-bottom feet from a fetus with trisomy 18. Note the prominent heels and somewhat convex profile of the soles of the feet. **C,** Pronounced radial deviation of hands (club hands) of the same infant as that in **B.** (Courtesy M. Barr, Ann Arbor, Mich.)

| TABLE 8-3 *Variations in Numbers of Sex Chromosomes* | | | |
|---|---|---|---|
| **Sex chromosome complement** | **Incidence** | **Phenotype** | **Clinical factors** |
| XO | 1:3000 | Immature female | Turner syndrome: short stature, webbed neck, high and arched palate (Fig. 8.8). |
| XX | | Female | Normal |
| XY | | Male | Normal |
| XXY | 1:1000 | Male | Klinefelter syndrome: small testes, infertility, often tall with long limbs |
| XYY | 1:1000 | Male | Tall, normal appearance; reputed difficulty with impulsive behavior |
| XXX | 1:1000 | Female | Normal appearance, mental retardation (up to one third of cases), fertile (in many cases) |

## Environmental Factors

Various environmental factors are linked with birth defects. These range from chemical teratogens and hormones to maternal infections and nutritional factors. Although the list of suspected teratogenic factors is long, relatively few are unquestionably teratogenic in humans.

### Maternal Infections

After the recognition in 1941 that rubella was the cause of a spectrum of developmental anomalies, several other maternal diseases have been implicated as direct causes of birth defects. With infectious diseases, however, it is important to distinguish those that cause malformations by interfering with early stages in the development of organs and structures from those that interfere by destroying structures already formed. The same pathogenic organism can cause lesions by interference with embryonic processes or by destruction of differentiated tissues, depending on when the organism attacks the embryo.

Most infectious diseases that cause birth defects are viral, with **toxoplasmosis** (caused by the protozoan

*Toxoplasma gondii*) and syphilis (caused by the spirochete *Treponema pallidum*) being notable exceptions. (A summary of the infectious diseases known to cause birth defects in humans is given in Table 8-5.)

The time of infection is very important in relation to the types of effects on the embryo. Rubella causes a high percentage of malformations during the first trimester, whereas cytomegalovirus infections usually kill the embryo during the first trimester. The agents of both syphilis and toxoplasmosis cross the placental barrier during the fetal period and to a large extent cause malformations by destroying existing tissues.

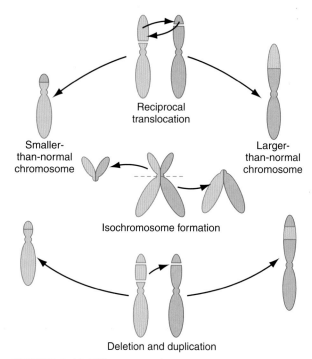

**FIGURE 8-11** Different types of structural errors of chromosomes.

| TABLE 8-4 *Genetic Mutations Leading to Abnormal Development* | |
|---|---|
| **Condition** | **Characteristics** |
| **AUTOSOMAL DOMINANT** | |
| Achondroplasia | Dwarfism caused mainly by shortening of limbs |
| Aniridia | Absence of iris (usually not complete) |
| Crouzon syndrome (craniofacial dysostosis) (Fig. 9-24) | Premature closure of certain cranial sutures, leading to flat face and towering skull |
| Neurofibromatosis | Multiple neural crest–derived tumors on skin, abnormal pigment areas on skin |
| Polycystic kidney disease (adult onset, type III) | Numerous cysts in kidneys |
| **AUTOSOMAL RECESSIVE** | |
| Albinism | Absence of pigmentation |
| Polycystic kidney disease (perinatal type I) (Fig. 16-16) | Numerous cysts in kidneys |
| Congenital phocomelia syndrome (Fig. 8-2) | Limb deformities |
| **X-LINKED RECESSIVE** | |
| Hemophilia | Defective blood clotting |
| Hydrocephalus (Fig. 11-38) | Enlargement of cranium |
| Ichthyosis | Scaly skin |
| Testicular feminization syndrome | Female phenotype caused by inability to respond to testosterone |

| TABLE 8-5 *Infectious Diseases that Can Cause Birth Defects* | | |
|---|---|---|
| **Infectious agent** | **Disease** | **Congenital defects** |
| **VIRUSES** | | |
| Rubella virus | German measles | Cataracts, deafness, cardiovascular defects, fetal growth retardation |
| Cytomegalovirus | Cytomegalic inclusion disease | Microcephaly, microphthalmia, cerebral calcification, intrauterine growth retardation |
| **SPIROCHETES** | | |
| *Treponema pallidum* (syphilis) | Syphilis | Dental anomalies, deafness, mental retardation, skin and bone lesions, meningitis |
| **PROTOZOA** | | |
| *Toxoplasma gondii* | Toxoplasmosis | Microcephaly, hydrocephaly, cerebral calcification, microphthalmia, mental retardation, prematurity |

## Chemical Teratogens

Many substances are known to be teratogenic in animals or are associated with birth defects in humans, but for only a relatively small number is there convincing evidence that links the substance directly to congenital malformations in humans (Table 8-6). This makes testing drugs for teratogenicity difficult, since what can cause a high incidence of severe defects in animal fetuses (e.g., cortisone and cleft palate in mice) may not cause malformations in other species of animals or in humans. Conversely, the classic teratogen thalidomide is highly teratogenic in humans, rabbits, and some primates but not in commonly used laboratory rodents.

### Folic Acid Antagonists

At one time, folic acid antagonists, which are known to be highly embryolethal, were used in clinical trials as **abortifacients** (agents causing abortion). Although three fourths of the pregnancies were terminated, almost a fourth of the embryos that survived to term were severely malformed. A classic example of an embryotoxic folic acid antagonist is **aminopterin**, which produces multiple severe anomalies such as anencephaly, growth retarda-

tion, cleft lip and palate, hydrocephaly, hypoplastic mandible, and low-set ears. These dramatic effects of folic acid antagonists underscore the importance of adequate amounts of folic acid in the diet to promote normal development.

### Androgenic Hormones

The administration of androgenic hormones to pregnant women either to treat tumors or to prevent threatened abortion resulted in the birth of hundreds of female infants with varying degrees of masculinization of the external genitalia. The anomalies consisted of clitoral hypertrophy and often varying amounts of fusion of the genital folds to form a scrotumlike structure (Figure 8-12).

### Anticonvulsants

Several commonly used anticonvulsants are known or strongly suspected to be teratogenic. Diphenylhydantoin produces a "fetal hydantoin syndrome" of anomalies, including growth anomalies, craniofacial defects, nail and digital hypoplasia, and mental retardation in up to a third of embryos exposed to hydantoin during pregnancy

| TABLE 8-6 Chemical Teratogens in Humans | |
|---|---|
| **Agent** | **Effects** |
| Alcohol | Growth and mental retardation, microcephaly, various malformations of face and trunk |
| Androgens | Masculinization of females, accelerated genital development in males |
| Anticoagulants (warfarin, dicumarol) | Skeletal abnormalities; broad hands with short fingers; nasal hypoplasia; anomalies of eye, neck, central nervous system |
| Antithyroid drugs (e.g., propyl-thiouracil, iodide) | Fetal goiter, hypothyroidism |
| Chemotherapeutic agents (methotrexate, aminopterin) | Variety of major anomalies throughout body |
| Diethylstilbestrol | Cervical and uterine abnormalities |
| Lithium | Heart anomalies |
| Organic mercury | Mental retardation, cerebral atrophy, spasticity, blindness |
| Phenytoin (Dilantin) | Mental retardation, poor growth, microcephaly, dysmorphic face, hypoplasia of digits and nails |
| Isotretinoin (Accutane) | Craniofacial defects, cleft palate, ear and eye deformities, nervous system defects |
| Streptomycin | Hearing loss, auditory nerve damage |
| Tetracycline | Hypoplasia and staining of tooth enamel, staining of bones |
| Thalidomide | Limb defects, ear defects, cardiovascular anomalies |
| Trimethadione and paramethadione | Cleft lip and palate, microcephaly, eye defects, cardiac defects, mental retardation |
| Valproic acid | Neural tube defects |

FIGURE 8-12 Ambiguous external genitalia in a newborn with pseudo-hermaphroditism. (From Reed GB, Claireaux AE, Bain AD: *Diseases of the fetus and newborn*, St Louis, 1989, Mosby.)

FIGURE 8-13 Face of an infant with fetal hydantoin syndrome. This infant has prominent eyes, hypertelorism (increased space between the eyes), micrognathia, and microcephaly. (From Wigglesworth JS, Singer DB: *Textbook of fetal and perinatal pathology*, 2 vols, Oxford, England, 1991, Blackwell Scientific.)

(Figure 8-13). Trimethadione also produces a syndrome of anomalies involving low-set ears, cleft lip and palate, and skeletal and cardiac anomalies.

### Sedatives and Tranquilizers

Thalidomide is highly teratogenic when administered even as infrequently as once during a very narrow window of pregnancy, especially between days 25 and 50, when even a single dose of 100 mg can be sufficient to cause birth defects. This represents the period when the primordia of most major organ systems are being established. The most characteristic lesions produced are gross malformations of the limbs, but the thalidomide syndrome also includes malformations of the cardiovascular system, absence of the ears, and assorted malformations of the urinary system, gastrointestinal system, and face. Despite years of intensive research, the mechanism by which thalidomide produces malformations is still unknown. Lithium carbonate, a commonly used agent for certain psychoses, is known to cause malformations of the heart and great vessels if administered early during pregnancy.

### Antineoplastic Agents

Several antineoplastic agents are highly teratogenic, in large part because they are designed to kill or incapaci-

tate rapidly dividing cells. Among these is aminopterin. Methotrexate and the combination of busulfan and 6-mercaptopurine cause severe anomalies of multiple organ systems. The use of these drugs during pregnancy is a difficult medical decision that must consider the lives of both the mother and the fetus.

### Alcohol

Accumulated evidence now leaves little doubt that maternal consumption of alcohol during pregnancy can lead to a well-defined constellation of developmental abnormalities that includes poor postnatal growth rate, mental retardation, heart defects, and hypoplasia of facial structures (Figure 8-14). This is now popularly known as **fetal alcohol syndrome**. Ingestion of as little as 3 ounces of alcohol in a day during the first 4 weeks of pregnancy can lead to extremely severe malformations of the **holoprosencephaly** type (see p. 337). Exposure to alcohol later in pregnancy is less likely to cause major anatomical defects in the fetus, but because of the complex course of physiological maturation in the brain throughout pregnancy, more subtle behavioral defects can result. Nevertheless, there are striking differences from normal in the shape of the corpus callosum, the main connecting link between the right and left sides of the brain, and although the IQ of an individual with fetal alcohol syndrome may be

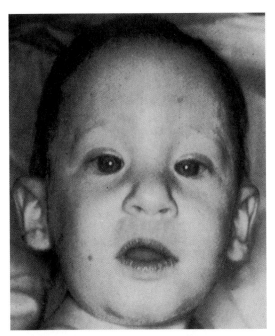

**FIGURE 8-14** Face of an infant with fetal alcohol syndrome showing a long and thin upper lip, shortened and upwardly slanting palpebral fissures, epicanthic folds, and mild hirsutism. (From Wigglesworth JS, Singer DB: *Textbook of fetal and perinatal pathology*, 2 vols, Oxford, England, 1991, Blackwell Scientific.)

normal, such individuals may show deficits in recognition of the consequences of actions or in planning into the future.

### Retinoic Acid (Vitamin A)

Derivatives of retinoic acid are used in the treatment of acne, but in recent years it has been established that retinoic acid acts as a potent teratogen when taken orally. Retinoic acid can produce a wide spectrum of defects, most of which are related to derivatives of the cranial neural crest (see page 280). These involve a variety of facial structures, the outflow tract of the heart, and the thymus.

Through a complex sequence of cytoplasmic binding proteins and nuclear receptors (see Figure 4-15), retinoic acid affects *Hox* genes, especially those expressed in the cranial and pharyngeal region (see Figure 11-11), resulting in alterations of the anterior rhombomeres and the neural crest cells derived from them.

As discussed later, neural crest cells emanating from rhombomeres are instrumental in patterning many structures of the face and neck and also contribute to the developing heart and thymus—hence the pattern of retinoic acid–induced defects previously outlined. In view of the increasing recognition that retinoic acid or its metabolites play an important role in pattern formation during early development, extreme caution

when using vitamin A in doses above those needed for basic nutritional requirements is recommended.

### Antibiotics

The use of two antibiotics during pregnancy is associated with birth defects. Streptomycin in high doses can cause inner ear deafness. Tetracycline given to the mother during late pregnancy crosses the placental barrier and seeks sites of active calcification in the teeth and bones of the fetus. Tetracycline deposits cause a yellowish discoloration of teeth and bones and, in high doses, can interfere with enamel formation.

### Other Drugs

A number of other drugs, such as the anticoagulant warfarin, are known to be teratogenic, and others are strongly suspected. However, firm proof of a drug's teratogenicity in humans is not easy to obtain. Several drugs, such as Agent Orange and some of the social drugs (e.g., LSD, marijuana), have often been claimed to cause birth defects, but the evidence to date is not entirely convincing. On the other hand, several studies have shown a variety of complications in pregnancy resulting from the use of cocaine, which can readily cross the placental barrier. In addition to structural malformations in organs such as the brain, cocaine use has been linked to intrauterine growth retardation, premature labor, and spontaneous abortion, as well as postnatal behavioral disturbances, such as attention deficit.

## Physical Factors

### Ionizing Radiation

Ionizing radiation is a potent teratogen, and the response is both dependent on the dose and related to the stage at which the embryo is irradiated. In addition to numerous animal studies, there is direct human experience based on survivors of the Japanese atomic bomb blasts and pregnant women who were given large doses of radiation (up to several thousand rads) for therapeutic reasons. There is no evidence that doses of radiation at diagnostic levels (only a few millirads) pose a significant threat to the embryo. Nevertheless, because ionizing radiation can cause breaks in DNA and is also known to cause mutations, it is prudent for a woman who is pregnant to avoid exposure to radiation if possible, although the dose in a diagnostic x-ray examination is so small that the risk is minimal.

Although ionizing radiation can cause a variety of anomalies in embryos (e.g., cleft palate; microcephaly; malformations of the viscera, limbs, and skeleton), defects of the central nervous system are very prominent in irradiated embryos. The spectrum runs from spina bifida to mental retardation.

### Other Physical Factors

A number of studies on the teratogenic effects of extremes of temperature and different concentrations of atmospheric gases have been conducted on experimental animals, but the evidence relating any of these factors to human malformations is still equivocal. One exception is the effect of excess concentrations of oxygen on prematurely born infants. When this was a common practice, **retrolental fibroplasia** developed in over 10% of premature infants weighing less than 3 pounds and in about 1% of those weighing between 3 and 5 pounds. When this was recognized, the practice of maintaining high concentrations of oxygen in incubators ceased, and this problem is now of only historical interest.

### Maternal Factors

A number of maternal factors have been implicated in the genesis of congenital malformations. **Maternal diabetes** is frequently associated with high birth weight and with stillbirths. Structural anomalies occur several times more frequently in infants of diabetic mothers than among the infants of mothers from the general population. Although there is a correlation between the duration and severity of the mother's disease and the effects on the fetus, the specific cause of interference with development has not been identified.

In general, maternal nutrition does not seem to be a major factor in the production of anomalies (folic acid being a notable exception), but if the mother is severely deficient in iodine, the newborn is likely to show the symptoms of cretinism (growth retardation, mental retardation, short and broad hands, short fingers, dry skin, and difficulty breathing).

There is now considerable evidence that **heavy smoking** by a pregnant woman leads to an increased risk of low birth weight and a low rate of growth after birth.

### Mechanical Factors

Although mechanical factors have been implicated in the genesis of congenital malformations for centuries, only in recent years has it been possible to relate specific malformations to mechanical causes. A number of the most common anomalies such as **clubfoot**, **congenital hip dislocations**, and even certain deformations of the skull can be attributed in large measure to abnormal intrauterine pressures imposed on the fetus. This can often be related to uterine malformations or a reduced amount of amniotic fluid (**oligohydramnios**).

Amniotic bands constricting digits or extremities of the fetus have been implicated as causes of intrauterine amputations (Figure 8-15). These bands form as the result of tears to the extraembryonic membranes during pregnancy. Chorionic villus sampling results in a low percentage of transverse limb defects, but the mechanism underlying the defective limb development is not well understood.

## DEVELOPMENTAL DISTURBANCES RESULTING IN MALFORMATIONS

### Duplications and Reversal of Asymmetry

The classic example of a duplication is identical twinning. Under normal circumstances, both members of the twin

A

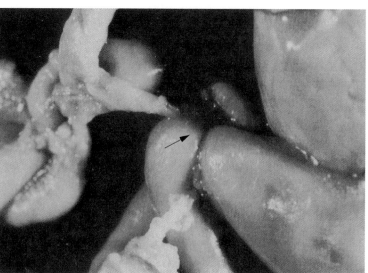

B

**FIGURE 8-15 A,** Digital amputations of the left hand presumably caused by amniotic bands. **B,** Amniotic bands involving the umbilical cord and limbs of a fetus. The arrow shows a constriction ring around the thigh. (**A** courtesy M. Barr, Ann Arbor, Mich. **B** from Wigglesworth JS, Singer DB: *Textbook of fetal and perinatal pathology*, 2 vols, Oxford, England, 1991, Blackwell Scientific.)

pair are completely normal, but rarely the duplication is not complete and **conjoined twins** result (see Figures 3-13 and 3-14). Twins can be conjoined at almost any site and to any degree. With modern surgical techniques, it is now possible to separate members of some conjoined pairs. A type of conjoined twinning is the condition of **parasitic twinning**, in which one member of the pair is relatively normal but the other is represented by a much smaller body, often consisting of just the torso and limbs, attached to an area such as the mouth or lower abdomen of the host twin (see Figure 3-15). In a high number of conjoined twins, one member of the pair has reversed asymmetry in relation to the other (see Figure 3-14).

In rare instances (approximately 1 in 10,000 births), an otherwise normal individual is found to have a partial or complete reversal of the asymmetry of the internal organs, a condition called **situs inversus**. Only recently has molecular research on early embryonic stages (see Figure 5-12) begun to provide a mechanistic explanation for this condition.

## Faulty Inductive Tissue Interactions

Absent or faulty induction early in development (e.g., induction of the central nervous system) is incompatible with life, but disturbances in later inductions can cause malformations. Absence of the lens (**aphakia**) or a kidney (**renal agenesis**) can result from an absent or abnormal inductive interaction.

## Absence of Normal Cell Death

Genetically or **epigenetically** (environmental influences imposed on the genetic background) controlled cell death is an important mechanism in sculpting a number of regions of the body. The absence of normal interdigital cell death has been implicated in **syndactyly** (webbed digits) (see Figure 10-20, *A*) and abnormal persistence of the tail (see Figure 9-20, *A*, for normal tail). The latter phenomenon has sometimes been considered an example of **atavism** (the persistence of phylogenetically primitive structures).

## Failure of Tube Formation

The formation of a tube from an epithelial sheet is a fundamental developmental mechanism. A classic case of failure of tube formation is seen in the family of spina bifida anomalies, which are based on the incomplete fusion of the neural tube (see Figure 11-42). (Some of the possible mechanisms involved in normal formation of the neural tube are given in Chapter 11.)

## Disturbances in Tissue Resorption

Some structures present in the early embryo must be resorbed for subsequent development to proceed normally. Good examples of this are the membranes that cover the future oral and anal openings. These membranes are composed of opposing sheets of ectoderm and endoderm, but if mesodermal cells become interposed between the two and this tissue becomes vascularized, breakdown typically fails to occur. **Anal atresia** is a common anomaly of this type (see Figure 15-16).

## Failure of Migration

Migration is an important developmental phenomenon that occurs at the level of cells or entire organs. The neural crest is a classic example of massive migrations at the cellular level, and disturbances in migration can cause abnormalities in any of the structures for which the neural crest is a precursor (e.g., thymus, outflow tracts of the heart, adrenal medulla). At the organ level, the kidneys undertake a prominent migration into the abdominal cavity from their origin in the pelvic region, and the testes migrate from the abdominal cavity into the scrotum. **Pelvic kidneys** (see Figure 16-14) and undescended testes (**cryptorchidism**) are not rare.

## Developmental Arrest

Early in the history of teratology, some malformations were recognized as the persistence of structures in a state that was normal at an earlier stage of development. Many of the patterns of **cleft lip** and **cleft palate** (see Figures 14-17 and 14-18) are examples of developmental arrest, although it is incorrect to assume that development has been totally arrested since the sixth to eighth weeks of embryogenesis.

Another example of the persistence of an earlier stage in development is a **thyroglossal duct** (see Figure 14-29), in which persisting epithelial cells mark the path of the thyroid gland as it migrates from the base of the tongue to its normal position.

## Destruction of Formed Structures

A number of teratogenic diseases or chemicals produce malformations by the destruction of structures already present. If the structure is in the early primordial stage, any tissues to which the primordium would normally give rise are missing or malformed. Interference with the blood supply of a structure can cause unusual patterns of malformations. For example, in the genesis of **phocomelia** (see Figure 8-2), damage to proximal blood vessels could destroy the primordia of the proximal limb segments, but the cells of the distal limb bud that give rise to the hands or feet could be spared if the distal microvasculature of the limb bud remained intact.

## Failure to Fuse or Merge

If two structures such as the palatal shelves fail to meet at the critical time, they are likely to remain separate. Similarly, the relative displacements of mesenchyme (**merging**) that are involved in the shaping of the lower jaw may not occur on schedule or in adequate amounts. This accounts for some malformations of the lower face.

## Hypoplasia and Hyperplasia

The normal formation of most organs and complex structures requires a precise amount and distribution of cellular proliferation. If cellular proliferation in a forming organ is abnormal, the structure can become too small (**hypoplastic**) or too large (**hyperplastic**). Even relatively minor growth disturbances can cause severe problems in complex regions such as the face. Occasionally, **gigantism** of a structure such as a digit or whole limb occurs. The mechanism underlying this excessive growth remains obscure.

## Receptor Defects

Some congenital malformations can be attributed to defects in specific receptor molecules. One of the earliest recognized is the **testicular feminization syndrome**, in which the lack of testosterone receptors results in the development of a typical female phenotype in a genetic male (see Figure 9-12).

## Defective Fields

Proper morphogenesis of many regions of the body is under the control of poorly understood morphogenetic fields. These regions of the body are under the control of an overall developmental blueprint. Disturbances in the boundaries or overall controls of fields can sometimes give rise to massive anomalies. One example is the fusion of lower limb fields, which is probably associated with a larger defect in the field controlling the development of the caudal region of the body. This mermaidlike anomaly is called sirenomelia (see Figure 8-1, *B*), an

extreme example of what is called the **caudal regression syndrome**.

## Effects Secondary to Other Developmental Disturbances

Because so much of normal development involves the tight interlocking of individual processes or building on completed structures, it is not surprising that a number of malformations are secondary manifestations of other disturbed embryonic processes. There are a number of examples in craniofacial development. Some cases of cleft palate have been attributed to a widening of the cranial base so that the palatal shelves, which may have been perfectly normal, are unable to make midline contact.

The single or widely separated tubular prosboscses that appear in certain major facial anomalies, such as **cyclopia** (Figure 8-16), are very difficult to explain unless it is understood that one of several primary defects, whether too much or too little tissue of the midface, prevented the two nasal primordia from joining in the midline. In the case of cyclopia, the primary defect is usually a deficiency of forebrain tissue, resulting from deficient sonic hedgehog signaling (see Clinical Correlation 14-1), and the facial defects are secondary to that.

**FIGURE 8-16** Cyclopia in a newborn. Note the fleshy proboscis above the partially fused eye. (Courtesy M. Barr, Ann Arbor, Mich.)

## Diagnosis and Treatment of Birth Defects

Only a few decades ago, birth defects were diagnosed only after the fact, and sometimes it was years after birth before certain defects could be discovered and treated. Although this can still happen today, technological changes have permitted the earlier diagnosis and treatment of certain congenital malformations.

One of the first advances was the technology associated with karyotyping and sex chromosome analysis. Initially these techniques were applied after birth to diagnose conditions based on abnormalities in chromosome number or structure. After the development of amniocentesis (the removal of samples of amniotic fluid during early pregnancy), chromosomal analysis could be applied to cells in the amniotic fluid. This was particularly useful in the diagnosis of Down syndrome, but it also permitted the prenatal diagnosis of the gender of the infant. Biochemical analysis of amniotic fluid has permitted the

diagnosis of a number of inborn errors of metabolism and neural tube defects (the latter through the detection of **S-100 protein**, which leaks through the open neural tube into the amniotic fluid).

More recently, techniques have been developed for the direct sampling of tissue from the chorionic villi. The risk-to-benefit ratio of this technique is still being debated.

With the development of modern imaging techniques such as ultrasound, computed tomography, and magnetic resonance imaging, visualization of fetal morphological structures is now possible (see Figures 18-11 to 18-14) These images can now serve as a direct guide to surgeons who are attempting to correct certain malformations by intrauterine surgery. Because surgical wounds in fetuses typically heal without scarring, there are distinct advantages to fetal corrective surgery (see Chapter 18).

---

**CLINICAL VIGNETTE**

A woman in her early forties who has chronic alcoholism, who smokes heavily, and who also occasionally uses cocaine gives birth to an infant with severe anencephaly. She had previously given birth to a child who had a less severe form of spina bifida. Another child, although small in stature, seemed normal but had a behavioral problem in school.

What is a likely basis for such a history?

## Germ Layer Defects

An understanding of normal development can explain the basis for a seemingly diverse set of anomalies. **Ectodermal dysplasias**, which are based on abnormalities in the ectodermal germ layer, can include malformations as diverse as thin hair, poorly formed teeth, short stature, dry and scaly skin, and hypoplastic nails. Other syndromes with diverse phenotypic abnormalities are related to defects of the neural crest (see Chapter 12).

## SUMMARY

⦿ Developmental disorders have been recognized for centuries, but a direct connection between environmental teratogens and human birth defects was not demonstrated until 1941.

⦿ Abnormal development is often the result of environmental influences imposed on genetic susceptibility. The

factors involved in abnormal development include age, race, country, nutrition, and time of year. The study of abnormal development is teratology, and an agent that causes abnormal development is a teratogen.

⦿ Genetic factors cause a significant number of birth defects. Abnormal chromosome numbers are associated with prenatal death and syndromes of abnormal structures. Common causes of abnormalities are monosomies and trisomies, which are often the result of nondisjunction during meiosis. Other malformations are based on abnormalities of chromosome structure. Certain malformations are based on genetic mutations.

⦿ Among the environmental factors leading to defective development are maternal infections, chemical teratogens, physical factors such as ionizing radiation, maternal factors, and mechanical factors.

⦿ A variety of disturbed developmental mechanisms may be involved in the production of a given congenital malformation. These include duplications, faulty inductive tissue interactions, absence of normal cell death, failure of tube formation, disturbances in tissue resorption, failure of migration, developmental arrest, destruction of an already formed structure, failure to fuse or merge, hypoplasia or hyperplasia, receptor defects, defective fields, effects secondary to other developmental disturbances, and germ cell layer defects.

⦿ With technological developments, it is now possible to diagnose increasing numbers of birth defects in utero. Some of the diagnostic techniques are karyotyping and sex chromosome analysis on cells obtained from amniotic fluid, biochemical analysis of amniotic fluid, biochemical and molecular analysis of cells obtained from amniotic fluid or chorionic villus sampling, and imaging techniques, especially ultrasonography. There have been a few attempts to correct malformations by surgery in utero.

## Review Questions

1. Phocomelia is most likely to be seen after maternal exposure to which teratogenic agent during the first trimester of pregnancy?
   A. Alcohol
   B. Aminopterin
   C. Androgens
   D. Ionizing radiation
   E. Thalidomide

2. Which of these anomalies can be attributed to a disturbance in tissue resorption?
   A. Pelvic kidney
   B. Cleft lip
   C. Anal atresia
   D. Renal agenesis
   E. Amputated digit in utero

3. Which of the following is responsible for the largest percentage of congenital malformations?
   A. Maternal infections
   B. Chemical teratogens
   C. Genetically based conditions
   D. Ionizing radiations
   E. Unknown factors

4. Folic acid deficiency is now felt to be a major cause of what class of malformations?
   A. Trisomies
   B. Neural tube defects
   C. Ambiguous genitalia
   D. Polyploidy
   E. Duplications

5. Cleft palate is the result of a defect in what developmental mechanism?
   A. Failure to fuse
   B. Failure to merge
   C. Faulty inductive tissue interaction
   D. Disturbance in tissue resorption
   E. Absence of normal cell death

6. An increased incidence of what condition is strongly associated with increasing maternal age?
   A. Trisomy 18
   B. Trisomy 21
   C. Trisomy 13
   D. Anencephaly
   E. Ambiguous external genitalia

7. A woman who was in a car accident and suffered abdominal bruising during the fourth month of pregnancy gave birth to an infant with a cleft palate. She sued the driver of the other car for expenses associated with treatment of the birth defect, claiming that it was caused by the accident. You are asked to be a witness for the defense. What is your case?

8. A woman who took a new sedative during the second month of pregnancy felt somewhat nauseated after ingestion of the drug and stopped taking it after a couple of weeks. She gave birth to an infant who had a septal defect of the heart and sued the manufacturer of the drug, saying the defect was caused by the drug that made her nauseated. You are asked to be a witness for the manufacturer. What is your case?

9. What is a likely cause for a badly turned-in ankle in a newborn?

10. A 3-year-old child is much smaller than normal, has sparse hair, and has irregular teeth. What is a likely basis for this constellation of defects?

## REFERENCES

Bookstein FL and others: Geometric morphometrics of corpus callosum and subcortical structures in the fetal alcohol-affected brain, *Teratology* 63:4–32, 2001.

Botto LD and others: Neural-tube defects, *N Engl J Med* 341:1509–1519, 1999.

Butterworth CE, Bendich, A: Folic acid and the prevention of birth defects, *Annu Rev Nutr* 16:73–97, 1996.

Buyse ML, ed: *Birth defects encyclopedia*, Dover, Mass, 1990, Centre for Birth Defects Information Services.

Catilla EE and others: Thalidomide, a current teratogen in South America, *Teratology* 54:273–277, 1996.

Coles CD: Prenatal alcohol exposure and human development. In Miller M, ed: *Development of the central nervous system: effects of alcohol and opiates*, New York, 1992, Wiley-Liss, pp 9–36.

Cooper MK and others: Teratogen-mediated inhibition of target tissue response to Shh signaling, *Science* 280:1603–1607, 1998.

Czeizel AE, Dudas I: Prevention of the first occurrence of neural-tube defects by periconceptional vitamin supplementation, *N Engl J Med* 327:1832–1835, 1992.

Erickson JD, ed: Congenital malformations surveillance report, *Teratology* 56:1–175, 1997.

Fanaroff A, Martin RJ: *Neonatal-perinatal medicine*, ed 6, St Louis, 1997, Mosby.

Frazer C: Of mice and children: reminiscences of a teratogeneticist, *Issues Rev Teratol* 5:1–75, 1990.

Ganapathy V, Leibach FH: Current topic: human placenta—a direct target for cocaine action, *Placenta* 15:785–795, 1994.

Hansen DK: The embryotoxicity of phenytoin: an update on possible mechanisms, *Proc Soc Exp Biol Med* 197:361–368, 1991.

Ikonomidou C and others: Ethanol-induced apoptotic neurodegeneration and fetal alcohol syndrome, *Science* 287:1056–1060, 2000.

Jones KL: *Smith's recognizable patterns of human malformation*, ed 4, Philadelphia, 1988, WB Saunders.

Kallen B, Mastroiacovo P, Robert E: Major congenital malformations in Down syndrome, *Am J Med Genet* 65:160–166, 1996.

Lacombe D: Transcription factors in dysmorphology, *Clin Genet* 55:137–143, 1999.

Marshall H and others: Retinoids and *Hox* genes, *FASEB J* 10:969–978, 1996.

Miller MM: Effects of prenatal exposure to ethanol on cell proliferation and neuronal migration. In Miller M, ed: *Development of the central nervous system: effects of alcohol and opiates,* New York, 1992, Wiley-Liss, pp 47–69.

Miller RK and others: Periconceptional vitamin A use: how much is teratogenic? *Reprod Toxicol* 12:75–88, 1998.

Mills JL and others: Vitamin A and birth defects, *Am J Obstet Gynecol* 177:31–36, 1997.

Mulder GB and others: Effects of excess vitamin A on development of cranial neural crest-derived structures: a neonatal and embryologic study, *Teratology* 62:214–226, 2000.

Munger RG and others: Maternal alcohol use and risk of orofacial cleft birth defects, *Teratology* 54:27–33, 1996.

Naeye RL: *Disorders of the placenta, fetus, and neonate,* St Louis, 1992, Mosby.

Nishimura H, Okamoto N: *Sequential atlas of human congenital malformations,* Baltimore, 1976, University Park Press.

Nyberg D, Mahony B, Pretorious D: *Diagnostic ultrasound of fetal anomalies,* St Louis, 1990, Mosby.

Paré A: *On monsters and marvels,* Chicago, 1982, University of Chicago Press.

Persaud TVN, Chudley AE, Skalko RG, eds: Basic concepts in teratology, New York, 1985, Liss.

Polifka JE, Friedman JM: Clinical teratology: identifying teratogenic risks in humans, *Clin Genet* 56:409–420, 1999.

Reed GB, Claireaux AE, Bain AD: *Diseases of the fetus and newborn,* St Louis, 1989, Mosby.

Soprano DR, Soprano KJ: Retinoids as teratogens, *Annu Rev Nutr* 15:111–132, 1995.

Stephens TD, Fillmore BJ: Hypothesis: thalidomide embryopathy—proposed mechanism of action, *Teratology* 61:189–195, 2000.

Sulik KK, Alles AJ: *Teratogenicity of the retinoids.* In Saurat J-H, ed: *Retinoids: 10 years on,* Basel, Switzerland, 1991, Karger, pp 282–295.

Volpe JJ: Effect of cocaine use on the fetus, *N Engl J Med* 327:399–407, 1992.

Warkany J: *Congenital malformations,* St Louis, 1971, Mosby.

Wigglesworth JS, Singer DB: *Textbook of fetal and perinatal pathology,* 2 vols, Oxford, England, 1991, Blackwell Scientific.

Willis RA: *The borderland of embryology and pathology,* ed 2, London, 1962, Butterworths.

Wilson GN: Genomics of human dysmorphogenesis, *Am J Med Genet* 42:187–196, 1992.

Wilson JG, Fraser FC, eds: *Handbook of teratology,* vols 1–4, New York, 1977, Plenum.

Zinn AR, Ross JL: Turner syndrome and haploinsufficiency, *Curr Opin Genet Devel* 8:322–327, 1998.

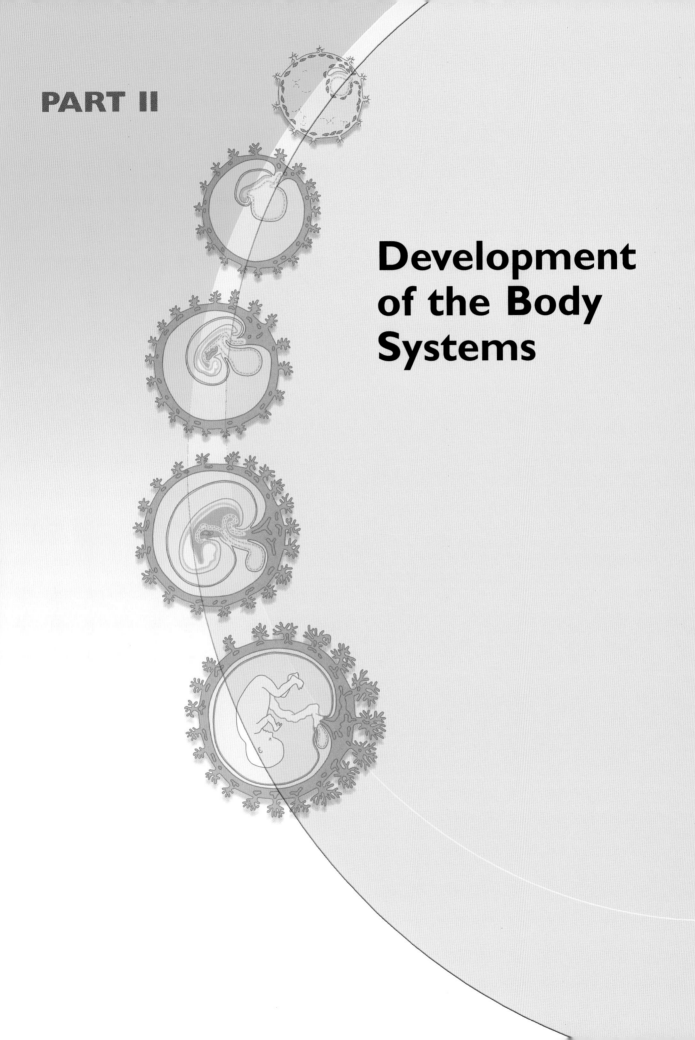

**PART II**

# Development of the Body Systems

# CHAPTER 9

# Integumentary, Skeletal, and Muscular Systems

The construction of the tissues of the body involves developmental phenomena at two levels of organization. One is the level of individual cells, in which the cells that make up a tissue undergo increasing specialization through a process called **cytodifferentiation** (see discussion of restriction, determination, and differentiation, p. 97). At the next level of complexity, various cell types develop in concert to form specific tissues through a process called **histogenesis**. This chapter will cover the development of three important tissues of the body: skin, bone, and muscle. The histogenesis of each of these tissues exemplifies important aspects of development.

## INTEGUMENTARY SYSTEM

The skin, consisting of the epidermis and dermis, is one of the largest structures in the body. The epidermis represents the interface between the body and its external environment, and its structure is well adapted for local functional requirements. Simple inspection of areas such as the scalp and palms shows that the structure of the integument varies from one part of the body to another. These local variations result from inductive interactions between the ectoderm and underlying mesenchyme. Abnormalities associated with the integumentary system are presented in Clinical Correlation 9-1, found near the end of this section.

## Epidermis

### Structural Development

The outer layer of the skin begins as a single layer of ectodermal cells (Figure 9-1, *A*). As development progresses, the ectoderm becomes multilayered, and regional differences in structure become apparent.

The first stage in epidermal layering is the formation of a thin outer layer of flattened cells known as the **periderm** at the end of the first month of gestation (Figure 9-1, *B*). Cells of the periderm, which is present in the epidermis of all amniote embryos, appear to be involved in the exchange of water, sodium, and possibly glucose between the amniotic fluid and the epidermis.

By the third month the epidermis becomes a three-layered structure, with a mitotically active **basal** (or **germinative**) **layer**, an intermediate layer of cells (Figure 9-1, *D*) that represent the progeny of the dividing stem cells of the basal layer, and a superficial layer of peridermal cells bearing characteristic surface blebs (Figure 9-2). Peridermal cells contain large amounts of glycogen, but its function remains uncertain.

During the sixth month, the epidermis beneath the periderm undergoes differentiation into the definitive layers characteristic of the postnatal epidermis. Many of the peridermal cells undergo programmed cell death (**apoptosis**) and are sloughed into the amniotic fluid. The epidermis becomes a barrier between the fetus and the outside environment instead of a participant in exchanges

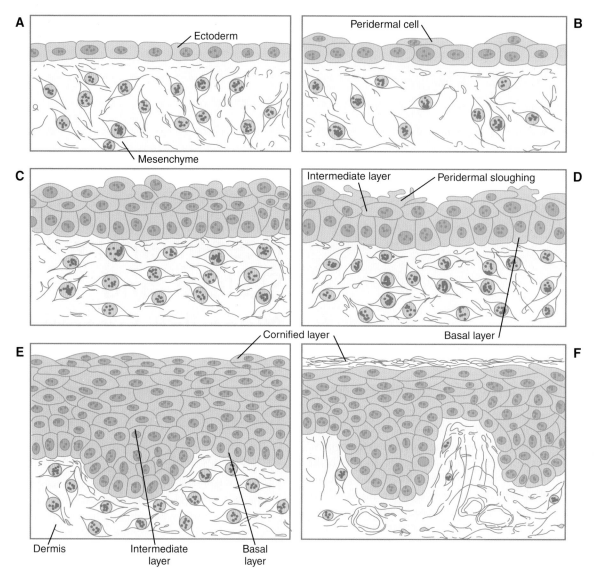

**FIGURE 9-1** Stages in the histogenesis of human skin. **A,** At **1 month. B,** At **2 months. C,** At **2½ months. D,** At **4 months. E,** At **6 months. F,** After birth. (Modified from Carlson B: *Patten's foundations of embryology,* ed 6, New York, 1996, McGraw-Hill.)

**FIGURE 9-2** Light micrograph *(left)* and scanning electron micrograph *(right)* of the epidermis of a **10-week-old** human embryo. The prominent surface blebs seen in the scanning micrograph are represented by the irregular surface of the periderm *(P)* in the light micrograph. The arrow in the figure on the left points to a melanocyte in the basal layer *(B)* of the epidermis. *I,* Intermediate layer of epidermis. (From Sybert VP, Holbrook KA. In Reed G, Claireaux A, Bain A: *Diseases of the fetus and newborn,* St Louis, 1989, Mosby.)

between the two. The change in function of the fetal epidermis may have adaptive value, since it occurs at about the time when urinary wastes begin to accumulate in the amniotic fluid.

### Immigrant Cells in the Epidermis

Despite its homogeneous histological appearance, the epidermis is really a cellular mosaic, with contributions from cells derived not only from surface ectoderm but also from other precursors, such as the neural crest or mesoderm. These cells play important specific roles in the function of the skin.

Early in the second month, **melanoblasts** derived from the neural crest migrate into the embryonic dermis; slightly later, they migrate into the epidermis. Although melanoblasts can be recognized early by staining with a monoclonal antibody (HMB-45, which reacts with a cytoplasmic antigen common to melanoblasts and **melanomas** [pigment cell tumors]), these cells do not begin to produce recognizable amounts of pigment until midpregnancy. This occurs earlier in heavily pigmented individuals than in those with light complexions. The differentiation of melanoblasts into mature **melanocytes** involves the formation of pigment granules called **melanosomes** from **premelanosomes**.

The number of pigment cells in the skin does not differ greatly among the various races, but the melanocytes of dark-skinned individuals contain more pigment granules per cell. **Albinism** is a genetic trait characterized by the lack of pigmentation, but albinos typically contain normal numbers of melanocytes in their skin. The melanocytes of albinos are generally unable to express pigmentation because they lack the enzyme **tyrosinase**, which is involved in the conversion of the amino acid tyrosine to **melanin**.

Late in the first trimester the epidermis is invaded by **Langerhans' cells**, which arise from precursors in the bone marrow. These cells are peripheral components of the immune system and are involved in the presentation of antigens; they cooperate with T lymphocytes (white blood cells involved in cellular immune responses) in the skin to initiate cell-mediated responses against foreign antigens. Langerhans' cells are present in low numbers (about 65 cells/mm² of epidermis) during the first two trimesters of pregnancy, but then their numbers increase several-fold to 2% to 6% of the total number of epidermal cells in the adult.

A third cell type in the epidermis, the **Merkel cell**, is of uncertain origin. Some evidence suggests that Merkel cells may differentiate from epidermal cell precursors, but experiments on birds involving the grafting of marked neural crest tissues indicate that precursors of Merkel cells migrate into the limb from the neural crest. These cells, which appear in palmar and plantar epidermis as early as 8 to 12 weeks of gestation, are associated with free nerve

terminals. They function as slow-adapting mechanoreceptors in the skin, but cytochemical evidence suggests that they may also function as neuroendocrine cells at some stage.

### Epidermal Differentiation

Once the multilayered epidermis becomes established, a regular cellular organization and sequence of differentiation appears within it (Figure 9-3). **Stem cells*** of the basal layer (**stratum basale**) divide and contribute daughter cells to the next layer, the **stratum spinosum**. The movement of epidermal cells away from the basal layer is preceded by a loss of adhesiveness to basal lamina components (e.g., fibronectin, laminin, and collagen types I and IV). These cellular properties can be explained by the loss of several **integrins** (membrane proteins that mediate the attachment of cells to extracellular matrix molecules). Cells of the stratum spinosum produce prominent bundles of **keratin** filaments, which converge on the patchlike desmosomes binding the cells to each other.

---

* Many types of tissues contain a population of **stem cells**, which have a high capacity for proliferation. Some of the daughter cells remain as stem cells, but other daughter cells become what in the epidermis are called **transit-amplifying cells**. These cells, which are located in the stratum basale and to some extent in the stratum spinosum, are capable of a few more mitotic divisions before permanently withdrawing from the cell cycle. The post-mitotic cells are sometimes called **committed cells**. In the epidermis, these are the cells that undergo keratinization.

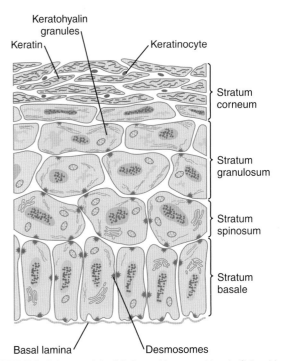

**FIGURE 9-3** Layers of the fully formed human epidermis. Cells arising in the stratum basale undergo terminal differentiation into keratinocytes as they move toward the surface. (Modified from Carlson B: *Patten's foundations of embryology*, ed 6, New York, 1996, McGraw-Hill.)

**Keratohyalin granules,** another marker of epidermal differentiation, begin to appear in the cytoplasm of the outer, postmitotic cells of the stratum spinosum and are prominent components of the stratum granulosum. Recent research has shown that keratohyalin granules are composed of two types of protein aggregates— one histidine rich and one sulfur rich—closely associated with bundles of keratin filaments. Because of their high content of keratin, epidermal cells are given the generic name **keratinocytes.** As the keratinocytes move into the stratum granulosum, their nuclei begin to show characteristic signs of terminal differentiation, such as a flattened appearance, dense masses of nuclear chromatin, and early signs of breaking up of the nuclear membrane. In these cells the bundles of keratin become more prominent, and the molecular weights of keratins that are synthesized are higher than in less mature keratinocytes.

As the cells move into the outer layer, the **stratum corneum,** they lose their nuclei and resemble very flattened bags densely packed with keratin filaments. The cells of this layer are interconnected by the histidine-rich protein **filaggrin,** which is derived from one of the granular components of keratohyalin. Depending on the region of the body surface, the cells of the stratum corneum accumulate to form approximately 15 to 20 layers of dead cells. In postnatal life, whether through friction or the degradation of the desmosomes and filaggrin, these cells are eventually shed (e.g., about 1300 cells/cm²/hr in the human forearm) and commonly accumulate as house dust.

Biochemical work has correlated the expression of keratin proteins (members of a complex family of proteins) with specific stages of epidermal differentiation (Figure 9-4). Keratins of the family of intermediate cellular filaments are first expressed in cells of the two-layered

**FIGURE 9-4** Expression of keratins and filaggrin during human fetal skin development. The lower figures show approximate stages in skin development at the times indicated. (Graph modified from Dale BA and others: *J Cell Biol* 101:1257–1269, 1985.)

epidermis during the second month of pregnancy. Three of the keratins (40-, 45-, and 52-kDa) are characteristic of simple epithelia, and the other two (50- and 58-kDa) are typically seen in stratified epithelia. As the epidermis begins to stratify (at 9 to 12 weeks' gestation), the outer cells of the intermediate layer begin to express small amounts of 56.5- and 67-kDa keratins, which are characteristic of keratinized epidermis. In succeeding weeks the amounts of these two keratins increase greatly, whereas the prominence of the simple epithelial keratins (40-, 45-, and 52-kDa) declines during the late fetal period. The expression of filaggrin, the intercellular binding protein, is closely correlated with the later differentiation of the outer cornified layers of the fetal epidermis.

The proliferation of basal epidermal cells is under the control of a variety of growth factors. Some of these stimulate and others inhibit mitosis (Box 9-1). Keratinocytes commonly spend about 4 weeks in their passage from the basal layer of the epidermis to ultimate desquamation, but in some skin diseases, such as **psoriasis**, epidermal cell proliferation is poorly controlled, and keratinocytes may be shed within a week after their generation.

One of the prominent features of the skin, particularly the thick skin of the palms and soles, is the presence of epidermal ridges and creases. On the tips of the digits, the ridges form loops and whorls in fingerprint patterns that are unique to the individual. These patterns form the basis for the science of **dermatoglyphics**, in which the patterns constitute the foundation for genetic analysis or criminal investigation.

The formation of epidermal ridges is closely associated with the earlier appearance of **volar pads** on the ventral

---

## Box 9-1　Peptide Factors that Affect Keratinocyte Proliferation

### STIMULATORS

Epidermal growth factor
Transforming growth factor-$\alpha$
Insulin
Insulin-like growth factors I and II
Fibroblast growth factor (FGF-1, FGF-2)
Interleukin-1/ETAF

### INHIBITORS

Transforming growth factor-$\beta_1$
Transforming growth factor-$\beta_2$
Interferon-$\alpha/\beta_1$
Interferon-$\beta_2$
Interferon
Tumor necrosis factor

---

surfaces of the fingers and toes (Figure 9-5). Volar pads first form on the palms at about $6\frac{1}{2}$ weeks, and by $7\frac{1}{2}$ weeks, they have formed on the fingers. The volar pads begin to regress by about $10\frac{1}{2}$ weeks, but while they are present, they set the stage for the formation of the epidermal ridges, which occurs between 11 and 17 weeks. Similar events in the foot occur approximately a week later than those in the hand.

**FIGURE 9-5** Scanning electron micrographs of the ventral surfaces of the hand **(A)** and the foot **(B)** of a human embryo at the **end of the second month.** Volar pads are prominent near the tips of the digits (*arrowheads*). (From Jirásek J: *Atlas of human prenatal morphogenesis*, Amsterdam, 1983, Martinus Nijhoff.)

The pattern of the epidermal ridges is correlated with the morphology of the volar pads when the ridges first form. If a volar pad is high and round, the epidermal ridges form a whorl; if the pad is low, an arch results. A pad of intermediate height results in a loop configuration of the digital epidermal ridges. The timing of ridge formation also appears to influence the morphology: early formation of ridges is associated with whorls and late formation with arches. The primary basis for dermatoglyphic patterns is still not understood.

When the epidermal ridges first form, the tips of the digits are still smooth, and the fetal epidermis is covered with peridermal cells. Beneath the smooth surface, however, epidermal and dermal ridges begin to take shape (Figure 9-6). Late in the fifth month of pregnancy the epidermal ridges become recognizable features of the surface landscape.

## Dermis

The dermis arises from several sources. In the trunk, dorsal dermis arises from the dermatome of the somites, whereas ventral and lateral dermis, as well as dermis of the limbs, is derived from the lateral mesoderm. In the face, much of the cranial skin, and anterior neck, dermal cells are descendants of cranial neural crest ectoderm (see Figure 12-10).

The future dermis is initially represented by loosely aggregated mesenchymal cells that are highly interconnected by focal tight junctions on their cellular processes. These early dermal precursors secrete a watery intercellular matrix rich in glycogen and hyaluronic acid.

Early in the third month the developing dermis undergoes a transition from the highly cellular embryonic form to a state characterized by the differentiation of the mesenchymal cells into fibroblasts and the formation of increasing amounts of a fibrous intercellular matrix. The principal types of fibers are types I and III collagen and elastic fibers. The dermis becomes highly vascularized, with an early capillary network transformed into layers of larger vessels. Shortly after the eighth week, sensory

nerves growing into the dermis and epidermis help complete reflex arcs, allowing the fetus to respond to pressure and stroking.

### Dermal/Epidermal Interactions

The transformation of simple ectoderm into a multilayered epidermis depends on continuing inductive interactions with the underlying dermis. Dermal/epidermal interactions are also the basis for the formation of a wide variety of epidermal appendages and the appearance of regional variations in the structure of the epidermis.

For example, early in development the epidermis covering the palms and soles becomes significantly thicker than that elsewhere on the body. These regions also do not produce hairs, whereas hairs of some sort, whether coarse or extremely fine, form in regular patterns from the epidermis throughout most of the rest of the body.

Tissue recombination experiments on a variety of vertebrate species have shown that the underlying dermis determines the course of development of the epidermis and its derivatives and that the ectoderm also influences the developmental course of the dermis. If the early ectodermal and mesenchymal components of the skin are enzymatically dissociated and grown separately, the ectodermal component remains simple ectoderm without differentiating into a multilayered epidermis with appropriate epidermal appendages. Similarly, isolated subectodermal mesenchyme retains its embryonic character without differentiating into dermis.

If ectoderm from one part of the body is combined with dermis from another area, the ectoderm differentiates into a regional pattern characteristic of underlying dermis rather than a pattern appropriate for the site of origin of the ectoderm (Figure 9-7). Cross-species recombination experiments have shown that even in distantly related animals, skin ectoderm and mesenchyme can respond to each other's inductive signals.

As in many other parts of the body, inductive interactions and subsequent morphogenesis of the skin and its appendages are mediated by the production and secretion

**A**    **B**    **C**

**FIGURE 9-6** Scanning electron micrographs of human digital palmar skin in a **14-week-old** fetus. **A,** Low-power view of the palmar surface of a digit. **B,** Epidermal surface of the dermis of the fingertip showing the primary dermal ridges. **C,** Basal surface of the epidermis showing the epidermal ridges. *Bars,* 100 μm. (From Misumi Y, Akiyoshi T: *Am J Anat* 119:419, 1991.)

**FIGURE 9-7** Recombination experiments illustrating the importance of tissue interactions in the differentiation of the skin. When separated **(A),** ectoderm and underlying mesenchyme do not differentiate. Recombinations (**B** and **C**) show that the dermis determines the nature of the ectodermal differentiation.

of common signaling molecules. Specific regional morphogenesis of the skin and its appendages appears to be patterned through the actions of transcription factors, probably functioning in concert with the still poorly understood influences of retinoic acid, which exerts powerful effects on the skin.

## Epidermal Appendages

As a result of inductive influences by the dermis, the epidermis produces a wide variety of appendages such as hair, nails, sweat and sebaceous glands, mammary glands, and even the enamel component of teeth. (The development of teeth is discussed in Chapter 14.)

### Hair

Hairs are specialized epidermal derivatives that arise as the result of inductive stimuli from the dermis. There are many types of hairs, ranging from the coarse hairs of the eyelashes and eyebrows to the barely visible hairs on the abdomen and back. Regional differences in morphology and patterns of distribution are imposed on the epidermis by the underlying dermis.

Hair formation is first recognizable at about the twelfth week of pregnancy as regularly spaced epidermal downgrowths associated with small condensations of dermal cells called **dermal papillae** (Figure 9-8). Under the continuing influence of a dermal papilla, the epidermal downgrowth continues over the next few weeks and forms an early **hair peg.** In succeeding weeks the epidermal peg overgrows the dermal papilla, resulting in the shaping of an early **hair follicle.** At this stage the hair follicle still does not protrude beyond the outer surface of the epidermis, but in the portion of the follicle that penetrates deeply into the dermis, two bulges (1) presage the formation of **sebaceous glands,** which secrete an oily skin lubricant (**sebum**), and (2) are the attachment site for the tiny **arrector pili muscle.** The arrector pili is a mesodermally derived smooth muscle that lifts the hair to a near-vertical position in a cold environment. In many animals, this increases the insulation properties of the hair. The developing hair follicle induces the adjacent

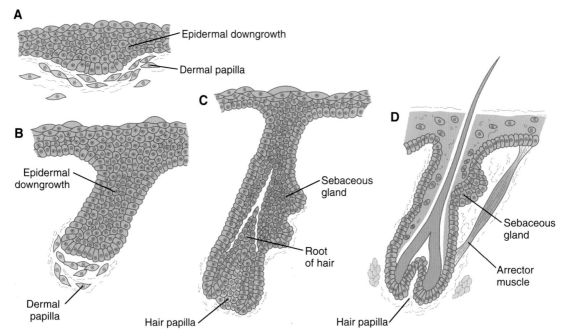

**FIGURE 9-8** Differentiation of a human hair follicle. **A,** Hair primordium **(12 weeks). B,** Early hair peg **(15 to 16 weeks). C,** Bulbous hair follicle **(18 weeks). D,** Adult hair.

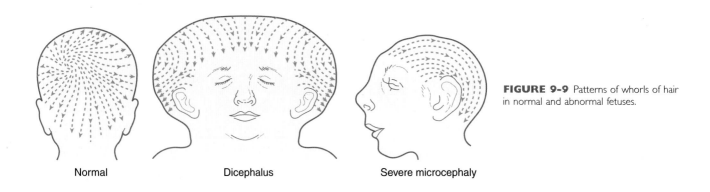

**FIGURE 9-9** Patterns of whorls of hair in normal and abnormal fetuses.

dermal mesoderm to form the smooth muscle cells of this muscle.

In hair formation, the establishment of an individual epidermal downgrowth (Figure 9-8, A) involves a stimulatory influence by **FGF-5** by the underlying mesenchyme (dermal papilla). Counteracting this is an inhibitory influence of **BMP-2** and **BMP-4,** which may regulate the spacing between adjacent downgrowths. Soon after its formation, the ectodermal downgrowth begins to express **sonic hedgehog,** which stimulates cell proliferation and growth of the follicle. In a number of developing systems the class of homeobox-containing genes, *Msx,* is produced at times and in places where epithelial-mesenchymal interactions and cellular proliferation are prominent. This is the case in the formation of skin appendages, in which the production of Msx by the thickened ectoderm is associated with intense proliferation of both the ectoderm and the underlying dermis. Interestingly, the homeobox gene *Hoxc-13* is expressed in hair

follicles throughout the body. In null mutants, the skin is essentially hairless, due to fragility of the newly forming hairs. In this case, *Hoxc-13* appears to be involved in some aspect of the keratinization process, a quite different function from that of the *Hox* genes early in development, when they are involved in setting up axial structures.

Erupted hairs are first seen on the eyebrows shortly after 16 weeks. Within a couple of weeks, they cover the scalp. The eruption of hairs follows a cephalocaudal gradient over the body. During the later stages of hair formation, the hair bulb becomes infiltrated with melanocytes, which provide color to the hair. Starting around the fifth month, the epidermal cells of the hair shaft begin to undergo keratinization, forming firm granules of **trichohyalin,** which imparts hardness to the hair.

Products of the fetal sebaceous glands accumulate on the surface of the skin as **vernix caseosa.** This substance may serve as a protective coating for the epidermis, which is continually exposed to amniotic fluid.

The first fetal hairs are very fine in texture and are close together. Known as **lanugo**, they are most prominent during the seventh and eighth months. Lanugo hairs are typically shed just before birth and are replaced by coarser definitive hairs, which arise from newly formed follicles.

The pattern of epidermal appendages such as hairs has been shown experimentally to relate to patterns generated in the dermis. Other studies have compared patterns of scalp hairs between normal embryos and those with cranial malformations (Figure 9-9) and have shown a correlation between whorls and the direction of hair growth and the tension on the epidermis at the time of formation of the hair follicles.

### Mammary Glands

As with many glandular structures, the mammary glands arise as epithelial (in this case, ectodermal) downgrowths into mesenchyme in response to inductive influences by the mesenchyme. The first morphological evidence of mammary gland development is the appearance of two bands of ectodermal thickenings called **milk lines** running along the ventrolateral body walls in embryos of both genders at about 6 weeks (Figure 9-10, *A*). The craniocaudal level and the extent along the milk lines at which mammary tissue develops vary among species. Comparing the location of mammary tissue in cows (caudal), humans (in the pectoral region), and dogs (along the length of the milk line) demonstrates the wide variation in location and number of mammary glands. In humans, supernumerary mammary tissue or nipples can be found anywhere along the length of the original milk lines (Figure 9-10, *B*).

Mammary ductal epithelial downgrowths (Figure 9-11) are associated with two types of mesoderm: fibroblastic and fatty. Experimental evidence suggests that inductive interactions with the fatty component of the connective tissue are responsible for the characteristic shaping of the mammary duct system. As with many developing glandular structures, the inductive message seems to be mediated to a great extent by the extracellular matrix of the connective tissue.

Although the mesoderm controls the branching pattern of the ductal epithelium, the functional properties of the mammary ducts are intrinsic to the epithelial component. An experiment in which mouse mammary ectoderm was combined with salivary gland mesenchyme illustrates this point. The mammary ducts developed a branching pattern characteristic of salivary gland epithelium, but despite this, the mammary duct cells produced one of the milk proteins, **α-lactalbumin.**

In keeping with their role as secondary sexual characteristics, mammary glands are extremely responsive to the hormonal environment. This has been shown by experiments conducted on mice. In contrast to the continued downgrowth of ductal epithelium in females, the

**FIGURE 9-10 A,** Milk lines *(blue)* in a generalized mammalian embryo. Mammary glands form along these lines. **B,** Common formation sites for supernumerary nipples or mammary glands along the course of the milk lines in the human.

mammary ducts in male mice respond to the presence of testosterone by undergoing a rapid involution. Female mammary ducts react similarly if they are exposed to testosterone. Further analysis has shown that the effect of testosterone is mediated through the mammary mesenchyme rather than acting directly on the ductal epithelium. Conversely, if male mammary ducts are allowed to develop in the absence of testosterone, they assume a female morphology.

The role of the mesoderm and **testosterone receptors** is well illustrated in experiments involving mice with a genetic mutant, **androgen insensitivity syndrome.** This is the counterpart of a human condition called the **testicular feminization syndrome,** in which genetic males lack testosterone receptors. Despite having high circulating levels of testosterone, these individuals develop female phenotypes, including typical female breast development (Figure 9-12, *A*), because without receptors, the tissue cannot respond to the testosterone.

In vitro recombination experiments on mice with androgen insensitivity have been instrumental in understanding the role of the mesoderm in mediating the effects of testosterone on mammary duct development (Figure 9-12, *B*). If mutant mammary ectoderm is combined with normal mesoderm in the presence of testosterone, the mammary ducts regress, but normal ectoderm combined with mutant mesoderm continues to form normal mammary ducts despite being exposed to high levels of testosterone. This shows that the genetic defect in testicular feminization is expressed in the mesoderm.

The postnatal development of female mammary gland tissue is also highly responsive to its hormonal environment. The simple mammary duct system that was laid down in the embryo remains in an infantile condition

**FIGURE 9-11** Stages in the embryonic development of the human mammary gland. **A, Sixth week. B, Seventh week. C, Tenth week. D, Fourth month. E, Sixth month. F, Eighth month.**

until it is exposed to the changing hormonal environment at the onset of puberty (Figure 9-13, A). Increasing levels of circulating estrogens and other, less prominent hormonal changes stimulate the proliferation of the mammary ducts and enlargement of the pad of fatty tissue that underlies it (Figure 9-13, B). As is the case with testosterone effects, estrogen effects on the epithelium of the mammary ducts are mediated via paracrine influences from the mammary connective tissue stroma, which contains the estrogen receptors. The next major change in the complete cycle of mammary tissue development occurs during pregnancy, although minor cyclical changes in mammary tissue are detectable in each menstrual cycle. During pregnancy, increased amounts of progesterone, along with prolactin and placental lactogen, stimulate the development of secretory alveoli at the ends of the branched ducts (Figure 9-13, C). With continuing development of the alveoli, the epithelial cells build up increased numbers of the cytoplasmic organelles,

such as rough endoplasmic reticulum and the Golgi apparatus, that are involved in protein synthesis and secretion.

Lactation involves a number of reciprocal influences between the mammary glands and the brain. (These are summarized in Figure 9-13, D). Stimulated by prolactin secretion from the anterior pituitary, the alveolar cells synthesize milk proteins (**casein** and **α-lactalbumin**) and lipids. In a rapid response to the suckling stimulus, the ejection of milk is triggered by the release of **oxytocin** by the posterior portion of the pituitary. Oxytocin causes the contraction of **myoepithelial cells**, which surround the alveoli. Suckling also causes an inhibition of the release of luteinizing hormone–releasing hormone by the hypothalamus, resulting in the inhibition of ovulation and a natural form of birth control.

With cessation of nursing, reduced prolactin secretion and the inhibitory effects of nonejected milk in the mammary alveoli result in the cessation of milk production. The mammary alveoli regress, and the duct system

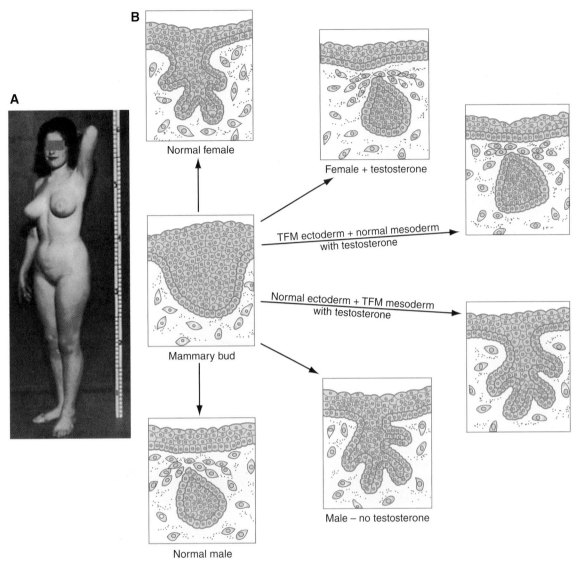

**FIGURE 9-12 A,** Testicular feminization, showing the female phenotype of a genetically male individual who had primary amenorrhea. Examination of the gonads after removal revealed immature testicular tubules. **B,** Roles of genetic specificity and testosterone in the development of mouse mammary gland tissue. With normal female mammary tissue *(top center),* the addition of testosterone causes prospective duct tissue to detach and regress as in normal male development. Conversely, in the absence of testosterone, male ductal primordia *(bottom center)* assume a female configuration. In the testicular feminization mutant *(TFM),* if normal mammary ectoderm is cultured with TFM mammary mesoderm in the presence of testosterone, mammary duct epithelium continues to develop *(lower right).* If normal male mammary mesoderm is combined with TFM ectoderm in the presence of testosterone, the normal male pattern of separation and regression of mammary duct epithelium occurs *(upper right),* showing that the genetic defect is expressed in TFM mesoderm. (**A** from Morris JM, Mahesh VB: *Am J Obstet Gynecol* 87:731, 1963. **B** based on studies by Kratochwil K: *J Embryol Exp Morphol* 25:141–153, 1971.)

of the mammary gland returns to the nonpregnant state (Figure 9-13, *E*).

## SKELETON

Skeletal tissue is present in almost all regions of the body, and the individual skeletal elements are quite diverse in morphology and tissue architecture. However, despite this diversity, there are some fundamental embryological commonalities.

All skeletal tissue arises from cells with a mesenchymal morphology, but the origins of the mesenchyme vary in different regions of the body. In the trunk the mesenchyme that gives rise to the segmented **axial skeleton** (i.e., vertebral column, ribs, sternum) originates from the sclerotomal portion of the mesodermal somites, whereas the appendicular skeleton (the bones of the limbs and their respective girdles) is derived from the mesenchyme of the lateral plate mesoderm.

The origins of the head skeleton are more complex. Some cranial bones (e.g., those making up the roof and

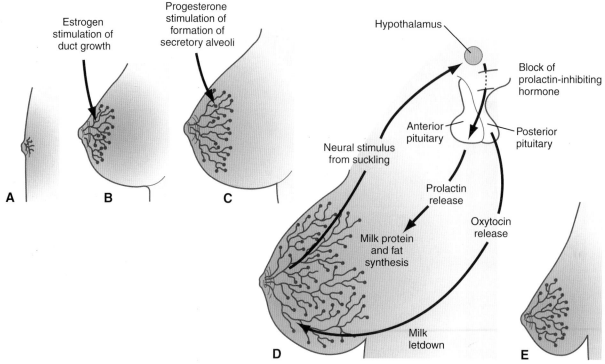

**FIGURE 9-13** Development of the mammary ducts and hormonal control of mammary gland development and function. **A,** Newborn. **B,** Young adult. **C,** Adult. **D,** Lactating adult. **E,** Adult after lactation.

## CLINICAL CORRELATION 9-1

### Abnormalities of Skin Development

Several types of anomalies affect the integumentary system. **Ectodermal dysplasia** is a germ layer defect that can affect a number of ectodermal derivatives depending on the type and severity of the condition. In addition to abnormalities of the epidermis itself, this syndrome can include the absence or abnormalities of hairs and teeth and short stature (caused by anterior pituitary gland maldevelopment).

A number of relatively rare conditions are included among the genetically transmitted disorders of keratinization. **Ichthyosis** is characterized by scaling and cracking of a hyperkeratinized epidermis. Disorders of sweat glands are commonly associated with this condi-

tion. A more severe autosomal recessive disorder is a **harlequin fetus**, in which epidermal platelike structures form, with deep cracks between the structures, because the skin cannot expand to accommodate the increasing bulk of the fetus. Infants with this condition typically do not survive longer than a few weeks.

**Angiomas** of the skin (birthmarks) are vascular malformations characterized by localized red or purplish spots ranging in size from tiny dots to formations many inches in diameter. Angiomas consist of abnormally prominent plexuses of blood vessels in the dermis, and they may be raised above the level of the skin or a mucous membrane.

much of the base of the skull) are mesodermal in origin, but the facial bones and some of the bones covering the brain arise from mesenchyme derived from the ectodermal neural crest.

The deep skeletal elements of the body typically first appear as cartilaginous models of the bones that will ultimately be formed (Figure 9-14). At specific periods during

embryogenesis, the cartilage is replaced by true bone through the process of **endochondral ossification**. In contrast, the superficial bones of the face and skull form by the direct ossification of mesenchymal cells without an intermediate cartilaginous stage (**intramembranous bone formation**). Microscopic details of both intramembranous and endochondral bone formation are

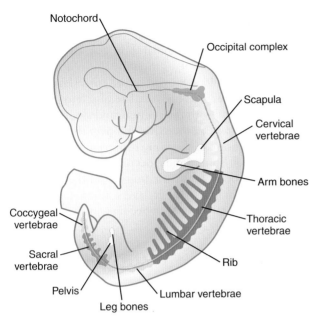

Notochord
Occipital complex
Scapula
Cervical vertebrae
Arm bones
Thoracic vertebrae
Coccygeal vertebrae
Rib
Sacral vertebrae
Pelvis
Lumbar vertebrae
Leg bones

**FIGURE 9-14** Precartilaginous primordia in the 9-mm long human embryo.

presented in the standard histology texts and are not repeated here.

A common element of many mesenchymal cell precursors of skeletal elements is their migration or relative displacement from their site of origin to the area where the bone will ultimately form. The displacement can be relatively minor, such as the aggregation of cells from the sclerotome of the receding somite around the notochord to form the body (**centrum**) of a vertebra, or it can involve extensive migrations of cranial neural crest cells to their final destinations as membrane bones of the face.

To differentiate into defined skeletal elements, the mesenchymal precursor cells must often interact with elements of their immediate environment—typically epithelia with associated basal laminae—or components of the neighboring extracellular matrix. Details of the interactions vary among regions of the body. In the limb, for example, a continuous interaction between the **apical ectodermal ridge** (see Chapter 10) and the underlying limb bud mesoderm is involved in the specification of the limb skeleton. An inductive interaction between the sclerotome and notochord or neural tube initiates skeletogenesis of the vertebral column. In the head, preskeletal cells of the neural crest may receive information at levels ranging from the neural tube itself, to sites along their path of migration, to the region of their final destination. Inductive interactions between regions of the brain and the overlying mesenchyme stimulate formation of the membrane bones of the cranial vault.

Regardless of the sources and types of environmental information that are used by the skeletal precursor cells, after they arrive at their final destinations, these cells typically undergo a local condensation before overt signs of differentiation occur. The condensation phase of bone formation is typically accompanied by the up-regulation of N-cadherin and N-CAM, which are molecules that mediate adhesion of the bone-forming cells and promote the establishment of a preskeletal condensation.

Skeletal tissues differentiate from pluripotent mesenchymal cells, which have the ability to differentiate into fibrous connective tissue, fat cells, muscle cells, cartilage, and bone. Specific transcription factors are known to direct the differentiation of mesenchymal cells into both adipocytes (fat cells) and muscle cells (see p. 197). **Sox-9**, a high mobility group transcription factor (see Figure 4-10), is a transcriptional activator of the *Col2α1* gene for **collagen IIA**, the expression of which marks the transition from condensed mesenchyme to precartilage. The transcription factor **Cbfa1 (core binding factor a1)**, a gene related to the pair-rule genes of *Drosophila*, has been shown to control the differentiation of mesenchymal cells into **osteoblasts** (bone-forming cells), but the formation of cartilage is independent of this gene. Mice bearing homozygous mutants of *Cbfa1* form the cartilaginous models of endochondral bones, but these bones never ossify; instead they undergo some calcification but remain as calcified cartilage. Intramembranous bones of the head and face do not form in these mice. **Bone morphogenetic proteins (BMPs)**, especially BMP-2, BMP-4, and BMP-7, are involved in embryonic bone formation. BMPs operate at several stages in the formation of bone, but some evidence suggests that an early function is to stimulate the expression of *Cbfa1*. The morphogenesis of individual skeletal elements is often under complex sets of controls, ranging from pattens of *Hox* gene expression in the somite stage of embryogenesis to inductive interactions between epithelia and mesenchymal precursor cells to mechanical influences that can act at any time from the early stages of morphogenesis to late postnatal life.

## Axial Skeleton

### Vertebral Column and Ribs

The earliest stages in establishing the axial skeleton were introduced in Chapter 6. Formation of the axial skeleton, however, is more complex than the simple subdivision of the paraxial mesoderm into somites and the medial displacement of sclerotomal cells to form primordia of the vertebrae. Each vertebra has a complex and unique morphology specified by controls operating at several levels and during several developmental periods.

According to the traditional view of vertebral development (see Figure 6-10), the sclerotomes split into cranial and caudal halves, and the densely packed caudal half of one sclerotome joins with the loosely packed cranial half of the next to form the centrum of a vertebra. Recent morphological research suggests that vertebral development is more complex than this model.

The vertebral column is divided into several general areas (see Figure 9-14): (1) an **occipital region**, which is incorporated into the bony structure of the base of the skull; (2) a **cervical region**, which includes the highly specialized **atlas** and **axis** that link the vertebral column to the skull; (3) the **thoracic region**, from which the true ribs arise; (4) the **lumbar region**; (5) a **sacral region**, in which the vertebrae are fused into a single **sacrum**; and (6) a **caudal region**, which represents the tail in most mammals and the rudimentary **coccyx** in humans. A

typical vertebra arises from the fusion of several cartilaginous primordia. The centrum, which is derived from the ventromedial sclerotomal portions of the paired somites (see Figure 6-9), surrounds the notochord and serves as a bony floor for the spinal cord (Figure 9-15). The **neural arches**, arising from lateral sclerotomal cells, fuse on either side with the centrum and along with other neural arches, form a protective roof over the spinal cord. Incomplete closure of the bony roof results in a common anomaly called **spina bifida occulta** (see Figure 11-42). The **costal process** forms the true ribs at the level of the thoracic vertebrae. At other levels along the vertebral column the costal processes become incorporated into the vertebrae proper.

**FIGURE 9-15 A,** Structure of a thoracic vertebra. **B** to **H,** Specific types of vertebrae, with homologous structures shown in the same color. **B,** Atlas with axis shown in its normal position beneath. **C,** Axis. **D,** Cervical vertebra. **E,** Thoracic vertebra. **F,** Lumbar vertebra. **G,** Sacrum. **H,** Coccyx.

Development of an individual vertebra begins with a sonic hedgehog–mediated induction by the notochord on the early somite to form the sclerotome. Under the continuing stimulus of shh, influencing the expression of Pax-1, the ventromedial portion of the somite will ultimately form the centrum of the vertebra. Formation of the dorsal part of the vertebra (the neural arch) is guided by a different set of developmental controls. An initial induction from the roof plate of the neural tube results in the expression of Pax-9 and the homeobox-containing genes *Msx-1* and *Msx-2*, which guide cells of the lateral sclerotome to form the neural arch.

The fundamental regional characteristics of the vertebrae are specified by the actions of discrete combinations of homeobox-containing genes (Figure 9-16). Expression of the *Hox* genes begins with the first appearance of the

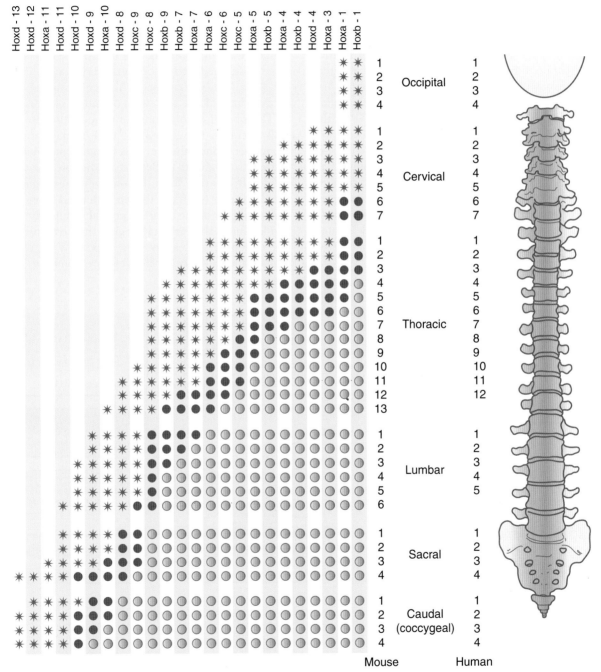

**FIGURE 9-16** *Hox* gene expression in relation to the development of the vertebral column of the mouse. Note that the vertebral column of the mouse *(left)* has one more thoracic and one more lumbar vertebra than does the vertebral column of the human. Green asterisks indicate levels at which there is definite expression of the *Hox* gene indicated at the top of the column. Purple circles represent the caudal border where expression fades out. Tan circles represent areas of no expression of the *Hox* gene. (Based on studies by Kessel M, Balling R, Gruss P: *Cell* 61:301–308, 1990.)

presomitic mesoderm and for most genes persists until chondrification begins in the primordia of the vertebrae. Formation of the normal segmental pattern along the craniocaudal axis of the vertebral column may be ensured by the fact that most vertebrae are specified by a unique combination of *Hox* genes. For example, in the mouse the atlas (C-1) is characterized by the expression of *Hoxa-1*, *Hoxa-3*, *Hoxb-1*, and *Hoxd-4*. The axis (C-2) is specified by these four genes plus *Hoxa-4* and *Hoxb-4*. **Retinoic acid** (vitamin A) can cause shifts in cranial or caudal levels in the overall segmental organization of the vertebrae if applied at specific developmental periods. For example, if administered early, retinoic acid results in a cranial shift (the last cervical vertebra is transformed into the first thoracic vertebra), and later administration causes a caudal shift (thoracic vertebrae extend into the levels of the first two lumbar vertebrae). Such shifts in level are called **homeotic transformations** and are representative of the broad family of homeotic mutants described in Chapter 6. In about 5% of humans, there are minor variations in the number or proportions of vertebrae. The **Klippel-Feil syndrome**, sometimes called **brevicollis**, is characterized by a short neck with a reduced number of cervical vertebrae, a low hairline, and other assorted anomalies. These variations in vertebral organization are likely related to imbalances of the expression of key homeobox-containing gene products.

Among the vertebrae, the axis and atlas have an unusual morphology and distinctive origin (Figure 9-17). The centrum of the atlas is deficient, but the area of the centrum is penetrated by the protruding **odontoid process** of the axis. The odontoid process consists of three fused centra that are presumably equivalent: (1) a half-segment from the centrum of a transitional bone (the **proatlas**) not found in humans, (2) the centrum that should have belonged to the atlas, and (3) the normal centrum of the axis. This arrangement permits a greater rotation of the head about the cervical spine. When the ubiquitously expressed *Hoxa-7* transgene was introduced into the germline of mice, the cranial part of the vertebral column was posteriorized. The base of the occipital bone was transformed into an occipital vertebra (the proatlas), and the atlas was combined with its centrum, resulting in an axis that did not possess an odontoid process.

The ribs arise from zones of condensed mesenchymal cells lateral to the centrum. The proximal part of a rib (head, neck, and tubercle) arises from ventromedial sclerotome (see Table 6-1). Because of the resegmentation of the somites as they form the vertebrae (see Figure 6-10), the distal part (shaft) of the rib is derived from the ventrolateral part of the adjacent cranial somite. By the time ossification in the vertebrae begins, the ribs separate from the vertebrae. **Accessory ribs**, especially in the upper lumbar and lower cervical levels, are common, but esti-

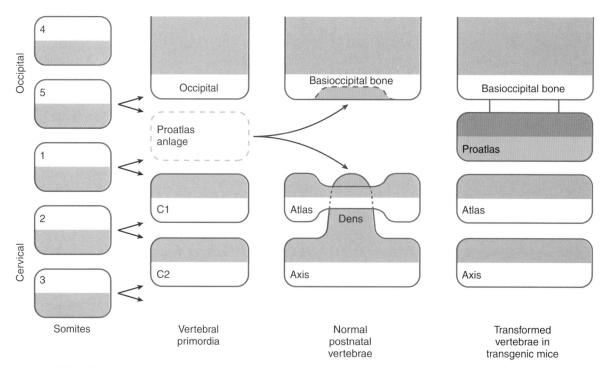

**FIGURE 9-17** Formation of the atlas and axis in normal and transgenic mice. In normal development, cells from a proatlas anlage contribute to the formation of the basioccipital bone and the dens of the axis. The normal atlas forms an anterior arch (only a transient structure in other vertebrae) instead of a centrum. The cells that would normally form the centrum at the level of the atlas instead fuse with the axis to form the dens of the axis. In mice containing the *Hoxa-7* (A7) transgene, a proatlas forms, and the atlas and axis have the form of typical vertebrae *(right column)*. (Based on studies by Kessel M, Balling R, Gruss P: *Cell* 61:301–308, 1990.)

mates of the incidence vary widely from one series to the next. Somewhat less than 1% may be a realistic estimate. These and other common rib anomalies (**forked** or **fused ribs**) are typically asymptomatic and are usually detected on x-ray examination. They are probably the result of misexpression of specific *Hox* genes.

The **sternum** arises as a pair of cartilaginous bands that converge at the ventral midline as the ventral body wall consolidates (Figure 9-18). After the primordial sternal bands come together, they reveal their true segmental nature by secondarily subdividing into craniocaudal elements. Such secondary segmentation follows an early morphological and molecular course that closely parallels the formation of synovial joints (see p. 223). Many of these ultimately fuse as they ossify to form a common unpaired body of the sternum. Several common anomalies of the sternum (e.g., **split xiphoid process**) are readily understood from its embryological development. Malformations of the xiphoid process are seen in mice mutant for both *Hoxc-4* and *Hoxa-5,* and mice mutant for *Hoxb-2* and *Hoxb-4* have split sternums.

The **clavicle** is sometimes considered to be part of the appendicular skeleton because it connects the sternum to the shoulder. The clavicle is one of the first bones in the body to become ossified, with ossification well advanced by the eighth week. Recent studies of mice heterozygous for the *Cbfa1* gene have shed light not only on the nature of the clavicle but also on a poorly understood human syndrome. Such heterozygotes exhibit hypoplasia of the clavicle, delayed ossification of membrane bones (e.g., of the skull), and open anterior and posterior fontanelles in the skull. **Cleidocranial dysplasia** in humans exhibits all of these conditions, as well as supernumerary teeth. Without clavicles, affected individuals can approximate their shoulders in the anterior midline (Figure 9-19). The findings in this mutant suggest that the clavicle is a purely membranous bone and may be a unique class of bone, being neither truly axial or appendicular in the usual sense.

Another late development is the disappearance of the notochord from the bodies of the vertebrae. Between the vertebrae the notochord expands into the condensed mesenchymal primordia of the intervertebral disks. In the adult the notochord persists as the **nucleus pulposus,** which constitutes the soft core of the disk. The bulk of the **intervertebral disk** consists of layers of fibrocartilage that differentiate from the rostral half of the sclerotome in the somite. *Pax-1* is expressed continuously during the development of intervertebral disks. In a mouse mutant, *undulated, Pax-1* expression is deficient, and fusion of the vertebral bodies results. It appears that *Pax-1* expression and the subsequent formation of the intervertebral disks

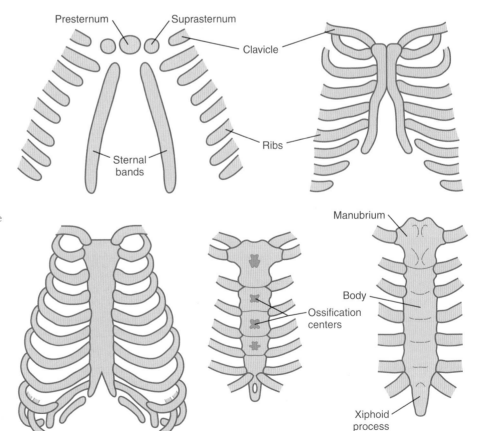

**FIGURE 9-18** Successive stages in the development of the sternum and clavicle.

**FIGURE 9-19** Drawing of a young woman with cleidocranial dysplasia. Because of the absence of clavicles, she can almost approximate her shoulders.

are important mechanisms in maintaining the individual segmental character of the vertebral column.

The caudal end of the axial skeleton is represented by a well-defined, tail-like appendage during much of the second month (Figure 9-20, A). During the third month, the tail normally regresses, largely through cell death and differential growth, to persist as the coccyx, but rarely a well-developed tail persists in newborns (Figure 9-20, B).

## Skull

The skull is a composite structure consisting of two major subdivisions: the **neurocranium**, which surrounds the brain, and the **viscerocranium**, which surrounds the oral cavity, pharynx, and upper respiratory passages. Each of

these subdivisions in turn consists of two components, one in which the individual bones are first represented by cartilaginous models and are subsequently replaced by bone through endochondral ossification and another in which bone arises directly through the ossification of mesenchyme.

The phylogenetic and ontogenetic foundation of the skull is represented by the **chondrocranium,** which is the cartilaginous base of the neurocranium (Figure 9-21, A). The fundamental pattern of the chondrocranium has been remarkably preserved in the course of phylogeny. It is initially represented by several sets of paired cartilages. One group (parachordals, hypophyseal cartilages, and trabeculae cranii) is closely related to midline structures. Caudal to the parachordal cartilages are four **occipital sclerotomes.** Along with the parachordal cartilages the occipital sclerotomes, which are homologous with precursors of the vertebrae, fuse to form the base of the occipital bone. More laterally, the chondrocranium is represented by pairs of cartilage that are associated with epithelial primordia of the sense organs (olfactory organ, eyes, and auditory organ).

The individual primordial elements of the chondrocranium undergo several patterns of growth and fusion to form the structurally complex bones of the basicranium (the occipital, sphenoid, and temporal bones as well as much of the deep bony support of the nasal cavity) (Figure 9-21, B). In addition, some of these bones (e.g., the occipital and temporal bones) incorporate membranous components during their development, so in their final form, they are truly composite structures (Figure 9-21, D). Other components of the neurocranium, such as the parietal and frontal bones, are purely membranous bones (Box 9-2).

Virtually all the bones of the neurocranium arise as the result of an inductive influence of an epithelial structure on the neighboring mesenchyme. These interactions are typically mediated by growth factors and the extracellular matrix. Immunocytochemical studies have shown the transient appearance of **type II collagen** (the principal collagenous component of cartilage) at the sites and times during which the interactions leading to the formation of the chondrocranium take place. In addition to type II collagen, a **cartilage-specific proteoglycan** also accumulates in areas of induction of chondrocranial elements. There is increasing evidence that epithelial elements in the head not only induce the skeleton but also control its morphogenesis. This contrasts with morphogenetic control of the appendicular skeleton, which is determined by the mesoderm rather than the ectoderm of the limb bud.

Elements of the membranous neurocranium (the paired parietal and frontal bones and the interparietal part of the occipital bone) arise as flat, platelike aggregations of bony spicules (trabeculae) from mesenchyme that has

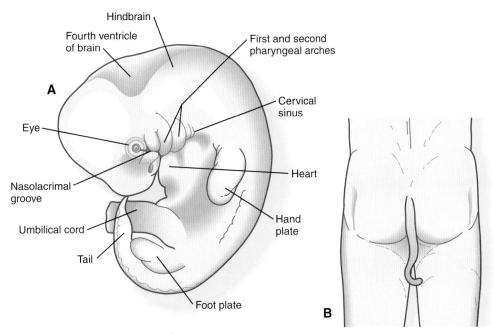

FIGURE 9-20 **A,** Drawing of a human embryo at the end of the **fifth week,** showing a prominent tail. Normally the tail regresses. **B,** Drawing of a persisting tail (9 inches long) in a **12-year-old boy. (B** modified from Patten BM: *Human embryology,* ed 3, New York, 1968, McGraw-Hill.)

## Box 9-2 Embryological Origins of Bones of the Cranium

NEUROCRANIUM

Chondrocranium
  Occipital
  Sphenoid
  Ethmoid
  Petrous and mastoid part of temporal
Membranous neurocranium
  Interparietal part of occipital
  Parietal
  Frontal
  Squamous part of temporal

VISCEROCRANIUM

**Pharyngeal Arch I**
Cartilaginous viscerocranium
  Meckel's cartilage
    Malleus
    Incus

Membranous viscerocranium
  Maxillary process (superficial)
    Squamous part of temporal
    Zygomatic
    Maxillary
    Premaxillary
    Nasal?
    Lacrimal?
  Maxillary process (deep)
    Palatine
    Vomer
    Pterygoid laminae
  Mandibular process
    Mandible
    Tympanic ring

PHARYNGEAL ARCH II

**Cartilaginous viscerocranium**
  Reichert's cartilage
  Stapes
  Styloid process

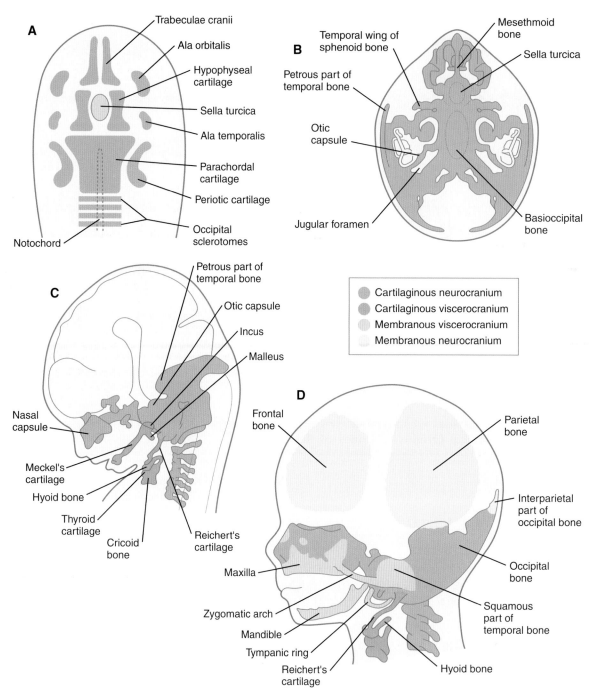

**FIGURE 9-21** Origins and development of the major skull bones. **A,** Basic skeletal elements of a **6-week-old** embryo viewed from above. **B,** Chondrocranium of an **8-week-old** embryo viewed from above. **C,** Lateral view of the embryo illustrated in **B. D,** Skull of a **3-month-old** embryo. (Modified from Carlson B: *Patten's foundations of embryology,* ed 6, New York, 1996, McGraw-Hill.)

been induced by specific parts of the developing brain. These bones remain separate structures during fetal development, and even at birth, they are separated by connective tissue sutures. Intersections between sutures where more than two bones meet are occupied by broader areas of connective tissue called **fontanelles.** The most prominent fontanelles are the **anterior fontanelle,** located at the intersection of the two frontal and two parietal bones, and the **posterior fontanelle,** located at the intersection of the parietal bones and the single occipital bone (Figure 9-22).

Like the neurocranium, the viscerocranium consists of two divisions: a **cartilaginous viscerocranium** and a **membranous viscerocranium.** In contrast to the neurocra-

**FIGURE 9-22** High-resolution computed tomographic scans of the skull of a **34½-week-old** fetus. **A,** Lateral view. **B,** Frontal view. The midline fissure in the forehead area is the metopic suture, which normally becomes obliterated after birth. The irregular black area above that is the anterior fontanelle, one of the "soft spots" in a newborn's head. (Courtesy R.A. Levy, H. Maher, and A.R. Burdi, Ann Arbor, Mich.)

nium, the bones of the viscerocranium originate largely from neural crest–derived mesenchyme. Phylogenetically, the viscerocranium is related to the skeleton of the **branchial arches** (gill arches). Each branchial arch (more commonly called a *pharyngeal arch* in humans) is supported by a cartilaginous rod, which gives rise to a number of definitive skeletal elements characteristic of that arch (see Box 9-2). (Details of the organization and derivatives of the noncranial pharyngeal arch cartilages are discussed in Chapter 14 [see Figure 14-22].)

The membranous viscerocranium consists of a series of bones associated with the upper and lower jaws and the region of the ear (see Figure 9-21, *D*). These arise in association with the first arch cartilage (**Meckel's cartilage**) and take over some of the functions originally subserved by Meckel's cartilage, as well as a number of new ones, such as sound transmission in the middle ear. Clinical Correlation 9-2 discusses conditions resulting from skull deformities.

### Appendicular Skeleton

The **appendicular skeleton** consists of the bones of the limbs and limb girdles. There are fundamental differences in organization and developmental control between the

axial and appendicular skeleton. The axial skeleton forms a protective casing around soft internal tissues (e.g., brain, spinal cord, pharynx), and the mesenchyme forming the bones is induced by the organs that the bones surround. In contrast, the bones of the appendicular skeleton form a central supporting core of the limbs. Although interaction with an epithelium (the apical ectodermal ridge of the limb bud [see Chapter 10]) is required for the formation of skeletal elements in the limb, morphogenetic control of the limb is inherent in the mesoderm, with the epithelium playing only a stimulatory role.

All components of the appendicular skeleton begin as cartilaginous models, which convert to true bone by endochondral ossification later during embryogenesis. (Details of the formation of the appendicular skeleton are given in Chapter 10.)

## MUSCULAR SYSTEM

Three types of musculature—skeletal, cardiac, and smooth—are formed during embryonic development. Virtually all skeletal musculature is derived from the paraxial mesoderm, specifically the somites or somitomeres (see Figure 6-7). Splanchnic mesoderm gives rise to the musculature of the heart (cardiac muscle) and the

## Conditions Resulting from Skull Deformities

A number of conditions are recognizable by gross deformities of the skull. Although many of these are true congenital malformations, others fall into the class of deformities that can be attributed to mechanical stress during intrauterine life or childbirth. Some malformations of the skull are secondary to disturbances in development of the brain. In this category are conditions such as **acrania** and **anencephaly** (see Figure 8-4), which are associated with severe malformations of the brain; **microcephaly** (see Figure 9-9), in which the size of the cranial vault accommodates to a very small brain; and **hydrocephaly** (see Figure 11-38), a greatly enlarged cranial vault that represents the response of the skeleton

of the head to an excessive buildup of cerebrospinal fluid.

One family of cranial malformations called **craniosynostosis** results from premature closure of certain sutures between major membrane bones of the neurocranium. Craniosynostosis is a feature of more than 100 human genetic syndromes and is seen in 1 in 3000 live births. One type, the Boston variant, is a dominant gain-of-function mutant of the homeobox-containing gene *Msx-2* expressed in both the mesenchymal tissue of the early sutures and the underlying neural tissue. Exactly how this mutation is translated into premature suture closure is not known. Premature closure of the **sagittal suture** between

**FIGURE 9-23** Frontal and lateral views of a boy with a narrow and elongated scaphocephalic skull. Note the high forehead and flat bridge of the nose. This patient had an associated facial palsy and mixed deafness. (From Goodman R, Gorlin R: *Atlas of the face in genetic disorders*, St Louis, 1977, Mosby.)

the two parietal bones produces a long, keel-shaped skull referred to as **scaphocephaly** (Figure 9-23).

**Oxycephaly,** or turret skull, is the result of premature fusion of the **coronal suture,** which is located between the frontal and parietal bones. A dominant genetic condition, **Crouzon's syndrome,** has a gross appearance quite similar to that of oxycephaly, but the malformation of the cranial vault is typically accompanied by malformations of the face, teeth, and ears and occasional malformations in other parts of the body (Figure 9-24).

**FIGURE 9-24** Lateral view of the flattened face of an individual with Crouzon's syndrome. (Courtesy A.R. Burdi, Ann Arbor, Mich.)

smooth musculature of the gut and respiratory tracts (Table 9-1). Other smooth muscle, such as that of the blood vessels and the arrector pili muscles, is derived from local mesoderm.

The development of muscle can be studied at several different levels, ranging from the determination and differentiation of individual muscle cells, to the histogenesis of muscle tissue, and finally to the formation (morphogenesis) of entire muscles. Skeletal muscle will be used as an example to illustrate how development occurs and is controlled at these different levels of organization.

## Skeletal Muscle

There is increasing evidence that certain cells of the epiblast are determined to become myogenic cells even before the somites are completely formed, but it is convenient to begin with the emergence of muscle precursor cells in the somites. For many decades the origin of the skeletal musculature was in question, with the somites and lateral mesoderm being likely candidates. This issue was finally resolved by tracing studies involving cellular markers (Box 9-3), and it is now known that virtually all of the skeletal muscle originates in somites or

TABLE 9-1 *Embryologic Origins of the Major Classes of Muscle*

| Embryologic origin | Derived muscle | Innervation |
|---|---|---|
| Somitomeres 1 through 3 and prechordal plate | Most extrinsic eye muscles | Cranial nerves III and IV |
| Somitomere 4 | Jaw-closing muscles | Cranial nerve V (mandibular branch) |
| Somitomere 5 | Lateral rectus muscle of eye | Cranial nerve VI |
| Somitomere 6 | Jaw-opening and other second-arch muscles | Cranial nerve VII |
| Somitomere 7 | Third-arch branchial muscles | Cranial nerve IX |
| Somites 1 and 2 | Intrinsic laryngeal muscles and pharyngeal muscles | Cranial nerve X |
| Occipital somites (1 through 7) | Muscles of tongue, larynx, and neck | Cranial nerves XI and XII, cranial cervical nerves |
| Trunk somites | Trunk muscles, diaphragm, and limb muscles | Spinal nerves |
| Splanchnic mesoderm | Cardiac muscle | Autonomic |
| Splanchnic mesoderm | Smooth muscles of gut and respiratory tract | Autonomic |
| Local mesenchyme | Other smooth muscle: vascular, arrector pili muscles | Autonomic |

From Carlson BM: *Patten's foundations of embryology,* ed 6, New York, 1996, McGraw-Hill.

somitomeres. Early steps in the determination of myogenic cells in somites are summarized in Figure 6-9.

### Determination and Differentiation of Skeletal Muscle

The mature skeletal muscle fiber is a complex multinucleated cell that is specialized for contraction. Precursors of most muscle lineages (**myogenic cells**) have been traced to the myotome of the somite (see Figure 6-8). Although these cells look like the mesenchymal cells that can give rise to many other cell types in the embryo, they have undergone a restriction event committing them to the muscle-forming line. Committed myogenic cells pass through several additional mitotic divisions before completing a terminal mitotic division and becoming **postmitotic myoblasts.**

Proliferating myogenic cells are kept in the cell cycle through the action of growth factors, such as **fibroblast growth factor** (FGF) and **transforming growth factor-β.** With the accumulation of myogenic regulatory factors (see next section), myogenic cells upregulate the synthesis of the cell cycle protein **p21**, which irreversibly removes them from the cell cycle. Then, under the influence of other growth factors, such as **insulin-like growth factor,** the postmitotic myoblasts begin to transcribe the mRNAs for the major contractile proteins **actin** and **myosin,** but the major event in the life cycle of a postmitotic myoblast is its fusion with other similar cells into a multinucleated **myotube** (Figure 9-26). The fusion of

myoblasts is a precise process involving their lining up and adhering by $Ca^{++}$-mediated recognition mechanisms, involving molecules such as M-cadherin, and the ultimate union of their plasma membranes.

Myotubes are intensively involved in mRNA and protein synthesis. In addition to forming actin and myosin, they synthesize a wide variety of other proteins, including the regulatory proteins of muscle contraction— **troponin** and **tropomyosin.** These proteins assemble into myofibrils, which are precisely arranged aggregates of functional contractile units called **sarcomeres.** As the myotubes fill with myofibrils, their nuclei, which had been arranged in regular central chains, migrate to the periphery of the myotube. At this stage the myotube is considered to have differentiated into a **muscle fiber,** the final stage in the differentiation of the skeletal muscle cell.

The development of a muscle fiber is not complete, however, with the peripheral migration of the nuclei of the myotube. The nuclei (**myonuclei**) of a multinucleated muscle fiber are no longer able to proliferate, but the muscle fiber must continue to grow in proportion to the rapid growth of the fetus and then the infant. Muscle fiber growth is accomplished by means of a population of myogenic cells, called **satellite cells,** which take up positions between the muscle fiber and the basal lamina in which each muscle fiber encases itself (see Figure 9-26). Operating under a poorly understood control mechanism, satellite cells divide slowly during the growth of an individual. Some of the daughter cells fuse with the muscle fiber so that the muscle fiber contains an adequate

## Box 9-3 Tracing Studies Involving Cellular Markers

The origins of many tissues in embryos have been identified by grafting tissues from quail embryos into homologous sites in chick embryos. The nuclei of quail cells contain a distinctive mass of dense chromatin and also react with a species-specific monoclonal antibody, enabling researchers to distinguish quail from chick cells with great reliability (Figure 9-25). If a putative precursor tissue is grafted from a quail into a chick embryo, the grafted quail tissue becomes well integrated into the chick host, and if cells migrate out of the graft, their pathway of migration into the host embryo can be clearly traced. Experiments involving this approach have been particularly useful in studies of muscle and the neural crest.

Chick cells

1. Remove brachial somatic mesoderm of chick

2. Replace with quail graft

Quail cells

3. Allow embryo to develop

Muscles

**FIGURE 9-25** Principle of quail/chick grafting for the tracing of cells. 1 and 2, Quail tissues are transplanted in place of the equivalent tissues removed from the chick embryo. The prominent nuclear chromatin mass in quail cells provides a permanent marker that can be used to trace the fate of the cells of the graft of quail tissue. 3, When quail somites are grafted into a chick embryo at the appropriate level, the muscles of the limb are derived from quail and not chick cells.

number of nuclei to direct the continuing synthesis of contractile proteins required by the muscle fiber. After muscle fiber damage, satellite cells proliferate and fuse to form regenerating muscle fibers.

A typical muscle is not composed of homogeneous muscle fibers. Instead, usually several types of muscle fibers are distinguished by their contractile properties and morphology and by their possession of different isoforms of the contractile proteins. For the purposes of this text, muscle fibers are considered to be either fast or slow.

### Muscle Transcription Factors

Myogenesis begins with a restriction event that channels a population of mesenchymal cells into a lineage of committed myogenic cells. The molecular basis for this commitment is the action of members of families of **myogenic regulatory factors** that, acting as master genetic regulators, turn on muscle-specific genes in the premuscle mesenchymal cells.

The first-discovered family of myogenic regulatory factors is a group of four basic helix-loop-helix tran-

**FIGURE 9-26** Stages in the morphological differentiation of a skeletal muscle fiber. Important subcellular elements in a muscle fiber are also shown.

scription factors, sometimes called the **MyoD family** (Figure 9-27). Another, more recently discovered regulatory factor, called **muscle enhancer factor-2** (MEF-2), appears to work downstream from or in concert with the MyoD family, but all of these myogenic regulatory factors are capable of converting nonmuscle cells (e.g., fibroblasts, adipocytes, chondrocytes, retinal pigment cells) to cells expressing the full range of muscle proteins.

As with many helix-loop-helix proteins, myogenic regulatory proteins of the MyoD family form dimers and

bind to a specific DNA sequence (CANNTG), called the **E box**, in the enhancer region of muscle-specific genes. The myogenic specificity of these proteins is encoded in the basic region (see Figure 9-27).

The regulatory activities of MyoD and other members of that family are themselves regulated by other regulatory proteins, which can modify their activities (Figure 9-28). For example, many cells contain a **transcriptional activator** designated E12. When a molecule of E12 forms a **heterodimer** with a molecule of MyoD, the complex

**FIGURE 9-27** Structural comparison of several myogenic regulatory factors. *H-L-H,* Homologous helix-loop-helix regions; *S-T,* homologous serine/threonine-rich region.

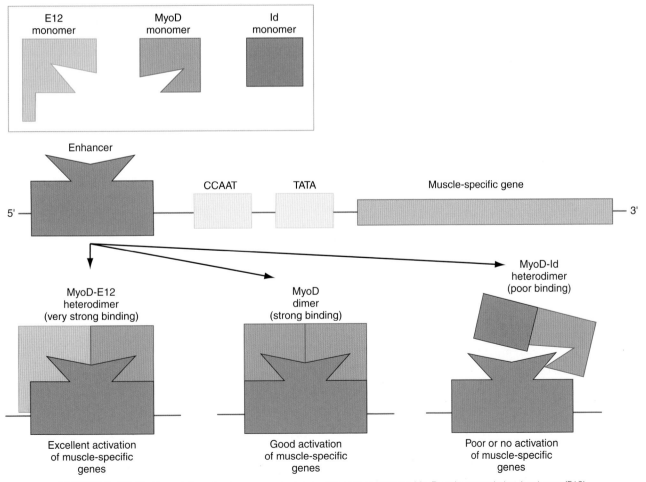

**FIGURE 9-28** MyoD regulation of early myogenesis, showing interactions between MyoD and a transcriptional activator *(E12)* and a transcriptional inhibitor *(Id).*

binds more tightly to the muscle-enhancer region of DNA than does a pure MyoD dimer. This increases the efficiency of transcription of the muscle genes. On the other hand, a **transcriptional inhibitor** called **Id** (inhibitor of DNA binding) can form a heterodimer with a molecule of MyoD. Id contains a loop-helix-loop region but no basic region, which is the DNA-binding part of the molecule. The Id molecule has a greater binding affinity for a MyoD molecule than another molecule of MyoD and can thus displace one of the units of a MyoD dimer, resulting in more Id-MyoD heterodimers. These bind very poorly to DNA and often fail to activate muscle-specific genes.

During muscle development, the myogenic regulatory factors of the MyoD family are expressed in a regular sequence (Figure 9-29). In mice the events leading to muscle formation begin in the somite, where both **Pax-3** and **myf-5**, working through apparently separate pathways, activate **MyoD**, causing certain cells of the dermomyotome to become committed to forming muscle. With increased levels of MyoD, the mononuclear cells withdraw from the mitotic cycle and begin to fuse into myotubes. At this stage **myogenin** is expressed. Finally, in maturing myotubes, **MRF-4** is expressed. Interestingly, in knockout mice, the absence of a single myogenic regulatory factor (e.g., myf-5, MyoD) alone does not prevent the formation of skeletal muscle (although there may be other minor observable defects), but when myf-5 and MyoD are knocked out simultaneously, muscle fails to form. Another very instructive double knockout of Pax-3 and myf-5 produces mice that are totally lacking in muscles of the trunk and limbs, but the head musculature remains intact. This shows that in the very earliest stages of determination, different regulatory pathways are followed by muscle-forming cells of the head and trunk.

This has been borne out by the recent recognition that the development of certain cranial muscles (primarily those derived from the first pharyngeal arch, see Chapter 14) is controlled by a different set of transcription factors, called **MyoR** and **capsulin**. In view of this, it is highly likely that a different set of transcription factors will be found to control development of the muscles of facial expression, which are derived from the second pharyngeal arch.

Muscle growth is negatively controlled, as well. **Myostatin**, a member of the TGF-β family of signaling molecules, arrests muscle growth once a muscle has attained its normal size. In the absence of myostatin function, animals develop a grossly hypertrophic musculature. Breeds of "double-muscled" cattle are known to have mutations of the myostatin gene.

Because each of the regulators, activators, and inhibitors is itself a protein, their formation is subject to similar positive and negative controls. The complex examples of the regulation of the first steps in myogenesis give some idea of the multiple levels of the control of gene expression and the stages of cytodifferentiation in mammals. Although the molecular aspects of myogenesis are better understood than the stages underlying the differentiation of most cell types, it is likely that similar sets of interlinked regulatory mechanisms operate in the differentiation of most cell types.

## Histogenesis of Muscle

Muscle as a tissue consists not only of muscle fibers but also of connective tissue, blood vessels, and nerves. Even the muscle fibers themselves are not homogeneous but can be separated into functionally and biochemically different types.

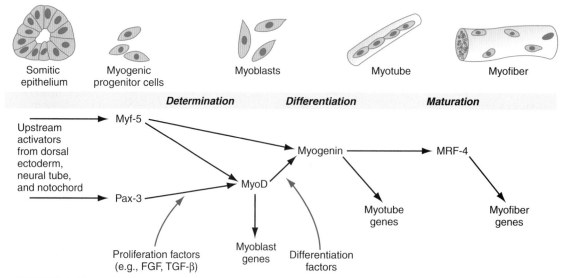

**FIGURE 9-29** Schematic representation of early myogenesis, showing the sequence of expression of myogenic regulatory factors and other influences on the myogenic process.

As muscles first form, the myoblasts are intermingled with future connective tissue mesenchyme. The role of the connective tissue in the morphogenesis of a muscle is discussed in the next section. Capillary sprouts grow into the forming muscle for nourishment, and motor nerve fibers enter shortly after the first myoblasts begin forming myotubes.

At one time, it was thought that all myoblasts were essentially identical and that their different characteristics (e.g., fast or slow) were imposed on them by their motor innervation. Recent research, however, has shown that in birds and several species of mammals, there are distinct populations of fast and slow muscle cells as early as the myoblast stage, well before nerve fibers reach the developing muscles.

Not only are there fast and slow myoblasts, but there are also early and late cellular isoforms of myoblasts, which have different requirements for serum factors and nerve interactions in their differentiation. When the earliest myoblasts fuse into myotubes, they give rise to **primary myotubes,** which form the initial basis for an embryonic muscle. The differentiation of primary myotubes occurs before motor nerve axons have entered the newly forming muscle. Subsequently, smaller **secondary myotubes** arising from late myoblasts form alongside the primary myotubes (Figure 9-30). By the time secondary myotubes form, early motor axons are present in the muscles, and there is evidence that the presence of nerves is required for the formation of secondary myotubes. A primary muscle fiber and its associated secondary muscle fibers are initially contained within a common basal lamina and are electrically coupled. These muscle fibers actively synthesize a wide variety of contractile proteins.

Early in their life history, embryonic muscle fibers are innervated by motor neurons. Although it has long been assumed that fast and slow motoneurons impose their own functional characteristics on the developing muscle fibers, it now appears that they may select muscle fibers of a compatible type through information contained on their cell surfaces. Initially, a motor nerve may terminate on both fast and slow muscle fibers, but ultimately, inappropriate connections are broken, so fast nerve fibers innervate only fast muscle fibers, and slow nerves innervate only slow muscle fibers.

The phenotypes of muscle fibers depend on the nature of the specific proteins that make up their contractile apparatus. There are qualitative differences between fast and slow muscle fibers in many of the contractile proteins, and within each type of muscle fiber, there is a succession of isoforms of major proteins during embryonic development. (The isoform transitions of **myosin** in a developing muscle fiber are used as an example.)

The myosin molecule is complex, consisting of two heavy chains and a series of four light chains (LCs) (Figure 9-31). Mature fast fibers have one LC1, two LC2, and one LC3 subunits; slow muscle myosin contains two LC1 and two LC2 subunits. In addition, there are fast and slow forms ($MHC_f$ and $MHC_s$) of the **myosin heavy chain** subunits. The myosin molecules possess adenosinetriphosphatase activity, and differences in this activity partly account for differences in the speed of contraction between fast and slow muscle fibers.

The myosin molecule undergoes a succession of isoform transitions during development. From the fetal period to maturity a series of three developmental isoforms of the myosin heavy chain (embryonic [$MHC_{emb}$],

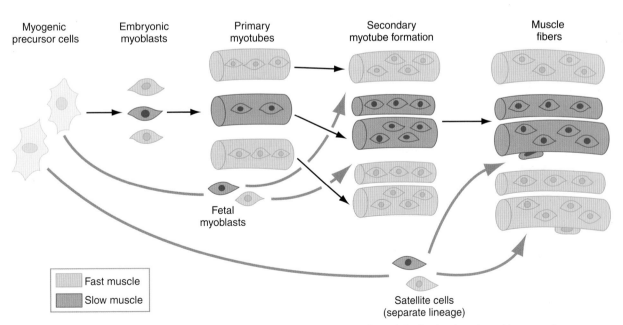

**FIGURE 9-30** Stages in the formation of primary and secondary muscle fibers. A family of embryonic myoblasts contributes to the formation of the primary myotubes, and fetal myoblasts contribute to secondary myotubes.

**Myosin molecule**

**FIGURE 9-31** Changes in myosin subunits during the development of a fast muscle fiber. A schematic representation of the myosin molecule is also shown.

neonatal [$MHC_{neo}$], and adult fast [$MHC_f$]) pass through a fast muscle fiber. (Developmental changes in the light and heavy chain subunits are summarized in Figure 9-31.) Other contractile proteins of muscle fibers (e.g., actin, troponin) pass through similar isoform transitions. After injury to muscle in the adult the regenerating muscle fibers undergo sets of cellular and molecular isoform transitions that closely recapitulate those occurring in normal ontogenesis.

The phenotype of muscle fibers is not irreversibly fixed. Even postnatal muscle fibers possess a remarkable degree of plasticity. They respond to exercise by undergoing hypertrophy or becoming more resistant to fatigue. On the other hand, they adapt to inactivity or denervation by becoming atrophic. All these changes are accompanied by various changes in gene expression. Many other types of cells can also modify their phenotypes in response to changes in the environment, but the molecular changes are not always as striking as those seen in muscle fibers.

## Morphogenesis of Muscle

At a higher level of organization, muscle development involves the formation of anatomically identifiable muscles. The overall form of a muscle is determined principally by its connective tissue framework rather than the myoblasts themselves. Experiments have shown that myogenic cells from somites are essentially interchangeable. For example, myogenic cells from somites that would normally form muscles of the trunk can participate in the formation of normal leg muscles. In contrast, the cells of the connective tissue component of the muscles appear to be imprinted with the morphogenetic blueprint.

## Muscles of the Trunk and Limbs

Quail/chick grafting experiments have clearly shown that the major groups of skeletal muscles in the trunk and limbs arise from myogenic precursors located in the somites. In the thorax and abdomen, the intrinsic muscles of the back (the **epaxial muscles**) are derived from cells arising in the dorsal myotomal lip, whereas ventrolateral muscles (**hypaxial muscles**) arise from epithelially organized ventral buds of the somites. In the limb regions, myogenic cells migrate from the epithelium of the ventrolateral dermomyotome early during development. More cranial myogenic cells originating in similar regions of the occipital somites migrate into the developing tongue and diaphragm. At the lumbar levels, precursors of the abdominal muscles also move out of the epithelium of ventrolateral somitic buds. Early specification of the future hypaxial musculature within the epithelial somite is initially regulated by dorsalizing (possibly a member of the Wnt family) and lateralizing (BMP-4) signals from the ectoderm and lateral mesoderm, respectively. This leads to a more intense expression of *Pax-3* and the expression of *Lbx-1*, a homeobox gene that is exclusively expressed in the lateral dermomyotomal lips. *Lbx-1* may prevent the premature differentiation of the hypaxial musculature. It is highly likely that the **prune-belly syndrome**, which is characterized by the absence of the abdominal musculature (Figure 9-32), will be found to be caused by a molecular deficiency in this population of myogenic cells.

Recent experiments have shown different cellular behavior in areas of the myotomes adjacent to limb and nonlimb regions. In thoracic segments, cells of the dermatome surround the lateral edges of the myotome. This is followed by an increase in the number of myotubes formed in the myotome and the penetration of the muscle primordia into the body wall. In contrast, at the levels of the limb buds, dermatome cells die before surrounding the early myotubes that form in the myotome. These myotubes neither increase significantly in number nor move out from the myotomes to form separate muscle primordia.

After their origin from the somites, the muscle primordia of the trunk and abdomen become organized into well-defined groups and layers (Figure 9-33). (Morphogenesis of the limb muscles is discussed in Chapter 10.) The results of a number of experiments have demonstrated fundamental differences in cellular properties between the cellular precursors of limb muscles and axial muscles. These are summarized in Table 9-2.

## Muscles of the Head and Cervical Region

The skeletal muscle of the head and neck is mesodermal in origin. Quail/chick grafting experiments have shown that the paraxial mesoderm, specifically the somitomeres, constitutes the main source of the cranial musculature,

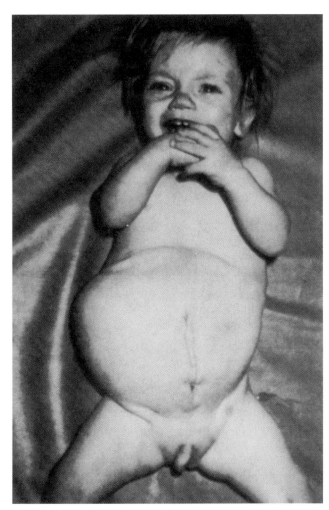

**FIGURE 9-32** Child with prune-belly syndrome. The abdominal musculature is absent or very hypoplastic. Urinary defects commonly accompany this defect. Note the characteristic dimples on the knees. (From Wigglesworth J, Singer D: *Textbook of fetal and perinatal pathology,* Oxford, England, 1991, Blackwell Scientific.)

**FIGURE 9-33** Groups and layers of trunk muscles.

**TABLE 9-2** *Differences between Cellular Precursors of Axial and Limb Muscles*

| Axial muscles | Limb muscles |
|---|---|
| Are mostly located in medial half of somite | Are located in lateral half of somite |
| Differentiate largely in situ | Migrate into limb buds before differentiating |
| Initial differentiation in mononucleate myocytes | Initial differentiation in multinucleate myotubes |
| Myogenic determination factors (Myf-5, MyoD) are expressed at or before the onset of myotome formation | Expression of myogenic determination genes is delayed until limb muscle masses begin to coalesce |
| Differentiation seems strongly influenced by neural tube and notochord | Migration and differentiation are little influenced by axial structures |

although some question still remains about the origin of the extraocular muscles. At least some of the cells that make up the extraocular muscles arise from the prechordal plate of the early embryo. There is increasing evidence that in some aspects, myogenesis in the head differs significantly from that in the trunk. Different controls at the level of myogenic determination between the head and the trunk have already been discussed. Also, a number of the craniofacial muscles have different phenotypic properties from trunk muscles (e.g., myosin isoforms and possibly elements of neuromuscular control of phenotype).

As with muscles in the trunk, muscles in the head and neck arise by the movement of myogenic cells away from the paraxial mesoderm through mesenchyme (either neural crest derived or mesodermal) on their way to their final destination. Morphogenesis of muscles in the cranial region appears to be determined by information inherent in the connective tissues that ensheathe the muscles. There is no early level specificity in the paraxial myogenic cells. This has been determined by grafting somites or somitomeres from one craniocaudal level to another. In these cases, the myogenic cells that leave the grafted structures form muscles normal for the region into which they migrate rather than muscles appropriate for the level of origin of the grafted somites.

Certain muscles of the head, in particular those of the tongue, arise from the occipital somites in the manner of trunk muscles and undergo extensive migration into the enlarging head. Their more caudal level of origin is evidenced by the innervation by the **hypoglossal nerve** (twelfth cranial nerve), which, according to some comparative anatomists, is a series of highly modified spinal nerves. Like the myogenic cells of the limb, precursor cells of the tongue musculature express *Pax-3* while they are migrating into the head. Despite their final location in the head, these muscles are subjected to the same types of early molecular regulation of myogenesis as trunk muscles.

### Anomalies of Skeletal Muscles

Variations and anomalies of skeletal muscles are common. Some, such as the absence of portions of the pectoralis major muscle, are associated with malformations of other structures. Further discussion of anomalies of specific muscles requires a level of anatomical knowledge beyond that assumed for this text.

**Muscular dystrophy** is a family of genetic diseases characterized by the repeated degeneration and regeneration of various groups of muscles during postnatal life. In Duchenne muscular dystrophy, which occurs in young boys, a membrane-associated protein called **dystrophin** is lacking from the muscle fibers. Its absence makes the muscle fibers more susceptible to damage when physically stressed.

## Cardiac Muscle

Although a striated muscle, cardiac muscle differs from skeletal muscles in many aspects of embryonic development. Derived from the splanchnic mesoderm of the early embryo, cardiac muscle cells arise from cells present in the myocardium. Differences between the differentiation of cardiac and skeletal muscle appear early, since MyoD and other common master regulators of skeletal muscle differentiation are not expressed in early cardiac muscle development. Yet, both cardiac and skeletal muscle precursors express the MADS (MCM1, Agamous, Deficiens, and serum response factor) box-containing transcription factor MEF-2, which in skeletal muscle, at least, dimerizes with other transcription factors to regulate the formation of some of the major contractile proteins of the myocytes. Early cardiac and skeletal muscle cells express isoforms of molecules that are characteristic of mature cells of the other type. For example, both cardiac and skeletal muscle cells in the embryo express high levels of cardiac $\alpha$-actin; however, after birth, expression of this molecule declines in skeletal muscle but remains high in cardiac muscle. Interestingly, in cardiac hypertrophy, mature cardiac muscle cells begin to express large amounts of skeletal $\alpha$-actin mRNA.

Even early cardiac myoblasts contain relatively large numbers of myofibrils in their cytoplasm, and they are capable of undergoing pronounced contractions. In the embryo the mononucleated cardiac myocytes face a difficult problem: the cells of the developing heart must continue to contract while the heart is increasing in mass. This functional requirement necessitates that cardiac myocytes undergo mitosis even though their cytoplasm

contains many bundles of contractile filaments (Figure 9-34). Cells of the body often lose their ability to divide when their cytoplasm contains structures characteristic of the differentiated state. Cardiac myocytes deal with this problem by partially disassembling their contractile filaments during mitosis. In contrast to skeletal muscle, cardiac myocytes do not undergo fusion but rather remain as individual cells, although they may become binucleated. Cardiac myocytes keep in close structural and functional contact through **intercalated disks**, which join adjacent cells to one another.

Later in development a network of cardiac muscle cells undergoes an alternative pathway of differentiation characterized by increased size, a reduction in the concentration of myofibrils, and a greatly increased concentration of glycogen in the cytoplasm. These cells form the **conducting system**, parts of which are called **Purkinje fibers**. Purkinje fibers also express a different profile of contractile protein isoforms from either atrial or ventricular myocytes.

## Smooth Muscle

As with cardiac muscle, much of the smooth muscle in the body arises from splanchnic mesoderm. Exceptions are the ciliary muscle and sphincter pupillae muscles of the eye, which are derived from neural crest ectoderm, and much of the vascular smooth muscle, which frequently arises from the local mesoderm. Very little is known about the morphology and mechanisms underlying the differentiation of smooth muscle cells.

## SUMMARY

○ The epidermis starts as a single layer of ectoderm, to which a single superficial layer of peridermal cells is added. As other layers are added, three cell types migrate from other sources: (1) melanoblasts (pigment cells) from the neural crest, (2) Langerhans' cells (immune cells) from precursors in the bone marrow, and (3) Merkel cells (mechanoreceptors), from the neural crest.

○ In the multilayered epidermis, unspecialized cells from the stratum basale differentiate as they move through the various layers toward the surface of the epidermis. The cells produce increasing amounts of intracellular keratins and filaggrin; the latter is involved in the interconnections of the keratinocytes, the final differentiated form of the epidermal cell.

○ In the trunk, the dermis arises from mesodermal cells derived from the dermatome of the somites. Dermal/epidermal interactions underlie the formation of epidermal appendages such as hairs. In mammary glands, hormonal influences are important in the development of the duct system after the ductal epithelium is induced.

**Precardiac mesoderm**

Myocytes in the wall of the cardiac tube

Dividing cell

Myocytes in later embryogenesis

Dividing cell

Postnatal myocytes

**FIGURE 9-34** Stages in the histogenesis of cardiac muscle. During mitosis, the contractile filaments undergo a partial disassembly. (Modified from Rumyantsev P: *Cardiomyocytes in processes of reproduction, differentiation and regeneration [in Russian]*, Leningrad, 1982, Nauka.)

## CLINICAL VIGNETTE

A pediatrician notices that a new patient, a 1½-year-old boy, has a shorter-than-normal neck and hair farther down the neck than usual. A family history produces no evidence of other similarly affected relatives. X-ray examination reveals that the boy's neck contains only six cervical vertebrae. The pediatrician then asks if the mother could remember taking or being exposed to certain compounds during early pregnancy.

1. Which of the following does the doctor suspect as possibly being related to the boy's condition?
    A. Folic acid
    B. Retinoic acid
    C. Cocaine
    D. Thalidomide
    E. Alcohol
2. A disturbance in what class of molecules is suspected to underlie this condition?
    A. *Hox* genes
    B. *Pax* genes
    C. Myogenic regulatory factors
    D. FGF
    E. Hedgehog proteins

○ Skeletal tissue arises from the mesenchyme of either mesodermal or neural crest origin. There are two major subdivisions of the skeleton: the axial skeleton of the trunk and the appendicular skeleton of the limbs.

○ The fundamental organization of the cranial components of the vertebral column is closely associated with expression of the homeobox-containing genes. Superimposed on this is the induction of many components of the axial skeleton by underlying ectodermal (usually neural) structures. Individual vertebrae are composite structures consisting of components derived from two adjoining somites.

○ The skull consists of two subdivisions: the neurocranium, which surrounds the brain, and the viscerocranium, which surrounds the oral cavity. The base of the neurocranium (chondrocranium) is initially represented by several sets of paired cartilage. These later become transformed into bone. Most bones surrounding the brain are formed by intramembranous bone, which differentiates directly from mesenchyme. The viscerocranium is also derived from cartilaginous and membranous components.

○ Skeletal muscle fibers undergo a sequence of differentiation from mononuclear myoblasts. First, they fuse to form multinucleated myotubes, and then they mature into skeletal muscle fibers. Mononucleated reserve cells (satellite cells) can proliferate and fuse to growing or mechanically stressed muscle fibers.

○ Pax-3 and myf-5 (a member of the MyoD transcription factor family) stimulate myogenic progenitor cells of the trunk to form myoblasts. Other regulatory factors can activate (e.g., E12) or inhibit (e.g., Id) the activities of muscle regulatory factors. Early myogenic cells are kept in the cell cycle by growth factors such as FGF and transforming growth factor-β. Myoblasts are characterized by the expression of MyoD, and growth factors such as insulin-like growth factor promote their fusion and differentiation into myotubes, which express myogenin.

○ The first multinucleated muscle fibers to form are primary myotubes. Secondary myotubes form around them. Innervation by motor nerve fibers is necessary for the full differentiation of muscle fibers. During the differentiative process, several sets of isoforms of myosin subunits and other contractile proteins appear in sequence in the muscle fibers.

○ Skeletal muscles of the limbs and trunk arise from cellular precursors in the somites. The cranial musculature arises from the somitomeres. Dorsal and ventral muscles of the trunk arise from precursors located in different regions of the somites. The limb musculature also arises from cells in the ventrolateral regions of the somites. These cells migrate into the limb buds and express *Pax-3* while migrating.

○ Cardiac muscle arises from splanchnic mesoderm. Cardiomyocytes differ from skeletal muscle cells in that they can divide mitotically after they are highly differentiated and contain contractile filaments.

## Review Questions

1. Satellite cells of muscle are activated under which of these conditions?
   A. Normal muscle fiber growth
   B. Muscle fiber regeneration
   C. Muscle fiber hypertrophy
   D. All of the above
   E. None of the above

2. Which cellular component of the epidermis is a peripheral outpost of the immune system and functions to present antigens to other immune cells?
   A. Merkel cells
   B. Keratinocytes
   C. Basal cells
   D. Melanocytes
   E. Langerhans' cells

3. Which structure is mesodermal in origin?
   A. Hair shaft
   B. Mammary duct
   C. Sebaceous gland
   D. Arrector pili muscle
   E. None of the above

4. Craniosynostosis is caused by an abnormal developmental course of the:
   A. Foramen magnum
   B. Cranial sutures
   C. Basicranium
   D. Jaws
   E. None of the above

5. Which myogenic regulatory factor is expressed latest in the development of a muscle fiber?
   A. Myogenin
   B. MyoD
   C. MRF-4
   D. myf-5
   E. Pax-3

6. In the let-down of milk during lactation, the myoepithelial cells contract in response to:
   A. Progesterone
   B. Oxytocin
   C. Estrogens
   D. Lactalbumin
   E. Casein

7. What component of the developing skin determines the nature of the hairs that form or the thickness of the epidermis in the fetus?

8. A male has two bilaterally symmetrical brownish spots about 8 mm in diameter located on the skin about 3 inches below each nipple. What is one explanation for them?

9. Why is cranial bone typically not found over an area where part of the brain is missing?

10. How was it determined that the limb musculature arises from the somites?

## REFERENCES

### Skin

Babler WJ: Embryologic development of epidermal ridges and their configurations, *Birth Defects* 27:95–112, 1991.

Chuong C-M and others: Early events during avian skin appendage regeneration: dependence on epithelial-mesenchymal interaction and order of molecular reappearance, *J Invest Dermatol* 107:639–646, 1996.

Chuong C-M and others: Sonic hedgehog signaling pathway in vertebrate epithelial appendage morphogenesis: perspectives in development and evolution, *Cell Mol Life Sci* 57:1672–1681, 2000.

Cummins H: The topographic history of the volar pads (walking pads; Tastballen) in the human embryo, *Carnegie Contr Embryol* 113:103–126, 1929.

Duboule D: Hox is in the hair: a break in colinearity? *Genes Devel* 12:1–4, 1998.

Duernberger H, Kratochwil K: Specificity of time interaction and origin of mesenchymal cells in the androgen response of the embryonic mammary gland, *Cell* 19:465–471, 1980.

Goldsmith LA, ed: *Physiology, biochemistry, and molecular biology of the skin*, ed 2, New York, 1991, Oxford University.

Halata Z, Grim M, Christ B: Origin of spinal cord meninges, sheaths of peripheral nerves, and cutaneous receptors, including Merkel cells, *Anat Embryol* 182:529–537, 1990.

Hall BK: Development of the clavicles in birds and mammals, *J Exp Zool* 289:153–161, 2001.

Holbrook KA: Structure and function of the developing human skin. In Goldsmith LA, ed: *Physiology, biochemistry, and molecular biology of the skin*, ed 2, New York, 1991, Oxford University, pp 63–110.

Imagawa W and others: Control of mammary gland development. In Knobil E, Neill JD, eds: *The physiology of reproduction*, ed 2, New York, 1994, Raven, pp 1033–1063.

Jones PH, Harper S, Watt FM: Stem cell patterning and fate in human epidermis, *Cell* 80:83–93, 1995.

Kimura S: Embryologic development of flexion creases, *Birth Defects* 27:113–129, 1991.

Krey AK and others: Morphogenesis and malformations of the skin, NICHD/NIADDK research workshop, *J Invest Dermatol* 88:464–473, 1987.

Manley NR and others: *Hobx2* and *Hoxb4* act together to specify ventral body wall formation, *Devel Biol* 237:130–144, 2001.

Millar S: The role of patterning genes in epidermal differentiation. In Cowin P, Klymkowsky MW, eds: *Cytoskeletal-membrane interactions and signal transduction*, Austin, Texas, 1997, Landes Bioscience, pp 87–102.

Olivera-Martinez and others: Dorsal dermis development depends upon a signal from the dorsal neural tube, which can be substituted by Wnt-1, *Mech Devel* 100:233–244, 2001.

Oro AE, Scott MP: Splitting hairs: dissecting roles of signaling systems in epidermal development, *Cell* 95:575–578, 1998.

Polakowska RR and others: Apoptosis in human skin development: morphogenesis, periderm, and stem cells, *Dev Dynam* 199:176–188, 1994.

Robinson GW, Karpf ABC, Kratochwil K: Regulation of mammary gland development by tissue interaction, *J Mamm Gland Biol Neoplasia* 4:9–19, 1999.

Sakakura T, Sakagami Y, Nishizuka Y: Dual origin of mesenchymal tissues participating in mouse mammary gland morphogenesis, *Dev Biol* 91:202–207, 1982.

Saxod R: Ontogeny of the cutaneous sensory organs, *Microscop Res Tech* 34:313–333, 1996.

Sengel P: *Morphogenesis of skin*, Cambridge, Mass, 1976, Cambridge University.

Strobl H and others: Epidermal Langerhans cell development and differentiation, *Immunobiology* 198:588–605, 1998.

### Skeleton

Balling R and others: Development of the skeletal system, *Ciba Found Symp* 165:132–143, 1992.

Bosma JF, ed: *Symposium on development of the basicranium*, DHEW Pub No (NIH) 76–989, Washington, DC, 1976, US Government Printing Office.

Cohen MM: Merging the old skeletal biology with the new, I and II, *J Craniofac Genet Dev Biol* 20:84–106, 2000.

Cohen MM: Craniofacial disorders caused by mutations in homeobox genes MSX1 and MSX2, *J Craniofac Genet Dev Biol* 20:19–25, 2000.

DeLise AM, Fischer L, Tuan RS: Cellular interactions and signaling in cartilage development, *Osteoarthrit Cart* 8:309–334, 2000.

Hall BK: Divide, accumulate, differentiate: cell condensation in skeletal development revisited, *Int J Devel Biol* 39:881–893, 1995.

Hanken J, Hall BK, eds: *The skull*, vol 1, *Development*, Chicago, 1993, University of Chicago.

Hehr U, Muenke M: Craniosynostosis syndromes: from genes to premature fusion of skull bones, *Mol Genet Metabol* 68:139–151, 1999.

Horan GSB and others: Mutations in paralogous Hox genes result in overlapping homeotic transformations of the axial skeleton: evidence for unique and redundant function, *Dev Biol* 169:359–372, 1995.

Huang R and others: Sclerotomal origin of the ribs, *Development* 127:527–532, 2000.

Karsenty G: Genetics of skeletogenesis, *Devel Genet* 22:301–313, 1998.

Kessel M: Molecular coding of axial positions by Hox genes, *Semin Dev Biol* 2:367–373, 1991.

Kessel M: Respecification of vertebral identities by retinoic acid, *Development* 115:487–501, 1992.

Kessel M, Balling R, Gruss P: Variations of cervical vertebrae after expression of a Hox-1.1 transgene in mice, *Cell* 61:301–308, 1990.

Liu YH and others: Premature suture closure and ectopic cranial bone in mice expressing msx2 transgenes in the development skull, *Proc Natl Acad Sci USA* 92:6137–6141, 1995.

Monsoro-Burq A-H and others: Heterogeneity in the development of the vertebra, *Proc Natl Acad Sci USA* 91:10435–10439, 1994.

Rodan GA, Harada S-I: The missing bone, *Cell* 89:677–680, 1997.

Schierhorn H: Ueber die Persistenz der embryonalen Schwanzknospe beim Menschen, *Anat Anz* 127:307–337, 1970.

Sensenig EC: The early development of the human vertebral column, *Carnegie Contr Embryol* 33:21–42, 1949.

Theiler K: Vertebral malformations, *Adv Anat Embryol Cell Biol* 112:1–99, 1988.

Verbout AJ: The development of the vertebral column, *Adv Anat Embryol Cell Biol* 90:1–122, 1985.

Vortkamp A and others: Regulation of rate of cartilage differentiation by Indian hedgehog and PTH-related protein, *Science* 273:613–622, 1996.

### Muscle

Arnold H-H, Braun T: Targeted inactivation of myogenic factor genes reveals their role during mouse myogenesis: a review, *Int J Dev Biol* 40:345–363, 1996.

Brand-Saberi B, Christ B: Genetic and epigenetic control of muscle development in vertebrates, *Cell Tissue Res* 296:199–212, 1999.

Christ B, Jacob M, Jacob HJ: On the origin and development of the ventrolateral abdominal muscles in the avian embryo: an experimental and ultrastructural study, *Anat Embryol* 166:87–102, 1983.

Currie PD, Ingham PW: The generation and interpretation of positional information within the vertebrate myotome, *Mech Devel* 73:3–21, 1998.

Dietrich S: Regulation of hypaxial muscle development, *Cell Tissue Res* 296:175–182, 1999.

Hans-Henning A, Braun T: Targeted inactivation of myogenic factor genes reveals their role during mouse myogenesis: a review, *Int J Dev Biol* 40:345–363, 1996.

Hughes SM, Salinas PC: Control of muscle fibre and motoneuron diversification, *Curr Opin Neurobiol* 9:54–64, 1999.

Kablar B and others: Myogenic determination occurs independently in somites and limb buds, *Devel Biol* 206:219–231, 1999.

Kieny M and others: Origin and development of avian skeletal musculature, *Reprod Nutr Dev* 28(3B):673–686, 1988.

Lu J-R and others: Control of facial muscle development by MyoR and capsulin, *Science* 298:2378–2381, 2002.

Ludolph DC, Konieczny SF: Transcription factor families: muscling in on the myogenic program, *FASEB J* 9:1595–1604, 1995.

Maroto M and others: Ectopic Pax-3 activates MyoD and myf-5 expression in embryonic mesoderm and neural tissue, *Cell* 89:139–148, 1997.

Molkentin JD, Olson EN: Defining the regulatory networks for muscle development, *Curr Opin Genet Devel* 6:445–453, 1996.

Noden DM: The embryonic origins of avian cephalic and cervical muscles and associated connective tissues, *Am J Anat* 168:257–276, 1983.

Rong PM and others: The neural tube/notochord complex is necessary for vertebral but not limb and body wall striated muscle differentiation, *Development* 115:657–672, 1992.

Rumyantsev PP: *Cardiomyocytes in processes of reproduction, differentiation and regeneration* (in Russian), Leningrad, 1982, Nauka.

Sabourin LA, Rudnicki MA: The molecular regulation of myogenesis, *Clin Genet* 57:16–25, 2000.

Sanes JR, Donoghue MJ, Merlie JP: Positional differences among adult skeletal muscle fibers. In Kelly AM, Blau HM, eds: *Neuromuscular development and disease*, New York, 1992, Raven, pp 195–209.

Sasson D: Myogenic regulatory factors: dissecting their role and regulation during vertebrate embryogenesis, *Dev Biol* 156:11–23, 1993.

Spiller MP and others: The myostatin gene is a downstream target gene of basic helix-loop-helix transcription factor MyoD, *Mol Cell Biol* 22:7066–7082, 2002.

Tajbakhsh S and others: Redefining the genetic hierarchies controlling skeletal myogenesis, *Cell* 89:127–138, 1997.

Walsh K, Perlman H: Cell cycle exit upon myogenic differentiation, *Curr Opin Genet Devel* 7:597–602, 1997.

Wigmore PM, Dunglison GF: The generation of fiber diversity during myogenesis, *Int J Devel Biol* 42:117–125, 1998.

# Limb Development

Limbs are remarkable structures that are designed almost solely for mechanical functions: motion and force. These functions are achieved through the coordinated development of various tissue components. No single tissue in the limb takes shape without reference to the other tissues with which it is associated. The limb as a whole develops according to a master blueprint that reveals itself sequentially with each successive stage in limb formation. Many of the factors that control limb development cannot be seen by examining morphology alone, but rather must be demonstrated by experimental means or through the localization of molecules. Despite remarkable recent progress in understanding the molecular basis of the tissue interactions that control limb development, many fundamental questions remain poorly understood. Important among these are what initiates the development of a limb, what determines the individual identity of the digits, and how a developing extremity turns out to be an arm or a leg. Limb anomalies are common and highly visible. Many of these are now known to be reflections of disturbances in specific cellular or molecular interactions that are fundamental to limb development. These are discussed in Clinical Correlation 10-1 at the end of the chapter.

## INITIATION OF LIMB DEVELOPMENT

Limb formation begins relatively late in embryonic development (at the end of the fourth week in humans) with the activation of a group of mesenchymal cells in the somatic lateral mesoderm (Figure 10-1). The initial stimulus for limb development remains incompletely understood, but it has been suggested that a signal from some axial structure leads to the expression of **fibroblast growth factor-10 (FGF-10)** in the prelimb lateral plate mesoderm. In FGF-10 knockout mice, limbs (and also lungs) do not form. Conversely, if a small porous bead containing FGF-10 is implanted into the mesoderm of the flank between the arm and the leg, a supernumerary limb is induced. The initial stimulus may also involve **retinoic acid,** because if the local synthesis and action of retinoic acid are inhibited, limb formation fails to occur. As will be seen later in this chapter, the early prelimb mesoderm also expresses molecules (Tbx-4 and Tbx-5) that specify whether the limb will be an arm or a leg and **Hoxb-8,** which is involved in establishing a major signaling center in the early limb bud (the zone of polarizing activity, see p. 215).

The mesodermal limb primordia form at discrete locations beneath a broad band of thickened ectoderm that encircles the ventrolateral aspect of the embryo (see Figure 6-23). In the earliest states of limb development the limb mesoderm, probably acting through FGF-10, is the prime mover. It stimulates the overlying ectoderm to produce **FGF-8** and to become a functional part of an interacting mesodermal-ectodermal primordium that has sufficient developmental information to form a limb even if isolated from the rest of the body (a so-called **self-differentiating system**).

The primacy of the early limb mesoderm was demonstrated long ago by transplantation experiments on

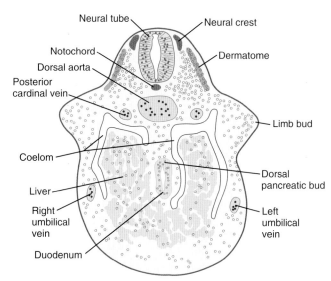

**FIGURE 10-1** Cross section through the trunk at an early stage of limb bud development, showing the position of the limb bud in relation to that of the somite (dermatome) and other major structures. The limb bud is an outgrowth of the body wall (lateral plate mesoderm).

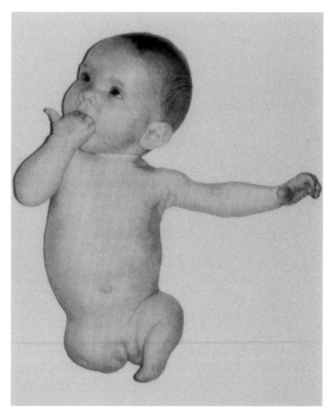

**FIGURE 10-2** Amelia of the right leg in an infant. Despite the absence of a foot, the left leg contains an upper and a lower leg segment. (From Connor JM, Ferguson-Smith MA: *Essential medical genetics*, ed 3, Oxford, England, 1991, Blackwell Scientific.)

amphibian embryos. If early limb mesoderm is removed, a limb fails to form. However, if the same mesoderm is transplanted to the flank of an embryo, a supernumerary limb grows at that site. In contrast, if the ectoderm overlying the normal limb mesoderm is removed, new ectoderm heals the defect, and a limb forms. If the original ectoderm that was removed is grafted to the flank, no limb forms. These experiments show that in *early* limb development, mesoderm is the primary bearer of the limb blueprint and ectoderm is only secondarily co-opted into the system.

In rare instances, individuals are born without one or sometimes all limbs (**amelia**) (Figure 10-2). In some cases this may reflect a disturbance in the production of the signaling molecules that initiate limb development or the cellular receptors for these molecules.

## REGULATIVE PROPERTIES AND AXIAL DETERMINATION

The early limb primordium is a highly regulative system, with properties very similar to those described for the cleaving embryo (see p. 48–49). These properties can be summarized with the following experiments (Figure 10-3):

1. If part of a limb primordium is removed, the remainder reorganizes to form a complete limb.

2. If a limb primordium is split into two halves and these are prevented from fusing, each half gives rise to a complete limb (the twinning phenomenon).

3. If two equivalent halves of a limb primordium are juxtaposed, one complete limb forms.

4. If two equivalent limb disks are superimposed, they reorganize to form a single limb (see section on tetraparental embryos, p. 49).

5. In some species, disaggregated limb mesoderm can reorganize and form a complete limb.

The organization of the limb is commonly related to the Cartesian coordinate system. The anteroposterior* axis runs from the first (anterior) to the fifth (posterior) digit. The back of the hand or foot is dorsal, and the palm or sole is ventral. The proximodistal axis extends from the base of the limb to the tips of the digits.

Experiments involving the transplantation and rotation of limb primordia in lower vertebrates have shown that these axes are fixed in a sequential order: anteroposterior to dorsoventral to proximodistal. Before all three axes are specified, a left limb primordium can be converted into a normal right limb simply by rotating it with respect to the normal body axes. These axes are important as reference points in several aspects of limb morphogenesis. Evidence indicates a similar sequence of axial specifications in certain other primordia, such as those of the retina and inner ear.

---

* Because of different conventions in the use of axial terms, some human embryologists would take exception to the axial terminology presented here. Specifically, according to strict human terminology, *anterior* means "ventral," and *posterior* means "dorsal." However, the axial terminology used in this chapter (*anterior* means "cranial," and *posterior* means "caudal") is so uniformly used in the experimental and comparative embryological literature that the student referring to the original literature in the field of limb development would find it very confusing to use human axial terminology.

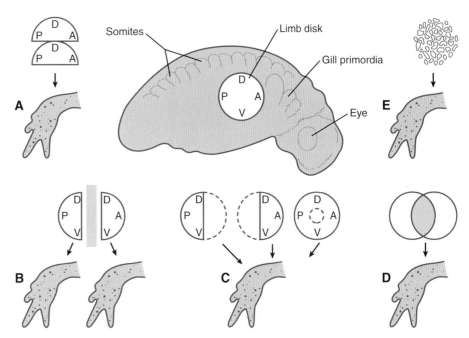

**FIGURE 10-3** Experiments demonstrating regulative properties of limb disks in amphibian embryos. **A,** Combining two identical halves of limb disks results in a single limb. **B,** Separation of two halves of a limb disk by a barrier results in each half forming a normal limb of the same polarity. **C,** After various types of tissue removal, the remaining limb tissue regulates to form a normal limb. **D,** Combining two disks results in the formation of a single normal limb. **E,** Mechanical disruption of a limb disk is followed by reorganization of the pieces and the formation of a normal limb. *A,* Anterior; *D,* dorsal; *P,* posterior, *V,* ventral. (Based on studies by Harrison RG: *J Exp Zool* 32:1–136, 1921; and Swett FH: *Q Rev Biol* 12:322–339, 1937.)

## OUTGROWTH OF LIMB BUD

Shortly after its initial establishment, the limb primordium begins to bulge from the body wall (late in the first month for the human upper extremity [Figure 10-4]). At this stage the limb bud consists of a mass of similar-looking mesodermal cells covered by a layer of ectoderm. Despite its apparently simple structure, the limb bud contains enough intrinsic information to guide its development, since if a mammalian limb bud is transplanted to another region of the body or is cultured in vitro, a recognizable limb forms.

A distinctive feature is the presence of a ridge of thickened ectoderm (**apical ectodermal ridge [AER]**) located along the anteroposterior plane of the apex of the limb bud (Figure 10-5). During much of the time when the AER is present, the hand- and foot-forming regions of the developing limb bud are paddle shaped, with the apical ridge situated along the rim of the paddle (Figure 10-6). Experiments have shown that the AER interacts with the underlying limb bud mesoderm to promote outgrowth of the developing limb. Other aspects of limb development, such as morphogenesis (the development of form), are guided by information contained in the mesoderm.

This section outlines many of the ways in which the limb bud mesoderm and ectoderm interact to control

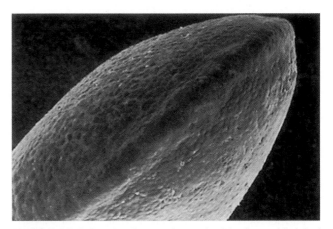

**FIGURE 10-4** Scanning electron micrograph of a **4-week** human embryo (5 mm), with 34 pairs of somites. Toward the lower left, the right arm bud protrudes from the body. (From Jirásek JE: *Atlas of human prenatal morphogenesis,* Amsterdam, 1983, Martinus Nijhoff.)

**FIGURE 10-5** Scanning electron micrograph of the flattened limb bud of a human embryo showing the prominent apical ectodermal ridge traversing the apical border. (From Kelley RO, Fallon JF: *Dev Biol* 51:241–256, 1976.)

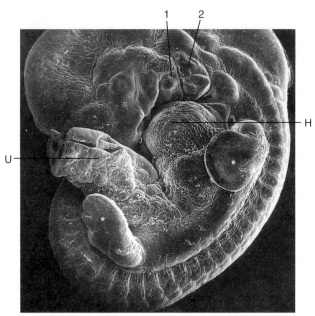

**FIGURE 10-6** Scanning electron micrograph of a **5-week** human embryo (10mm). The arm and leg buds (*asterisks*) are in the flattened paddle stage. *H*, Heart; *U*, umbilical cord; *1*, *2*, pharyngeal arches 1 and 2. (From Jirásek JE: *Atlas of human prenatal morphogenesis*, Amsterdam, 1983, Martinus Nijhoff.)

limb development. Recognition of these developmental mechanisms is important in understanding the genesis of a number of limb malformations.

## Apical Ectodermal Ridge

The earliest limb bud begins to form before an AER is present, but soon a thickened AER appears along the border between dorsal and ventral limb ectoderm. Molecular studies have shown that the position of the AER corresponds exactly to the border between dorsal ectoderm that expresses the signaling molecule **radical fringe** and **ventral ectoderm**, which expresses the transcription factor, **Engrailed-1 (En-1)** (see Figure 10-14, *A*).

Although the AER had been recognized for years, its role in limb development was not understood until it was subjected to experimental analysis. Removal of the AER results in an arrest of limb development, leading to distal truncation of the limb (Figure 10-7). In the *limbless* mutant in chickens, early limb development is normal; later the AER disappears and further limb development ceases. If mutant ectoderm is placed over normal limb bud mesoderm, limb development is truncated, whereas combining mutant mesoderm with normal ectoderm results in more normal limb development, suggesting that the ectoderm is defective in this mutant.

Further analysis has shown that in the *limbless* mutant the entire ectoderm of the limb bud displays a dorsal character, that is, radical fringe and other "dorsal" molecules are expressed in both dorsal and ventral

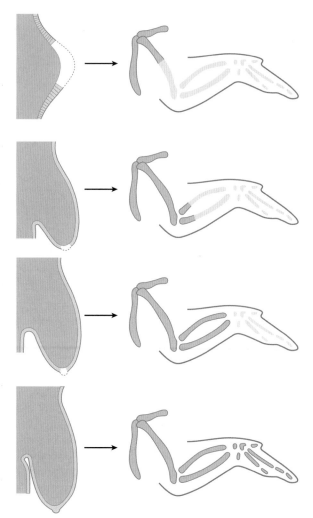

**FIGURE 10-7** *Top three*, Effect of removing the apical ectodermal ridge at successively later stages on the development of the avian wing bud. The more mature the wing bud, the more skeletal elements form after apical ridge removal. Missing structures are shown in light gray. *Bottom*, Normal development of an untouched wing bud. (Based on Saunders JW: *J Exp Zool* 108:363–403, 1948.)

ectoderm; correspondingly, En-1 is not expressed in ventral ectoderm. In the absence of the juxtaposition of ectoderm with dorsal and ventral properties an AER cannot be maintained.

The power of the AER is demonstrated by experiments or mutants that result in the formation of two AERs on the limb bud. This results in the formation of a supernumerary limb, as is illustrated by the mutants **eudiplopodia** in the chicken and **diplopodia** in the human (Figure 10-8).

Recent studies have shown that the outgrowth-promoting signal produced by the AER is FGF. In the earliest stages of limb formation, the lateral ectoderm begins to produce FGF-8 as it thickens to form an AER. As the limb bud begins to grow out, the apical ridge also produces FGF-2 throughout its entire length and FGF-4 in its posterior half (see Figure 10-14). If the AER is removed, outgrowth of limb bud mesoderm can be supported by the local application of either FGF-2 or

FIGURE 10-8 **A,** Duplicated wing bud in a chick with eudiplopodia. Under the influence of a secondary apical ectodermal ridge, a supernumerary limb bud forms. **B,** Diplopodia in the human. Dorsal and ventral views of the right foot, where duplication has occurred along the anteroposterior axis. (**A** from Goetinck P: *Dev Biol* 10:71–79, 1964. **B** courtesy D. Hootinck, Buffalo, NY.)

FGF-4. Other studies have shown that in mutants characterized by deficient or absent outgrowth of the limb, the mutant ectoderm fails to produce FGF. The effects of the FGF produced by the apical ectoderm on the underlying mesoderm are discussed later in this chapter.

## Mesoderm of Early Limb Bud

### Structure and Composition

The mesoderm of the early limb bud consists of homogeneous mesenchymal cells supplied by a well-developed vascular network. The mesenchymal cells are embedded in a matrix consisting of a loose meshwork of collagen fibers and ground substance, with hyaluronic acid and glycoproteins being prominent constituents of the latter. There are no nerves in the early limb bud.

It is not possible to distinguish different cell types within the early limb bud mesenchyme by their morphology alone. Nevertheless, mesenchymal cells from several sources are present (Figure 10-9). Initially the limb bud mesenchyme consists exclusively of cells derived from the lateral plate mesoderm. These cells give rise to the skeleton, connective tissue, and some blood vessels.

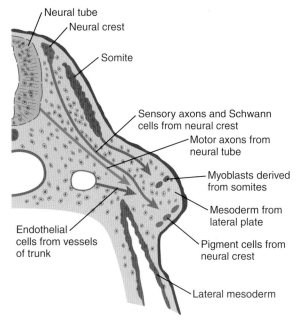

**FIGURE 10-9** The different types of cells that enter the limb bud.

Neural tube
Neural crest
Somite
Sensory axons and Schwann cells from neural crest
Motor axons from neural tube
Myoblasts derived from somites
Mesoderm from lateral plate
Pigment cells from neural crest
Endothelial cells from vessels of trunk
Lateral mesoderm

Mesenchymal cells derived from the somites migrate into the limb bud as precursors of muscle cells. Another population of migrating cells is that from the neural crest, which ultimately form the Schwann cells of the nerves and pigment cells (**melanocytes**).

### Mesodermal-ectodermal Interactions and the Role of Mesoderm in Limb Morphogenesis

Limb development occurs as the result of continuous interactions between the mesodermal and ectodermal components of the limb bud. The apical ectoderm stimulates outgrowth of the limb bud by promoting mitosis and preventing differentiation of the distal mesodermal cells of the limb bud. Although the AER promotes outgrowth, its own existence is reciprocally controlled by the mesoderm. If an AER from an old limb bud is transplanted onto the mesoderm of a young wing bud, the limb grows normally until morphogenesis is complete. However, if old limb bud mesoderm is covered by young apical ectoderm, limb development ceases at a time appropriate for the age of the mesoderm and not that of the ectoderm.

Similar reciprocal transplantation experiments have been used to demonstrate that the overall shape of the limb is determined by the mesoderm and not the ectoderm. This is most dramatically represented by experiments done on birds because of the great differences in morphology between the extremities. For example, if leg bud mesoderm in the chick embryo is covered with wing bud ectoderm, a normal leg covered with scales develops.

In a somewhat more complex example, if chick leg bud ectoderm is placed over duck wing bud mesoderm, a duck wing covered with chicken feathers forms. Such experiments, which have sometimes involved mosaics of avian and mammalian limb bud components, show that the overall morphology of the limb is determined by the mesodermal component and not the ectoderm. In addition, the regional characteristics of ectodermal appendages (e.g., scalp hair versus body hair in the case of mammals) is also dictated by the mesoderm. Cross-species grafting experiments, however, show that the nature of the ectodermal appendages formed (e.g., hair versus feathers) is appropriate for the species from which the ectoderm was derived.

**Polydactyly** is a condition characterized by supernumerary digits and exists as a mutant in birds. Reciprocal transplantation experiments between mesoderm and ectoderm have shown that the defect is inherent in the mesoderm and not the ectoderm. Polydactyly in humans (Figure 10-10) is typically inherited as a genetic recessive trait and is commonly found in populations such as certain American Amish communities, where the total genetic pool is relatively restricted.

**FIGURE 10-10** Ultrasound images of normal **(A)** and polydactylous (six digit) **(B)** hands of human fetuses **16** and **31 weeks old.** In both cases the digits are imaged in cross section. *Arrow,* Thumb; *F,* face; *I,* thumb; *2 to 6,* fingers on polydactylous hand. (**A** from Bowerman R: *Atlas of normal fetal ultrasonographic anatomy,* St Louis, 1992, Mosby. **B** from Nyberg D and others: *Diagnostic ultrasound of fetal anomalies,* St Louis, 1990, Mosby.)

## Zone of Polarizing Activity and Morphogenetic Signaling

During the course of experiments investigating programmed cell death in the limb bud, researchers grafted mesodermal cells from the posterior base of the avian wing bud into the anterior margin. This manipulation resulted in the formation of a supernumerary wing, which was a mirror image of the normal wing (Figure 10-11). Much subsequent experimentation has shown that this posterior region, called the **zone of polarizing activity (ZPA)**, acts as a signaling center along the anteroposterior axis of the limb. The signal itself has been shown to be **sonic hedgehog (shh)** (see Figure 10-15), a molecule that mediates a wide variety of tissue interactions in the embryo (see Table 4-3). As will be seen later in this chapter, shh not only organizes tissues along the anteroposterior axis but also maintains the structure and function of the AER. In the absence of the ZPA or shh, the apical ridge regresses.

Cross-species grafting experiments have demonstrated that mammalian (including human) limb buds also contain a functional ZPA. A transplanted ZPA acts on the AER, eliciting a growth response from the mesenchymal cells just beneath the part of the ridge adjacent to the transplanted ZPA. As few as 50 cells from the ZPA can stimulate supernumerary limb formation. Other structures, such as pieces of Hensen's node, notochord, and even feather germs have been shown to stimulate the formation of supernumerary limbs if grafted into the anterior margin of the limb. Since these experiments were conducted, all of the effective implanted tissues have been found to be sources of sonic hedgehog.

The ZPA is already established by the time the limb bud begins to grow out from the body wall. There is now evidence that in the forelimb the position of the ZPA is determined by the location of the highest concentration of *Hoxb-8* expression along the body axis. Experiments have shown that in response to the localized application of retinoic acid along the anterior margin of the forelimb bud, *Hoxb-8* expression is induced within 30 minutes. This suggests a cascade beginning with retinoic acid signaling, leading to *Hoxb-8* expression, which in turn determines the location of the ZPA.

Members of the **Gli** family of zinc-finger transcription factors have recently been recognized to play a major role in regulating morphogenesis along the anteroposterior axis of the limb bud. **Gli-1** is expressed adjacent to sources of shh (e.g., the ZPA) and may be an important mediator of the shh signal. **Gli-3**, in contrast, is expressed in the anterior part of the limb bud and represses shh signaling there. *Gli-3* mutants are characterized by polydactyly, which is a reflection of the

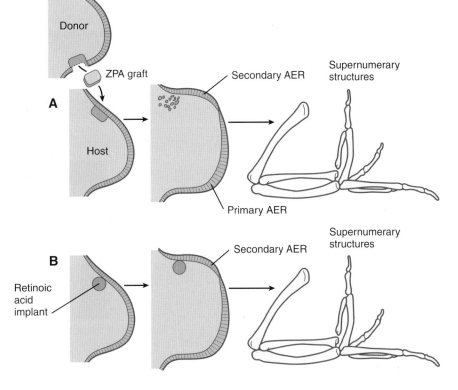

**FIGURE 10-11 A,** Grafting of the zone of polarizing activity (*ZPA*) into the anterior border of the avian limb bud results in the formation of a secondary apical ectodermal ridge and a supernumerary limb. **B,** Implantation of a bead soaked in retinoic acid into the anterior border of the limb bud also stimulates the formation of a supernumerary limb. *AER,* Apical epidermal ridge.

Donor

ZPA graft

Secondary AER

Supernumerary structures

**A**

Host

Primary AER

Retinoic acid implant

**B**

Secondary AER

Supernumerary structures

ectopic expression of shh in the anterior part of the limb bud in the absence of the repressive activity of the absent Gli-3.

## Progress Zone

The AER acts as the organizing center for the proximodistal axis of the limb by stimulating the proliferation of the underlying cells. Just beneath the AER is a several-hundred-micron-thick region of distal mesoderm called the **progress zone** (Figure 10-12). Cells in the progress zone divide actively and are not morphogenetically determined. As the limb bud grows out, however, mesodermal cells that are proximal enough to escape the influence of the AER become fixed in their ultimate morphogenetic fate so that cells leaving the progress zone early ultimately form proximal skeletal elements (e.g., humerus, femur) and cells leaving later form elements of the forearm or hand in the upper limb.

Cells in the progress zone are characterized by their expression of the *Msx-1* gene, and as they leave the

progress zone, expression of this gene ceases. There is something about the environment of the progress zone that stimulates *Msx-1* expression, because if mesodermal cells that have left the progress zone (and consequently cease the production of *Msx-1*) are transplanted back into the progress zone, they reexpress that molecule (Figure 10-12, *B*). In addition, they are now capable of forming more distal structures than they would have become had they been left in their original positions before transplantation.

## MORPHOGENETIC CONTROL OF EARLY LIMB DEVELOPMENT

Shortly after the prelimb mesoderm expresses FGF-10, which stimulates the production of FGF-8 by the overlying prelimb ectoderm, the same mesoderm begins to express transcription factors that determine whether that limb will become a forelimb (arm) or a hindlimb (leg). Two of these are members of the **T-box** family (T locus, see page 93). **Tbx-5** is expressed exclusively in the forelimb, whereas **Tbx-4** is expressed only in the hindlimb (Figure 10-13). In the hindlimb, another transcription factor, **Pitx-1**, acts upstream of Tbx-4 in specifying limb identity. At present, we do not know what influences lead to the localized expression of Tbx-5 in the forelimb region or Tbx-4 and Pitx-1 in the future hindlimb, nor is it known how expression of these transcription factors is translated into the morphology that distinguishes an arm from a leg.

As the limb bud begins to grow out from the body wall, its fundamental axial characteristics are controlled by interacting signaling centers for each of the three cardinal axes (Figure 10-14). We have already discussed the ZPA, which through the secretion of shh is important in controlling development along the anteroposterior axis, and the AER, which stimulates outgrowth of the limb along the proximodistal axis by secreting members of

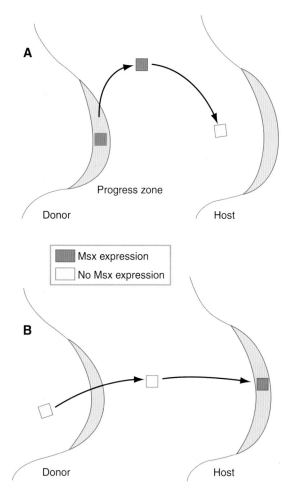

**FIGURE 10-12** Msx-1 expression and the progress zone. **A,** If Msx-1–expressing tissue from the progress zone is transplanted into more proximal regions of the limb bud, it soon stops expressing that molecule. **B,** If proximal mesenchyme that has already stopped expressing Msx-1 is transplanted back into the progress zone, it reexpresses the molecule.

Stage 29

**FIGURE 10-13** Whole mount in situ hybridization preparations of stage 29 chick embryos showing the localized expression of the mRNAs to Tbx4 in the hindlimb and Tbx5 in the forelimb. (Courtesy H-G Simon, Northwestern University Medical School.)

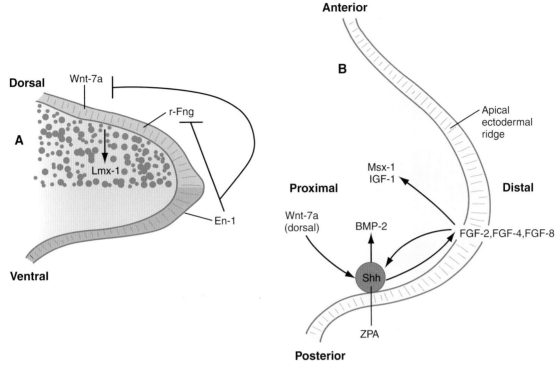

**FIGURE 10-14** Schematic representations of molecular control of limb development. **A,** Molecular control of the dorsoventral axis. En-1 inhibits both Wnt-7a and r-Fng. **B,** Molecular control along the anteroposterior and proximodistal axes. *r-Fng*, Radical fringe; *ZPA*, zone of polarizing activity.

the FGF family (Figure 10-15). Organization of the dorsoventral axis of the limb begins when the dorsal ectoderm produces the signaling molecule, **Wnt-7a**, which stimulates the underlying limb bud mesenchyme to express the transcription factor, **Lmx-1b**, a molecule that imparts a dorsal character to the mesoderm underlying the dorsal ectoderm. Ventral ectoderm produces

**En-1**, which represses the formation of Wnt-7a and consequently the formation of Lmx-1b in what will become ventral limb mesoderm, possibly by a default pathway (see Figure 10-14, *A*). The AER marks the border between dorsal and ventral limb bud ectoderm, and this border is characterized by an expression boundary between another signaling factor, **radical fringe**, secreted by dorsal ectoderm, and the En-1 formed in the ventral ectoderm. Further ventral spread of radical fringe expression is held in check by En-1.

All three axial signaling centers (Table 10-1) interact in the early limb bud. Wnt-7a from the dorsal ectoderm has a stimulating effect upon the ZPA (See Figure 10-14, *B*), whereas the shh from the ZPA is required for the production of FGFs from the AER, which in turn, provide additional positive feedback to the ZPA.

Simultaneous with the establishment of the ZPA, an orderly sequence of the homeobox-containing genes,

**FIGURE 10-15** Whole-mount preparation (double in situ hybridization) of a chick embryo showing the expression of FGF-4 in the apical ectodermal ridge *(arrows)* and somites. In addition to the bases of the limb buds (dark spots indicated by *asterisks*), sonic hedgehog is expressed in the notochord, floor plate, gut, some branchial arches, midbrain, and forebrain. (Courtesy A. López-Martínez and J.F. Fallon, Madison, Wis.)

| TABLE 10-1 *Axial Control in the Developing Limb* | | |
|---|---|---|
| **Axis** | **Signaling center** | **Molecular signal** |
| Proximodistal | AER | FGF-2, FGF-4, FGF-8 |
| Anteroposterior | ZPA | Sonic hedgehog |
| Dorsoventral | Dorsal ectoderm | Wnt-7a (dorsal) |
|  | Ventral ectoderm | En-1 (ventral) |

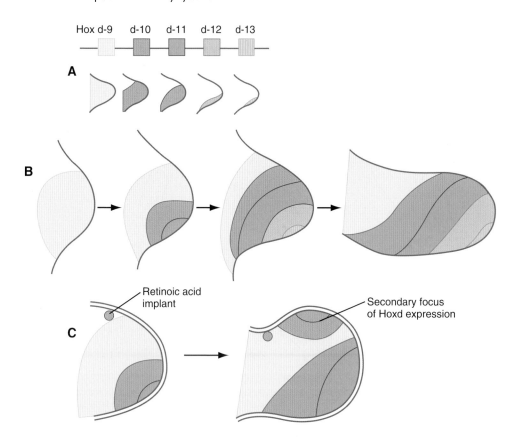

Hox d-9   d-10   d-11   d-12   d-13

A

B

C

Retinoic acid
implant

Secondary focus
of Hoxd expression

FIGURE 10-16 *Hoxd* gene expression in the chick limb bud. **A,** Map of this gene family and distribution of individual gene products. **B,** Development of the aggregate pattern of *Hoxd* gene expression over time in the normal limb bud. **C,** The development of a secondary focus of *Hoxd* gene expression in the area of supernumerary limb formation caused by an implant of retinoic acid. (Based on Tabin CJ: *Development* 116:289–296, 1992.).

*Hoxd-9* to *Hoxd-13* (Figure 10-16), as well as certain of the *Hoxa* genes, occurs in the early limb bud. What stimulates the expression of the *Hox* genes in the limb is presently not understood, but Gli-3 is involved in confining *Hox* gene expression to the more posterior parts of the limb bud. The *Hox* genes are involved in patterning the proximodistal axis of the limb (Figure 10-17). Studies on mice and the analysis of certain human mutants have shown that certain defects in limb regions correspond to absent expression of specific *Hox* gene paralogues. For example, mutations of *Hoxa-13* and *Hoxd-13* cause characteristic reduction defects of the digits resulting from shortness of the phalanges (Figure 10-18).

## Cell Death and Development of Digits

Although it may seem paradoxical, genetically programmed **cell death (apoptosis)** is important in the development of a number of structures in the body. In the forelimb, it is prominently manifested in the anterior limb margin, the future axillary region, between the radius and ulna, and in the interdigital spaces (Figure 10-19). Experiments on avian embryos have shown that, to a certain stage, mesodermal cells scheduled to die could be spared by transplanting them to areas in which cell death did not

normally occur. However, after a certain time, a "death clock" was set (an example of determination), and the cells could no longer be rescued.

As limb development proceeds, changes become apparent in the AER. Instead of remaining continuous around the entire apex of the limb, the ridge begins to break up, leaving intact segments of thickened ridge epithelium covering the emerging digital rays (cartilaginous models of the digital bones). Between the digits, the ridge regresses (see Figure 10-19, *A*). As the digital primordia continue to grow outward, cell death sculpts the interdigital spaces (see Figure 10-19, *C*). **Bone morphogenetic protein-2 (BMP-2)**, BMP-4, and BMP-7 and the transcription factors **Msx-1** and **-2** are strongly expressed in the interdigital spaces. The exact mechanism of interdigital cell death is still not entirely clear, but the BMPs, especially BMP-4 acting under the mediation of Msx-2, are the prime movers in initiating interdigital cell death. The FGFs produced by the AER seem to play a dual role in interdigital cell death. On the one hand, FGF-2 antagonizes the death-inducing effects of the BMPs, but on the other, the FGFs promote the production of Msx-2, which cooperates with the BMPs in inducing interdigital cell death.

If interdigital cell death does not occur, a soft tissue web connects the digits on either side. This is the basis for the development of webbed feet on ducks and the abnormal formation of **syndactyly** (Figure 10-20, *A*) in

Hoxa, Hoxd

9 10 11 12 13

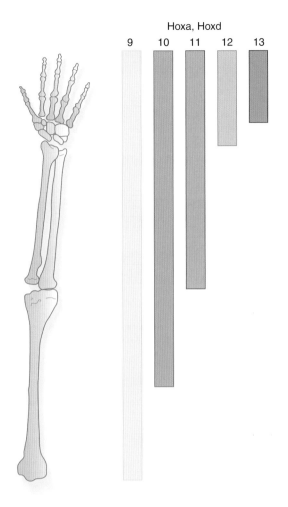

**FIGURE 10-17** Levels of *Hox* gene expression in relation to skeletal components of the limb. Molecular data from the mouse are superimposed on the human limb skeleton.

humans. BMP is not found in the interdigital mesoderm in developing duck feet, although it is found in other regions of cell death in the duck limb.

There is more, however, to the development of digits than simply sculpting the interdigital spaces by cell death. Well before cell death becomes evident, other events in the interdigital spaces specify the nature of each digit. A future digit is first recognizable as a longitudinal condensation of mesenchyme, which soon begins to lay down a precartilaginous matrix. The early digital ray then undergoes segmentation (see Figure 10-24) to form specific phalangeal segments. Each digit will develop its own character, as determined by the number of phalangeal segments or its specific size and shape. The underlying basis for the development of digital form is just becoming understood.

According to recent experiments, the newly formed digital rays are yet unspecified as to digital identity. Signals from the interdigital mesoderm, probably BMPs, act on the digital rays to specify which digits they will become. The concentration of BMP appears to be an important determinant of digital identity, with increasing concentrations of BMP specifying successively more posterior digits. According to this model, the highest concentrations of BMP are present in the interdigital mesoderm between digits 4 and 5, and this concentration specifies the nature of the fourth digit. How the identity of digit 5 is determined remains unclear. In each case, the BMP concentration in the interdigital mesoderm specifies the nature of the more anterior digit bordering that mesoderm (Figure 10-21). If a digital ray is divided longitudinally by an impermeable barrier, the anterior half of the ray, under the influence of the interdigital mesoderm adjacent to it, becomes transformed to a ray of the next most anterior type (e.g., an anterior half of ray 3 becomes a

**FIGURE 10-18** Hands and feet of a person with a mutation of the *Hoxa-13* gene. Both thumbs and great toes are more proximally situated than normal. In addition, some phalanges are shortened, and the nails are hypoplastic. (Courtesy J.W. Innis, Ann Arbor, Mich.)

## Limb Anomalies

Because they are so obvious, limb anomalies have attracted attention for centuries and have been subject to many systems of classification. Until recently, most classification schemes have been based upon morphology alone, usually from the perspective of surgeons or rehabilitation specialists. Only in recent decades has it been possible to assign genetic or mechanistic causes to some of the known limb malformations. A summary of the common types of morphological limb defects is presented in Table 10-2. Many of the most common limb malformations are the result of still poorly understood developmental disturbances. Although an increasing number of limb malformations can be attributed to genetic causes (Table 10-3), the means by which many gene mutations are translated into defective development are not well understood.

Some of the most frequently encountered limb anomalies are due to causes that do not involve classical development mechanisms. Several are due to mechanical causes. **Intrauterine amputations** by amniotic bands, presumably caused by tears in the amnion, can result in the loss of parts of digits or even hands or feet (see Figure 8-15). Other deformities, such as **clubfoot** (**talipes equinovarus**) and some causes of congenital dislocations, have been attributed to persistent mechanical pressures of the uterine wall on the fetus, particularly in cases of **oligohydramnios** (see Chapter 7).

A very rare limb deformity is **macromelia** (or **macrodactyly**), in which a limb or a digit is considerably enlarged over the normal size. Such abnormalities are sometimes associated with neurofibromatosis, and the neural crest may be involved in this defect.

**TABLE 10-2** *Common Structural Types of Limb Malformations*

| Term | Description |
| --- | --- |
| Amelia (ectromelia) | Absence of an entire limb |
| Acheiria, apodia | Absence of hands, feet |
| Phocomelia | Absence or shortening of proximal limb segments |
| Hemimelia | Absence of pre- or postaxial parts of limb |
| Meromelia | General term for absence of part of a limb |
| Ectrodactyly | Absence of any number of digits |
| Polydactyly | Excessive number of digits |
| Syndactyly | Presence of interdigital webbing |
| Brachydactyly | Shortened digits |
| Split hand or foot | Absence of central components of hand or foot |

**TABLE 10-3** *Genetic Conditions Causing Primary Patterning Defects of the Limb*

| Type of molecule | Gene | Syndrome | Limb defect |
| --- | --- | --- | --- |
| Transcription factor | GLI-3 | Greig | Polydactyly, syndactyly, cephalopolysyndactyly |
| | GLI-3 | Pallister-Hall | Posterior polydactyly |
| | TBX-3 | Ulnar-mammary | Upper limb deficiencies and posterior duplications |
| | TBX-5 | Holt-Oram | Upper limb deficiencies and anterior duplications |
| | HOXA-13 | Hand-foot-genital | Brachydactyly |
| | HOXD-13 | Synpolydactyly | Syndactyly, insertional polydactyly, brachydactyly |
| | PAX-3 | Waardenburg I & III | Syndactyly |
| | SOX-9 | Campomelic dysplasia | Bowing of long bones |
| Signaling protein | CDMP1 | Hunter-Thompson | Brachydactyly |
| | CDMP1 | Grebe | Severe brachydactyly |

Adapted from Bamshad M and others: *Pediatr Res* 45:291–299, 1999.

| Type of molecule | Gene | Syndrome | Limb defect |
|---|---|---|---|
| Receptor protein | FGFR-1 or -2 | Pfeiffer | Brachydactyly, syndactyly |
| | FGFR-2 | Apert | Syndactyly |
| | FGFR-2 | Jackson-Weiss | Syndactyly, brachydactyly |
| Unknown | — | Split-hand/foot | Distal syndactyly, fusion |
| | — | Tarsal-carpal coalition | Brachydactyly, bony fusions |
| | — | Nagar | Posterior limb deficiencies |
| | — | Ectrodactyly | Median limb deficiencies |
| | — | Triphalangeal thumb | Additional segment in thumb |
| | — | Posterior polydactyly | Extra digits |
| | — | Polysyndactyly | Interdigital webbing |

TABLE 10-3 *Genetic Conditions Causing Primary Patterning Defects of the Limb (Continued)*

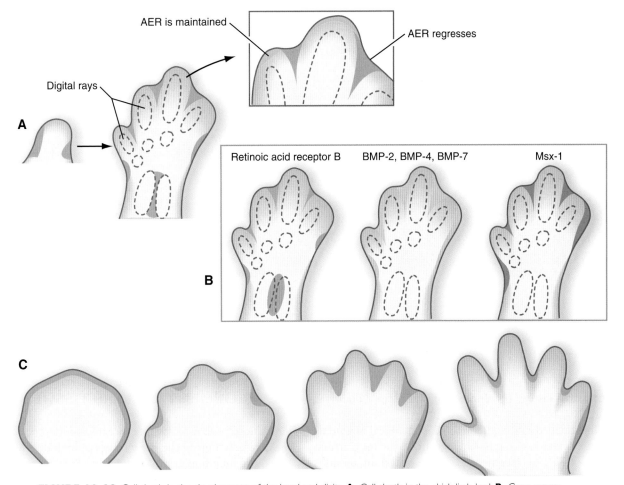

FIGURE 10-19 Cell death in the development of the hand and digits. **A,** Cell death in the chick limb bud. **B,** Gene expression in zones of cell death of the chick embryo. **C,** Cell death in the developing human hand. *AER,* Apical ectodermal ridge; *BMP,* bone morphogenetic protein.

**FIGURE 10-20 A,** Syndactyly in the human. **B,** Triphalangeal thumb in a human fetus. (**A** from Connor J, Ferguson-Smith M: *Essential medical genetics,* ed 2, Oxford, England, 1987, Blackwell Medical. **B** courtesy M. Barr, Ann Arbor, Mich.)

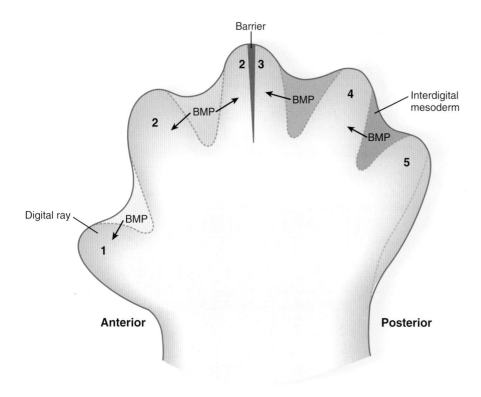

**FIGURE 10-21** According to a new model of digital specification (Dahn and Fallon, 2000), the concentration of BMP in the interdigital mesenchyme determines the identity of the adjacent digits. In the normal limb, the highest concentration of BMP (darkest color) specifies the fifth digit, and the lowest (lightest color) specifies that the first digit will form. When a barrier separates the normal third digital ray into two halves, the posterior half of that digital ray becomes a third digit and the anterior half becomes a supernumerary second digit.

second digit instead of a component of the third digit (see Figure 10-21).

All human digits contain three phalangeal segments except for the first digits (thumb and great toe), which consist of only two segments. On rare occasions, an individual is born with a triphalangeal thumb (Figure 10-20, *B*). Why digits have different numbers of phalangeal segments is still not understood.

## DEVELOPMENT OF LIMB TISSUES

The morphogenetic events previously described take place largely during the early stages of limb development when the limb bud consists of a homogeneous-appearing mass of mesodermal cells covered by ectoderm. The differentiation and histogenesis of the specific tissue components of the limb are later developmental events that build on the morphogenetic blueprint already established.

## Skeleton

The skeleton is the first major tissue of the limb to show signs of overt differentiation. Its gross morphology, whether normal or abnormal, closely reflects the major pattern-forming events that shape the limb as a whole. Formation of the skeleton can be first seen as a condensation of mesenchymal cells in the central core of the proximal part of the limb bud. Even before undergoing condensation, these cells are determined to form cartilage, and if they are transplanted to other sites or into culture, they differentiate only into cartilage. However, other mesenchymal cells that would normally form connective tissue retain the capacity to differentiate into cartilage if they are transplanted into the central region of the limb bud.

The ectoderm of the limb bud exerts an inhibitory effect on cartilage differentiation, so cartilage does not form in the region just beneath the ectoderm. In vitro studies suggest that the inhibition is mediated by a diffusible material secreted by the ectoderm. Whether this is the same mechanism that maintains the integrity of the progress zone remains to be determined.

The condensed cells comprising the precartilaginous aggregates express both BMP-2 and BMP-4. As skeletal development continues, their expression becomes progressively restricted to the cells that will become the perichondrium or periosteum surrounding the bones. BMP-3 transcripts are first seen in cartilage, rather than precartilage, but this growth factor also becomes ultimately located in the perichondrium. The translocation of expression of these BMP molecules to the perichondrium reflects their continuing role in the earliest phases of differentiation of skeletal tissues.

In contrast, another BMP (BMP-6) is expressed only in areas of maturing (hypertrophying) cartilage within the limb bones. **Indian hedgehog**, a molecule related to sonic hedgehog, is also expressed in the same regions of hypertrophying cartilage (which is also marked by the presence of type X collagen), and this signaling molecule may actually induce the expression of BMP-6.

Differentiation of the cartilaginous skeleton occurs in a proximodistal sequence, and in mammals the postaxial structures of the distal limb segments differentiate before the preaxial structures. For example, the sequence of formation of the digits is from the fifth to the first (Figure 10-22). The postaxial skeleton of the arm is considered to be the humerus, ulna, digits 2–5 and their corresponding carpal and metacarpal elements. The preaxial portion of the limb bud becomes progressively reduced during limb outgrowth and contributes only to the radius and possibly the first digital ray. Certain limb defects,

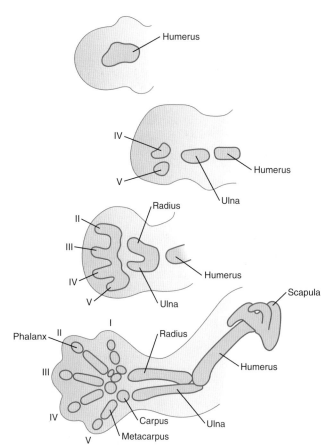

**FIGURE 10-22** Formation of the skeleton in the mammalian forelimb.

sometimes called **hemimelias**, are characterized by deficiencies of preaxial or postaxial limb components (Figure 10-23).

One of the characteristic features in differentiation of the limb skeleton is the formation of joints. Joint formation occurs by the transverse splitting of precartilaginous rods rather than by the apposition of two separate skeletal elements. Joint formation is first apparent when transverse strips of highly condensed cells cross a precartilaginous rod (Figure 10-24). Formation of the zone of cell density is induced by **Wnt-14**, which in turn stimulates the formation of **growth differentiation factor-5 (Gdf-5)**, a member of the BMP family, in the region of the future joint. BMP activity, which is strongly involved in cartilage formation, must be excluded from the region of the developing joint. **Noggin**, an antagonist of BMP, plays an important role in joint formation, because in its absence BMP is expressed throughout the region where the joint should form, and the digital rays develop into solid rods of cartilage without joints.

Condensation is followed by cell death and matrix changes in the region of the future joint. Then the skeletal elements on either side of the joint form articular cartilage, and a fluid-filled gap forms between them. Additional condensations of mesenchymal cells form the

**FIGURE 10-23** Radial hemimelia (absent radius) in a **27-week-old** fetus. **A,** Ultrasound image showing a thumb *(arrow)* but no radius. **B,** Postnatal x-ray image confirming the absent radius. *u,* ulna; *h,* humerus. (From Nyberg D and others: *Diagnostic ultrasound of fetal anomalies,* St Louis, 1990, Mosby.)

joint capsule, ligaments, and tendons. During later development, muscular activity is required to maintain the integrity of the joint, but early joint development is completely independent of muscular activity. A well-known mutant, called **brachypodism,** involves a shortening of the limb and the lack of development of certain joints, specifically those between the proximal and middle phalanges. In this mutant, Gdf-5 expression is absent in these joint regions.

## Musculature

The musculature of the limb is derived from myogenic cells that migrate into the very early limb bud from the ventral part of the dermomyotome of the somite. Each somite in the limb region contributes 30 to 100 migratory precursor cells to the future limb musculature. These cells are stimulated to leave the somite and migrate toward the limb through the stimulus of **scatter factor (hepatic growth factor),** which is produced by the proximal cells of the limb-forming area. Before migrating, the premuscle cells in the somite express **c-met,** which is a specific receptor for scatter factor. The premyogenic cells, which are morphologically indistinguishable from the other mesenchymal cells but which express Pax-3, spread throughout the limb bud. In the splotch mutant, which is characterized by the absence of Pax-3 expression, muscle cells do not populate the limb bud. Migrating premuscle cells also express the cell adhesion molecule **N-cadherin,** which is important in correctly distributing them throughout the limb bud mesenchyme. The migrating premuscle cells keep pace with the elongation of the limb bud, although cells expressing characteristic muscle molecules (e.g., MyoD) are not seen in the progress zone. Some experimental evidence suggests that premyogenic cells are not present in the progress zone; other experiments have shown that the environment of the progress zone suppresses the expression of MyoD and other muscle-specific molecules, possibly through the mitosis-promoting influence of the FGFs in that area.

Shortly after the condensations of the skeletal elements take shape, the myogenic cells themselves begin to coalesce into two common muscle masses: one the precursor of the flexor muscles and the other giving rise to the extensor muscles. The next stage in muscle formation is the splitting of the **common muscle masses** into anatomically recognizable precursors of the definitive muscles of the limb. Little is known about the mechanisms that guide the splitting of the common muscle masses. The fusion of myoblasts into early myotubes begins to occur during these early stages of muscle development.

Considerable evidence suggests that myogenic precursor cells do not possess intrinsic information guiding their morphogenesis. Rather, the myogenic cells follow the lead of connective tissue cells, which are the bearers and effectors of the morphogenetic information required to form anatomically correct muscles. In experiments in which the somites normally associated with a limb bud are removed and replaced by somites from elsewhere along the body axis, myogenic cells are morphogenetically neutral. Muscle morphogenesis is typically normal even though the muscle fiber precursors are derived from abnormal sources.

Through the removal of somites, the use of x-radiation, and the analysis of certain mutants such as *wingless,* it has been shown that the tendons and connective tissue components of a muscle are derived from the limb bud mesoderm, whereas the muscle fibers

**FIGURE 10-24** Sequence of the formation of the joints in the limbs.

themselves are somite derived. In situations in which myogenic cells are prevented from entering the limb bud, morphologically appropriate tendons still form, but these tendons are not attached to "muscles." In the same limbs, other connective tissue cells form a model of the muscle, even though it does not contain muscle fibers.

Depending on the specific muscle, the migration, fusion, or displacement of muscle primordia may be involved in the genesis of the final form of the muscle. In one case, genetically programmed cell death, apoptosis, is responsible for the disappearance of an entire muscle layer (the **contrahentes muscle**) in the flexor side of the human hand. The myogenic cells differentiate to the myotube stage; they then accumulate with glycogen and soon degenerate. The contrahentes muscle layer is preserved in most of the great apes. The reason it degenerates in the human hand at such a late stage in its differentiation is not understood.

Although limb muscles assume their definitive form in the very early embryo, they must undergo considerable growth in both length and cross-sectional area to keep up with the overall growth of the embryo. This is accomplished by the division of the satellite cells (see p. 196) and the fusion of their progeny with the muscle fibers. The added satellite cell nuclei increase the potential of the muscle fiber to produce structural and contractile proteins, which increase the cross-sectional area of each muscle fiber. Accompanying this addition to the nuclear complement of the muscle fibers is their lengthening by

the addition of more sarcomeres, usually at the ends of the muscle fibers. The formation of new muscle fibers typically ceases at or shortly after birth. Although the muscles are capable of contracting in the early fetal period, their physiological properties continue to mature until after birth.

## Innervation

Motor axons originating in the spinal cord enter the limb bud at an early stage of development (during the fifth week) and begin to grow into the dorsal and ventral muscle masses before the latter have split up into primordia of individual muscles (Figure 10-25). Tracing studies have shown a high degree of order in the projection of motor neurons into the limb. Neurons located in medial positions in the spinal cord send axons to the ventral muscle mass, whereas those located more laterally in the spinal cord supply the dorsal muscle mass. Similarly, a correlation exists between the craniocaudal position of neurons in the cord with the anteroposterior pattern of innervation of limb muscles within the common muscle masses. For example, the rostralmost neurons innervate the most anterior muscle primordia.

Local cues at the base of the limb bud guide the entering pathways of nerve fibers into the limb bud. If a segment of the spinal cord opposite the area of limb bud outgrowth is reversed in the craniocaudal direction, the

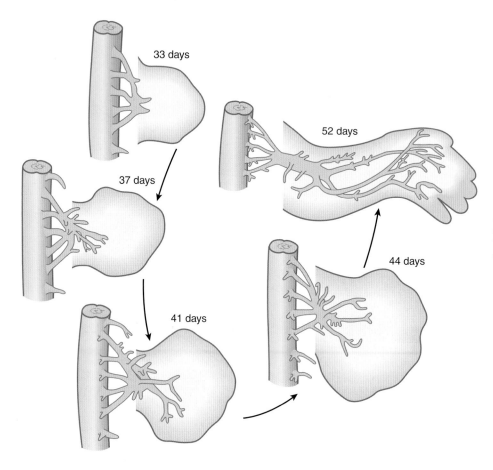

33 days

37 days

41 days

44 days

52 days

**FIGURE 10-25** Development of the nerve pattern of the human upper extremity. (Based on Shinohara H and others: *Acta Anat* 138:265–269, 1990.)

motor neurons change the direction of their outgrowth and enter the limb bud in their normal positions (Figure 10-26). If larger segments of spinal cord are reversed and the neurons are at considerable distances from the level of the limb bud, their axons do not find their way to their normal locations in the limb bud. The muscles themselves apparently do not provide specific target cues to the ingrowing axons, since if muscle primordia are prevented from forming, the main patterns of innervation in the limb are still normal.

Sensory axons enter the limb bud after the motor axons. Similarly, neural crest cell precursors of Schwann cells lag slightly behind the outgrowth of motor axons into the limb bud. Cells of the neural crest surround both motor and sensory nerve fibers to form the coverings of the nerves in the limbs. By the time digits have formed in developing limbs, the basic elements of the gross pattern of innervation in the adult limb have been established.

## Vasculature

The earliest vasculature of the limb bud is derived from endothelial cells arising from several segmental branches of the aorta and the cardinal veins and to some extent

from **angioblasts** (endothelial cell precursors) endogenous to the limb bud mesoderm. Initially, the limb vasculature consists of a fine capillary network, but soon, some channels are preferentially enlarged, resulting in a large central artery that supplies blood to the limb bud (Figure 10-27). From the central artery, the blood is distributed to the periphery via a mesh of capillaries and then collects into a **marginal sinus**, which is located beneath the AER. Blood in the marginal sinus drains into peripheral venous channels, which carry it away from the limb bud.

Even in the earliest limb bud there is a peripheral avascular zone of mesoderm within about $100\,\mu$m of the ectoderm of the limb bud (Figure 10-28, *A*). The avascular region persists until the digits have begun to form. Angioblasts are present in the avascular zone, but they are isolated from the functional capillaries. Experimental studies have clearly shown that the proximity of ectoderm is inhibitory to vasculogenesis in the limb bud mesoderm. If the ectoderm is removed, vascular channels form to the surface of the limb bud mesoderm, and if a piece of ectoderm is placed into the deep limb mesoderm, an avascular zone forms around it (Figure 10-28, *B*). Degradation products of hyaluronic acid, which is secreted by the ectoderm, appear to be the inhibitory agents.

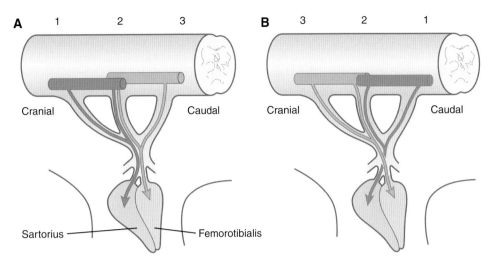

**FIGURE 10-26** Pathways taken by axons from specific pools of motoneurons in the spinal cord to limb muscles in the hindlimb of the chick embryo. **A,** Normal limb. **B,** After reversal of three segments of the embryonic spinal cord, axons originating from the spinal cord pass through abnormal pathways to innervate the muscles that they were originally destined to innervate. (Modified from Brown M and others: *Essentials of neural development,* Cambridge, Mass, 1990, Cambridge University Press.)

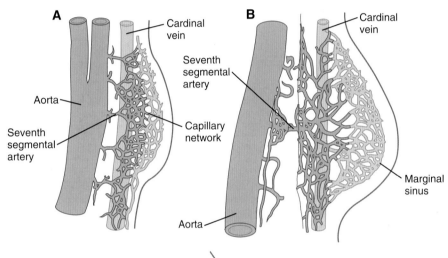

**FIGURE 10-27** Early stages in the development of the vascular pattern in the mammalian limb bud. **A,** Equivalent of a **4-week-old** human embryo. **B,** Equivalent of **5-week-old** human embryo. **C,** Equivalent of a **6-week-old** human embryo.

**FIGURE 10-28 A,** Photomicrograph of a quail wing bud with ink-injected blood vessels. **B,** Experiments illustrating the inhibitory effect of limb ectoderm on vascularization of the subjacent mesoderm. *Left,* Normal limb bud with an avascular zone beneath the ectoderm. *Upper right,* After removal of a piece of ectoderm, capillaries grow to the edge of the mesoderm in the region of removal. *Lower right,* A zone of avascularity appears around a piece of implanted ectoderm. (**A** courtesy R. Feinberg. Based on Feinberg RN, Noden DM: *Anat Rec* 231:136–144, 1991.)

Just before the skeleton begins to form, avascular zones appear in the areas where the cartilaginous models of the bones will take shape. Neither the stimuli for the disappearance of the blood vessels nor the fate of the endothelial cells that were present in these regions is understood at this time.

The pattern of the main vascular channels changes constantly as the limb develops, probably from the expansion of preferred channels within the capillary network that perfuses the distal part of the developing limb. With the establishment of the digital rays, the apical portion of the marginal sinus breaks up, but the proximal channels of the marginal sinus persist into adulthood as the **basilic** and **cephalic veins** of the arm (see Figure 10-27, *C*).

Similar major changes take place in the arterial channels that course through the developing limb (Figure 10-29). Preferred channels connected to the primary axial artery ultimately take ascendancy, especially in the forearm, leaving the original primary axial artery a relatively minor vessel (the **interosseous artery**) in the forearm.

## SUMMARY

○ Limbs arise from the lateral mesoderm and the overlying ectoderm under the influence of an inductor (possibly FGF-10 from the axial mesoderm). The early limb bud is a highly regulative system that can compensate for a variety of surgical disturbances and still form a normal limb. The axes of the limb are fixed in an anteroposterior, dorsoventral, and proximodistal sequence.

○ The early limb bud mesoderm stimulates the overlying ectoderm to form an AER that stimulates the outgrowth of the limb through proliferation of the underlying mesodermal cells. FGF-2 and FGF-4 are secreted by the apical ridge and can induce outgrowth in the absence of the ridge. The overall morphogenesis of the limb is determined by properties of the mesoderm, whereas the ectoderm acts in a more permissive sense.

○ Cell death is an important mechanism in normal limb development. Regions of programmed cell death include the axillary region and the interdigital spaces. In the absence of interdigital cell death, syndactyly results.

○ A ZPA located in the posterior mesoderm acts as a biological signaler and plays an important role in the anteroposterior organization of the limb by releasing sonic hedgehog. Wnt-7a, which is released by dorsal ectoderm, is the organizer of dorsoventrality in the limb bud. According to the concept of positional information, cells in the developing limb are exposed to positional cues (such as the signal from the ZPA) that allow them to determine their relative position within the limb bud. The cells then process this information and differentiate accordingly. Proximodistal control of morphogenesis may reside in the progress zone, a narrow band of mesoderm beneath the AER.

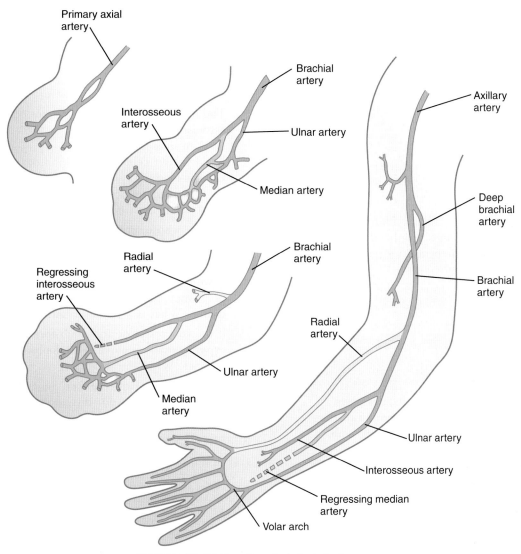

**FIGURE 10-29** Formation of arteries in the human arm.

○ Early forelimb buds are characterized by the expression of Tbx-5, whereas hindlimb buds express Tbx-4 and Pit-1. These may represent master control genes for the development of arms and legs.

○ Retinoic acid exerts a profound effect on limb morphogenesis and can cause the formation of a supernumerary limb if applied to the anterior border of the limb bud, but its exact role in limb development remains obscure. Expression of a variety of homeobox-containing genes follows well-defined patterns in the normally developing limb. Some patterns of gene expression are profoundly altered in limbs treated with retinoic acid.

○ The skeleton of the limb arises from lateral mesoderm. The ectoderm of the limb bud inhibits cartilage formation in the mesoderm cells immediately beneath it. This could explain the reason the skeleton of the vertebrate limb forms in a central position.

○ Limb muscles arise from cells derived from somitic mesoderm. These cells express Pax-3 during their migration into the limb bud. Myogenic cells first form dorsal and ventral common muscle masses, which later split into primordia of individual muscles. Morphogenetic control of muscles resides in the associated connective tissue rather than in the muscle cells themselves. Later stages in muscle development may involve cell death, the fusion of muscle primordia, and the displacement of muscle primordia to other areas.

○ Nerves grow into the developing limb bud and become associated with the common muscle masses as they split into individual muscles. Local cues are important in guiding growing axons into the developing limb.

○ The vasculature of the limb bud arises from cells budding off the aorta and cardinal veins as well as from endogenous mesodermal cells. The early vascular pattern

## CLINICAL VIGNETTE

After a normal pregnancy and labor, a 32-year-old woman gives birth to a 7-lb boy who has a duplication of his right foot along the anteroposterior axis. To the left of a single big toe (hallux) are four additional toes arranged in a mirror-symmetrical fashion so that the pattern of digits in that foot is 543212345, with 1 being the common hallux. Two older siblings are normal.

How can you explain this malformation on the basis of developmental mechanisms learned in this chapter?

consists of a central artery, which drains into a peripheral marginal sinus and then into peripheral venous channels. Blood vessels do not form beneath the ectoderm or in the central cartilage-forming regions.

○ Limb anomalies can form as the result of genetic mutations, drug effects, disturbed tissue interactions, and purely mechanical effects.

# Review Questions

1. Which of the following molecules plays an important role in the determination of the dorsoventral axis of the developing limb?
   A. Msx-1
   B. Wnt-7a
   C. Hoxd-13
   D. Pax-1
   E. FGF-8

2. What molecule is associated with myogenic cells migrating into the limb bud from the somites?
   A. Shh
   B. BMP-7
   C. FGF-4
   D. Pax-3
   E. En-1

3. What is the principal function of the AER?
   A. Stimulating outgrowth of the limb bud
   B. Setting up the anteroposterior axis of the limb bud
   C. Determining the specific characteristics of the ectodermal appendages of the limb
   D. Determining the pattern of neural ingrowth into the limb
   E. Attracting the subcutaneous plexus of capillaries in the limb bud

4. In the developing limb the sonic hedgehog (shh) gene product is produced in the:
   A. Progress zone
   B. Region of interdigital cell death
   C. ZPA
   D. AER
   E. Common muscle mass

5. The connective tissue of the limb arises from the:
   A. Paraxial mesoderm
   B. Neural crest
   C. Intermediate mesoderm
   D. Somitic mesoderm
   E. Lateral mesoderm

6. The formation of clubfoot (talipes equinovarus) is associated with:
   A. A misplaced ZPA
   B. Defective cellular migration from somites
   C. Thalidomide
   D. Oligohydramnios
   E. A neural crest defect

7. A baby whose mother underwent chorionic villus sampling during pregnancy was born with the tips of two digits missing. What is a possible cause?

8. A woman who underwent amniocentesis during pregnancy gave birth to a child with a duplicated thumb. What is a possible cause?

9. If the somites close to a limb-forming region are experimentally removed, the limbs form without muscles. Why?

10. A child is born with webbed fingers (syndactyly). What is the reason for this anomaly?

## REFERENCES

Bamshad M and others: Reconstructing the history of human limb development: lessons from birth defects, *Pediatr Res* 45:291–299, 1999.

Brand-Saberi B and others: Scatter factor/hepatocyte growth factor (SF/HGF) induces emigration of myogenic cells at interlimb level in vivo, *Dev Biol* 179:303–308, 1996.

Brunet LJ and others: Noggin, cartilage morphogenesis, and joint formation in the mammalian skeleton, *Science* 280:1455–1457, 1998.

Chen Y, Zhao X: Shaping limbs by apoptosis, *J Exp Zool* 282:691–702, 1998.

Christ B, Jacob HJ, Jacob M: Experimental analysis of the origin of the wing musculature in avian embryos, *Anat Embryol* 150:171–186, 1977.

Cihák R: Ontogenesis of the skeleton and intrinsic muscles of the human hand and foot, *Adv Anat Embryol Cell Biol* 46:1–194, 1972.

Coelho CND and others: Altered expression of the chicken homeobox-containing genes GHox-7 and GHox-8 in the limb buds of *limbless* mutant chick embryos, *Development* 113:1487–1493, 1991.

Dahn RD, Fallon JF: Interdigital regulation of digit identity and homeotic transformation by modulated BMP signaling, *Science* 289:438–441, 2000.

Dealy CN, Kosher RA: IGF-1, insulin and FGFs induce outgrowth of the limb buds of amelic mutant chick embryos, *Development* 122:1323–1330, 1996.

Dylevsky I: Connective tissue of the hand and foot, *Acta Univ Carol [Med Mongr]* 127:1–195, 1988.

Dylevsky I: Growth of the human embryonic hand, *Acta Univ Carol [Med Monogr]* 114:1–139, 1986.

Feinberg RN: Vascular development in the embryonic limb bud. In Feinberg RN, Sherer GK, Auerbach R, eds: *The development of the vascular system*, Basel, Switzerland, 1991, Karger, pp 136–148.

Feinberg RN, Noden DM: Experimental analysis of blood vessel development in the avian wing bud, *Anat Rec* 231:136–144, 1991.

Fernandez-Teran M and others: Limb initiation and development is normal in the absence of the mesonephros, *Dev Biol* 189:246–255, 1997.

Ganan Y and others: Role of TGFβs and BMPs as signals controlling the position of the digits and the areas of interdigital cell death in the developing chick autopod, *Development* 122:2349–2357, 1996.

Goodman FR: Limb malformations and the human *Hox* genes, *Am J Med Genet* 112:256–265, 2002.

Grieshammer U and others: The chick limbless mutation causes abnormalities in limb bud dorsal-ventral patterning: implications for the mechanism of apical ridge formation, *Development* 122:3851–3861, 1996.

Grim M, Wachtler F: Muscle morphogenesis in the absence of myogenic cells, *Anat Embryol* 183:67–70, 1991.

Harrison RG: On relations of symmetry in transplanted limbs, *J Exp Zool* 32:1–136, 1921.

Hartmann C, Tabin CJ: Wnt-14 plays a pivotal role in inducing synovial joint formation in the developing appendicular skeleton, *Cell* 104:341–351, 2001.

Heymann S and others: Regulation and function of SF/HGF during migration of limb muscle precursor cells in chicken, *Dev Biol* 180:566–578, 1996.

Hinchliffe JR, Johnson DR: *The development of the vertebrate limb*, Oxford, England, 1980, Clarendon.

Izpisua-Belmonte J-C, Duboule D: Homeobox genes and pattern formation in the vertebrate limb, *Dev Biol* 152:26–36, 1992.

Johnson RL, Tabin CJ: Molecular models for vertebrate limb development, *Cell* 90:979–990, 1997.

Laufer E and others: Expression of radical fringe in limb-bud ectoderm regulates apical ectodermal ridge formation, *Nature* 386:366–373, 1997.

Logan C and others: The role of engrailed in establishing the dorsoventral axis of the chick limb, *Development* 124:2317–2324, 1997.

Logan M, Tabin CJ: Role of Pitx1 upstream of Tbx4 in specification of hindlimb identity, *Science* 283:1736–1739, 1999.

Lu H-C and others: Retinoid signaling is required for the establishment of a ZPA and for the expression of Hoxb-8, a mediator of ZPA formation, *Development* 124:1643–1651, 1997.

Marigo A and others: Conservation in hedgehog signaling: induction of a chicken patched homolog by sonic hedgehog in the developing limb, *Development* 122:1225–1233, 1996.

Michaud JL, Lapointe F, Le Douarin NM: The dorsoventral polarity of the presumptive limb is determined by signals produced by the somites and by the lateral somatopleure, *Development* 124:1453–1463, 1997.

Mrázková O: Blood vessel ontogeny in upper extremity of man as related to developing muscles, *Acta Univ Carol [Med Monogr]* 115:1–114, 1986.

Muragaki Y and others: Altered growth and branching patterns in synpolydactyly caused by mutations in Hoxd 13, *Science* 272:548–551, 1996.

Nelson CE and others: Analysis of Hox gene expression in the chick limb bud, *Development* 122:1449–1466, 1996.

Niswander L and others: Function of FGF-4 in limb development, *Mol Reprod Dev* 39:83–89, 1994.

Ohuchi H and others: Correlation of wing-leg identity in ectopic FGF-induced chimeric limbs with the differential expression of chick *Tbx5* and *Tbx4*, *Development* 125:51–60, 1998.

Ohuchi H, Noji S: Fibroblast-growth-factor-induced additional limbs in the study of initiation of limb formation, limb identity, myogenesis, and innervation, *Cell Tissue Res* 296:45–56, 1999.

Pizette S, Niswander L: BMPs negatively regulate structure and function of the limb apical ectodermal ridge, *Development* 123:883–894, 1999.

Riddle RD and others: Sonic hedgehog mediates the polarizing activity of the ZPA, *Cell* 75:1401–1416, 1993.

Rijli FM, Chambon P: Genetic interactions of Hox genes in limb development: learning from compound mutants, *Curr Opin Genet Dev* 7:481–487, 1997.

Robert B and others: The apical ectodermal ridge regulates Hox-7 and Hox-8 gene expression in developing limb buds, *Genes Dev* 5:2363–2374, 1991.

Robert E, Harris J, Kallen BAJ: The epidemiology of preaxial limb formations, *Reprod Toxicol* 11:653–662, 1997.

Rodriguez-Esteban C and others: The T-box genes *Tbx4* and *Tbx5* regulate limb outgrowth and identity, *Nature* 398:814–818, 1999.

Rodriguez-Niedenfuehr M and others: Development of the arterial pattern in the upper limb of staged human embryos: normal development and anatomical variations, *J Anat* 199:407–417, 2001.

Ros MA and others: Apical ridge dependent and independent mesodermal domains of and GHox-8 expression in chick limb buds, *Development* 116:811–818, 1992.

Ros MA and others: The limb field mesoderm determines initial limb bud anteroposterior asymmetry and budding independent of sonic hedgehog or apical ectodermal gene expressions, *Development* 122:2319–2330, 1996.

Rubin L, Saunders JW: Ectodermal-mesodermal interactions in the growth of limb buds in the chick embryo: constancy and temporary limits of the ectodermal induction, *Dev Biol* 28:94–112, 1972.

Sanders EJ, Wride MA: Programmed cell death in development, *Internat Rev Cytol* 163:105–173, 1995.

Saunders JW: The proximodistal sequence of origin on the parts of the chick wing and the role of the ectoderm, *J Exp Zool* 108:363–403, 1948.

Saunders JW, Gasseling MT: Ectodermal-mesenchymal interactions in the origin of limb symmetry. In Fleischmajer R, Billingham RE, eds: *Epithelial-mesenchymal interactions*, Baltimore, 1968, Williams & Wilkins, pp 78–97.

Saunders JW, Gasseling MT, Saunders LC: Cellular death in morphogenesis of the avian wing, *Dev Biol* 5:147–178, 1962.

Schaller SA and others: Cell biology of limb patterning, *Internat Rev Cytol* 203:483–517, 2001.

Seichert V: Significance of the differential growth, relative tissue shifts and the vascular bed in limb development, *Acta Univ Carol [Med Monogr]* 125:1–162, 1988.

Sekine K and others: FGF10 is essential for limb and lung formation, *Nature Genet* 21:138–141, 1999.

Shinohara H and others: Development of innervation patterns in the upper limb of staged human embryos, *Acta Anat* 138:265–269, 1990.

Simon H-G: T-box genes and the formation of vertebrate forelimb- and hindlimb-specific pattern, *Cell Tissue Res* 296:57–66, 1999.

Stephens TD: The wolffian ridge: history of a misconception, *Isis* 73:254–259, 1982.

Storm EE, Kingsley DM: Joint patterning defects caused by single and double mutations in members of the bone morphogenetic protein (BMP) family, *Development* 122:3969–3979, 1996.

Storm, EE, Kingsley DM: GDF5 coordinates bone and joint formation during digit development, *Devel Biol* 209:11–27, 1999.

Stratford TH, Kostakopoulou K, Maden M: *Hoxb-8* has a role in establishing early anterior-posterior polarity in chick forelimb but not hindlimb, *Development* 124:4225–4234, 1997.

Stratford T, Horton C, Maden M: Retinoic acid is required for the initiation of outgrowth in the chick limb bud, *Curr Biol* 6:1124–1133, 1996.

Stratford TH, Kostakopoulou K, Maden M: Hoxb-8 has a role in establishing early anterior-posterior polarity in chick forelimb but not hindlimb, *Development* 124:4225–4234, 1997.

Summerbell D, Lewis JW, Wolpert L: Positional information in chick limb morphogenesis, *Nature* 244:492–496, 1973.

Swett FH: Determination of limb-axes, *Q Rev Biol* 12:322–339, 1937.

Tanaka M and others: Induction of additional limb at the dorsal-ventral boundary of a chick embryo, *Dev Biol* 182:191–203, 1997.

Theil T and others: *Gli* genes and limb development, *Cell Tissue Res* 296:75–83, 1999.

Tickle C, Eichele G: Vertebrate limb development, *Annu Rev Cell Biol* 10:121–152, 1994.

Wang G, Scott SA: Independent development of sensory and motor innervation patterns in embryonic chick hindlimbs, *Devel Biol* 208:324–336, 1999.

Wilkie AOM and others: FGF's, their receptors, and human limb malformations: clinical and molecular correlations, *Am J Med Genet* 112:266–278, 2002.

Wolpert L: Positional information revisited, *Development* 107(suppl):3–12, 1989.

Xu X and others: Fibroblast growth factor receptors (FGFRs) and their roles in limb development, *Cell Tissue Res* 296:33–43, 1999.

Yang Y, Niswander L: Interaction between the signalling molecules Wnt-7a and shh during vertebrate limb development: dorsal signals regulate anteroposterior patterning, *Cell* 80:939–947, 1995.

Zakany J, Duboule D: Hox genes in digit development and evolution, *Cell Tissue Res* 296:19–25, 1999.

Zwilling E: Limb morphogenesis, *Adv Morphogen* 1:301–330, 1961.

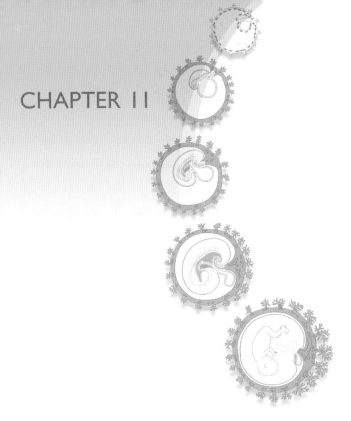

# CHAPTER 11

# Nervous System

Many fundamental developmental processes are involved in the formation of the nervous system. Some of these dominate certain stages of embryogenesis; others occur only at limited times and in restricted locations. The major processes follow:

1. **Induction**, including both primary induction of the nervous system by the underlying notochord and secondary inductions driven by neural tissues themselves

2. **Proliferation**, first as a response of the neuroectodermal cells to primary induction and later to build up critical numbers of cells for virtually all aspects of morphogenesis of the nervous system

3. **Pattern formation**, in which cells respond to genetic or environmental cues in forming the fundamental subdivisions of the nervous system

4. **Determination** of the identity of specific types of neuronal or glial cells

5. **Intercellular communication** and the adhesion of like cells

6. **Cell migration**, of which there are a variety of distinct patterns in the nervous system

7. **Cellular differentiation** of both neurons and glial cells

8. Formation of specific connections or **synapses** between cells

9. **Stabilization** or **elimination** of specific interneuronal connections, sometimes associated with massive episodes of cell death of unconnected neurons

10. Progressive **development of integrated patterns** of neuronal function, which results in coordinated reflex movements

## ESTABLISHMENT OF NERVOUS SYSTEM

As described in Chapter 5, primary induction of the nervous system results in the formation of a thickened ectodermal **neural plate** overlying the notochord. Much of the dorsal ectoderm in gastrulating embryos produces the signaling protein **bone morphogenetic protein-4 (BMP-4)**, which inhibits the dorsal ectoderm from forming neural tissue. Instead of sending positive signals to the overlying ectoderm, the neural inducers, **noggin** and **chordin** block the inhibitory influence of BMP-4, thus allowing the dorsal ectoderm to form neural tissue (the neural plate [see Figure 5-10]).

Shortly following neural induction, further signals from the notochord and head organizing regions (prechordal plate and anterior visceral endoderm) result in the expression of the transcription factor **Otx-2** in the forebrain/midbrain region and **Gbx2** in the hindbrain region. The expression boundary between these two transcription factors forms the **isthmic organizer**. The signaling molecules fibroblast growth factor-8 (**FGF-8**) and **Wnt-1** diffuse from this boundary and are instrumental in setting

233

up the pattern for forming the midbrain and hindbrain. Then, under the influence of specific combinations of *Hox* genes and other transcription factors, the hindbrain undergoes a highly regular segmentation into **rhombomeres**, which presage the overall organization of the entire facial and cervical region (see Figure 11-11).

The neural tube, which is the morphological manifestation of the earliest stages in establishing the nervous system, is a prominent structure. In the human, it dominates the cephalic end of the embryo (see Figure 6-1). This chapter describes how the early neural tube develops into the major morphological and functional components of the mature nervous system.

## EARLY SHAPING OF NERVOUS SYSTEM

Closure of the neural tube first occurs in the region where the earliest somites appear; closure spreads both cranially and caudally (see Figure 6-10). The unfused regions of the neural tube are known as the **cranial** and **caudal neuropores**. Even before the closure of the neuropores (24 days' gestation for the cranial neuropore and 26 days' gestation for the caudal neuropore), some fundamental subdivisions in the early nervous system have become manifest. The future spinal cord and brain are recognizable, and within the brain the forebrain (**prosencephalon**), midbrain (**mesencephalon**), and hindbrain (**rhombencephalon**) can be distinguished (Figure 11-1, *A*).

A prominent force in shaping the early nervous system is the overall bending of the cephalic end of the embryo into a **C**-shape. Associated with this bending is the appearance at the end of the third week of a prominent **cephalic flexure** of the brain at the level of the mesencephalon (see Figure 11-1, *A*). Soon the brain almost doubles back on itself at the cephalic flexure. At the beginning of the fifth week a **cervical flexure** appears at the boundary between the hindbrain and the spinal cord.

By the fifth week the original three-part brain has become further subdivided into five parts (Figures 11-1, *B*, and 11-2). The prosencephalon gives rise to the **telencephalon** (endbrain), with prominent lateral outpocketings that ultimately form the cerebral hemispheres, and a more caudal **diencephalon**. The diencephalon is readily recognizable because of the prominent lateral **optic vesicles** that extend from its lateral walls. The mesencephalon, which is sharply bent by the cephalic flexure, remains undivided and tubular in its overall structure. The roof of the rhombencephalon becomes very thin, and there are early indications of the subdivision of the rhombencephalon into a **metencephalon** and a more caudal **myelencephalon**. These five subdivisions of the early brain represent a fundamental organization that persists through adulthood. Many further structural and functional components give added layers of complexity to the brain over the next several weeks of embryonic life.

## HISTOGENESIS WITHIN THE CENTRAL NERVOUS SYSTEM

### Proliferation Within the Neural Tube

Shortly after induction, the thickening neural plate and early neural tube organize into a pseudostratified epithelium (Figure 11-3). In this type of epithelium the nuclei appear to be located in several separate layers within the elongated neuroepithelial cells. The nuclei undertake extensive shifts of position within the cytoplasm of the neuroepithelial cells.

The neuroepithelial cells are characterized by a high degree of mitotic activity, and the position of the nuclei

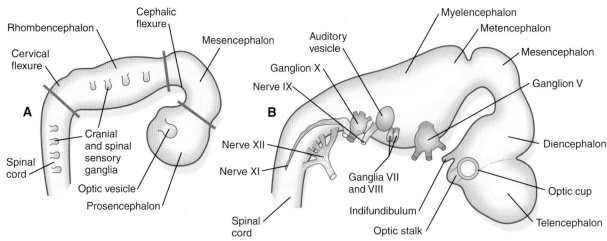

**FIGURE 11-1** Basic anatomy of the three-part (**A**) and five-part (**B**) human brain.

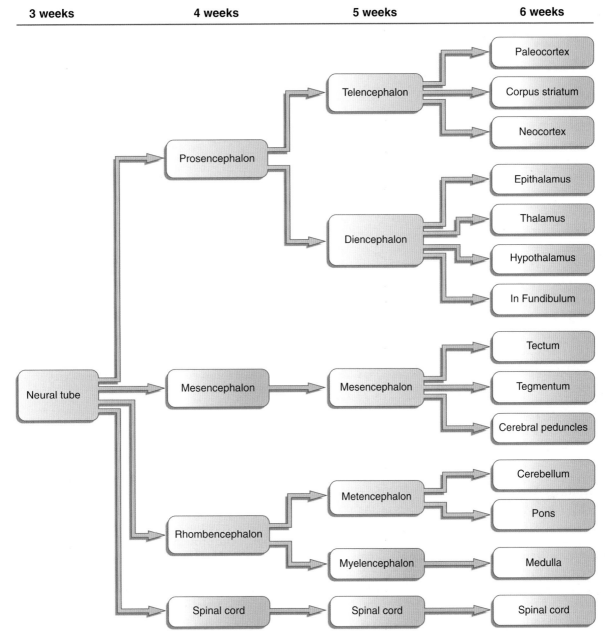

| 3 weeks | 4 weeks | 5 weeks | 6 weeks |
|---|---|---|---|

**FIGURE 11-2** Increasing levels of complexity of the developing human brain.

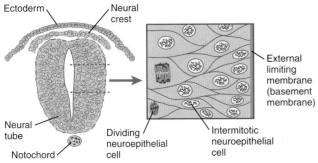

**FIGURE 11-3** *Left,* Cross section through the early neural tube. *Right,* Higher magnification of a segment of the wall of the neural tube.

within the neural tube and their stage in the mitotic cycle are closely correlated (Figure 11-4). DNA synthesis occurs in nuclei located near the **external limiting membrane** (the basal lamina surrounding the neural tube). As these nuclei prepare to go into mitosis, they migrate within the cytoplasm toward the lumen of the neural tube, where they will undergo mitotic division. The orientation of the mitotic spindle during this division determines the fate of the daughter cells. If the metaphase plate (plane of cleavage) is perpendicular to the apical (inner) surface of the neural tube, the two daughter cells slowly migrate in tandem back toward the outer side of the neural tube, where they prepare for another round of

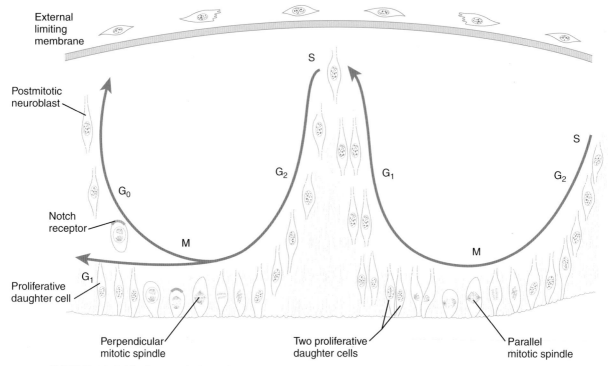

External
limiting
membrane

Postmitotic
neuroblast

S

S

$G_2$

$G_1$

$G_2$

$G_0$

Notch
receptor

M

M

$G_1$

Proliferative
daughter cell

Perpendicular
mitotic spindle

Two proliferative
daughter cells

Parallel
mitotic spindle

**FIGURE 11-4** Mitotic events in the early neural tube. In the pseudostratified epithelial cells that constitute the early neural tube, nuclei that synthesize DNA (S phase) are located near the external limiting membrane. These nuclei move toward the inner margin of the neural tube, where mitosis occurs. If the mitotic spindle is parallel to the inner margin, the two daughter cells both remain in a proliferative state and migrate back toward the external limiting membrane for another round of DNA synthesis. If in the next mitosis the mitotic spindle is oriented perpendicular to the inner margin, one daughter cell remains in the proliferative state. The other daughter cell, which expresses Notch, leaves the mitotic cycle to become a neuroblast.

DNA synthesis (Figure 11-4). In contrast, if the plane of cleavage is parallel with the inner surface of the neural tube, the daughter cells undergo dramatically different fates. The daughter cell that is closer to the inner surface migrates away very slowly and remains a proliferative progenitor cell that is capable of mitosis. The daughter cell that is closer to the basal surface (external limiting membrane) inherits a high concentration of the Notch receptor on its surface and quickly moves away from the apical surface as a **postmitotic neuroblast** (see Figure 11-4). The neuroblasts, cellular precursors of neurons, begin to produce cell processes that ultimately become axons and dendrites.

## Cell Lineages in Histogenesis of the Central Nervous System

The origins of most cells found in the mature central nervous system can be traced to **multipotential stem cells** within the early neuroepithelium (Figure 11-5). These cells undergo numerous mitotic divisions before maturing into **bipotential progenitor cells**, which give rise to either neuronal or glial progenitor cells. This developmental bifurcation is accompanied by a change in gene expression. Multipotential stem cells express an inter-

mediate filament protein called **nestin**. Nestin is downregulated as descendants of bipolar progenitor cells separate into neuronal progenitor cells, which express **neurofilament protein**, and glial progenitor cells, which express **glial fibrillary acidic protein**.

The **neuronal progenitor cells** give rise to a series of neuroblasts. The earliest **bipolar neuroblasts** possess two slender cytoplasmic processes that contact both the external limiting membrane and the central luminal border of the neural tube. By retracting the inner process, a bipolar neuroblast loses contact with the inner luminal border in the process of becoming a **unipolar neuroblast**. The unipolar neuroblasts accumulate large masses of rough endoplasmic reticulum (**Nissl substance**) in their cytoplasm and then begin to send out several cytoplasmic processes. At this point, they are known as **multipolar neuroblasts**. Their principal developmental activities are to send out axonal and dendritic processes and to make connections with other neurons or end organs.

The other major lineage stemming from the bipotential progenitor cells is the glial line. **Glial progenitor cells** continue to undergo mitosis, and their progeny split into several lines. One, the **O-2A progenitor cell** (see Figure 11-5), is a precursor to two lines of glial cells that ultimately form the **oligodendrocytes** and **type-2 astrocytes**.

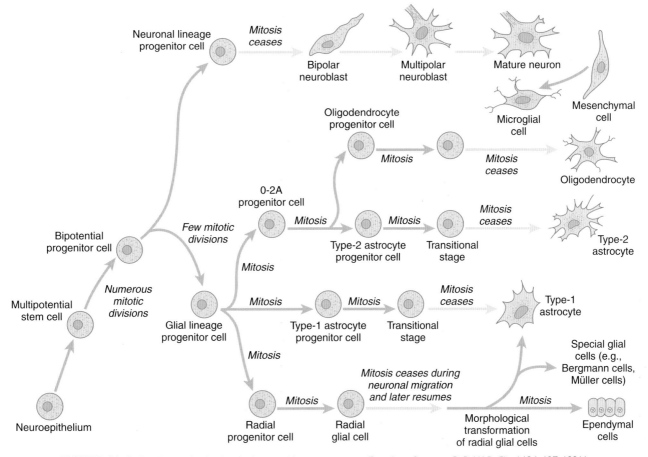

**FIGURE 11-5** Cell lineages in the developing central nervous system. (Based on Cameron R, Rakić P: *Glia* 4:124–127, 1991.)

Another glial lineage gives rise to **type-1 astrocytes**. The origin of oligodendrocytes has long been a matter for debate, but studies have shown that human oligodendrocytes arise from progenitor cells located in the ventral ventricular zone (see Figure 11-6) alongside the floor plate. From there, they spread throughout the brain and spinal cord and ultimately form the myelin coverings around neuronal processes in the white matter. The formation of oligodendrocyte precursors depends on an inductive signal from the notochord (sonic hedgehog). If notochord is transplanted alongside dorsal neural tube, oligodendrocyte precursors differentiate there, showing that cells with the potential to form oligodendrocytes reside in that area, but normally do not develop because of the lack of an adequate inductive signal.

The third glial lineage has a more complex history. Radial progenitor cells give rise to **radial glial cells**, which act as guide wires in the brain for the migration of young neurons (see Figure 11-22). When the neurons are migrating along the radial glial cells during midpregnancy, they inhibit the proliferation of the radial glial cells. After neuronal cell migration, the radial glial cells, now free from the inhibitory influence of the neurons, reenter the mitotic cycle. Their progeny can transform into a number

of cell types. Some can seemingly cross lineage lines and differentiate into type-1 astrocytes (see Figure 11-5). Other progeny differentiate into various specialized glial cell types or even into **ependymal cells**. According to some authors, the remaining neuroepithelial cells represent another source of ependymal cells.

Not all cells of the central nervous system originate in the neuroepithelium. **Microglial cells**, which serve a phagocytic function after damage to the brain, are mesodermally derived immigrant cells. Microglia are not found in the developing brain until it is penetrated by blood vessels.

## Fundamental Cross-Sectional Organization of the Developing Neural Tube

The developing spinal cord is a useful prototype for studying the overall structural and functional features of the central nervous system because it preserves its fundamental organization through much of development. With the beginning of cellular differentiation in the neural tube, the neuroepithelium thickens and appears layered.

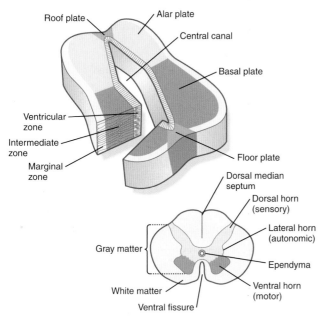

**FIGURE 11-6** Major regions in cross sections of the neural tube *(top)* and spinal cord *(bottom)*.

The layer of cells closest to the lumen (**central canal**) of the neural tube remains epithelial and is called the **ventricular zone** (the **ependymal zone** in older literature). This zone, which still contains mitotic cells, ultimately becomes the **ependyma**, a columnar epithelium that lines the ventricular system and central canal of the central nervous system (Figure 11-6). Farther from the ventricular zone is the **intermediate** (formerly called **mantle**) **zone**, which contains the cell bodies of the differentiating postmitotic neuroblasts. As the neuroblasts continue to produce axonal and dendritic processes, the processes form a peripheral **marginal zone** that contains neuronal processes but not neuronal cell bodies.

As the spinal cord matures, the intermediate zone becomes the gray matter, in which the cell bodies of the neurons are located. The marginal zone is called the **white matter** because of the color imparted by the numerous tracts of myelinated nerve fibers in that layer (see Figure 11-6). During development, the proliferating progenitor cell populations in the ventricular zone become largely exhausted, and the remaining cells differentiate into the epithelium of the ependymal layer.

Once the basic layers in the spinal cord are established, a number of important topographical features can be recognized in cross sections of the cord. A **sulcus limitans** within the central canal divides the cord into a dorsal **alar plate** and a ventral **basal plate** on each side of the central canal. The right and left alar plates are connected dorsally over the central canal by a thin **roof plate**, and the two basal plates are connected ventrally by a **floor plate**.

The basal plate represents the motor component of the spinal cord. Axons arising from neurons located in the

**ventral horn** of the gray matter exit the spinal cord as **ventral motor roots** of the spinal nerves (see Figure 11-14). The gray matter of the alar plate, called the **dorsal horn**, is associated with sensory functions. Sensory axons from the spinal ganglia (neural crest derivatives) enter the spinal cord as dorsal roots and synapse with neurons in the dorsal horn. A small projection of gray matter between the dorsal and ventral horns at spinal levels T1 to L2 contains cell bodies of autonomic neurons. This projection is called the **lateral horn** or sometimes the **intermediolateral gray column** (see Figure 11-6).

The floor plate is far more than an anatomical connection between the right and left basal plates. Cells of the future floor plate are the first to differentiate in the neural plate after primary induction of the nervous system. Experimental work has demonstrated a specific inductive influence of the notochord on the neuroepithelial cells that overly it. If an extra notochord is grafted along the lateral surface of the neural tube, the neuroepithelial cells closest to it acquire the properties of floor plate cells (Figure 11-7). Conversely, if a segment of normal notochord is removed, the neuroepithelial cells overlying it do not acquire the properties of floor plate cells. Through its action on the floor plate, the notochord also exerts a profound effect on the organization of the dorsal and ventral roots that enter and leave the spinal cord. If the notochord is absent, the neural tube closes, but recognizable dorsal and ventral roots are absent. Numerous ectopic nerve fibers appear in their place (Figure 11-8). If the future floor plate is split, the side of the neural tube on which the notochord is located develops normal dorsal and ventral roots, whereas the side lacking these structures gives off ectopic nerves (see Figure 11-7, C).

Recent studies have provided a molecular basis for cross-sectional pattern formation within the early neural plate and neural tube (Figure 11-9). In the early neural plate the homeobox-containing transcription factors, Pax-3, Pax-7, Msx-1, and Msx-2, are expressed throughout the neural plate. Even before the neural plate has folded over to become the neural tube, the notochord, which is adherent to the midline neural plate at this stage, releases **sonic hedgehog**. Local hedgehog signaling stimulates the neural plate cells directly above the notochord to transform into **floor plate**. One of the first stages of this transformation is the repression of Pax-3 and Pax-7 expression, which allows the neuroectodermal cells near the midline of the neural plate to adopt a ventral fate (i.e., floor plate or basal plate). Cells of the floor plate itself then become sites of production of sonic hedgehog.

Development of the overall cross-sectional organization of the neural tube involves not only a ventralizing influence from the notochord, but also an opposing dorsalizing influence from the epidermal ectoderm adjacent to the developing neural tube. In the lateral regions of the neural plate (future dorsal region of the neural tube)

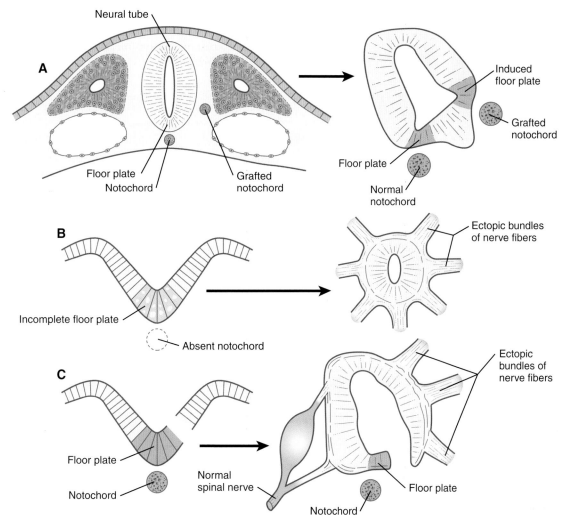

**FIGURE 11-7** Experiments illustrating the influence of the notochord on development of the floor plate and exit sites of nerves from the spinal cord. **A,** Grafting an extra notochord near the neural tube induces a secondary floor plate. **B,** In the absence of a notochord, a very incomplete floor plate forms, and nerve fibers exit from multiple sites around the spinal cord. **C,** Slitting the neural plate on one side of the floor plate removes the wall of the neural tube from the influence of the notochord, allowing the disorganized exit of nerve fibers from that part of the spinal cord. (Modified from Hirano S, Fuse S, Sohal GS: *Science* 251:310–313, 1991.)

BMP-4 and BMP-7, expressed by nonneural ectoderm at the ectodermal-lateral neural plate junction, exert a dorsalizing inductive effect on the neuroectodermal cells by elevating levels of Pax-3, Pax-7, Msx-1, and Msx-2. This results in the formation of the **roof plate** and the alar plate (see Figure 11-9). After closure of the neural tube, the BMP influence induces the formation of sensory interneurons in the dorsal half (alar plate) of the spinal cord.

While the broader regions of the cross-section of the spinal cord are being set in place, a tightly controlled molecular grid forms the basis for specification of the major types of neurons found in the ventral part of the spinal cord. Within the basal plate is an array of five types of neurons—**motoneurons** and four types of **interneurons**—that are arranged in a well-defined dorsoventral pattern. These classes of neurons are specified by specific combinations of homeodomain transcription factors, whose pattern of expression is set by a gradient of sonic hedgehog emanating from the floor plate (Figure 11-10). Some of these transcription factors (class I) are repressed at varying dorsoventral levels by the shh gradient, whereas others (class II) are induced by shh (Figure 11-10). The net result is that a different combination of the transcription factors at each dorsoventral level specifies each of the five types of neurons, which in turn are characterized by their own unique molecular signature. One in particular, **islet-1**, is characteristic of motoneurons. Shortly after the production of motoneurons has ceased, a shift in regulatory factors stimulates the production of **glial progenitor cells** from the ventral neuroepithelium. This leads to the formation of the oligodendrocytes that become closely associated with the neurons.

**FIGURE 11-8 A,** Photomicrograph of a normal embryonic quail spinal cord. **B,** In an experiment in which the notochord was absent, the spinal cord is disorganized and has multiple exit sites of nerve fibers (see Figure 12-7, B). Arrowheads indicate ectopic spinal nerves. *D,* Dorsal; *V,* ventral; *DR,* dorsal root; *VR,* ventral root; *N,* notochord; *F,* floor plate. (From Hirano S, Fuse S, Sohol GS: *Science* 251:310–313, 1991.)

In addition to inducing motor neurons, the floor plate plays other roles in the developing nervous system. A number of groups of neuronal processes cross from one side of the central nervous system to the other through the floor plate as **commissural axons.** These axons, leading from neuronal cell bodies located in the dorsal half of the neural tube, are attracted to the floor plate by specific molecules produced in that region, (e.g., **netrin 1**). In mutant animals lacking netrin 1, commissural axons are disorganized and do not cross to the other side through the floor plate. Not only does the floor plate attract certain types of axons, but it also repels others. A specific example is the trochlear nerve (cranial nerve IV), whose axons do not cross to the other side from their cell bodies of origin because of some yet undefined repellent molecules present in the floor plate.

## CRANIOCAUDAL PATTERN FORMATION AND SEGMENTATION

Through neural induction, the early central nervous system becomes organized into broad regions that will develop cranial, middle, and caudal characteristics (see p. 91). This is soon followed by the appearance of the morphological subdivisions outlined in Figure 11-2. At an even finer level, segments called **rhombomeres** appear in the region of the hindbrain (see Figure 6-3), and a less distinct series of subdivisions called **prosomeres** appears in the forebrain.

## Patterning in the Hindbrain and Spinal Cord Regions

The rhombomeres, which were introduced in Chapter 6, are the morphological reflection of a highly segmentally ordered pattern of expression of a variety of developmentally prominent transcription factors (Figure 11-11). The establishment of the isthmic organizer and the pathways that set up this pattern were discussed in Chapter 6 (see pp. 105–107).

The correspondence between the rhombomeres of the developing hindbrain and other structures of the cranial and pharyngeal arch region is remarkable (see Chapter 14). The cranial nerves, which have a highly ordered pattern by which they supply structures derived from the pharyngeal arches and other structures in the head, have an equally highly ordered origin with respect to the rhombomeres (Figure 11-12). For example, cranial nerve V innervates structures derived from the first pharyngeal arch. Cranial nerves VII and IX innervate the second and third arch structures, respectively. In embryos of birds, the species studied most extensively, cell bodies of the motor components of cranial nerves V, VII, and IX are initially found exclusively in rhombomeres 2, 4, and 6. Dye injection studies have shown that the progeny of a single neuroblast remain within the rhombomere containing the injected cell, suggesting that rhombomeres have the properties of cellular compartments. Axons contributing to a cranial nerve extend laterally within the rhombomere and converge on a common exit site in the craniocaudal midpoint of the rhombomere. At a slightly later stage in development, motor neurons originating in the next more posterior rhombomere (3, 5, 7) extend axons laterally. However, before the axons reach the margin of the rhombomere, they cross into rhombomeres 2, 4, or 6 and converge on the motor axon exit site in the even-numbered rhombomere. Comparative studies indicate species differences in the relationship between rhombomeres and origins of the cranial nerves. Relationships between neuromeres and cranial nerves are outlined in Table 11-1.

The cell bodies (within the central nervous system the collection of cell bodies of a single cranial nerve is called a **nucleus**) of the cranial nerves that innervate the pharyngeal arches arise in register along the craniocaudal axis. The motor nuclei of other cranial nerves that innervate somatic structures (e.g., extraocular muscles or the tongue) arise in a different craniocaudal column along the hindbrain and do not occupy contiguous rhombomeres (see Figure 11-12).

**Neural plate**

Slug

**A**

BMP-4,
BMP-7

Shh

**Future neural crest**

BMP-4,
BMP7

**Notochord**

**Roof plate**

BMPs

**C**

**Neural crest**

Slug

**Alar plate**

Pax-3
Pax-7

**Basal plate**

Pax-6

Shh

**Motoneurons**

**Floor plate**

Shh

BMPs

Slug

**Neural crest**

**B**

Pax-3, Pax7
Msx-1, Msx-2

Shh

**Floor plate**

Shh

**FIGURE 11-9** Dorsal and ventral signaling in the early central nervous system. **A,** Signals from sonic hedgehog *(Shh)* *(orange arrows)* in the notochord induce the floor plate. **B,** In the dorsal part of the future neural tube, BMP-4 and BMP-7 *(green arrows)* from the ectoderm adjacent to the neural tube induces slug in the future neural crest and maintains *Pax-3* and *Pax-7* expression dorsally. Ventrally, sonic hedgehog, now produced by the floor plate, induces motoneurons. **C,** Sonic hedgehog, produced by the floor plate, suppresses the expression of dorsal *Pax* genes *(Pax-3 and Pax-7)* in the ventral half of the neural tube.

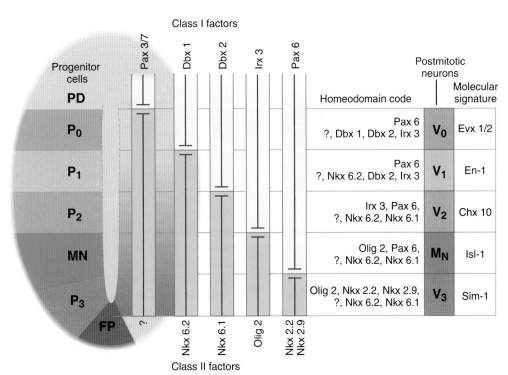

Class I factors

Pax 3/7  Dbx 1  Dbx 2  Irx 3  Pax 6

Progenitor cells

Postmitotic neurons

Molecular signature

Homeodomain code

| Progenitor cells | | Homeodomain code | Postmitotic neurons | Molecular signature |
|---|---|---|---|---|
| PD | | | | |
| P₀ | | Pax 6 ?, Dbx 1, Dbx 2, Irx 3 | V₀ | Evx 1/2 |
| P₁ | | Pax 6 ?, Nkx 6.2, Dbx 2, Irx 3 | V₁ | En-1 |
| P₂ | | Irx 3, Pax 6, ?, Nkx 6.2, Nkx 6.1 | V₂ | Chx 10 |
| MN | | Olig 2, Pax 6, ?, Nkx 6.2, Nkx 6.1 | Mₙ | Isl-1 |
| P₃ | | Olig 2, Nkx 2.2, Nkx 2.9, ?, Nkx 6.2, Nkx 6.1 | V₃ | Sim-1 |
| FP | | | | |

?  Nkx 6.2  Nkx 6.1  Olig 2  Nkx 2.2 Nkx 2.9

Class II factors

**FIGURE 11-10** The molecular basis for the specification of neurons throughout the cross-section of the neural tube. At the left, various classes of progenitor neurons are given labels beginning in P. At the right of the neural tube, a decreasing concentration gradient of sonic hedgehog is indicated by the fading red-brown background. The class I factors (upper bars) are repressed by shh, whereas the class II factors are induced by shh. To the right of the bars is the set of homeodomain codes that specify the various levels of precursor neurons, and at the far right is the molecular signature of the neurons. *FP,* floor plate; *MN,* motoneuron precursors.

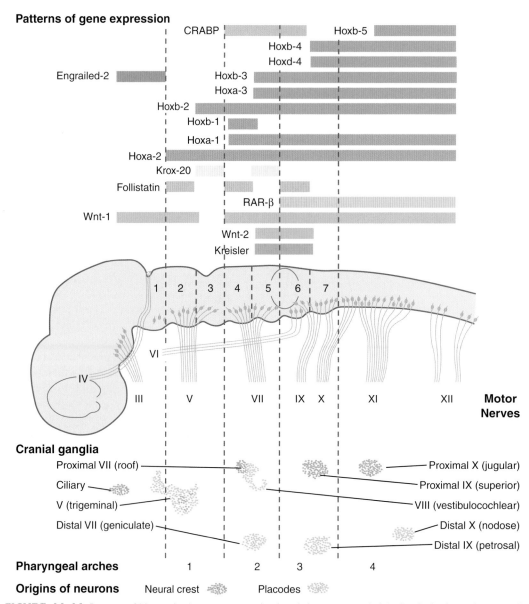

**Patterns of gene expression**

**FIGURE 11-11** Patterns of Hox and other gene expression in relation to anatomical landmarks in the early mammalian embryo. The bars refer to craniocaudal levels of expression of a given gene product. Cranial sensory nerves derived from the neural crest and placodal precursors are laid out in proper register. *CRABP,* Cytoplasmic retinoic acid–binding protein; *RAR,* retinoic acid receptor. (Modified from Noden DM: *J Craniofac Genet Dev Biol* 11:192–213, 1991.)

Direct and indirect evidence indicates that properties of the walls of the rhombomeres prevent axons from straying into inappropriate neighboring rhombomeres. One cellular property, which is also characteristic of regions of somites that restrict the movement of neural crest cells, is the ability of cells of the wall of the rhombomere to bind specific lectins. In apparent contradiction to the compartmentalization just described, processes growing from sensory neuroblasts and from nerves of a tract called the **medial longitudinal fasciculus** are free to cross rhombomeric boundaries. Blood vessels first enter the hindbrain in the region of the floor plate soon after the emergence of the motor axons and spread within the

interrhombomeric junctions. The way the vascular branches recognize the boundaries of the rhombomeres is not known.

In contrast to the hindbrain, the pattern of nerves emanating from the spinal cord does not appear to be determined by craniocaudal compartmentalization within the cord. Rather, the segmented character of the spinal nerves is dictated by the somitic mesoderm along the neural tube. Outgrowing motor neurons from the spinal cord and migrating neural crest cells can easily penetrate the anterior mesoderm of the somite, but they appear to be repulsed by the posterior half of the somite. This results in a regular pattern of spinal nerve outgrowth,

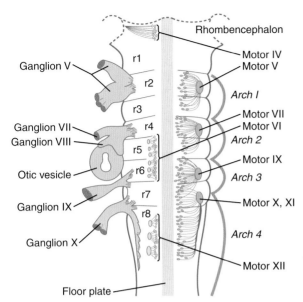

**FIGURE 11-12** Origin of cranial nerves in relation to rhombomeres (r) in the developing chick brain. (Based on Lumsden A, Keynes R: *Nature* 337:424–428, 1989.)

with one bilateral pair of spinal nerves per body segment. Rotating the early neural tube about its craniocaudal axis does not result in an abnormal pattern of spinal nerves. This further strengthens the viewpoint that the pattern of spinal nerves is not generated within the neural tube itself.

## Patterning in the Midbrain Region

One of the fundamental patterning mechanisms in the midbrain region is a molecular signaling center (**isthmic organizer**) located at the border between the mesencephalon and metencephalon (see Figure 6-4). The principal signaling molecule is **FGF-8**, which is expressed in a narrow ring at the anterior border of the first rhombomere, a subdivision of the metencephalon. Acting with **Wnt-1**, FGF-8 induces the expression of engrailed genes **En-1** and **En-2**, as well as **Pax-2** and **Pax-5**, which are expressed in decreasing concentrations at increasing distances from the FGF-8 signaling center (see Figure 6-4). The isthmic organizer induces and polarizes the dorsal midbrain region and the cerebellum. Grafts of the isthmic organizer or beads releasing FGF-8 alone into more cranial regions of the forebrain of the avian embryo induce a second tectum (dorsal mesencephalon or colliculi in mammals). Similarly, isthmic grafts into regions of the hindbrain can induce supernumerary cerebellar structures.

One byproduct of the recent molecular studies is the realization that in some species, at least, the boundary between the future midbrain and hindbrain does not correspond to the anatomical constriction between the mesencephalon and rhombencephalon. Instead, it is located cranial to that constriction in a plane marked by the posterior limit of expression of the homeobox-containing gene, **Otx-2**.

**TABLE 11-1** *Relationship Among Neuromeres, Pharyngeal Arches, Cranial Nerves, and the Neural Crest*

| Primary neuromeres | Secondary neuromeres | Exits of Cranial Nerves | | | Neural crest | Pharyngeal arches |
| | | SSA | SVE | GSE | | |
|---|---|---|---|---|---|---|
| P | T / D1 / D2 | I / II | | | | |
| M | M1 / M2 / Isthmus | | | III / IV | Mesencephalic | |
| Rh A | r1 / r2 / r3 | | V | | Trigeminal | 1 |
| Rh B | r4 | VIII | VII | | Otic | 2 |
| Rh C | r5 / r6 / r7 | | IX / X, XI | VI | Glossopharyngeal / Vagal | 3 / 4–6 |
| Rh D | r8 | | | XII | Hypoglossal | |

Adapted from Müller F, O'Rahilly R: *Acta Anat* 158:83–99, 1997.
*SSA*, Special somatic afferent; *SVE*, special visceral efferent; *GSE*, general somatic efferent; *P*, prosencephalon; *T*, telencephalon; *D*, diencephalon; *M*, mesencephalon; *Rh*, rhombencephalon; *r*, rhombomere.

Like the spinal cord, the midbrain is also highly patterned along its cross-sectional (dorsoventral) axis, and ventrally secreted sonic hedgehog is the molecular basis for much of this patterning, which is represented by five arc-shaped territories of gene expression. If a point source of shh is introduced into a more dorsal region of the midbrain, an additional ectopic set of five corresponding territorial arcs is produced. In addition to promoting neuronal development in the basal plate of the midbrain, shh restricts ventral expression of molecules, such as **Pax-7**, which are characteristic of the alar plate.

Cranially, the midbrain is separated from the forebrain (diencephalon) through a different set of molecular interactions. The alar plate of the diencephalon is characterized by the expression of **Pax-6**, a molecule that among other things acts as the master gene underlying eye formation (see Chapter 13). The mesencephalon, on the other hand, is a domain of **En-1** expression. Through the action of intermediate negative regulators, Pax-6 inhibits en-1 expression, whereas En-1 directly inhibits Pax-6 expression. The craniocaudal level at which each of these molecules inhibits the other becomes a sharp diencephalic-mesencephalic border.

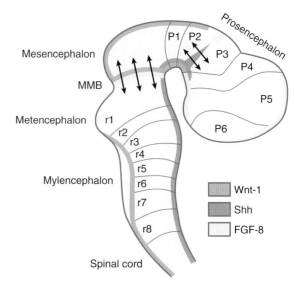

**FIGURE 11-13** Generalized brain of a vertebrate embryo showing segmentation in the hindbrain (rhombomeres [r]) and forebrain (prosomeres [P]) and the distribution of major signaling molecules. The midbrain/hindbrain signaling region is indicated by the arrows just rostral to the first rhombomere. The arrows between the second and third prosomeres represent a hypothetical signaling region in the forebrain. *MMB*, Mesencephalic-metencephalic border. (Adapted from Bally-Cuif L, Wassef M: *Curr Opin Genet Dev* 5:450–458, 1995.)

## Patterning in the Forebrain Region

Although much less apparent than in the hindbrain, the neuromeric organization of the early brain appears to extend into the forebrain region as a set of six **prosomeres**, which extend from the midbrain-forebrain boundary to the tip of the forebrain (Figure 11-13). Prosomeres 1 to 3 (p1 to p3), the most posterior prosomeres, become incorporated into the diencephalon, with p2 and p3 respectively forming the dorsal and ventral **thalamus,** which serves as a major relay station for transmitting neural signals between the cerebral cortex and the body. P4 to p6 contribute to both diencephalic and telencephalic structures. Within the domain of p4 to p6, the basal plate develops into the major regions of the hypothalamus, the structure that integrates autonomic nervous functions and controls endocrine release from the pituitary. The alar plate in this domain is the precursor of the **cerebral cortex,** the **basal ganglia** (collectively the telencephalon), and the **optic vesicles** (diencephalic structures that take the lead in formation of the eyes). As development progresses, p4 to p6 become sharply folded beneath p2 to p3, and in humans the enormous outgrowth of the alar plates of p4 to p6 envelops the other prosomeres as the **telencephalic vesicles** (future cerebral cortex).

Discrete patterns of gene expression also mirror the basic regional organization of the forebrain. Early in development, **FGF-8**, secreted by the anterior neural ridge (see Figure 6-4, *B*), induces the expression of **BF-1** (brain factor-1), which regulates development of the telencephalon and optic vesicles. Within the forebrain a thin

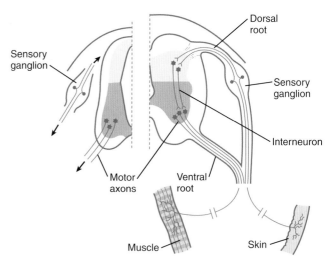

**FIGURE 11-14** Development of a peripheral nerve. *Left*, Early embryo. *Right*, Fetus.

rim of expression of the transcription factor **Nkx 2.2** marks the border between alar and basal plate. Along the dorsoventral axis, the alar plates are characterized by the expression of *Emx-1* & *Emx-2* and *Pax-6*, important regulators of regional identity within the cerebral cortex. In an intermediate region of the prosencephalic alar plate, *Emx* expression drops out, leaving *Pax-6* to function as the master gene controlling eye development (see Chapter 13). In the more ventral area that will eventually form the basal ganglia, *Dlx* (distalless) is a dominant expressed gene.

Like the spinal cord, the ventral forebrain is induced and organized by **sonic hedgehog**, secreted by midline axial structures. In the absence of shh signaling in this area, the tissues of the ventral forebrain are greatly reduced, leading sometimes to midline fusion of the optic vesicles and a general reduction of the growth of the midface region. This results in a type of anomaly called **holoprosencephaly** (see p. 337), which in extreme cases is accompanied by **cyclopia**.

A narrow band of sonic hedgehog expression at the border between the future dorsal (p2) and ventral (p3) thalamus has been suggested to be a forebrain signaling center, but more research is necessary to verify that hypothesis.

## PERIPHERAL NERVOUS SYSTEM

### Structural Organization of a Peripheral Nerve

The formation of a peripheral nerve begins with the outgrowth of axons from motor neuroblasts located in the basal plate (the future ventral horn of the gray matter) of the spinal cord (Figure 11-14). Near the dorsal part of the spinal cord, thin processes also begin to grow from neural crest–derived neuroblasts that have aggregated to form the spinal ganglia. **Dendrites**, which conduct impulses toward the nerve cell body, grow from the sensory neurons toward the periphery. **Axons**, which conduct impulses away from the cell body, penetrate the dorsolateral aspect of the spinal cord and terminate in the dorsal horn (the gray matter of the alar plate). Within the gray matter, short interneurons connect the terminations of the sensory axons to the motor neurons. These three connected neurons (motor, sensory, and interneuron) constitute a simple **reflex arc** through which a sensory stimulus can be translated into a simple motor response. Autonomic nerve fibers are also associated with typical spinal nerves.

Within a peripheral nerve the neuronal processes can be myelinated or unmyelinated. At the cellular level, **myelin** is a multilayered spiral sheath consisting largely of phospholipid material that is formed by individual **Schwann cells** (neural crest derivatives) wrapping themselves many times around a nerve process like a jelly roll (Figure 11-15). This wrapping serves as a form of insulation that determines to a great extent the character of the electrical impulse (action potential) traveling along the neuronal process. **Unmyelinated nerve fibers** are also embedded in the cytoplasm of Schwann cells, but they lack the characteristic spiral profiles of myelinated processes (see Figure 11-15).

The Schwann cells that surround myelinated and unmyelinated axons are different not only in their morphology but also, not surprisingly, in their patterns of gene expression. Through the actions of a family of growth factor–like proteins (**neuregulins**), the axon associated with a Schwann cell precursor promotes the differentiation of the Schwann cell and helps determine whether it will produce myelin or form a nonmyelinating Schwann cell. Schwann cell precursors that are not associated with axons do not receive neuregulin support and undergo programmed cell death, a mechanism that preserves an appropriate ratio of Schwann cells to axons.

Within the central nervous system the color of the white matter is the result of its high content of myelinated nerve fibers, whereas the gray matter contains unmyelinated fibers. Schwann cells are not present in the central nervous system; instead, myelination is accomplished by oligodendrocytes. Although one Schwann cell in a myelinated peripheral nerve fiber can wrap itself around only one axon or dendrite, a single oligodendroglial cell can myelinate several nerve fibers in the central nervous system.

### Patterns and Mechanisms of Neurite Outgrowth

The outgrowth of **neurites** (axons or dendrites) involves many factors both intrinsic and extrinsic to the neurite. Although similar in many respects, the outgrowth of axons and dendrites differs in fundamental ways.

An actively elongating neurite is capped by a **growth cone** (Figure 11-16). Growth cones are characterized by an expanded region of cytoplasm with numerous spikelike projections called **filopodia**. In vitro and in vivo studies of living nerves show that the morphology of an active growth cone is in a constant state of flux, with filopodia regularly extending and retracting as if testing the local environment. Growth cones contain numerous cytoplasmic organelles, but much of the form and function of the filopodia depends on the large quantities of **actin** microfilaments that fill these processes. In the presence of agents that disrupt actin filaments, the filopodia retract and the growth cones cease to function normally.

Whether growth cones progress forward, remain static, or change directions depends in large measure on their interactions with the local environment. If the environment is favorable, a filopodium remains extended and adheres to the substrate around it, whereas other filopodia on the same growth cone retract. Depending on the location of the adhering filopodia, the growth cone may lead the neurite to which it is attached straight ahead or change its direction of outgrowth. This outgrowth appears to be guided by four broad types of environmental influences: **chemoattraction**, **contact attraction**, **chemorepulsion**, and **contact repulsion**. It now appears that outgrowing nerve processes find themselves in different environments every couple hundred microns and

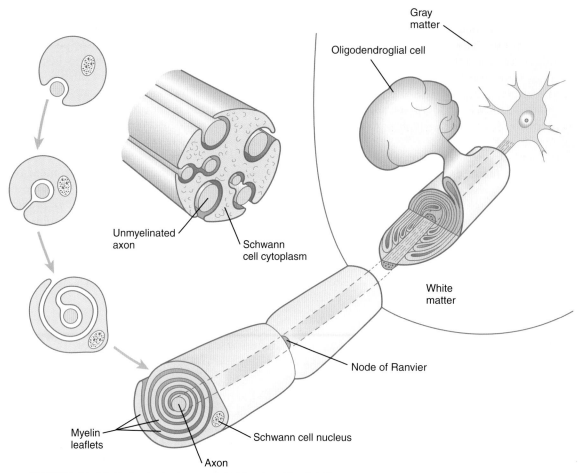

**FIGURE 11-15** Myelination in the central *(right)* and peripheral *(left)* nervous systems. Within the central nervous system, myelin is formed by oligodendroglial cells. In the peripheral nervous system, Schwann cells wrap around individual axons. The inset shows a segment through a region of unmyelinated nerve fibers embedded in the cytoplasm of a single Schwann cell.

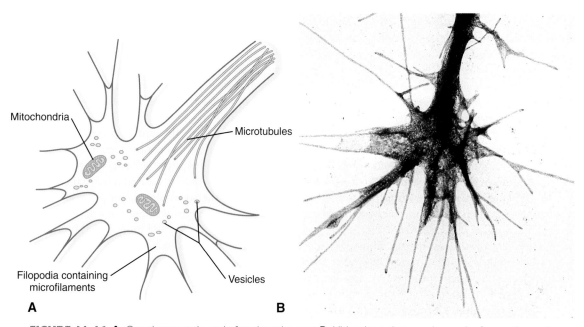

**FIGURE 11-16 A,** Growth cone at the end of an elongating axon. **B,** High-voltage electron micrograph of a growth cone in culture. (**A** from Landis S: *Annu Rev Physiol* 45:567–580, 1983. **B** courtesy K. Tosney, Ann Arbor, Mich.)

that some environments give them signals to continue extending forward, whereas other environments may act as "stop" signals or "turn" signals.

Growth cones can respond to concentration gradients of diffusible substances (e.g., nerve growth factor) or to weak local electrical fields. A major family of chemoattractant molecules is called the **netrins**. The repulsive counterparts to the netrins are members of a family of secreted proteins called **semaphorins**. The various growth cone attractants produce their effects by stimulating signal transduction machinery that results in elevated levels of cyclic nucleotide second messengers (cAMP or cGMP), whereas repulsants exert their effects through decreased levels of these second messengers.

Growth cones can also respond to fixed physical or chemical cues from the microenvironment immediately surrounding them. For example, the caudal half of the somite repulses the ingrowth of motor axons and of neural crest cells into that area. Repulsion is manifested by the collapse of the growth cone and the retraction of the filopodia. On the other hand, extracellular matrix glycoproteins such as **fibronectin** and especially **laminin** strongly promote the adhesion and outgrowth of neurites. Integral membrane proteins (**integrins**) on the neurites bind specifically to arginine-glycine-asparagine sequences on the glycoproteins and promote adhesion to the substrate containing these molecules.

Other molecules, such as **N-cadherin, E-cadherin,** and **L1**, are involved in intercellular adhesion at various stages of cell migration or neurite elongation. N-cadherin, which uses $Ca^{++}$ as an ionic agent to bind two like molecules together, is heavily involved in the intercellular binding of cells in neuroepithelia. It also plays a role in the adhesion of parallel outgrowing neurites. In a peripheral nerve, one **pioneering axon** typically precedes the others in growing toward its target. Other axons then follow, forming **fascicles** (bundles) of axons. Fasciculation is facilitated by intercellular adhesion proteins such as L1, which help bind parallel nerve fibers. If antibodies to the L1 protein are administered to an area of neurite outgrowth, fasciculation is disrupted. N-CAM is present on the surfaces of most embryonic nerve processes and muscle fibers and is involved in the initiation of neuromuscular contacts. Antibodies to N-CAM interfere with the development of neuromuscular junctions in embryos. Outgrowing neurites interact with many other molecules, the full extent of which is just becoming apparent.

Although the growth cone can be thought of as the director of neurite outgrowth, other factors are important for the elongation of axons. Essential to the growth and maintenance of axons and dendrites is **axonal transport**. In this intracellular process, materials produced in the cell body of the neuron are carried to the ends of these neurites, which can be several feet long in humans.

The cytoskeletal backbone of an axon is an ordered array of microtubules and neurofilaments. **Microtubules** are long, tubular polymers composed of **tubulin** subunits. As an axon extends from its cell body, tubulin subunits are transported down the axon and polymerize onto the distal end of the microtubule. The assembly of **neurofilaments** is organized in a similar polarized manner. The site of these cytoskeletal additions is close to the base of the growth cone, meaning that the axon elongates by being added to distally rather than being pushed out by an addition to its proximal end near the neuronal cell body. A characteristic accompaniment of axonal growth is the production of large amounts of **growth-associated proteins (GAPs)**. Particularly prominent among these is **GAP-43**, which serves as a substrate for protein kinase C and is concentrated in the growth cone.

Outgrowing axons and dendrites differ in several important ways. In contrast to axons, dendrites contain microtubules with polarity running in both directions (Figure 11-17). Another prominent difference is the absence of GAP-43 protein in growing dendrites. One of the first signs of polarity of a developing neuron is the concentration of GAP-43 in the outgrowing axon and its disappearance from the dendritic processes.

## Neurite/Target Relations During Development of a Peripheral Nerve

Developing neurites continue to elongate until they have contacted an appropriate end organ. In the case of motor neurons, that end organ is a developing muscle fiber. Dendrites of sensory neurons relate to a number of types of targets. The end of the neurite must first recognize its appropriate target, and then it must make a functional connection with it.

In the case of motor neurons, evidence that very specific cues guide individual nerves and axons to their muscle targets is increasing. Tracing and transplantation studies have shown that outgrowing motor nerves to limbs supply the limb muscles in a well-defined order and that after minor positional dislocations, they will seek out the correct muscles (see Figure 10-26). Recent evidence suggests that even at the level of neurons, "fast" axons are attracted to the precursors of fast muscle fibers and "slow" axons to those of slow muscle fibers. There are many similar examples of target specificity in dendrites in the peripheral nervous system and of both dendrites and axons in the central nervous system. Even within a single developing muscle fiber, an aggregation of muscle-specific tyrosine kinase receptor molecules determines the exact site at which the outgrowing axonal terminal connects with the muscle fiber.

When a motor axon and a muscle fiber meet, a complex series of changes in both the nerve and muscle fibers marks the formation of a functional **synapse**, in this case called a **neuromuscular junction** (Figure 11-18). The early changes consist of (1) the cessation of outgrowth of

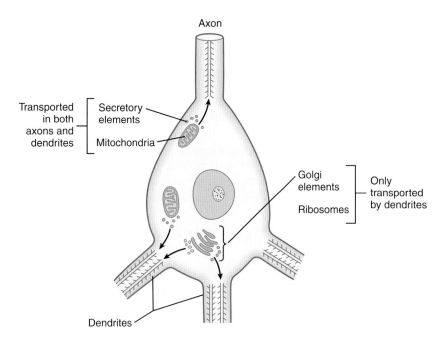

the axon, (2) the preparation of the nerve terminal for the ultimate release of appropriate neurotransmitter molecules, and (3) modifications of the muscle fibers at the site of nerve contact so that the neural stimulus can be received and translated into a contractile stimulus. Both neural and muscular components of the neuromuscular junction are involved in stabilizing the morphological and functional properties of this highly specialized synapse.

One of the first signs of specialization at an incipient neuromuscular junction is the formation of synaptic vesicles, which is caused by an influence of the muscle fiber. These vesicles store and ultimately release the neurotransmitter substance **acetylcholine** from the nerve ter-

minal (see Figure 11-18). Before the developing muscle fiber is contacted by the motor neuron, **acetylcholine receptors** (nonjunctional type) are scattered throughout the length of the muscle fiber. After initial nerve contact, myonuclei in the vicinity of the neuromuscular junction produce junction-specific acetylcholine receptors that reside on nerve-induced postjunctional folds of the muscle fiber membrane, and the scattered nonjunctional receptors disappear. Between the nerve terminal and the postsynaptic apparatus of the muscle fiber lies a basal lamina containing molecules that stabilize the acetylcholine receptors at the neuromuscular junction and also **acetylcholinesterase**, an enzyme produced by the muscle fiber.

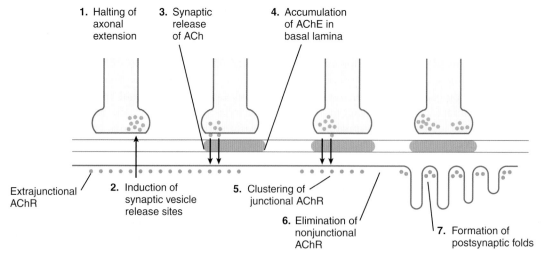

**FIGURE 11-18** Major steps in the formation of a neuromuscular junction. *ACh*, Acetylcholine; *AChE*, acetylcholinesterase; *AChR*, acetylcholine receptors.

## Factors Controlling Numbers and Kinds of Connections Between Neurites and End Organs in the Peripheral Nervous System

At many stages in the formation of a peripheral nerve, interactions between the outgrowing neurites and the target structure influence the numbers and quality of either the nerve fibers or the targets. The existence of such mechanisms was demonstrated in the early 1900s by transplanting limb buds onto flank regions. The motor nerves and sensory ganglia that supplied the grafted limbs were substantially larger than the contralateral spinal nerves, which innervated only structures of the body wall. Examination of the spinal cord at the level of the transplant revealed larger ventral horns of gray matter containing more motor neurons than normal for levels of the spinal cord that supply only flank regions.

Additional experiments of this type cast light on normal anatomical relations, which show relatively larger volumes of gray matter and larger nerves at levels from which the normal limbs are innervated. Deletion experiments, in which a limb bud is removed before neural outgrowth, or the congenital absence of limbs results in deficient numbers of peripheral neurons and reduced volumes of gray matter in the affected regions.

Neuronal **cell death (apoptosis)** plays an important role in normal neural development. For example, when a muscle is first innervated, far more than the normal adult number of neurons supply it. At a critical time in development, massive numbers of neurons die. There seem to be a number of reasons for this seemingly paradoxical phenomenon, including the following:

1. Some axons fail to reach their normal target, and cell death is a way of eliminating them.
2. Cell death could be a way of reducing the size of the neuronal pool to something appropriate to the size of the target.
3. Similarly, cell death could compensate for a presynaptic input that is too small to accommodate the neurons in question.
4. Neuronal cell death may also be a means of eliminating connection errors between the neurons and their specific end organs.

All of these reasons for neuronal cell death may be part of a general biological strategy that reduces superfluous initial connections to ensure that enough correct connections have been made. The other developmental strategy, which seems to be much less used, is to control the outgrowth and connection of neurites with their appropriate end organs so tightly that there is little room for error from the beginning. Because of the overall nature of mammalian development, such tight developmental controls would rob the embryo of the overall flexibility it needs to compensate for genetically or environmentally induced variations in other aspects of development.

The mechanisms by which innervated target structures prevent the death of the neurons that supply them are only beginning to be understood. A popular hypothesis is that the target cells release chemical **trophic factors** that neurites take up, usually by binding to specific receptors. The trophic factor then sustains the growth of the neurite. The classic example of a trophic factor is **nerve growth factor**, which supports the outgrowth and prevents the death of sensory neurons. Several other well-characterized molecules are also candidates for trophic factors.

## AUTONOMIC NERVOUS SYSTEM

The autonomic nervous system is the component of the peripheral nervous system that subserves many of the involuntary functions of the body, such as glandular activity and motility within the digestive system, heart rate, vascular tone, and sweat gland activity. It is divided into two major divisions, the sympathetic and parasympathetic nervous systems. Components of the **sympathetic nervous system** arise from the thoracolumbar levels (T1 to L2) of the spinal cord, whereas the **parasympathetic nervous system** has a widely separated dual origin from the cranial and sacral regions. Both components of the autonomic nervous system consist of two tiers of neurons: **preganglionic** and **postganglionic**. Postganglionic neurons are derivatives of the neural crest (see Chapter 12).

### Sympathetic Nervous System

Preganglionic neurons of the sympathetic nervous system arise from the **intermediate horn** (visceroefferent column) of the gray matter in the spinal cord. At levels from T1 to L2, their myelinated axons grow from the cord through the ventral roots, paralleling the motor axons that supply the skeletal musculature (Figure 11-19). Shortly after the dorsal and ventral roots of the spinal nerve join, the preganglionic sympathetic axons, which are derived from the neuroepithelium of the neural tube, leave the spinal nerve via a **white communicating ramus**. They soon enter one of a series of **sympathetic ganglia** to synapse with neural crest–derived postganglionic neurons.

The sympathetic ganglia, the bulk of which are organized as two chains running ventrolateral to the vertebral bodies, are laid down by neural crest cells that migrate from the closing neural tube along a special pathway (see Figure 12-4). Once the **migrating sympathetic neuroblasts** have reached the site at which the

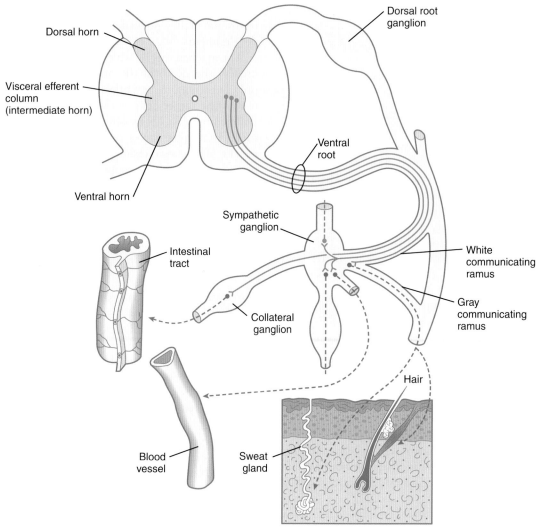

**FIGURE 11-19** Organization of the autonomic nervous system at the level of the thoracic spinal cord. First-order sympathetic neurons are indicated by solid blue lines; second-order sympathetic neurons are indicated by dashed green lines.

**sympathetic chain ganglia** form, they spread both cranially and caudally until the extent of the chains approximates that seen in the adult. Some of the sympathetic neuroblasts migrate farther ventrally than the level of the chain ganglia to form a variety of other **collateral ganglia** (e.g., **celiac** and **mesenteric ganglia**), which occupy somewhat variable positions within the body cavity. The **adrenal medulla** can be broadly viewed as a highly modified sympathetic ganglion.

The outgrowing preganglionic sympathetic neurons either terminate within the chain ganglia or pass through on their way to more distant sympathetic ganglia to form synapses with the cell bodies of the second-order postganglionic sympathetic neuroblasts (see Figure 11-19). Axons of some postganglionic neuroblasts, which are unmyelinated, leave the chain ganglia as a parallel group and reenter the nearest spinal nerve through the **gray** **communicating ramus.** Once in the spinal nerve, these axons continue to grow until they reach appropriate peripheral targets, such as sweat glands, arrector pili muscles, and walls of blood vessels. Axons of other postganglionic sympathetic neurons leave their respective ganglia as tangled **plexuses** of nerve fibers and grow toward other visceral targets.

## Parasympathetic Nervous System

Although also organized on a preganglionic and postganglionic basis, the parasympathetic nervous system has a distribution quite different from that of the sympathetic system. Like those of the sympathetic nervous system, preganglionic parasympathetic neurons originate in the visceroefferent column of the central nervous system.

However, the levels of origin of these neuroblasts are in the midbrain and hindbrain (specifically associated with cranial nerves III, VII, IX, and X) and in the second to fourth sacral segments of the developing spinal cord. Axons from these preganglionic neuroblasts grow long distances before they meet the neural crest–derived postganglionic neurons. These are typically embedded in scattered small ganglia or plexuses in the walls of the organs that they innervate.

The neural crest precursors of the postganglionic neurons often undertake extensive migrations (e.g., from the hindbrain to final locations in the walls of the intestines). The migratory properties of the neural crest precursors of parasympathetic neurons are impressive, but this population of cells also undergoes a tremendous expansion until the final number of enteric neurons approximates the number of neurons in the spinal cord. Evidence is increasing that factors in the gut wall stimulate the mitosis of the neural crest cells migrating there. A striking demonstration of the stimulatory powers of the gut is the ability of pieces of gut wall transplanted

**FIGURE 11-20** Influence of the gut on growth of the neural tube. A graft of quail duodenum was placed between the neural tube and somites of a chick embryo host. The spinal cord on the side near the graft of gut has greatly enlarged, causing secondary distortion of the musculoskeletal structures near it. *cy,* Cyst of donor endoderm. (From Rothman TP and others: *Dev Biol* 124:331–346, 1987.)

along the neural tube to cause a great expansion of the region of the neural tube closest to the graft (Figure 11-20).

## Differentiation of Autonomic Neurons

At least two major steps are involved in the differentiation of autonomic neurons. The first is the determination of certain migrating neural crest cells to differentiate into autonomic neurons instead of the other possible neural crest derivatives.

At early stages the neural crest cells have the option of becoming components of either the sympathetic or parasympathetic system. This was demonstrated by level-shift transplantations of neural crest cells in birds. For example, when the cephalic neural crest, which would normally form parasympathetic neurons, was transplanted to the level of somites 18 to 24, the transplanted cells migrated and settled into the adrenal medulla as **chromaffin cells,** which are part of the sympathetic nervous system. Conversely, trunk neural crest cells transplanted into the region of the head often migrated into the lining of the gut and differentiated into postganglionic parasympathetic neurons.

A second major step in the differentiation of autonomic neurons involves the choice of the neurotransmitter that the neuron will use. Typically, parasympathetic postganglionic neurons are **cholinergic** (i.e., they use acetylcholine as a transmitter), whereas sympathetic neurons are **adrenergic** (noradrenergic) and use norepinephrine as a transmitter.

As they arrive at their final destinations, autonomic neurons are noradrenergic. They then enter a phase during which they select the neurotransmitter substance that will characterize their mature state. Considerable experimental evidence suggests that the choice of transmitter proceeds independently of other concurrent events, such as axonal elongation and the innervation of specific target organs.

At surprisingly late stages in their development, autonomic neurons still retain flexibility in their choice of neurotransmitter. For example, sympathetic neurons in newborn rats are normally adrenergic, and if grown in standard in vitro culture conditions, they produce large amounts of norepinephrine and negligible amounts of acetylcholine. If the same neurons are cultured in a medium that has been conditioned by the presence of cardiac muscle cells, they undergo a functional conversion and instead produce large amounts of acetylcholine (Figure 11-21).

An example of a natural transition of the neurotransmitter phenotype from noradrenergic to cholinergic occurs in the sympathetic innervation of sweat glands in

**FIGURE 11-21** Experiment illustrating the effect of the environment on the choice of transmitter by differentiating sympathetic neurons. In standard medium, they become adrenergic; in medium conditioned by cardiac muscles, they become cholinergic. Levels of norepinephrine are in red; levels of acetylcholine are in blue. (Based on Patterson PH and others: *Sci Am* 239[1]:50–59, 1978.)

the rat. Neurotransmitter transitions depend on target-derived cues. One such cue is **cholinergic differentiation factor,** a glycosylated basic 45-kDa protein. This molecule, which is present in cardiomyocyte-conditioned medium, is one of a number of chemical environmental factors that can exert a strong influence on late phases of differentiation of autonomic neurons.

## Congenital Aganglionic Megacolon (Hirschsprung's Disease)

If a newborn exhibits symptoms of complete constipation in the absence of any demonstrable physical obstruction, the cause is usually an absence of parasympathetic ganglia from the lower (sigmoid) colon and rectum. This condition, commonly called **aganglionic megacolon** or **Hirschsprung's disease** (see p. 367), is normally attributed to the absence of colonization of the wall of the lower colon by neural crest–derived parasympathetic neuronal precursors, probably of cranial origin. In rare cases, greater parts of the colon lack ganglia.

## LATER STRUCTURAL CHANGES IN CENTRAL NERVOUS SYSTEM*

### Histogenesis Within the Central Nervous System

A major difference between the brain and spinal cord is the organization of the gray and white matter. In the spinal cord the gray matter is centrally located, with white matter surrounding it (see Figure 11-6). In many parts of the brain, this arrangement is reversed, with a large core of white matter and layers of gray matter situated superficial to this core.

One of the fundamental processes in histogenesis within the brain is cell migration. From their sites of origin close to the ventricles in the brain, neuroblasts migrate toward the periphery following set patterns.

---

* The later changes in the central nervous system are so extensive that an exhaustive treatment of even one aspect, such as morphology, is well beyond the scope of this book. This section instead stresses fundamental aspects of the organization of the central nervous system and summarizes the major changes in the organization of the brain and spinal cord.

These patterns often result in a multilayering of the gray substance of the brain tissue. Key players in the migratory phenomenon are radial glial cells, which extend long processes from cell bodies located close to the ventricular lumen toward the periphery of the developing cortex (Figure 11-22). Young postmitotic neurons, which are typically simple bipolar cells, wrap themselves around the radial glial cells and use them as guides on their migrations from their sites of origin to the periphery.

In areas of brain cortex characterized by six layers of gray matter, the large neurons populating the innermost layer migrate first. The remainder of the layers of gray matter are formed by smaller neurons migrating through the first layer and other previously formed layers to set up a new layer of gray matter at the periphery. With this pattern of histogenesis, the outermost layer of neurons is the one formed last, and the innermost is the layer formed first. In a mouse mutant called **weaver**, specific behavioral defects are related to abnormal function of the cerebellum. The morphological basis for this mutant is an abnormality of the radial glial cells in the cerebellum and a consequent abnormal migration of the cells that normally form the granular layer of the cerebellar cortex. Another mutant, called **reeler**, is characterized by abnormal behavior and the absence of normal cortical layering. Recently an extracellular protein, called **reelin**, has been shown to be defective in the reeler mutant. Its exact cellular function has not yet been determined, but it may serve as a stop signal for radial neuronal migration or as an insertional signal for migrating neurons.

Not all neuronal migration within the central nervous system follows the inside-out pattern described earlier. Neuronal migration parallel to the surface occurs during early development of the cerebellum, and in contrast to the cerebral cortex, within the three layers of gray matter in the hippocampus and superior colliculi the neurons in the outer layer are the oldest and those of the innermost layer the youngest.

Increasing evidence indicates that the seemingly featureless cerebral cortex is a matrix of discrete **columnar radial units** that consist of radial glial cells and the neuroblasts that migrate along them. There may be as many as 200 million radial units in the human cerebral cortex. The radial units begin as proliferative units, with most cortical neurons generated between days 40 and 125. As with many aspects of neural differentiation, the number of radial units seems to be sensitive to their own neural input. For example, in cases of **congenital anophthalmia** (the absence of eyes), neural input from visual pathways to the area of the occipital cortex associated with vision is reduced. This results in both gross and microscopic abnormalities of the visual cortex, principally related to a reduced number of radial units in that region.

## Spinal Cord

In the spinal cord, inputs from many peripheral sensory nerves are distributed as local reflex arcs or are channeled to the brain through tracts of axons. Also, motor messages originating in the brain are distributed to appropriate peripheral locations via motor tracts and ventral (motor) roots of individual spinal nerves. Although several aspects of spinal cord organization were discussed earlier in this chapter, some are briefly reviewed because of their value in understanding basic brain organization.

The early spinal cord is divided into alar and basal plate regions, which are precursors for the sensory and motor regions of the cord (see Figure 11-6). The mature cord has a similar organization, but these regions are further subdivided into somatic and visceral components. Within the brain, still another layer of input and output is added with "special" components. These are summarized in Box 11-1.

A gross change of the spinal cord that is of clinical significance is the relative shortening of the cord in relation to the vertebral column (Figure 11-23). In the first trimester the spinal cord extends the entire length of the body, and the spinal nerves pass through the intervertebral spaces directly opposite their site of origin. In later months, growth of the posterior part of the body outstrips that of both the vertebral column and the spinal cord, but growth of the cord lags significantly behind that of the vertebral column. This disparity is barely apparent in the cranial and thoracic regions, but at birth the spinal

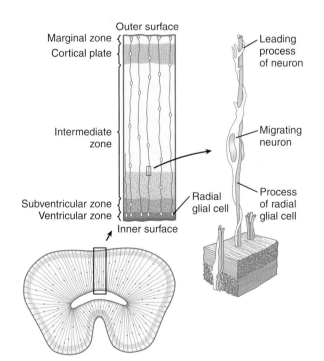

**FIGURE 11-22** Radial glial cells and their association with peripherally migrating neurons during the development of the brain. (Based on Rakić P: *Birth Defects Orig Article Series* II[7]:95–129, 1975.)

## Box 11-1    Functional Regions in the Spinal Cord and Brain

### ALAR PLATE (AFFERENT OR SENSORY)

General somatic afferent: sensory input from the skin, joints, and muscles

Special visceral afferent: sensory input from the taste buds and pharynx

General visceral afferent: sensory input from the viscera and heart

### BASAL PLATE (EFFERENT: MOTOR OR AUTONOMIC)

General visceral efferent: autonomic (two-neuron) links from the intermediate horn to the viscera

Special visceral efferent: motor nerves to striated muscles of the pharyngeal arches

General somatic efferent: motor nerves to the striated muscles other than those of the pharyngeal arches

**FIGURE 11-23** *Top,* Changes in the level of the end of the spinal cord in relation to bony landmarks in the vertebral column during fetal development. *Bottom,* Development of the curvature of the spine.

cord terminates at the level of L3. By adulthood, the cord terminates at the L2.

The consequence of this growth disparity is the considerable elongation of the lumbar and sacral dorsal and ventral spinal nerve roots to accommodate the increased distance between their point of origin and the appropriate intervertebral space. This gives them the collective appearance of a horse's tail (hence their name, **cauda equina**). A thin, filament-like **filum terminale** extending from the end of the spinal cord proper to the base of the vertebral column marks the original excursion of the spinal cord. This arrangement is convenient for the clinician because the space below the termination of the cord is a safe place from which to withdraw cerebrospinal fluid for analysis.

## Myelencephalon

The **myelencephalon**, the most caudal subdivision of the rhombencephalon (see Figures 11-1 and 11-2), develops into the **medulla oblongata** of the adult brain (Figure 11-24). It is in many respects a transitional structure between the brain and spinal cord, and the parallels between its functional organization and that of the spinal cord are readily apparent (Figure 11-25). Much of the medulla serves as a conduit for tracts that link the brain with input and output nodes in the spinal cord, but it also contains centers for the regulation of vital functions such as the heart beat and respiration.

The fundamental arrangement of alar and basal plates with an intervening sulcus limitans is retained almost unchanged in the myelencephalon. The major topographical change from the spinal cord is a pronounced expansion of the roof plate to form the characteristic thin roof overlying the expanded central canal, which in the myelencephalon is called the **fourth ventricle** (see Figure 11-37). (Details of the ventricles and the coverings of the brain and spinal cord are presented later in this chapter.)

Special visceral **afferent** (leading toward the brain) and **efferent** (leading from the brain) columns of nuclei (aggregations of neuronal cell bodies in the brain) appear in the myelencephalon to accommodate structures derived from the pharyngeal arches.

## Metencephalon

The **metencephalon**, the more cranial subdivision of the hindbrain, consists of two main parts: the **pons**, which is directly continuous with the medulla, and the **cerebellum**, a phylogenetically newer and ontogenetically later-appearing component of the brain (see Figure 11-24). The formation of these structures depends on the functioning of engrailed-1 in the early midbrain/hindbrain region.

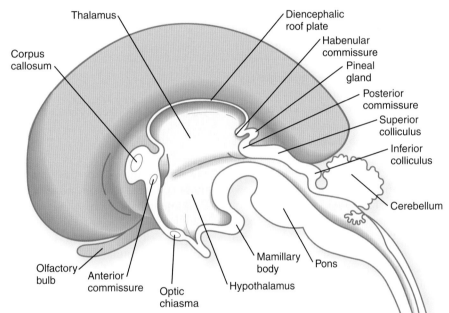

**FIGURE 11-24** Anatomy of the brain in **9-week-old** *(top)* and **16-week-old** *(bottom)* human embryos.

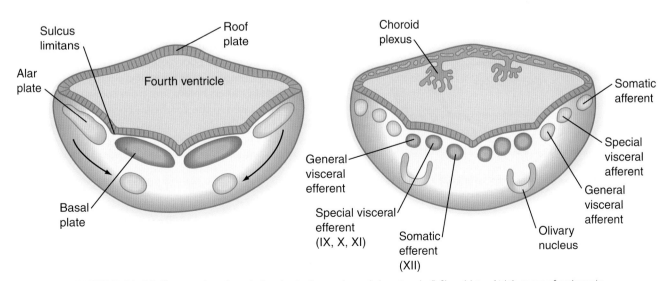

**FIGURE 11-25** Cross sections through the developing myelencephalon at early *(left)* and later *(right)* stages of embryonic development. Motor tracts (from the basal plate) are shown in green; sensory tracts (from the alar plate) are orange. (Modified from Sadler T: *Langman's medical embryology,* ed 6, 1990, Williams & Wilkins.)

As its name implies, the pons, derived from the basal plate, serves as a bridge that carries tracts of nerve fibers between higher brain centers and the spinal cord. Its fundamental organization remains like that of the myelencephalon, with three sets of afferent and efferent nuclei (Figure 11-26). In addition to these, other special pontine nuclei, which originated from alar plate–derived neuroblasts, are present in the ventral white matter. The caudal part of the pons also has an expanded roof plate similar to that of the myelencephalon.

The cerebellum, an alar plate derivative, is structurally and functionally complex, but phylogenetically it arose as a specialization of the vestibular system and was involved with balance. Other functions, such as the orchestration of general coordination and involvement in auditory and visual reflexes, were later superimposed.

The future site of the cerebellum is first represented by the rhombic lips of the 5- to 6-week embryo. The rhombic lips represent the somewhat diamond (rhombus)-shaped border between the thin roof plate and the main body of the rhombencephalon (Figure 11-27). The rhombic lips, situated from rhombomeres 1 to 8 (r1 to r8) are the product of an inductive interaction between the roof plate (through BMP signaling) and the neural tube within the original rhombencephalon. The cerebellum proper arises from the anterior (cerebellar) rhombic lips (r1), whereas the posterior rhombic lips (r2 to r8) give rise to the migratory precursors of a variety of ventrally situated nuclei (e.g., olivary and pontine nuclei—see Figures 11-25 and 11-26) that are located in the metencephalon and rhombencephalon. Soon after the induction of the rhombic lips, precursors of **granule cells** migrate anteriorly along the dorsal region of r1 from the cerebellar rhombic lips to form a transient germinal epithelium called the **external granular layer** (Figure 11-28). After terminal mitotic divisions, the postmitotic external granule cells undergo a second radial migration

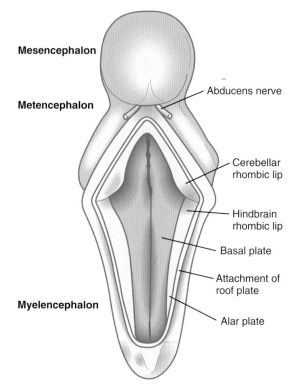

**FIGURE 11-27** Dorsal view of the midbrain and hindbrain of a **5-week-old** embryo. The roof of the fourth ventricle has been opened.

toward the interior of the future cerebellum. En route, these cells pass through a layer of precursors of the larger **Purkinje cells**, which are migrating radially in the opposite direction. Once past the Purkinje cells, the migrating granule cells settle in the **inner granular layer**, simply called the **granular layer** in the mature cerebellum (see Figures 11-28 and 11-29, *E*).

Until the end of the third month, the expansion of the cerebellar rhombic lips is mainly anterior and inward, but thereafter the rapid growth in volume of the cerebellum is directed outward (Figure 11-29). As the volume of the developing cerebellum expands, the two lateral rhombic lips join in the midline, giving the early cerebellar primordium a dumbell appearance. The cerebellum then enters a period of rapid development and external expansion. As the complex process of cerebellar histogenesis porceeds, many fibers emanating from the vast number of neurons generated in the cerebellar cortex leave the cerebellum through a pair of massive **superior cerebellar peduncles**, which grow into the mesencephalon.

## Mesencephalon

The **mesencephalon, or midbrain,** is structurally a relatively simple part of the brain in which the fundamental relationships between the basal and alar plates are essentially preserved (Figure 11-30). As in the spinal cord,

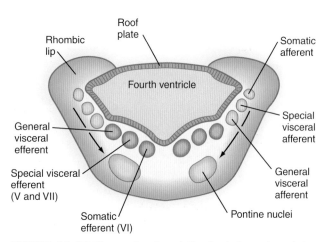

**FIGURE 11-26** Cross section through the developing metencephalon. Motor tracts are green; sensory tracts are orange. (Modified from Sadler T: *Langman's medical embryology,* ed 6, 1990, Williams & Wilkins.)

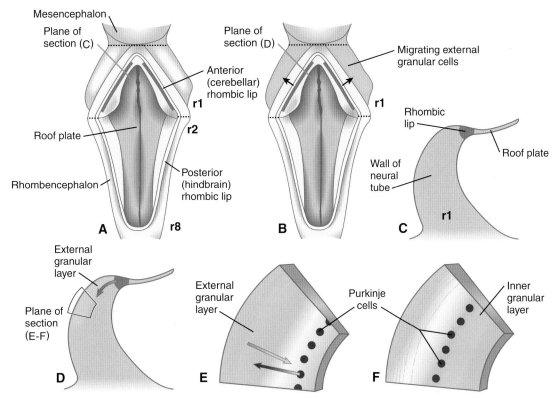

**FIGURE 11-28** Origin and migrations of cerebellar precursor cells. **A,** Dorsal view of the hindbrain. **B,** Dorsal view of the early migration of the external granular cells. **C,** Cross-sectional view of the premigratory stage, indicated by the red line in **A. D,** Cross-sectional view of the early migratory stage, indicated by the red line in **B. E, F,** Cross-sectional views of later stages of inward migration of the external granular cells and the outward migration of the Purkinje cells.

dorsoventral organization within the midbrain is largely based upon sonic hedgehog signaling from the floor, which in addition to promoting neuronal development within the basal plate, suppresses the expression of molecules characteristic of the alar plate.

The basal plates form the neuron-rich area, called the **tegmentum,** in which are located the somatic efferent nuclei of cranial nerves III and IV, which supply most of the extrinsic muscles of the eye. A small visceroefferent nucleus, the **Edinger-Westphal nucleus,** is responsible for innervation of the pupillary sphincter of the eye.

The alar plates form the sensory part to the midbrain, which subserves the functions of vision and hearing. Neuroblasts migrating toward the roof form two prominent pairs of bulges, collectively called the **corpora quadrigemina.** The caudal pair, called the **inferior colliculi,** are relatively simple in structure and are functionally part of the auditory system. The **superior colliculi** take on a more complex layered architecture through the migration patterns of the neuroblasts that give rise to it. The superior colliculi are an integral part of the visual system, and they serve as an important synaptic relay station between the optic nerve and the visual areas of the cerebral (occipital) cortex. Connections between the superior and inferior colliculi help coordinate visual and auditory reflexes.

The third major region of the mesencephalon is represented by prominent ventrolateral bulges of white matter called the **cerebral peduncles** (crus cerebri, see Figure 11-30). A number of the major descending fiber tracts pass through these structures on their way from the cerebral hemispheres to the spinal cord.

## Diencephalon

Cranial to the mesencephalon, the organization of the developing brain becomes so highly modified that it is difficult to relate later morphology to the fundamental alar plate/basal plate plan. In fact, it is widely believed that the forebrain structures (diencephalon and telencephalon) are highly modified derivatives of the alar plates and roof plate without significant representation by basal plates.

Development of the early diencephalon is characterized by the appearance of two pairs of prominent swellings on the lateral walls of the **third ventricle.** These swellings line the greatly expanded central canal in this region (see Figure 11-24). The largest pair of masses represents the developing **thalamus,** in which neural tracts from higher brain centers synapse with those of other regions of the brain and brainstem. Among the many thal-

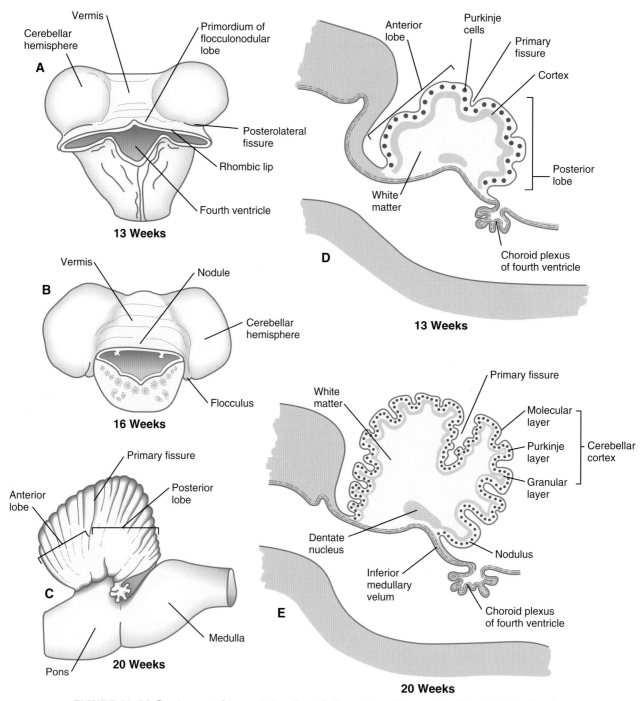

**FIGURE 11-29** Development of the cerebellum. **A** and **B,** Dorsal views. **C,** Lateral view. **D** and **E,** Sagittal sections.

amic nuclei are those that receive input from the auditory and visual systems and transmit them to the appropriate regions of the cerebral cortex. In later development the thalamic swellings may thicken to the point where they meet and fuse in the midline across the third ventricle. This connection is called the **massa intermedia.**

Ventral to the thalamus, the swellings of the incipient **hypothalamus** are separated from the thalamus by the **hypothalamic sulcus.** As mentioned earlier, the hypo-

thalamus receives input from many areas of the central nervous system. It also acts as a master regulatory center, controlling many basic homeostatic functions such as sleep, temperature control, hunger, fluid and electrolyte balance, emotions, and rhythms of glandular secretion (e.g., of the pituitary). A number of its functions are neurosecretory; therefore the hypothalamus serves as a major interface between the neural integration of sensory information and the humoral environment of the body.

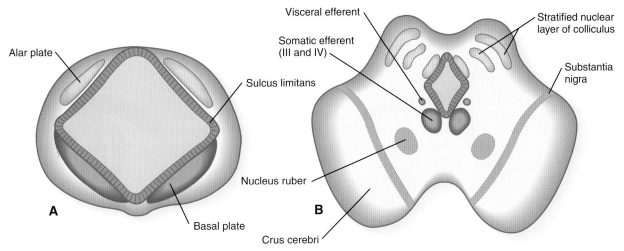

**FIGURE 11-30** Cross sections through the early and later developing mesencephalon. Motor tracts are green; sensory tracts are orange. (Modified from Sadler T: *Langman's medical embryology,* ed 6, 1990, Williams & Wilkins.)

In early embryos (specifically, those around 7 to 8 weeks' gestational age), a pair of less prominent bulges dorsal to the thalamus mark the emergence of the **epithalamus** (see Figure 11-24), a relatively poorly developed set of nuclei relating to masticatory and swallowing functions. The most caudal part of the diencephalic roof plate forms a small diverticulum that becomes the **epiphysis (pineal body),** a phylogenetically primitive gland that often serves as a light receptor. Under the influence of light/dark cycles, the pineal gland secretes (mainly at night) **melatonin,** a hormone that inhibits function of the pituitary-gonadal axis of hormonal control.

The **hypophysis** (pituitary gland) develops from two initially separate ectodermal primordia that secondarily unite. One of the primordia, called the **infundibular process,** forms as a ventral downgrowth from the floor of the diencephalon. The other primordium is **Rathke's pouch,** a midline outpocketing from the stomodeal ectoderm that extends toward the floor of the diencephalon as early as the fourth week. An inductive event from the overlying diencephalon, mediated by BMP-4 first and then FGF-8, stimulates the formation of a **Rathke's pouch primordium** in the dorsal stomodeal ectoderm. Through the action of *Rpx* (Rathke's pouch homeobox-containing gene) and the Lim-type homeobox-containing genes *Lhx-3* and *Lhx-4*, Rathke's pouch primordium forms the definitive Rathke's pouch (Figure 11-31). Experimental evidence from a number of species indicates that in the early embryo the cells in Rathke's pouch originate in the anterior ridge of the neural plate.

The infundibular process is intimately related to the hypothalamus (see Figure 1-14), and certain hypothalamic neurosecretory neurons send their processes into the infundibular process, which ultimately becomes the **neural lobe of the hypophysis.** Throughout development, the histological structure of the infundibulum retains a neural character.

As development proceeds, Rathke's pouch elongates toward the infundibulum (see Figure 11-31). While its blind end partially enfolds the infundibulum like a double-layered cup, the stalk of Rathke's pouch begins to regress. The outer wall of the cup thickens and assumes a glandular appearance in the course of its differentiation into the **pars distalis** (anterior lobe) of the hypophysis. The inner layer of the cup, which is closely adherent to the neural lobe, becomes the **pars intermedia.** It remains separated from the anterior lobe by a slitlike **residual lumen,** which represents all that remains of the original lumen of Rathke's pouch.

With the progression of pregnancy, the hypophysis undergoes a phase of cytodifferentiation. Late in the fetal period, specific cell types begin to produce small amounts of hormones. Molecular cascades underlying the differentiation of specific cell types in the pituitary are being discovered (Box 11-2).

Although Rathke's pouch normally begins to lose its connections to the stomodeal epithelium by the end of the second month, portions of the tissue may occasionally persist along the pathway of the elongating stalk. If the tissue is normal, it is called a **pharyngeal hypophysis.** Sometimes, however, the residual tissue becomes neoplastic and forms hormone-secreting tumors called **craniopharyngiomas.**

The **optic cups** are major outpocketings of the diencephalic wall during early embryogenesis. Earlier in development the ventral diencephalon constitutes a single optic field, characterized by the expression of Pax-6. Then the single optic field is separated into left and right optic primordia by anterior movements of ventral diencephalic cells, which depend upon the expression of the gene *cyclops*. Further development of the optic cups and the optic nerves (cranial nerve II) is discussed in Chapter 13.

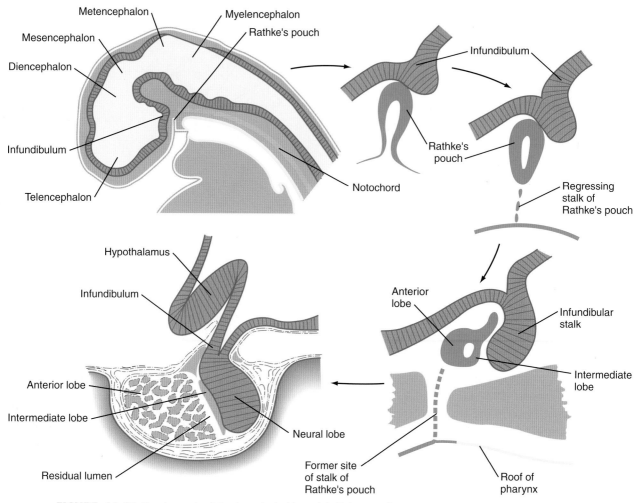

**FIGURE 11-31** Development of the hypophysis. *Upper left,* Reference diagram showing a sagittal section through a **4-week-old** human embryo.

## Box 11-2   Cytodifferentiation of Secretory Cells in the Adenohypophysis

Cytodifferentiation of four of the five major secretory cells in the adenohypophysis (thyrotrophs, gonadotrophs, lactotrophs, and somatotrophs) appears to depend on the expression of a Lim homeobox-containing gene (*Lhx3* in the mouse). Corticotrophs arise from a cell lineage that is independent of Lhx3. Lhx3 mutant mice do not form the anterior or intermediate lobes of the hypophysis. A transcriptional activator, **Pit-1**, a member of the POU homeodomain family, is expressed before the differentiation of any pituitary cell types, and it is required for the differentiation of cells of the somatotroph, lactotroph, and thyrotroph lineages. Further downstream, each cell type of the pituitary requires its own set of molecular activators so that it can differentiate.

## Telencephalon

Development of the **telencephalon** is dominated by the tremendous expansion of the bilateral **telencephalic vesicles**, which ultimately become the cerebral hemispheres (see Figure 11-24). The walls of the telencephalic vesicles surround the expanded lateral ventricles, which are outpocketings from the midline third ventricle located in the diencephalon (see Figure 11-37). Although the cerebral hemispheres first appear as lateral structures, the dynamics of their growth cause them to approach the midline over the roofs of the diencephalon and mesencephalon (Figure 11-32). The two cerebral hemispheres never actually meet in the dorsal midline because they are separated by a thin septum of connective tissue (part of the dura mater) known as the **falx cerebri**. Below this septum the two cerebral hemispheres are connected by the ependymal roof of the third ventricle.

Although the cerebral hemispheres expand greatly during the early months of pregnancy, their external sur-

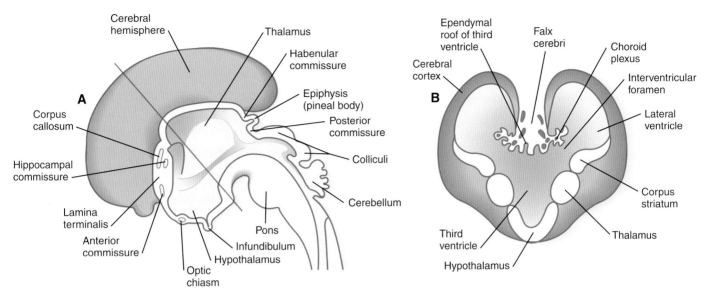

**FIGURE 11-32** Early formation of the cerebral hemispheres in a **10-week-old** embryo. **A,** Sagittal section through the brain. **B,** Cross section through the level indicated by the red line in **A.** (Modified from Moore K, Persaud T: *The developing human,* ed 5, Philadelphia, 1993, WB Saunders.)

faces remain smooth until the fourteenth week. With continued growth, the cerebral hemispheres undergo folding at several levels of organization. The most massive folding involves the large **temporal lobes,** which protrude laterally and rostrally from the caudal part of the cerebral hemispheres. From the fourth to the ninth month of pregnancy, the expanding temporal lobes and the frontal and parietal lobes completely cover areas of the cortex known as the **insula** (island) (Figure 11-33). While these major changes in organization are occurring, other precursors of major surface landmarks of the definitive cerebral cortex are being sculpted. Several major sulci and fissures begin to appear as early as the sixth month. By the eighth month the **sulci** (grooves) and **gyri** (convolutions) that characterize the mature brain take shape.

Internally, the base of each telencephalic vesicle thickens to form the comma-shaped **corpus striatum** (Figure 11-34). Located dorsal to the thalamus, the corpus striatum becomes more **C**-shaped as development progresses. With histodifferentiation of the cerebral cortex, many fiber tracts converge on the area of the corpus striatum, which becomes subdivided into two major nuclei: the **lentiform nucleus** and the **caudate nucleus.** These structures, which are components of the complex aggregation of nuclei known as the **basal ganglia,** are involved in the unconscious control of muscle tone and complex body movements.

Although the grossly identifiable changes in the developing telencephalic vesicles are very prominent, a multitude of internal cellular events determine the functionality of the telencephalon. Specific details are beyond the scope of this text, but for many parts of the brain the general sequence of events begins with early regionaliza-

tion of the telencephalon. This is followed by the generation and directed migration of neuronal precursors and the formation of the various layers of the cerebral cortex or the formation of aggregates of neurons in internal structures of the telencephalon or diencephalon, such as the thalamus or the hippocampus. Once the neuronal cell bodies are properly positioned, axonal or dendritic processes growing from them undergo tightly guided outgrowth to specific targets, for example, the pyramidal cells of the cerebral cortex. The pyramidal cells, in turn, send out long processes that may leave the telencephalon as massive fiber bundles, such as the pyramids, which are the gross manifestations of the corticospinal tracts that are part of the circuitry controlling coordinated movement.

Aside from the telencephalic vesicles, the other major component of the early telencephalon is the **lamina terminalis,** which forms its median rostral wall (Figure 11-35 and see Figure 11-37, *A*). Initially the two cerebral hemispheres develop separately, but toward the end of the first trimester of pregnancy, bundles of nerve fibers begin to cross from one cerebral hemisphere to the other. Many of these connections occur through the lamina terminalis.

The first set of connections to appear in the lamina terminalis becomes the **anterior commissure** (see Figure 11-24, *B*), which connects olfactory areas from the two sides of the brain. The second connection is the **hippocampal commissure (fornix).** The third commissure to take shape in the lamina terminalis is the **corpus callosum,** the most important connection between the right and left halves of the brain. It initially forms (see Figure 11-32, *A*) at 74 days as a small bundle in the lamina terminalis but expands greatly to form a broad band connecting a large part of the base of the cerebral hemispheres (see Figure

**FIGURE 11-33** Lateral views of the developing brain.

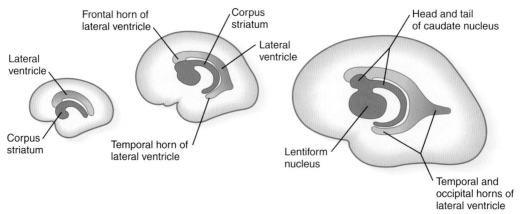

**FIGURE 11-34** Development of the corpus striatum and lateral ventricles. (Modified from Moore K: *The developing human,* ed 4, Philadelphia, 1988, WB Saunders.)

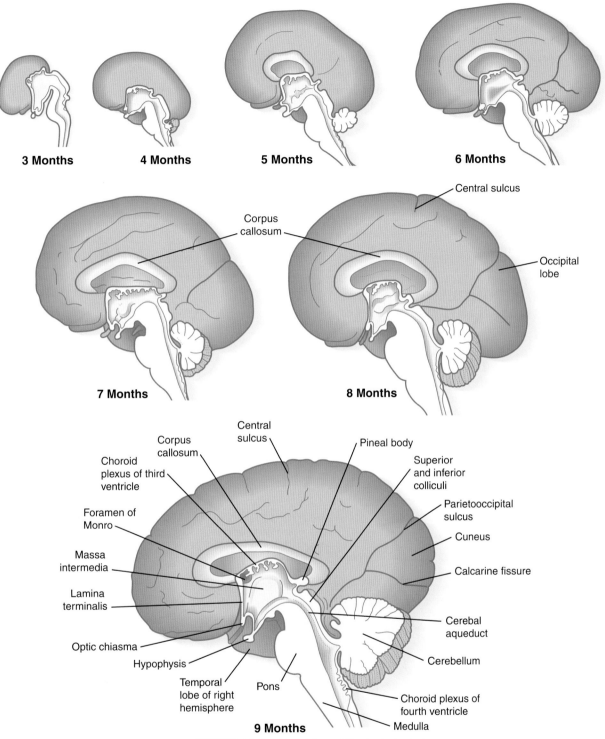

**3 Months**  **4 Months**  **5 Months**  **6 Months**

Central sulcus

Corpus
callosum

Occipital
lobe

**7 Months**

**8 Months**

Central
sulcus

Corpus
callosum

Pineal body

Choroid
plexus of third
ventricle

Superior
and inferior
colliculi

Parietooccipital
sulcus

Foramen of
Monro

Cuneus

Massa
intermedia

Calcarine fissure

Lamina
terminalis

Cerebal
aqueduct

Optic chiasma

Cerebellum

Hypophysis

Temporal
lobe of right
hemisphere

Pons

Choroid plexus of
fourth ventricle

**9 Months**

Medulla

**FIGURE 11-35** Medial views of the developing brain.

11-35). Formation of the corpus callosum is complete by 115 days. In mutations of the homeobox gene, ***EMX-2,*** the corpus callosum fails to form, leading to an anomaly sometimes called **schizencephaly** (split brain). Other commissures not related to the lamina terminalis are the **posterior** and **habenular commissures** (see Figure 11-32), which are located close to the base of the pineal gland,

and the **optic chiasma**, the region in the diencephalon where parts of the optic nerve fibers cross to the other side of the brain.

Neuroanatomists subdivide the telencephalon into several functional components that are based on the phylogenetic development of this region. The oldest and most primitive component is called the **rhinencephalon** (also the **archicortex** and **paleocortex**). As the name implies, it is heavily involved in olfaction. The morphologically dominant cerebral hemispheres are called the **neocortex**. In early development, much of the telencephalon is occupied by rhinencephalic areas (Figure 11-36), but with the expansion of the cerebral hemispheres, the neocortex takes over as the component occupying most of the mass of the brain.

The **olfactory nerves** (cranial nerve I), arising from paired ectodermal placodes in the head, send fibers back into the **olfactory bulbs,** which are outgrowths from the rhinencephalon. A subpopulation of cells from the olfactory placode migrates along the olfactory nerve into the brain, ultimately settling in the hypothalamus, where these cells become the cells that secrete luteinizing hormone–releasing hormone.

## VENTRICLES, MENINGES, AND CEREBROSPINAL FLUID FORMATION

The ventricular system of the brain represents an expansion of the central canal of the neural tube. As certain parts of the brain take shape, the central canal expands into well-defined **ventricles**, which are connected by thinner channels (Figure 11-37). The ventricles are lined by ependymal epithelium and filled with clear cere-

**FIGURE 11-36** Decrease in the prominence of the rhinencephalic areas *(green)* of the brain as the cerebrum expands.

**FIGURE 11-37** Development of the ventricular system of the brain. **A,** Section from an early embryo. **B,** Ventricular system during expansion of the cerebral hemispheres. **C,** Postnatal morphology of the ventricular system.

brospinal fluid. Cerebrospinal fluid is formed in specialized areas called **choroid plexuses**, which are located in specific regions in the roof of the third, fourth, and lateral ventricles. Choroid plexuses are highly vascularized structures that project into the ventricles (see Figure 11-32, *B*) and secrete cerebrospinal fluid into the ventricular system.

Cerebrospinal fluid has a well-characterized circulatory path. As it forms, it flows from the lateral ventricles into the third and ultimately the fourth ventricle. Much of it then escapes through three small holes in the roof of the fourth ventricle and enters the **subarachnoid space** between two layers of meninges. A significant portion of the fluid leaves the skull and bathes the spinal cord as a protective layer.

If an imbalance exists between the production and resorption of cerebrospinal fluid or if its circulation is blocked, the fluid may accumulate within the ventricular system of the brain and through increased mechanical pressure, resulting in a massive enlargement of the ventricular system. This in turn causes a thinning of the walls of the brain and a pronounced increase in the diameter of the skull, a condition known as **hydrocephalus** (Figure 11-38). The blockage of fluid can result from a congenital **stenosis** (narrowing) of the narrow parts of the ventricular system, or it can be the result of certain fetal viral infections.

A specific malformation leading to hydrocephalus is the **Arnold-Chiari malformation**, in which parts of the cerebellum herniate into the foramen magnum, thereby mechanically preventing the escape of cerebrospinal fluid from the skull. This condition can be associated with some form of closure defect of the spinal cord or vertebral column. The underlying cause of the several anatomic forms of Arnold-Chiari malformation remains unknown.

In the early fetal period, two layers of mesenchyme appear around the brain and spinal cord. The thick outer layer, which is of mesodermal origin, forms the tough **dura mater** as well as the membrane bones of the calvarium. A thin inner layer of neural crest origin later subdivides into a thin **pia mater**, which is closely apposed to the neural tissue, and a middle **arachnoid layer**. Spaces that form within the pia-arachnoid layer fill with cerebrospinal fluid.

## CRANIAL NERVES

Although based on the same fundamental plan as the spinal nerves, the cranial nerves (Figure 11-39) have lost their regular segmental arrangement and have become highly specialized (Table 11-2). One of the major differences is the tendency of many cranial nerves to be either sensory (dorsal root based) or motor (ventral root based) rather than mixed, as is the case with the spinal nerves.

The cranial nerves can be subdivided into several categories on the basis of their function and embryological origin. Cranial nerves I and II (olfactory and optic) are often regarded as extensions of brain tracts rather than true nerves. Cranial nerves III, IV, VI, and XII are pure motor nerves that appear to have evolved from primitive ventral roots. Nerves V, VII, IX, and X are mixed nerves with both motor and sensory components, and each nerve supplies derivatives of a different pharyngeal arch (Table 11-2 and Figures 11-40 and 14-21).

The sensory components of the nerves supplying the pharyngeal arches (V, VII, IX, and X) and the auditory nerve (VIII) have a multiple origin from both the neural

**FIGURE 11-38** Fetus with pronounced hydrocephalus. (Courtesy M. Barr, Ann Arbor, Mich.)

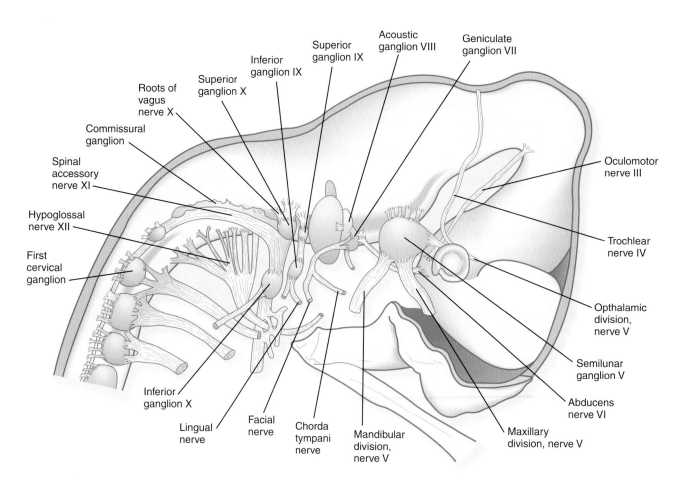

**FIGURE 11-39** Reconstruction of the brain and cranial nerves of a 12-mm pig embryo.

**TABLE 11-2** *Cranial Nerves*

| Cranial nerve | Associated component of central nervous system | Functional components | Distribution |
|---|---|---|---|
| Olfactory (I) | Telencephalon/olfactory placode | Special sensory (olfaction) | Olfactory area of nose |
| Optic (II) | Diencephalon (evagination) | Special sensory (vision) | Retina of eye |
| Oculomotor (III) | Mesencephalon | Motor, autonomic (minor) | Intraocular and four extraocular muscles |
| Trochlear (IV) | Mesencephalon (isthmus) | Motor | Superior oblique muscle of eye |
| Trigeminal (V) | Metencephalon (r2, r3, [pharyngeal arch 1]) | Sensory, motor (some) | Derivatives of branchial arch I |
| Abducens (VI) | Metencephalon (r5, r6) | Motor | Lateral rectus muscle of eye |
| Facial (VII) | Metencephalic/myelencephalic junction (r4 [pharyngeal arch 2]) | Motor Sensory (some) Autonomic (minor) | Derivatives of branchial arch II |
| Auditory (VIII) | Metencephalic/myelencephalic junction (r4–6, otic placode) | Special sensory (hearing, balance) | Inner ear |
| Glossopharyngeal (IX) | Myelencephalon (r6, r7 [pharyngeal arch 3]) | Sensory, motor (some) | Derivatives of pharyngeal arch III |
| Vagus (X) | Myelencephalon (r7, r8 [pharyngeal arch 4]) | Sensory, motor, autonomic (major) | Derivatives of pharyngeal arch IV |
| Accessory (XI) | Myelencephalon (r7, r8 [pharyngeal arch 4]) Spinal cord | Motor Autonomic (minor) | Gut, heart, visceral organs Some neck muscles |
| Hypoglossal (XII) | Myelencephalon (r8 [arch 4]) | Motor | Tongue muscles |

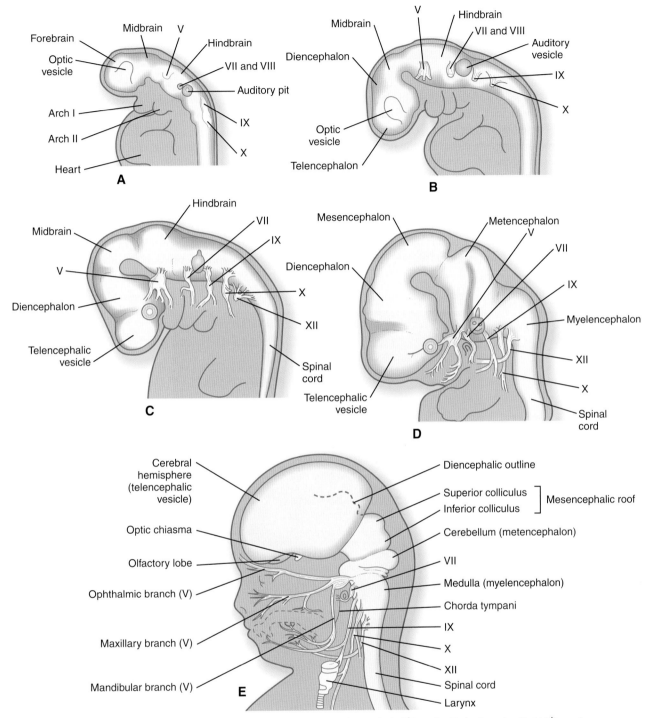

**FIGURE 11-40** Development of the cranial nerves in human embryos. **A,** At **3½ weeks. B,** At **4 weeks. C,** At **5½ weeks. D,** At **7 weeks. E,** At **11 weeks.**

crest and the ectodermal placodes, which are located along the developing brain (see Figure 13-1). These nerves have complex, often multiple sensory ganglia. Neurons in some parts of the ganglia are of neural crest origin and those of other parts or ganglia arise from placodal ectoderm. (Ectodermal placodes are discussed on p. 108.)

## DEVELOPMENT OF NEURAL FUNCTION

During the first 5 weeks of embryonic development, there is no gross behavioral evidence of neural function. Primitive reflex activity can first be elicited at the sixth week, when touching the perioral skin with a fine bristle is

## Congenital Malformations of the Nervous System

In an organ system as prominent and complex as the nervous system, it is not surprising that the brain and spinal cord are subject to a wide variety of congenital malformations. These range from severe structural anomalies resulting from incomplete closure of the neural tube to functional deficits caused by unknown factors acting late in pregnancy.

### DEFECTS IN CLOSURE OF THE NEURAL TUBE

Failure of the neural tube to close occurs most commonly in the anterior and posterior neuropore, but failure to close in other locations is also possible. In this condition the spinal cord or brain in the affected area is splayed open, with the wall of the central canal or ventricular system constituting the outer surface. A number of the closure defects can be diagnosed by the detection of elevated levels of α-**fetoprotein** in the amniotic fluid or by ultrasound scanning. A closure defect of the spinal cord is called **rachischisis**, and a closure defect of the brain is called **cranioschisis**. A patient with cranioschisis dies. Rachischisis (Figures 11-41 and 11-42, *A*) is associated with a wide variety of severe problems, including chronic infection, motor and sensory deficits, and disturbances in

**FIGURE 11-41** Fetus with a severe case of rachischisis. The brain is not covered by cranial bones, and the light-colored spinal cord is totally exposed. (Courtesy M. Barr, Ann Arbor, Mich.)

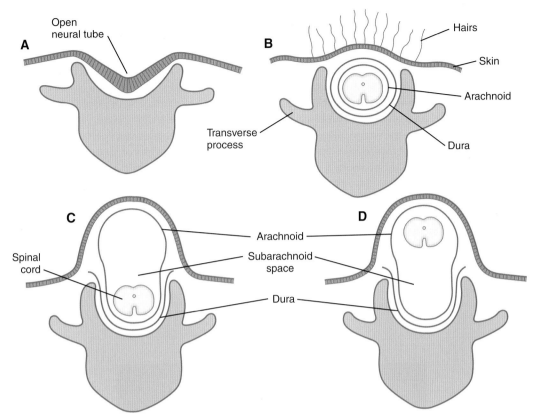

**FIGURE 11-42** Varieties of closure defects of the spinal cord and vertebral column. **A,** Rachischisis. **B,** Spina bifida occulta, with hair growth over the defect. **C,** Meningocele. **D,** Myelomeningocele.

bladder function. These defects commonly accompany anencephaly (see Fig. 8-4), in which there is a massive deficiency of cranial structures.

## OTHER CLOSURE DEFECTS

A defect in the formation of the bony covering overlying either the spinal cord or brain can result in a graded series of structural anomalies. In the spinal cord the simplest defect is called **spina bifida occulta** (Figure 11-42, *B*), which occurs in at least 5% of the population. The spinal cord and meninges remain in place, but the bony covering (neural arch) of one or more vertebrae is incomplete. Sometimes the defect goes unnoticed for many years. The neural arches are induced by the roof plate of the neural tube, with the mediation of Msx-2. Thus spina bifida occulta probably results from a local defect in induction. The site of the defect in the neural arches is often marked by a tuft of hair. This localized hair formation may result from exposure of the developing skin to other inductive influences from the neural tube or its coverings. Normally the neural arches act as a barrier to such influences.

The next most severe category of defect is a **meningocele,** in which the dura mater may be missing in the area of the defect and the arachnoid layer bulges prominently beneath the skin (Figure 1-42, *C*). The spinal cord, however, remains in place, and neurological symptoms are often minor. The most severe condition is a **myelomeningocele,** in which the spinal cord bulges or is entirely displaced into the protruding subarachnoid space (Figures 11-42, *D*, and 11-43). Because of problems associated with displaced spinal roots, neurological problems are commonly associated with this condition.

*Continued*

A similar spectrum of anomalies is associated with cranial defects (Figures 11-44 and 11-45). A **meningocele** is typically associated with a small defect in the skull, whereas brain tissue alone (**meningoencephalocele**) or brain tissue containing part of the ventricular system (**meningohydroencephalocoele**) may protrude through a larger opening in the skull. Depending on the nature of the protruding tissue, these malformations may be associated with neurological deficits. The mechanical circumstances may also lead to secondary hydrocephalus in some cases.

**Microcephaly** is a relatively uncommon condition characterized by the underdevelopment of both the brain and the cranium (see Figure 9-9). Although it can result from premature closure of the cranial sutures, in most cases, its etiology is uncertain.

Many of the functional defects of the nervous system are poorly characterized, and their etiology is not understood. Studies on mice with genetically based defects of movement or behavior caused by abnormalities of cell migration or histogenesis in certain regions of the brain suggest the probability of a parallel spectrum of human defects. A good example is **lissencephaly**, a condition characterized by a smooth brain surface instead of the gyri and sulci that characterize the normal brain. Underlying this gross defect is abnormal layering of cortical neurons in a manner reminiscent of the pathology seen in reeler mice (see p. 253). **Mental retardation** is common and can be attributed to many causes, both genetic and environmental. The timing of the insult to the brain may be late in the fetal period.

**FIGURE 11-43** Infant with a myelomeningocele and secondary hydrocephalus. (Courtesy M. Barr, Ann Arbor, Mich.)

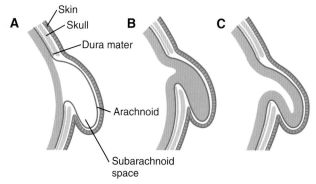

**FIGURE 11-44** Herniations in the cranial region. **A,** Meningocele. **B,** Meningoencephalocele. **C,** Meningohydroencephalocele.

**FIGURE 11-45** Fetuses with an occipital meningocele **(A)** and a frontal encephalocele **(B)**. (Courtesy M. Barr, Ann Arbor, Mich.)

followed by contralateral flexion of the neck. Over the next 6 to 8 weeks, the region of skin sensitive to tactile stimulation spreads from the face to the palms of the hands and the upper chest; by 12 weeks, the entire surface of the body except for the back and top of the head is sensitive. As these sensitive areas expand, the nature of the reflexes elicited matures from generalized movements to specific responses of more localized body parts. There is a general craniocaudal sequence of appearance of reflex movements.

Spontaneous uncoordinated movements typically begin when the embryo is somewhat more than 7 weeks old.

Later coordinated movements (see Figure 18-7) are the result of the establishment of motor tracts and reflex arcs within the central nervous system. Behavioral development during the last trimester, which has been revealed by studying prematurely born infants, is often subtle and reflects the structural and functional maturation of neuronal circuits.

The development of functional circuitry can be illustrated by the spinal cord. Several stages of structural and functional maturation can be identified (Figure 11-46). The first is a pre-reflex stage, which is characterized by the initial differentiation (including axonal and dendritic growth) of the neurons according to a well-defined sequence, starting with motor and followed by sensory and finally including the interneurons that connect the two (see Figures 11-14 and 11-46, *A*). The second stage consists of closure of the primary circuit, which allows the expression of local segmental reflexes. While the local circuit is being set up, other axons are growing down descending tracts in the spinal cord or are crossing from the other side of the cord. When these axons make contact with the components of the simple reflex that was established in the second stage, the anatomical basis for intersegmental and cross-cord reflexes is set up. Later in the fetal period, these more complex circuits are completed, and the tracts are myelinated by oligodendrocytes.

The functional maturation of individual tracts, as indicated by their myelination, takes place over a broad time span and is not completed until early adulthood. Particularly in early postnatal life, the maturation of functional tracts in the nervous system can be followed by clinical neurological examination.

Myelination begins in the peripheral nervous system, with motor roots becoming myelinated before sensory roots (which occurs in the second through fifth months). Myelination begins in the spinal cord at about 11 weeks and proceeds according to a craniocaudal gradient. During the third trimester, myelination begins to occur in the brain, but there, in contrast to the peripheral nervous system, myelination is first seen in sensory tracts (e.g., in the visual system). Myelination in complex association pathways in the cerebral cortex occurs after birth. In the **corticospinal tracts**, the main direct connection between the cerebral cortex and the motor nerves emanating from the spinal cord, myelination extends caudally only to the level of the medulla by 40 weeks. Myelination continues after birth, and its course can be appreciated by the increasing mobility of infants during their first year of life.

## SUMMARY

⦿ While the neural tube is closing, its open ends are the cranial and caudal neuropores. The newly formed brain consists of three parts: the prosencephalon, the mesencephalon, and the rhombencephalon. The prosencephalon later subdivides into the telencephalon and the diencephalon, and the rhombencephalon forms the metencephalon and myelencephalon.

⦿ Within the neural tube, neuroepithelial cells undergo active mitotic proliferation. Their daughter cells form neuronal or glial progenitor cells. Among the glial cells, radial glial cells act as guide wires for the migration of neurons from their sites of origin to definite layers in the brain. Microglial cells arise from mesoderm.

⦿ The neural tube divides into ventricular, intermediate, and marginal zones. Neuroblasts in the intermediate zone (future gray matter) send out processes that collect principally in the marginal zone (future white matter). The

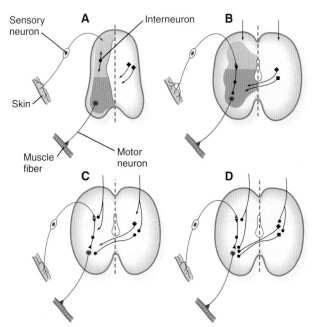

**FIGURE 11-46** Stages in the development of neural circuitry. **A,** Presynaptic stage. **B,** Closure of the primary reflex circuit. **C,** Connections with longitudinal and lateral inputs. **D,** Completion of circuits and myelination. (Based on Bodian D. In Quartan GC, Melnechuk T, Adelman G, eds: *The neurosciences: second study program*, New York, 1970, Rockefeller University Press, pp 129–140.

**CLINICAL VIGNETTE**

An infant is born with rachischisis of the lower spine. During succeeding weeks, his head also begins to increase in size. Radiological imaging reveals that the infant's ventricular system is greatly dilated and the walls of the brain itself are thinned.

Assuming that the infant lives, what are some of the clinical problems that he faces in later life?

neural tube is also divided into a dorsal alar plate and a ventral basal plate. The basal plate represents the motor component of the spinal cord, and the alar plate is largely sensory.

○ Through an induction by the notochord, mediated by sonic hedgehog, a floor plate develops in the neural tube. Further influences of sonic hedgehog, produced by both the notochord and floor plate, result in the induction of motoneurons in the basal plate.

○ Much of the early brain is a highly segmented structure. This is reflected structurally in the rhombomeres and molecularly in the patterns of expression of homeobox-containing genes. Neurons and their processes developing within the rhombomeres follow specific rules of behavior with respect to rhombomere boundaries. Nerve processes growing from the spinal cord react to external cues provided by the environment of the somites. Neurons and neural crest cells can readily penetrate the anterior but not the posterior mesoderm of the somite.

○ The midbrain and metencephalic structures are specified by a signaling center, the isthmic organizer, at the midbrain/hindbrain border. FGF-8 is one of the major signaling molecules. The forebrain is divided into six segments called prosomeres. FGF-8, secreted by the anterior neural ridge, induces the expression of BF-1, which regulates development of the telencephalon and optic vesicles. Sonic hedgehog, secreted by midline axial structures, organizes the ventral forebrain.

○ A peripheral nerve forms by the outgrowth of motor axons from the ventral horn of the spinal cord. The outgrowing axons are capped by a growth cone. This growing tip continually samples its immediate environment for cues that guide the amount and direction of axonal growth. The motor component of a peripheral nerve is joined by the sensory part, which is based on neural crest–derived cell bodies in dorsal root ganglia along the spinal cord. Axons and dendrites from the sensory cell bodies penetrate the spinal cord and also grow peripherally with the motor axons. Connections between the nerve and end organs are often mediated through trophic factors. Neurons that do not establish connections with peripheral end organs often die.

○ The autonomic nervous system consists of two components: the sympathetic and parasympathetic nervous systems. Both components contain preganglionic neurons, which arise from the central nervous system, and postganglionic components, which are of neural crest origin. Typically, sympathetic neurons are adrenergic and parasympathetic neurons are cholinergic. However, the normal choice of transmitter can be overridden by environmental factors so that a sympathetic neuron, for example, can secrete acetylcholine.

○ The spinal cord functions as a pathway for organized tracts of nerve processes as well as an integration center for local reflexes. During the fetal period, growth in the length of the spinal cord lags behind that of the vertebral column, pulling the nerve roots and leaving the end of the spinal cord as a cauda equina.

○ Within the brain, the myelencephalon retains an organizational similarity to the spinal cord with respect to the tracts passing through, but centers that control respiration and heart rate also form at the site. The metencephalon contains two parts: the pons (which functions principally as a conduit) and the cerebellum (which integrates and coordinates many motor movements and sensory reflexes). In the cerebellum, which forms from the rhombic lips, the gray matter forms on the outside. The ventral part of the mesencephalon is the region through which the major tracts of nerve processes that connect centers in the cerebral cortex with specific sites in the spinal cord pass. The dorsal part of the mesencephalon develops the superior and inferior colliculi, which are involved with the integration of visual and auditory signals, respectively.

○ Both the diencephalon and the telencephalon represent modified alar plate regions. Many important nuclei and integrating centers develop in the diencephalon, among them the thalamus, hypothalamus, neural hypophysis, and pineal body. The eyes also arise as outgrowths from the diencephalon. In humans, the telencephalon ultimately overgrows other parts of the brain. Like the cerebellum, it is organized with the gray matter in layers outside the white matter. Neuroblasts migrate through the white matter to these layers by using radial glial cells as their guides.

○ Within the central nervous system, the central canal expands to form a series of four ventricles in the brain. Specialized vascular plexuses form cerebrospinal fluid, which circulates throughout the central nervous system. Around the brain and spinal cord, two layers of mesenchyme form the meninges.

○ The cranial nerves are organized on the same fundamental plan as the spinal nerves, but they have lost their regular segmental pattern and have become highly specialized. Some are purely motor, others are purely sensory, and still others are mixed.

○ Many congenital malformations of the nervous system are based on incomplete closure of the neural tube or associated skeletal structures. In the spinal cord the spectrum of defects ranges from a widely open neural tube (rachischisis) to relatively minor defects in the neural arch over the cord (spina bifida occulta). A similar spectrum of defects is seen in the brain.

○ Neural function appears in concert with the structural maturation of various components of the nervous system. The first reflex activity is seen in the sixth week. During successive weeks, the reflex movements become more complex, and spontaneous movements appear. Final functional maturation coincides with myelination of the tracts and is not completed until many years after birth.

# Review Questions

1. What molecule produced by the notochord is instrumental in inducing the floor plate of the neural tube?
   A. Hoxa-5
   B. Retinoic acid
   C. Pax-3
   D. Msx-1
   E. Sonic hedgehog

2. The cell bodies of the motor neurons of a spinal nerve arise from the:
   A. Basal plate
   B. Marginal zone
   C. Floor plate
   D. Roof plate
   E. Alar plate

3. A young patient with a tuft of hair over the lumbar region of the vertebral column undergoes surgery for a congenital anomaly in that region. During surgery, it was found that the dura and arachnoid layers over the spinal cord were complete but that the neural arches of several vertebrae were missing. What condition did the infant have?
   A. Meningocoele
   B. Meningomyelocoele
   C. Encephalocoele
   D. Spina bifida occulta
   E. Rachischisis

4. Growth cones adhere strongly to a substrate containing:
   A. Acetylcholine
   B. Laminin
   C. Epinephrine
   D. Norepinephrine
   E. Sonic hedgehog

5. Complete failure of the neural tube to close in the region of the spinal cord is:
   A. Spina bifida occulta
   B. Meningocele
   C. Cranioschisis
   D. Rachischisis
   E. Myelomeningocele

6. Rhombomeres are segmental divisions of the:
   A. Forebrain
   B. Midbrain
   C. Hindbrain
   D. Spinal cord
   E. None of the above

7. Pregnant women typically first become aware of fetal movements during what month of pregnancy?
   A. Second
   B. Third
   C. Fourth
   D. Sixth
   E. Eighth

8. Rathke's pouch arises from the:
   A. Diencephalon
   B. Stomodeal ectoderm
   C. Mesencephalon
   D. Pharyngeal endoderm
   E. Infundibulum

9. In the early days after birth, an infant does not pass fecal material and develops abdominal swelling. An anal opening is present. What is the probable condition?

10. What is the likely appearance of the spinal cord and brachial nerves in an infant who was born with the congenital absence of one arm (amelia)?

## REFERENCES

Agarwala S, Sanders TA, Ragsdale CW: Sonic hegehog control of size and shape in midbrain pattern formation, *Science* 291:2147–2150, 2001.

Altman J, Bayer SA: *Development of the Human Spinal Cord,* New York, 2001, Oxford University Press.

Arber S, Burden SJ, Harris AJ: Patterning of skeletal muscle, *Curr Opin Neurobiol* 12:100–103, 2002.

Armstrong CL, Hawkes R: Pattern formation in the cerebellar cortex, *Biochem Cell Biol* 78:551–562, 2000.

Black IB: Stages of neurotransmitter development of autonomic neurons, *Science* 215:1198–1204, 1982.

Breedlove SM: Sexual dimorphism in the vertebrate central nervous system, *J Neurosci* 12:4133–4142, 1992.

Briscoe J and others: A homeodomain protein code specifies progenitor cell identity and neuronal fate in the ventral neural tube, *Cell* 101:435–445, 2000.

Briscoe J Ericson J: Specification of neuronal fates in the ventral neural tube, *Curr Opin Neurobiol* 11:43–49, 2001.

Brown MC, Hopkins WG, Keynes RJ: Essentials of neural development, Cambridge, England, 1991, Cambridge University Press.

Cameron RS, Rakić P: Glial cell lineage in the cerebral cortex: a review and synthesis, *Glia* 4:124–137, 1991.

Caroni P: Driving the growth cone, *Science* 281:1465–1466, 1998.

Carpenter EM: Hox genes and spinal cord development, *Dev Neurosci* 24:24–34, 2002.

Chenn A, McConnell SK: Cleavage orientation and the asymmetric inheritance of Notchl immunoreactivity in mammalian neurogenesis, *Cell* 82:631–641, 1995.

Colello RJ, Pott U: Signals that initiate myelination in the developing mammalian nervous system, *Mol Neurobiol* 15:83–100, 1997.

Cordes SP: Molecular genetics of cranial nerve development in the mouse, *Nature Revs: Neuroscience* 2:611–623, 2001.

Cowan WM, Jessell TM, Zipursky SL: *Molecular and Cellular Approaches to Neural Development*, New York, 1997, Oxford University Press.

Crossley PH, Martinez S, Martin GR: Midbrain development induced by FGF8 in the chick embryo, *Nature* 380:66–68, 1996.

Dickson BJ: Molecular mechanisms of axon guidance, *Science* 298:1959–1964, 2002.

Dubois PM, El Amraoui A: Embryology of the pituitary gland, *Trends Endocrinol Metab* 6:1–7, 1995.

Echelard Y and others: Sonic hedgehog, a member of a family of putative signaling molecules, is implicated in the regulation of CNS polarity, *Cell* 75:1417–1430, 1993.

Eickholt BJ and others: Rhombomere interactions control segmental differentiation of hindbrain neurons, *Mol Cell Neurosci* 18:141–148, 2001.

Ferrer I and others: Cell death and removal in the cerebral cortex during development, *Prog Neurobiol* 39:1–43, 1992.

Gassmann M, Lemke G: Neuregulins and neuregulin receptors in neural development, *Curr Biol* 7:87–92, 1997.

Gershon M: Genes and lineages in the formation of the enteric nervous system, *Curr Opin Neurobiol* 7:101–109, 1997.

Hajihosseini M, Tham TN, Dubois-Dalcq M: Origin of oligodendrocytes within the human spinal cord, *J Neurosci* 16:7981–7994, 1996.

Hatten ME: New directions in neuronal migration, *Science* 297:1660–1663, 2002.

Inoue T, Nakamura S, Osumi N: Current topics in comparative developmental biology of vertebrate brains, *Neurosci Res* 39:371–376, 2001.

Joyner AL: Engrailed, Wnt and Pax genes regulate midbrain-hindbrain development, *Trends Genet* 12:15–20, 1996.

Kageyama R, Nakanishi S: Helix-loop-helix factors in growth and differentiation of the vertebrate nervous system, *Curr Opin Genet Dev* 7:659–665, 1997.

Kessaris N, Pringle N, Richardson WD: Ventral neurogenesis and the neuron-glial switch, *Neuron* 31:677–680, 2001.

Keynes RJ and others: Spinal nerve segmentation in higher vertebrates: axon guidance by repulsion and attraction, *Semin Neurosci* 8:339–345, 1996.

Lambert de Rouvroit C, Goffinet AM: Neuronal migration, *Mech Devel* 105:47–56, 2001.

Lance-Jones C and others: *Hoxd10* induction and regionalization in the developing lumbosacral spinal cord, *Development* 128:2255–2268, 2001.

Landmesser LT, ed: *The assembly of the nervous system*, New York, 1989, Liss.

Le Douarin NM, Catala M, Batini C: Embryonic neural chimeras in the study of vertebrate brain and head development, *Int Rev Cytol* 175:241–309, 1997.

Lumsden A, Keynes R: Segmental patterns of neuronal development in the chick hindbrain, *Nature* 337:424–428, 1989.

Lumsden A, Krumlauf R: Patterning the vertebrate neuraxis, *Science* 274:1109–1115, 1996.

Marquardt T, Pfaff SL: Cracking the transcriptional code for cell specification in the neural tube, *Cell* 106:1–4, 2001.

McMahon AP: Neural patterning: the role of *Nkx* genes in the ventral spinal cord, *Genes Devel* 14:2261–2264, 2000.

Millet S and others: The caudal limit of OTX2 gene expression as a marker of the midbrain/hindbrain boundary: a study using in situ hybridization and chick/quail homotopic grafts, *Development* 122:3785–3797, 1996.

Müller F, O'Rahilly RO: The timing and sequence of appearance of neuromeres and their derivatives in staged human embryos, *Acta Anat* 158:83–99, 1997.

Norman MG: Malformations of the brain, *J Neuropath Exp Neurol* 55:133–143, 1996.

O'Rahilly R, Müller F: *The Embryonic Human Brain*, New York, 1994, Wiley-Liss.

Oppenheim RW: Cell death during development of the nervous system, *Annu Rev Neurosci* 14:453–501, 1991.

Orentas DM, Miller RH: The origin of spinal cord oligodendrocytes is dependent on local influences from the notochord, *Dev Biol* 177:43–54, 1996.

Patten I, Placzek M: The role of sonic hedgehog in neural tube patterning, *Cell Mol Life Sci* 57:1695–1708, 2000.

Parks JS, Adess ME, Brown MR: Genes regulating hypothalamic and pituitary development, *Acta Paediatr Suppl* 423:28–32, 1997.

Placzek M, Dodd J, Jessell TM: Discussion point. The case for floor plate induction by the notochord, *Curr Opin Neurobiol* 10:15–22, 2000.

Ragsdale CW, Grove EA: Patterning the mammalian cerebral cortex, *Curr Opin Neurobiol* 11:50–58, 2001.

Rakić P: Radial versus tangential migration of neuronal clones in the developing cerebral cortex, *Proc Natl Acad Sci USA* 92:11323–11327, 1995.

Rakić P: Specification of cerebral cortical areas, *Science* 241:170–176, 1988.

Robinson SR, Smotherman WP: Fundamental motor patterns of the mammalian fetus, *J Neurobiol* 23:1574–1600, 1992.

Rothman TP and others: The effect of back-transplants of the embryonic gut wall on growth of the neural tube, *Dev Biol* 124:331–346, 1987.

Rubenstein JLR and others: The embryonic vertebrate forebrain: the prosomeric model, *Science* 266:578–580, 1994.

Sanes, DH, Reh TA, Harris WA: *Development of the Nervous System*, San Diego, 2000, Academic Press.

Sarnat HB: Molecular genetic classification of central nervous system malformations, *J Child Neurol* 15:675–687, 2000.

Seitanidou T and others: Krox-20 is a key regulator of rhombomere-specific gene expression in the developing hindbrain, *Mech Dev* 65:31–42, 1997.

Serafini T and others: Netrin-1 is required for commissural axon guidance in the developing nervous system, *Cell* 87:1001–1014, 1996.

Sheng HZ and others: Multistep control of pituitary organogenesis, *Science* 278:1809–1812, 1997.

Sheng HZ and others: Specification of pituitary cell lineages by the LIM homeobox gene *Lhx3*, *Science* 272:1004–1007, 1996.

Shimamura K, Rubenstein JLR: Inductive interactions direct early regionalization of the mouse forebrain, *Development* 124:2709–2718, 1997.

Takuma H and others: Formation of Rathke's pouch requires dual induction from the diencephalon, *Development* 125:4835–4840, 1998.

Tarozzo G, Peretto P, Fasolo A: Cell migration from the olfactory placode and the ontogeny of the neuroendocrine compartments, *Zool Sci* 12:367–383, 1995.

ten Donkelaar HJ: Major events in the development of the forebrain, *Europ J Morphol* 38:301–308, 2000.

Tessier-Lavigne M, Goodman CS: The molecular biology of axon guidance, *Science* 274:1123–1133, 1996.

Theil T and others: Segmental expression of the EpphA4 (Sek-1) receptor tyrosine kinase in the hindbrain is under direct transcriptional control of Krox-20, *Development* 125:443–452, 1998.

Tosney KW: Cells and cell-interactions that guide motor axons in the developing chick embryo, *Bioessays* 13:17–23, 1991.

Varga ZM, Wegner J, Westerfield M: Anterior movement of ventral diencephalic precursors separates the primordial eye field in the neural plate and requires *cyclops*, *Development* 126:5533–5546, 1999.

Vettivel S: Vertebral level of the termination of the spinal cord in human fetuses, *J Anat* 179:149–161, 1991.

Watkins DE, Camper SA: How many homeobox genes does it take to make a pituitary gland? *Trends Genet* 14:284–290, 1998.

Wingate RJT: The rhombic lip and early cerebellar development, *Curr Opin Neurobiol* 11:82–88, 2001.

Zorick TS, Lemke G: Schwann cell differentiation, *Curr Opin Cell Biol* 8:870–876, 1996.

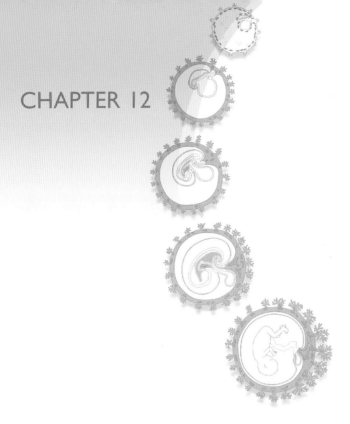

# CHAPTER 12

# Neural Crest

Although its existence has been recognized for more than a century, not until adequate methods of marking neural crest cells became available—first with isotopic labels and subsequently with stable biological markers, monoclonal antibodies, intracellular dyes, and genetic markers—did the neural crest become one of the most widely studied components of the vertebrate embryo. Most studies on the neural crest have been conducted on the avian embryo because of its accessibility and the availability of specific markers. Recent research suggests that except for relatively minor structural details information learned from birds can be directly applied to mammalian embryos. Congenital malformations of the neural crest are presented in Clinical Correlation 12-1, at the end of this chapter.

## ORIGINS OF NEURAL CREST

The neural crest originates from cells located along the lateral margins of the neural plate. Neural crest cells are specified as the result of an inductive action by the non-neural ectoderm (possibly mediated by a gradient of bone morphogenetic protein-4 [BMP-4] and BMP-7 as well as Wnt) on the lateral cells of the neural plate. The induced neural crest cells express **slug**, a transcription factor of the zinc finger family, which characterizes cells that break away from an embryonic epithelial layer and subsequently migrate as mesenchymal cells.*

Neural crest cells break free from the neural plate or neural tube by changing their shape and properties from those of typical neuroepithelial cells to those of mesenchymal cells. In the head region, incipient neural crest cells send out processes that penetrate the basal lamina underlying the neuroepithelium well before neural tube closure (Figure 12-1). After the basal lamina is further degraded, the neural crest cells, which by this time have assumed a mesenchymal morphology, pass through the remnants of the basal lamina and embark on a remarkable series of migrations.

Another significant change accompanying the epithelial-to-mesenchymal transformation of the neural crest cells is a loss of cell-to-cell adhesiveness. This is accompanied by the loss of cell adhesion molecules (CAMs) characteristic of the neural tube (e.g., N-CAM and N-cadherin) on the neural crest cells during their migratory phase. After neural crest cells have completed their migrations and differentiated into certain structures (such as spinal ganglia), CAMs are often reexpressed.

In the trunk, neural crest cells do not leave the neuroepithelium until after the neural tube has formed. They do not, however, have to contend with penetrating a basal lamina because the dorsal part of the neural tube does not form a basal lamina until after emigration of the crest cells.

---

* Slug is also expressed during gastrulation by cells of the epiblast after they have entered the walls of the primitive streak and are about to leave as mesenchymal cells of the mesoderm germ layer.

**FIGURE 12-1** Early migration of neural crest cells from the lateral margin of the neural plate.

## MIGRATIONS OF NEURAL CREST

After leaving the neuroepithelium, the neural crest cells first encounter a relatively cell-free environment rich in extracellular matrix molecules (Figure 12-2). In this environment they undergo extensive migrations along several well-defined pathways. These migrations are determined by both intrinsic properties of the neural crest cells and features of the external environment encountered by the migrating cells.

Neural crest migration is influenced by a variety of molecules residing in the extracellular matrix. Although the presence of a basal lamina can inhibit their emigration from the neural tube, neural crest cells often prefer to migrate along basal laminae, such as those of the surface ectoderm or neural tube, after they have left the neural tube. Components of the extracellular matrix permissive for migration include molecules found in basal

**FIGURE 12-2** Scanning electron micrograph of a chick embryo, showing the early migration of neural crest cells (*arrow*) out of the neural tube (*NT*). The subectodermal pathway of neural crest migration (*) is relatively cell free but contains a fine mesh of extracellular matrix molecules. *N,* Notochord; *S,* somite. (Courtesy K. Tosney, Ann Arbor, Mich.)

laminae, such as fibronectin, laminin, and type IV collagen (Figure 12-3). Attachment to and migration over these substrate molecules is mediated by the family of attachment proteins called **integrins**. Other molecules, such as chondroitin sulfate proteoglycans, are not good substrates for neural crest cells and inhibit their migration.

The somite is a good example of the effect of the environment on neural crest cell migration. Neural crest cells enter only the anterior parts of the somites, where many of them settle to form the sensory ganglia. They do not penetrate the posterior regions of the somites, which have elevated concentrations of chondroitin sulfate. This substance is also produced by the notochord, which compounds the inhibitory effect.

Neural crest cells in the head and trunk follow different migratory pathways. These will be described later in this chapter.

## DIFFERENTIATION OF NEURAL CREST CELLS

Neural crest cells ultimately differentiate into an astonishing array of adult structures (Table 12-1). What controls their differentiation is one of the principal questions of neural crest biology. Two opposing hypotheses have been proposed. According to one, all neural crest cells are equal in developmental potential, and their ultimate differentiation is entirely determined by the environment through which they migrate and into which they finally settle. The other suggests that premigratory crest cells are already programmed for different developmental fates and that certain stem cells are favored while others are inhibited from further development during migration. Recent research indicates that the real answer can be found somewhere between these two positions.

Increasing evidence shows a correlation between the time of migration of neural crest cells from the neural tube and their developmental potential. For example, the cells that first begin to migrate have the potential to differentiate into several different types of cells. Crest cells that begin to migrate later are capable of forming only derivatives characteristic of more dorsal locations (e.g., spinal ganglia) but not sympathetic neurons or adrenal medullary cells. Those that leave the neural tube last can form only pigment cells.

Several experiments have shown that the fates of neural crest cells are not irreversibly fixed along a single pathway. One type of experiment involves the transplantation of neural crest cells from one part of the body to another. For example, many neural crest cells from the trunk differentiate into sympathetic neurons that produce norepinephrine as the transmitter. In the cranial region, however, neural crest cells give rise to parasympathetic neurons, which produce acetylcholine. If thoracic neural

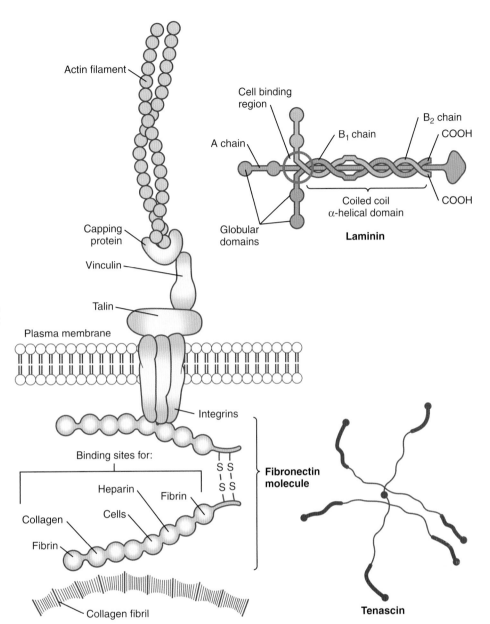

**FIGURE 12-3** Structure of some of the common extracellular matrix molecules.

crest cells are transplanted into the head, some cells differentiate into cholinergic parasympathetic neurons instead of the adrenergic sympathetic neurons normally produced. Conversely, cranial neural crest cells grafted into the thoracic region respond to their new environment by forming adrenergic sympathetic neurons. A more striking example is the conversion of cells of the periocular neural crest mesenchyme, which in birds would normally form cartilage, into neurons if they are associated with embryonic hindgut tissue in vitro. Many of the regional influences on the differentiation of local populations of neural crest cells are now recognized to be interactions between the migrating neural crest cells and specific tissues that they encounter during migration. Some examples of tissue interactions that promote the

differentiation of specific neural crest derivatives are given in Table 12-2.

The plasticity of differentiation of neural crest cells can be demonstrated by cloning single neural crest cells in culture. In the same medium and under apparently the same environmental conditions, the progeny of the single cloned cells frequently differentiate into neuronal and nonneuronal (e.g., pigment cell) phenotypes. Similarly, if individual neural crest cells are injected in vivo with a dye, over 50% of the injected cells give rise to progeny with two to four different phenotypes containing the dye. By exposing cloned neural crest precursor cells to specific environmental conditions in vitro, one can begin to understand the mechanisms that determine phenotype in vivo. For example, in one experiment, rat neural crest cells

**TABLE 12-1** *Major Derivatives of the Neural Crest*

| | Trunk crest | Cranial and circumpharyngeal crests |
|---|---|---|
| **Nervous system** | | |
| Sensory nervous system | Spinal ganglia | Ganglia of trigeminal nerve (V), facial nerve (VII), glossopharyngeal nerve (superior ganglion) (IX), vagus nerve (jugular ganglion) (X) |
| Autonomic nervous system | Sympathetic chain ganglia, collateral ganglia: celiac and mesenteric<br>Parasympathetic ganglia: pelvic and visceral plexuses<br>Satellite cells of sensory ganglia, Schwann cells of peripheral nerves, enteric glial cells | Parasympathetic ganglia: ciliary, ethmoidal, sphenopalatine, submandibular, visceral<br>Satellite cells of sensory ganglia, Schwann cells of peripheral nerves, leptomeninges of prosencephalon and part of mesencephalon |
| **Pigment cells** | Melanocytes | Melanocytes |
| **Endocrine and paraendocrine cells** | Adrenal medulla, neurosecretory cells of heart and lungs | Carotid body (type I cells), parafollicular cells (thyroid) |
| **Mesectodermal cells** | | |
| Skeleton | None | Cranial vault (squamosal and part of frontal), nasal and orbital, otic capsule (part), palate and maxillary, sphenoid (small contribution), trabeculae (part), visceral cartilages, external ear cartilage (part) |
| Connective tissue | None | Dermis and fat of skin; cornea of eye (fibroblasts of stroma and corneal endothelium); dental papilla (odontoblasts); connective tissue stroma of glands: thyroid, parathyroid, thymus, salivary, lacrimal; outflow tract (truncoconal region) of heart; cardiac semilunar valves; walls of aorta and aortic arch–derived arteries |
| Muscle | None | Ciliary muscles, dermal smooth muscles, vascular smooth muscle, minor skeletal muscle elements (?) |

grown under standard in vitro conditions differentiated into neurons, but if they were exposed to glial growth factor, they differentiated into Schwann cells because the glial growth factor suppressed their tendency to differentiate into neurons. Similarly, the growth factors BMP-2 and BMP-4 cause cultured neural crest cells to differentiate into autonomic neurons, whereas exposure of these cells to transforming growth factor-β causes them to differentiate into smooth muscle.

Not all types of transformations among possible neural crest derivatives can occur. For example, crest cells from the trunk transplanted into the head cannot form cartilage or skeletal elements, although this is normal for cells of the cranial neural crest. Most experiments suggest that early neural crest cells segregate into intermediate lineages that preserve the option of differentiating into several but not all types of individual phenotypes. In the chick embryo, some neural crest cells are antigenically different from others even before they have left the neural tube.

A number of neural crest cells are bipotential, depending on signals from their local environment for cues to

their final differentiation. Cultured heart cells secrete a protein that converts postmitotic sympathetic neurons from an adrenergic (norepinephrine transmitter) phenotype to a cholinergic (acetylcholine-secreting) phenotype (see Figure 11-21). During normal development, the sympathetic neurons that innervate sweat glands are catecholaminergic until their axons actually contact the sweat glands. At that point, they become cholinergic.

## MAJOR DIVISIONS OF NEURAL CREST

The neural crest arises from a wide range of craniocaudal levels, from the prosencephalon to the future sacral region. For many years it was traditional to subdivide the neural crest into trunk and cranial components. In recent years, however, it has become increasingly apparent that the neural crest in the posterior rhombencephalic region, often called the circumpharyngeal crest, represents another major subdivision seeding cells into the pharyngeal region, the outflow tract of the heart and

**TABLE 12-2** *Environmental Factors Promoting Differentiation of Neural Crest Cells*

| Neural crest derivative | Interacting structure |
|---|---|
| Bones of cranial vault | Brain |
| Bones of base of skull | Notochord, brain |
| Pharyngeal arch cartilages | Pharyngeal endoderm |
| Meckel's cartilage | Cranial ectoderm |
| Maxillary bone | Maxillary ectoderm |
| Mandible | Mandibular ectoderm |
| Palate | Palatal ectoderm |
| Otic capsule | Otic vesicle |
| Dentine of teeth | Oral ectoderm |
| Glandular stroma: thyroid, parathyroid, thymus, salivary | Local epithelium |
| Adrenal medullary chromaffin cells | Glucocorticoids secreted by adrenal cortex |
| Enteric neurons | Gut wall |
| Sympathetic neurons | Spinal cord, notochord, somites |
| Sensory neurons | Peripheral target tissue |
| Pigment cells | Extracellular matrix along pathway of migration |

great vessels, and much of the gut-associated crest derivatives.

## Trunk Neural Crest

The neural crest of the trunk extends from the level of the sixth somite to the most caudal somites. Within much of the trunk, three main migratory pathways of neural crest cells can be seen in cross section (Figure 12-4). One is a dorsolateral pathway between the ectoderm and the somites. The cells that elect this pathway disperse beneath the ectoderm and ultimately enter the ectoderm as pigment cells (melanocytes).

The second pathway of migration is a ventral one, along which the neural crest cells initially move into the space between the anterior half of the somites and the neural tube. It continues just under the ventromedial surface of the somite until the cells reach the dorsal aorta. Cells that follow this branch belong to the sympathoadrenal lineage. These cells contribute to the formation of the adrenal medulla and elements of the sympathetic nervous system.

A third ventrolateral pathway leads into the anterior halves of the somites. The cells that follow this route form the segmentally arranged sensory ganglia.

The sympathoadrenal lineage is derived from a committed sympathoadrenal progenitor cell that has already passed a number of restriction points so that it can no longer form sensory neurons, glia, or melanocytes. This progenitor cell gives rise to four types of cellular progeny: (1) adrenal chromaffin cells, (2) small, intensely fluorescent cells found in the sympathetic ganglia, (3) adrenergic sympathetic neurons, and (4) a small population of cholinergic sympathetic neurons.

Somewhat farther down this cellular lineage is a bipotential progenitor cell that can give rise to either adrenal chromaffin cells or sympathetic neurons. The bipotential progenitor cell already possesses some neuronal traits, but final differentiation depends on the environment surrounding these cells. In the presence of fibroblast growth factor (FGF) and nerve growth factor in early sympathetic ganglia, these precursors differentiate into definitive sympathetic neurons. On the other hand, precursor cells in the developing adrenal medulla encounter glucocorticoids secreted by adrenal cortical cells. Under this hormonal influence, they lose their neuronal properties and differentiate into chromaffin cells. This differentiative choice, however, is not absolutely fixed, since chromaffin cells can be stimulated after birth to transdifferentiate into neurons if they are exposed to nerve growth factor in vitro.

The entire length of the gut is populated by neural crest–derived parasympathetic neurons and associated cells, the enteric glia. These arise from neural crest cells in the cervical (vagal) and sacral levels and, under the influence of **glial-derived neurotrophic factor** (GDNF), undertake extensive migrations along the developing gut. Sacral neural crest cells colonize the hindgut, but even there they form only a minority of the enteric neurons. The rest are derived from vagal crest. Within the gut the neural crest cells form the enteric nervous system, which in many respects acts like an independent component of the nervous system. The number of enteric neurons nearly matches the number of neurons in the spinal cord, and most of them are not directly connected to the brain or spinal cord. This independence explains how the bowel can maintain reflex activity in the absence of input from the central nervous system.

Neural crest cells are not committed to form gut-associated nervous tissue before leaving the spinal cord. If vagal crest is replaced by the neural crest of the trunk, which normally does not give rise to gut-associated derivatives, the gut is colonized by the transplanted trunk-level neural crest cells. Evidence that the pathways of migration affect differentiation is seen in the neurotransmitters produced by these transplanted crest cells. Parasympathetic neurons differentiated from trunk cells produce serotonin but not catecholamines in the gut. If they had

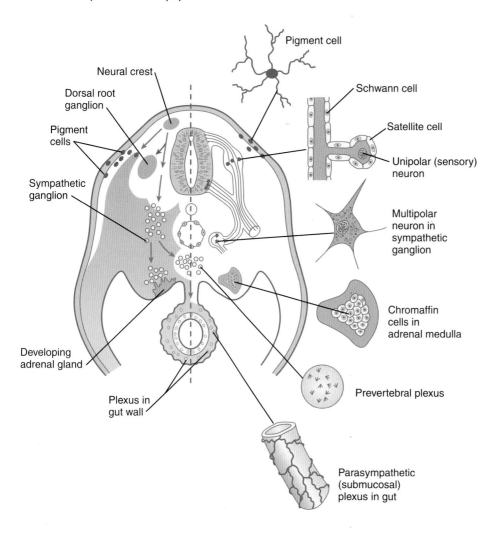

Pigment cell

Neural crest

Dorsal root
ganglion

Pigment
cells

Sympathetic
ganglion

Developing
adrenal gland

Plexus in
gut wall

Schwann cell

Satellite cell

Unipolar (sensory)
neuron

Multipolar
neuron in
sympathetic
ganglion

Chromaffin
cells in
adrenal medulla

Prevertebral plexus

Parasympathetic
(submucosal)
plexus in gut

**FIGURE 12-4** Major neural crest migratory pathways and derivatives in the trunk. *Left,* Pathways in the early embryo. The dorsolateral pathway is indicated by the green arrow; the ventral (sympathoadrenal) pathway is indicated by the red arrow; and the ventrolateral pathway is indicated by the purple arrow. *Right,* Derivatives of the trunk neural crest.

differentiated in their normal sites in the trunk, these neurons would have produced catecholamines and not serotonin.

Despite the strong influence of the environment of the gut on the differentiation of neural crest cells exposed to its influences, neural crest cells retain a surprising degree of developmental flexibility. If crest-derived cells already in the gut of avian embryos are retransplanted into the trunk region of younger embryos, they seem to lose the memory of their former association with the gut. They enter the pathways (e.g., adrenal or peripheral nerve) common to trunk crest cells (except that they cannot enter pigment cell pathways) and differentiate accordingly.

Most neural crest precursors of gut-associated parasympathetic neurons express the basic helix-loop-helix transcription factor, Mash 1, which is also expressed in the precursors of sympathetic but not sensory neurons. Expression of Mash 1 in these cells is stimulated by the growth factors BMP-2 and BMP-4, and Mash 1 appears to maintain the competence of the postmigratory cells in the gut to differentiate into neurons. Other environmen-

tal factors are required for complete commitment of these cells to form autonomic neurons.

Compared with the cranial neural crest, the trunk neural crest has a relatively limited range of differentiation options. The derivatives of the trunk neural crest are summarized in Table 12-1.

## Circumpharyngeal Neural Crest

The circumpharyngeal neural crest arises in the posterior rhombencephalic region, and in the lower part of the pharynx, emigrating circumpharyngeal crest cells pass behind the sixth pharyngeal arch (Figure 12-5). Ventral to the pharynx it sweeps cranially, providing the pathway through which the hypoglossal nerve (XII) and its associated skeletal muscle precursor cells pass. The circumpharyngeal crest marks the pathway of migration of enteric (vagal) crest cells toward the gut and cardiac neural crest cells into the cardiac outflow tract. Neural crest cells from the anterior rhombencephalon to the level of somite 5 emigrate from the circumpharyngeal

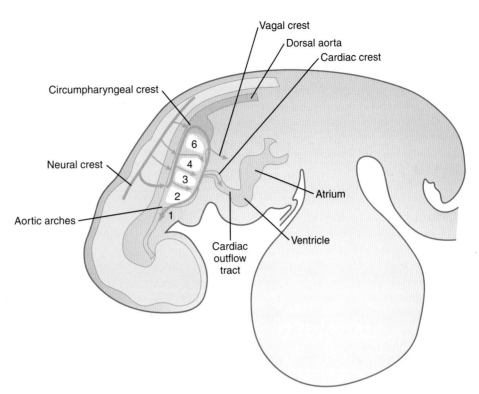

**FIGURE 12-5** Migration of circumpharyngeal neural crest cells (*green lines* and *arrows*) through the pharyngeal region and into the aortic arches and the outflow tract of the heart.

crest as a stream, called the **cardiac crest,** toward the developing heart and aortic arches, while other neural crest cells from the levels of somites 1 to 7 constitute the **vagal crest** and migrate into the developing gut as precursors of the parasympathetic innervation of the digestive tract. Still other cells in the anterior rhombencephalon migrate into the pharyngeal arches.

The cardiac crest surrounds the endothelial precursors of the third, fourth, and sixth aortic arches, and it contributes massively to the truncoconal folds that separate the outflow tract of the heart into aortic and pulmonary segments (see Chapter 17). Cardiac crest cells migrate toward the heart and contribute to the leaflets of the semilunar valves at the base of the outflow tract, and in the bird, at least, they may even penetrate the interventricular septum. Studies on mammalian embryos have shown a contribution of cardiac neural crest to the walls of the proximal coronary arteries near their attachment to the ascending aorta. Recent research suggests that the cardiac neural crest also interacts with pharyngeal endoderm to modify the signals leading to the normal differentiation of myocardial cells.

While much of the cardiac crest contributes to the outflow tract of the heart and the great vessels, portions of the cardiac neural crest population become associated with the newly forming thymus, parathyroid, and thyroid glands. In mammalian embryos a relatively massive presence of cardiac neural crest in early embryogenesis becomes attenuated in later development, but its importance in early organogenesis is demonstrated by abnor-malities of the above organs when the cardiac neural crest is deficient.

Circumpharyngeal neural crest cells migrate ventral to the pharynx in bilateral streams accompanying the somite-derived myoblasts that are migrating cranially to form the intrinsic muscles of the tongue and the hypopharyngeal muscles. This is the only known case in which somite-derived muscles are invested with neural crest–derived connective tissue. The cardiac neural crest also supplies the Schwann cells that are present in the hypoglossal and other cranial nerves.

A disturbance in this region of neural crest can result in cardiac septation defects (**aorticopulmonary septum**), as well as glandular and craniofacial malformations. The **DiGeorge syndrome,** which is associated with a deletion on chromosome 22, is characterized by hypoplasia and reduced function of the thymus, thyroid, and parathyroid glands and cardiovascular defects, such as persistent truncus ateriosus and abnormalities of the aortic arches. Hoxa-3 mutant mice show a similar spectrum of pharyngeal defects. The common denominator for this constellation of pathology is a defect of the cardiac crest supplying the third and fourth pharyngeal arches and cardiac outflow tract. Similar defects have been described in human embryos exposed to excessive amounts of retinoic acid early in embryogenesis.

The other component of the population that gives rise to the circumpharyngeal crest is the stream of cells known as the **vagal crest.** These cells, which arise at levels from somites 1 to 7, exit the main circumpharyngeal crest pathway caudal to the sixth pharyngeal arch and become closely associated with the embryonic foregut. The vagal crest cells enter the anterior region of the foregut and migrate caudally until they populate the entire length of the gut. When they first colonize the gut, these cells express no neuronal markers, but soon a wave of differentiation passes down the gut, and the cells synthesize neurofilament proteins and initially express catecholaminergic traits. These cells form the myenteric plexuses.

## Cranial Neural Crest

The cranial neural crest is a major component of the cephalic end of the embryo. Comparative anatomical and developmental research suggests that the cranial neural crest may represent the major morphological substrate for the evolution of the vertebrate head. Largely because of the availability of precise cellular marking methods, the understanding of the cranial neural crest has increased dramatically. The majority of studies on the cranial neural crest have been conducted on avian embryos; however, the properties and role of the neural crest in mammalian cranial development are quite similar to those in birds.

In the mammalian head, neural crest cells leave the future brain well before closure of the neural folds (Figure 12-6). Although the pathways of migration of the cranial neural crest in mammals are not nearly as well delineated as in birds, there nevertheless appear to be distinct but somewhat overlapping migratory territories in the embryonic mammalian head (Figure 12-7). Because of the distribution of primary mesenchymal cells and extracellular matrix molecules in the mammalian head, the neural crest cells migrate in diffuse streams throughout the cranial mesenchyme to reach their final destinations.

A major functional subdivision of cranial neural crest occurs at the boundary between rhombomeres 2 (r2) and 3 (r3). Those neural crest cells emerging from the diencephalon posteriorly through r2 do not express any *Hox* genes, whereas those emerging from the hindbrain region from r3 and posteriorly express a well-ordered sequence of *Hox* genes (see Figure 12-9).

There is remarkable specificity in the relationship among the origins of the neural crest in the hindbrain, its

**FIGURE 12-6** Neural crest migration in the head of a seven-somite rat embryo. In this scanning electron micrograph the ectoderm was removed from a large part of the side of the head, exposing migrating neural crest (*NC*) cells cranial (to the left) to the preotic sulcus (*PS*). Many of the cells are migrating toward the first pharyngeal arch (*I*). The area between the preotic sulcus and the first somite (*S₋₁*) is devoid of neural crest cells because in this region they have not begun to migrate from the closing neural folds. The white bar at the bottom represents 100 μm. (Based on Tan SS, Morriss-Kay G: *Cell Tissue Res* 204:403–416, 1985.)

**FIGURE 12-7** Major cranial neural crest migration routes in the mammal. (Based on Morriss-Kay G, Tuckett F: *J Craniofac Genet Dev Biol* 11:181–191, 1991.)

For a number of years it was thought that neural crest cells did not migrate from r3 or r5 despite the fact that neural crest cells form in these areas. It is known that some of the neural crest cells associated with r3 and r5 undergo apoptosis because of the presence of the apoptosis-inducing molecule **BMP-4,** but recent research has shown that the mesenchyme lateral to r3 and r5 exerts a repulsive effect on neural crest cells that try to enter these areas. Instead, surviving neural crest cells from r3 diverge into small streams that enter the first and second pharyngeal arches, and those from r5 behave similarly, merging with the streams of neural crest cells emanating from r4 and r6. The mesenchyme opposite r3 and r5 exerts a repulsive effect on any neural crest cells trying to enter these areas. It appears that influences from both the epithelium of the neural tube and the overlying ectoderm in these areas are required for the mesenchyme to maintain its repulsive properties. This complex mechanism is probably required to maintain the separate streams of neural crest cells that populate the pharyngeal arches.

ultimate destination within the pharyngeal arches, and the expression of certain gene products (Figures 12-8 and 12-9). Neural crest cells associated with rhombomeres 1 and 2 migrate into and form the bulk of the first pharyngeal arch, those of rhombomere 4 into the second arch, and those of rhombomeres 6 and 7 into the third arch as three separate streams of cells.

A close correlation exists between the pattern of migration of the rhombomeric neural crest cells and the expression of products of the Hoxb gene complex. Hoxb-2, Hoxb-3, and Hoxb-4 products are expressed in a regular sequence in both the neural tube and the neural crest–derived mesenchyme of the second, third, and fourth pharyngeal arches. Hoxb is not expressed in rhombomere 2 or in the first pharyngeal arch mesenchyme. Only after the pharyngeal arches become populated with neural crest cells does the ectoderm overlying the arches

**FIGURE 12-8** Migration pathways of neural crest cells from rhombomeres 2, 4, and 6 into the first three pharyngeal arches. Small contributions from rhombomeres 1, 3, and 5 are indicated by arrows.

**FIGURE 12-9** Spread of *Hox* gene expression from the neural plate (*far left*) into the migrating neural crest (*middle*) and into tissues of the pharyngeal arches (*right*). Arrows in the middle diagram indicate directions of neural crest migration. *C.N.,* Cranial nerve; *r,* rhombomere. (Modified from Hunt P and others: *Development* 1[suppl]:187–196, 1991.)

express a similar pattern of Hoxb gene products (see Figure 12-9). These *Hoxb* genes may play a role in positionally specifying the neural crest cells with which they are associated. Furthermore, interactions between the neural crest cells and the surface ectoderm of the pharyngeal arches may specify the ectoderm of the arches.

The molecular control of pharyngeal arch identity remains incompletely understood, but considerable evidence suggests that ***Hoxa-2*** may act as a selector gene for patterning the second arch.

Determining how level-specific patterns in cranial neural crest–derived structures are generated and maintained has had a complex history. For many years it was assumed that, in contrast to trunk neural crest, cranial neural crest cells were preprogrammed with morphogenetic instructions before they left the neural tube and that these instructions were firmly imprinted on the cells. A major basis for this concept was an experiment in which early first arch neural crest was transplanted to the level of more posterior rhombomeres. When the transplanted crest cells arrived into the more posterior pharyngeal arch, that arch assumed the morphological characteristics of the first arch, such as mandibular structures. This type of experiment served as the principal basis for the notion of preprogramming of cranial neural crest cells within the neural tube.

Subsequent experimental work has shown that environmental factors play a much more prominent role in the determination of cell fate in the cranial neural crest than was earlier supposed. A reexamination of the earlier neural crest transplantation experiments suggests that the

basis for the transformation of the second pharyngeal arch into the first arch may not have been so much due to the immutable properties of the transplanted crest, but rather the presence of isthmic organizer tissue (see Figure 6-4) along with the graft. Isthmic tissue emits a high concentration of FGF-8, which suppresses *Hoxa-2,* the selector gene for determining the character of the second arch. The introduction of FGF-8 alone into the region of the future second arch also suppresses its formation, and it takes on the character of the first arch. Why forming a first arch is a default response by the cells normally forming the second arch is not understood.

Other research has shown that transplanted individual or small groups of cranial neural crest cells can adapt to their new environment, whereas larger groups of cells retain their original characteristics. The cranial mesoderm is presently suspected of playing a formerly unexpected role in regulating the fate of migrating cranial neural crest cells. According to our present understanding, it appears that upon emigrating from the neural tube, neural crest cells from the hindbrain region are to a certain extent preprogrammed to form specific pharyngeal arches, but that interactions with the local cranial mesoderm are important in maintaining and expressing that information.

Cranial neural crest cells differentiate into a wide variety of cell and tissue types (see Table 12-1), including connective tissue and skeletal tissues. These tissues constitute much of the soft and hard tissues of the face (Figure 12-10). (Specific details of morphogenesis of the head are presented in Chapter 14.)

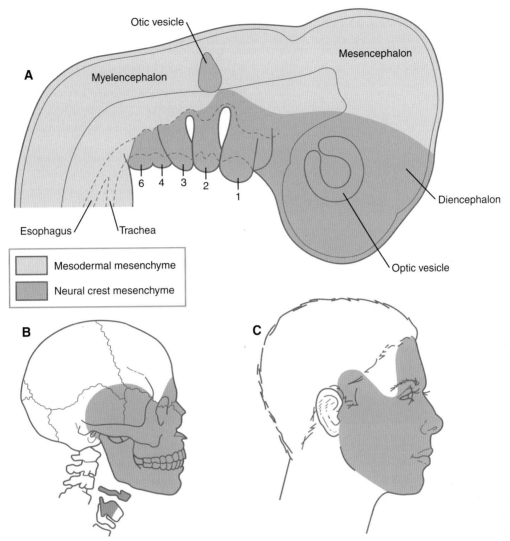

**FIGURE 12-10** Neural crest distribution in the human face and neck. **A,** In the early embryo. **B** and **C,** In the adult skeleton and dermis.

**CLINICAL VIGNETTE**

A newborn is diagnosed as having an incomplete separation between the aorta and pulmonary artery (a mild form of persistent truncus arteriosus). Later, after corrective heart surgery, she has more colds and sore throats than her siblings. After testing, her physician tells the parents that there is evidence of immunodeficiency. The doctor also tells the parents that it would be a good idea to check her levels of parathyroid hormone.

What is the basis for this suggestion?

## SUMMARY

⚪ The neural crest arises from neuroepithelial cells along the lateral border of the neural plate. Having left the neural tube, neural crest cells migrate to peripheral locations throughout the body. Some substrates, such as those containing chondroitin sulfate molecules, are not favorable for neural crest cell migration.

⚪ Neural crest cells differentiate into many types of adult cells, such as sensory and autonomic neurons, Schwann cells, pigment cells, and adrenal medullary cells. Cells from the cranial and circumpharyngeal neural crest also differentiate into bone, cartilage, dentin, dermal fibroblasts, selected smooth muscle, the connective tissue stroma of pharyngeal glands, and several regions of the heart and great vessels.

⚪ The control of differentiation of neural crest cells is diverse, with some cells being determined before they begin to migrate and others responding to environmental cues along their paths of migration. Trunk neural crest cells cannot differentiate into skeletal elements.

⚪ Neural crest cells in the trunk follow three main paths of migration: (1) a dorsolateral pathway for pigment cells, (2) a ventral path for cells of the sympathoa-

## Box 12-1 Major Neurocristopathies

### DEFECTS OF MIGRATION OR MORPHOGENESIS

**Trunk Neural Crest**

Hirschsprung's disease (aganglionic megacolon)

**Cranial Neural Crest**

Aorticopulmonary septation defects of heart

Anterior chamber defects of eye

Cleft lip, cleft palate, or both

Frontonasal dysplasia

DiGeorge syndrome (hypoparathyroidism, thyroid deficiency, thymic dysplasia leading to immunodeficiency,
defects in cardiac outflow tract and aortic arches)

Certain dental anomalies

**Trunk and Cranial Neural Crest**

CHARGE association

Waardenburg's syndrome

### TUMORS AND PROLIFERATION DEFECTS

Pheochromocytoma: tumor of chromaffin tissue of
adrenal medulla

Neuroblastoma: tumor of adrenal medulla, autonomic
ganglia, or both

Medullary carcinoma of thyroid: tumor of parafollicular
(calcitonin-secreting) cells of thyroid

Carcinoid tumors—tumors of enterochromaffin cells of
digestive tract

Neurofibromatosis (von Recklinghausen's disease):
peripheral nerve tumors

### GENETIC DEFECT INVOLVING NEURAL CREST CELLS

Albinism

---

### CLINICAL CORRELATION 12-1

## Neurocristopathies

Because of the complex developmental history of the neural crest, a variety of congenital malformations are associated with its defective development. These have commonly been subdivided into two main categories—defects of migration or morphogenesis and tumors of neural crest tissues (Box 12-1). Some of these defects involve only a single component of the neural crest; others affect multiple components and are recognized as syndromes.

Several syndromes or associations of defects are understandable only if the wide distribution of derivatives of the neural crest is recognized. For example, one association called **CHARGE** consists of coloboma (see Chapter 13), *h*eart disease, *a*tresia of nasal choanae, retardation of development, *g*enital hypoplasia in males, and anomalies of the *e*ar.

Types I and III of **Waardenburg's syndrome**, which is caused by Pax-3 mutations, involve various combinations of pigmentation defects (commonly a white stripe in the hair and other pigment anomalies in the skin), deafness, cleft palate, and **ocular hypertelorism** (increased space between the eyes). One variant (type I) of Waardenburg's syndrome is also characterized by hypoplasia of the limb muscles, which is not surprising considering the important association between Pax-3 and myogenic cells migrating into the limb buds from the somites. Pax-3 is similarly expressed in migrating cardiac neural crest cells, but is downregulated when the cells settle in the walls of the cardiac outflow tract or aortic arches. Cardiovascular defects in these areas are also seen in Pax-3 mutants.

The **DiGeorge syndrome**, which is associated with a deletion on chromosome 22 that encompasses up to 15 genes, is characterized by hypoplasia and reduced function of the thymus, thyroid, and parathyroid glands, as well as cardiovascular defects, such as persistent truncus arteriosus and abnormalities of the aortic arches. *Hoxa-3* mutant mice show a similar spectrum of pharyngeal defects. The common denominator for this constellation of pathology is a defect of the neural crest supplying the third and fourth pharyngeal arches and the cardiac outflow tract. Similar defects have been described in human embryos exposed to excessive amounts of retinoic acid early in embryogenesis.

**Neurofibromatosis** (von Recklinghausen's disease) is a common genetic disease manifested by multiple tumors of neural crest origin. Common features are **café au lait spots** (light brown pigmented lesions) on the skin, multiple (often hundreds) **neurofibromas** (peripheral nerve tumors), occasional gigantism of a limb or digit, and various other conditions. Neurofibromatosis occurs in approximately 1 of 3000 live births, and the gene is a very large one and subject to a high mutation rate.

Because of the massive contribution of the neural crest to the face and other parts of the head and neck, various malformations in the craniofacial region involve neural crest derivatives. A wide spectrum of facial abnormalities lumped together under the term **frontonasal dysplasia** (see Chapter 13) heavily involve neural crest–derived tissues.

drenal lineage, and (3) a ventrolateral pathway leading through the anterior halves of the somites for sensory ganglion–forming cells.

○ Cells of the cranial neural crest form many tissues of the facial region. In the pharyngeal region the pathways of crest cell migration are closely correlated with regions of expression of products of the *Hoxb* gene complex. Cells of the cranial crest may be patterned with level-specific instructions, whereas those of the trunk crest are not.

○ Several genetic diseases and syndromes are associated with disturbances of the neural crest. Neurofibromatosis is often characterized by multiple tumors and pigment disturbances. Disturbances of the cardiac neural crest can result in septation defects in the heart and outflow tract.

# ◖ Review Questions

1. Which of these cell and tissue types arises from cranial but not trunk neural crest cells?
    A. Sensory ganglia
    B. Adrenal medulla
    C. Melanocytes
    D. Schwann cells
    E. None of the above

2. Which molecule is a poor substrate for migrating neural crest cells?
    A. Laminin
    B. Chondroitin sulfate
    C. Fibronectin
    D. Type IV collagen
    E. Hyaluronic acid

3. Neural crest cells arise from the:
    A. Somite
    B. Dorsal nonneural ectoderm
    C. Neural tube
    D. Splanchnic mesoderm
    E. Yolk sac endoderm

4. A 6-month-old infant exhibits multiple congenital defects, including a cleft palate, deafness, ocular hypertelorism, and a white forelock but otherwise dark hair on his head. The probable diagnosis is:
    A. CHARGE association
    B. von Recklinghausen's disease
    C. Hirschsprung's disease
    D. Waardenburg's syndrome
    E. None of the above

5. What molecule is involved in the migration of neural crest cells from the neural tube?
    A. Slug
    B. BMP-2
    C. Mash 1
    D. Norepinephrine
    E. Glial growth factor

6. Which is not a derivative of the neural crest?
    A. Sensory neurons
    B. Motor neurons
    C. Schwann cells
    D. Adrenal medulla
    E. Dental papilla

7. What maintains the competence of neural crest cells to differentiate into autonomic neurons?
    A. Sonic hedgehog
    B. Acetylcholine
    C. Mash 1
    D. Glial growth factor
    E. Transforming growth factor-β

8. If trunk neural crest cells are transplanted into the cranial region, they can form all of the following types of cells except:
    A. Pigment cells
    B. Schwann cells
    C. Sensory neurons
    D. Cartilage
    E. Autonomic neurons

9. How does the segmental distribution of the spinal ganglia occur?

10. What are three major differences between cranial and trunk neural crests?

## REFERENCES

Anderson DJ: Cellular and molecular biology of neural crest lineage determination, *Trends Genet* 13:276–280, 1997.
Anderson DJ: Genes, lineages and the neural crest: a speculative review, *Phil Trans Roy Soc Lond B* 355:953–964, 2000.
Aybar MJ, Mayor R: Early induction of neural crest cells: lessons learned from frog, fish and chick, *Curr Opin Genet Devel* 12:452–458, 2002.
Barald KF: Culture conditions affect the cholinergic development of an isolated subpopulation of chick mesencephalic neural crest cells, *Dev Biol* 135:349–366, 1989.
Birgbauer E and others: Rhombomeric origin and rostrocaudal reassortment of neural crest cells revealed by intravital microscopy, *Development* 121:935–945, 1995.
Bronner-Fraser M: Rostrocaudal differences within the somites confer segmental pattern to trunk neural crest migration, *Curr Top Devel Biol* 47:279–296.
Conway SJ, Henderson DJ, Copp AJ: Pax3 is required for cardiac neural crest migration in the mouse: evidence from the splotch (Sp2H) mutant, *Development* 124:505–514, 1997.
Epstein JA: Pax3, neural crest and cardiovascular development, *Trends Cardiovasc Med* 6:255–261, 1996.
Erickson CA: Morphogenesis of the neural crest. In Browder LW, ed: *Developmental biology*, vol 2, New York, 1986, Plenum, pp 481–543.
Farrell M and others: A novel role for cardiac neural crest in heart development, *Trends Cardiac Med* 9:214–219, 1999.
García-Castro MI, Marcelle C, Bronner-Fraser M: Ectodermal Wnt function as a neural crest inducer, *Science* 297:848–851, 2002.
Gershon MD: Genes and lineages in the formation of the enteric nervous system, *Curr Opin Neurobiol* 7:101–109, 1997.
Golding JP, Dixon M, Gassmann: Cues from neuroepithelium and surface ectoderm maintain neural crest-free regions within cranial mesenchyme of the developing chick, *Development* 129:1095–1105, 2002.
Hall BK, Hörstadius S: *The neural crest*, London, 1988, Oxford University Press.
Hunt P, Wilkinson D, Krumlauf R: Patterning the vertebrate head: murine Hox 2 genes mark distinct subpopulations of premigratory and migratory cranial neural crest, *Development* 112:43–50, 1991.

Imai H and others: Contribution of early-emigrating midbrain crest cells to the dental mesenchyme of mandibular molar teeth in rat embryos, *Dev Biol* 176:151–165, 1996.

Johnston MC, Vig KWL, Ambrose LJH: Neurocristopathy as a unifying concept: clinical correlations. In Riccardi VM, Mulvihill JJ, eds: *Neurofibromatosis (von Recklinghausen disease)*, New York, 1981, Raven, pp 97–104.

Jones MC: The neurocristopathies: reinterpretation based upon the mechanism of abnormal morphogenesis, *Cleft Palate J* 27:136–140, 1990.

Kirby ML, Waldo KL: Neural crest and cardiovascular patterning, *Circ Res* 77:211–215, 1995.

Knecht AK, Bronner-Fraser M: Induction of the neural crest: a multigene process, *Nature Revs, Genet* 3:453–461, 2002.

Kulesa PM, Fraser SE: In ovo time-lapse analysis of chick hindbrain neural crest cell migration shows cell interactions during migration to the branchial arches, *Development* 127:1161–1172, 2000.

Kuratani S: Spatial distribution of postotic crest cells defines the head/trunk interface of the vertebrate body: embryological interpretation of peripheral nerve morphology and evolution of the vertebrate head, *Anat Embryol* 195:1–13, 1997.

Kuratani SC, Kirby ML: Initial migration and distribution of the cardiac neural crest in the avian embryo: an introduction to the concept of the circumpharyngeal crest, *Am J Anat* 191:215–227, 1991.

Kuratani SC, Kirby ML: Migration and distribution of circumpharyngeal crest cells in the chick embryo, *Anat Rec* 234:263–280, 1992.

LaBonne C, Bronner-Fraser M: Molecular mechanisms of neural crest formation, *Annu Rev Cell Dev Biol* 15:81–112, 1999.

Le Douarin NM, Kalcheim C: *The Neural Crest*, 2nd ed, Cambridge, England, 1999, Cambridge University Press.

Liem KF and others: Dorsal differentiation of neural plate cells induced by BMP-mediated signals from epidermal ectoderm, *Cell* 82:969–979, 1995.

Lumsden A: Multipotent cells in the avian neural crest, *Trends Neurosci* 12:81–83, 1989.

Lumsden A, Guthrie S: Alternating patterns of cell surface properties and neural crest cell migration during segmentation of the chick hindbrain, *Development* 2(suppl):9–15, 1991.

Manley NR, Capecci MR: The role of Hoxa-3 in mouse thymus and thyroid development, *Development* 121:1989–2003, 1995.

Maschhoff KL, Baldwin HS: Molecular determinants of neural crest migration, *Am J Med Genet* 97:280–288, 2000.

Morell R and others: Three mutations in the paired homeodomain of PAX3 that cause Waardenburg syndrome type 1, *Hum Hered* 47:38–41, 1997.

Morriss-Kay G, Tan S-S: Mapping cranial neural crest cell migration pathways in mammalian embryos, *Trends Genet* 3:257–261, 1987.

Newgreen DF, Erickson CA: The migration of neural crest cells, *Int Rev Cytol* 103:89–143, 1986.

Nieto MA and others: Control of cell behavior during vertebrate development by *Slug*, a zinc finger gene, *Science* 264:835–839, 1994.

Noden DM: Origins and patterning of craniofacial mesenchymal tissues, *J Craniofac Genet Dev Biol* 2(suppl):15–31, 1986.

Noden DM: The role of the neural crest in patterning of avian cranial skeletal, connective and muscle tissues, *Dev Biol* 96:144–165, 1983.

Oakley PA and others: Glycoconjugates mark a transient barrier to neural crest migration in the chicken embryo, *Development* 120:103–114, 1994.

Patterson PH: Control of cell fate in a vertebrate neurogenic cell lineage, *Cell* 62:1035–1038, 1990.

Quevedo C, Holstein TJ: Molecular genetics and the ontogeny of pigment patterns in mammals, *Pigment Cell Res* 5:328–334, 1992.

Scammbler PJ: DiGeorge syndrome and related birth defects, *Semin Dev Biol* 5:303–310, 1994.

Sechrist J and others: Segmental migration of the hindbrain neural crest does not arise from its segmental generation, *Development* 118:691–703, 1993.

Selleck MAJ and others: Origins of neural crest diversity, *Dev Biol* 159:1–11, 1993.

Shah NM and others: Glial growth factor restricts mammalian neural crest stem cells to a glial fate, *Cell* 77:349–360, 1994.

Trainor PA, Ariza-McNaughton, Krumlauf R: Role of the isthmus and FGFs in resolving the paradox of neural crest plasticity and prepatterning, *Science* 295:1288–1291, 2002.

Trainor P, Krumlauf R: Plasticity in mouse neural crest cells reveals a new patterning role for cranial mesoderm, *Nature Cell Biol* 2:96–102, 2000.

Trainor PA, Krumlauf R: *Hox* genes, neural crest cells and branchial arch patterning, *Curr Opin Cell Biol* 13:698–705, 2001.

Weston JA: Phenotypic diversification in neural crest–derived cells: the time and stability of commitment during early development, *Curr Topics Dev Biol* 20:195–210, 1986.

# CHAPTER 13

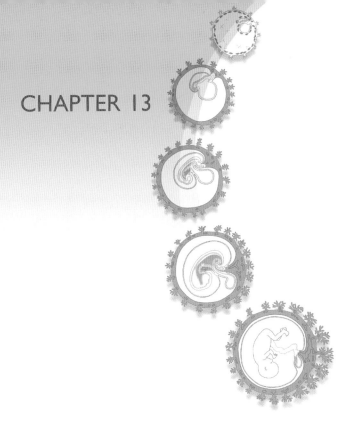

# Sense Organs

The major sense organs arise in large measure from the thickened ectodermal placodes that appear lateral to the neural plate in the early embryo (see Figure 6-5). The following descriptions begin with the most cranial placodes and continue to the most caudal. The midline **hypophyseal placode**, located in the anterior neural ridge (see Figure 6-5, *B*), will become the primordium of Rathke's pouch (the precursor of the adenohypophysis). This arises adjacent to the neural tissue that will ultimately form the neurohypophysis. Arising also from the anterior neural region, bilateral **olfactory placodes** (see Figure 6-5) are the precursors of the olfactory epithelium. They give rise to olfactory neurons and their supporting cells and also to glial cells and neuroendocrine cells that migrate from the placode into the brain. Closely associated with the olfactory placodes is the preneural tissue that will form the functionally associated olfactory bulbs of the brain. The bilateral **lens placodes**, associated with the optic vesicles (future retina) extending outward from the diencephalic part of the brain, are the lens precursors.

Next in line are the paired **trigeminal placodes** (cranial nerve V), each of which arises from two placodal precursors—the opthalmic and maxillomandibular (see Figure 6-5, *C*). The **otic placodes** (precursors of the inner ear) in the human are the remaining representatives of the **dorsolateral series** of placodes, all of which produce vibration-detecting organs. In fishes and some amphibians, the other members of the dorsolateral series give rise to the lateral line organs,

which serve as vibration and electroreceptors in aquatic vertebrates.

The caudalmost group constitutes the **epibranchial placodes**, which are located just dorsal to the region where the first through third pharyngeal pouches abut the cervical ectoderm (see Figure 6-5, *A*). These placodes produce sensory neurons that supply visceral structures. The first epibranchial placode produces neurons (geniculate ganglion of cranial nerve VII, Figure 13-1, *B*) that innervate taste buds. Similarly, neurons arising from the second epibranchial placode (inferior [petrosal] ganglion of cranial nerve IX) innervate taste buds as well, but also the heart and other visceral organs. The third epibranchial placode contributes to the inferior (nodose) ganglion of the vagus (X) nerve, and its neurons innervate the heart, stomach, and other viscera. Of cranial nerves V, VII, IX, and X, the proximal sensory ganglia are derived largely from neural crest cells, and the distal ganglia are principally placodal in origin (Figure 13-1, *B*). The placode-derived neurons (those in the distal ganglia) begin to establish peripheral and central connections before axons emerge in the neural crest–derived neuronal precursors in the proximal ganglia.

This chapter concentrates on the development of the eyes and ears, the most complex and important sense organs in humans. Discussion of the organs of smell and taste is deferred to Chapter 14, since their development is intimately associated with that of the face and pharynx. The sensory components of the cranial nerves are discussed in Chapter 11.

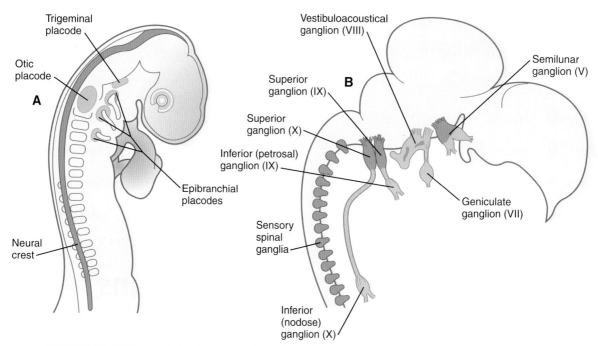

**FIGURE 13-1** Ectodermal placodes and neural crest in the formation of sensory ganglia of cranial and spinal nerves in the chick embryo. **A,** At 2 days. **B,** At 8 days. Neural crest is shown in green, placodes in blue. (Modified from LeDouarin N and others: *Trends Neurosci* 9[4]:175–180, 1986.)

## EYE

The eye is a very complex structure that originates from constituents derived from a number of sources, including the wall of the diencephalon, the overlying surface ectoderm, and migrating cranial neural crest mesenchyme. Two basic themes occur throughout ocular development. One is an ongoing series of inductive signals that result in the initial establishment of the major components of the eye. The other is the coordinated differentiation of many of these components.

For normal vision to occur, many complex structures within the eye must properly relate to neighboring structures. For example, the cornea and lens must both become transparent and properly aligned to provide an appropriate pathway for light to reach the retina. The retina in turn must be configured to both receive concrete visual images and transmit patterned visual signals to the proper parts of the brain through neural processes extending from the retina into the optic nerve.

### Early Events in the Establishment of the Eye

The early eye fields are Pax-6–expressing areas on either side of the diencephalon. A combination of sonic hedgehog (shh) expression by the prechordal plate plus ventral forebrain and midline cell movement repress Pax-6 expression in the ventral midline of the diencephalon and

keeps the two optic fields separate. In the absence of the influence of the prechordal plate, forebrain tissue is deficient, the optic fields converge, and **cyclopia** results (see Figure 8-16).

Development of the eye is first evident at about 22 days' gestation, when the lateral walls of the diencephalon begin to bulge out as **optic grooves** (Figure 13-2). Within a few days the optic grooves enlarge to form **optic vesicles**, which terminate very close to the overlying surface ectoderm. Apposition of the outer wall of the optic vesicle to the surface ectoderm is essential for the transmission of an important inductive message that stimulates the surface ectodermal cells to thicken and begin forming the lens (Figure 13-3).

The interaction between the optic vesicle and overlying ectoderm was one of the first recognized inductive processes. It was initially characterized by deletion and transplantation experiments conducted on amphibian embryos. When the optic vesicles were removed early, the surface ectoderm differentiated into ordinary ectodermal cells instead of lens fibers. Conversely, when optic vesicles were combined with certain types of ectoderm other than eye, the ectoderm was stimulated to form lens fibers. Subsequent research on amphibian embryos has shown that a series of preparatory inductions from neural plate and underlying mesoderm condition the ectoderm for its final induction into lens by the optic vesicle. In mammals an important mechanism underlying the severe **microphthalmia** (tiny eyes) or **anophthalmia** (absence of eyes) seen in the *small eye* and *fidget* mutants is a distur-

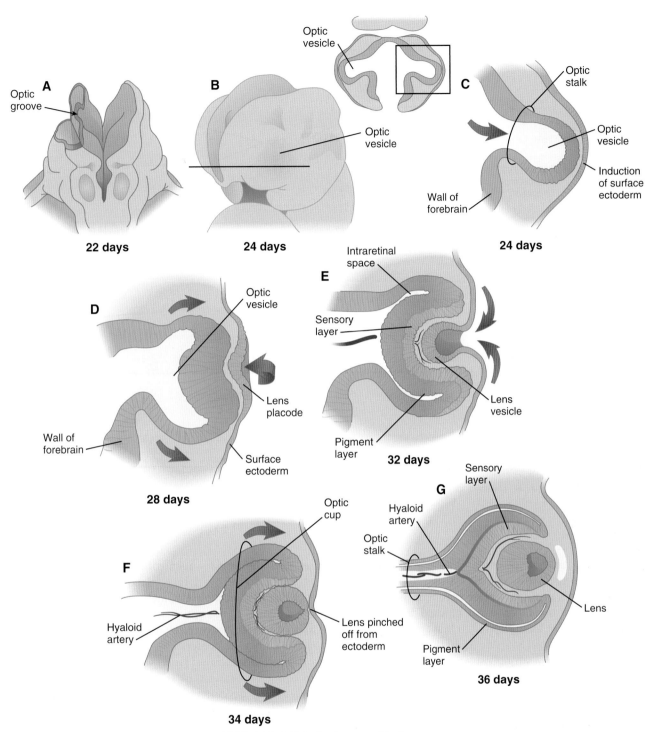

**FIGURE 13-2** Early development of the human eye.

bance in the apposition of optic vesicles and surface ecto-derm, which interferes with lens induction.

The paired box gene **Pax-6** plays a prominent role throughout early eye development and at a number of later stages of development of the retina and lens. Pax-6 is initially expressed in both the lens and nasal placodes as well as much of the diencephalon. In *Drosophila*, Pax-6

has been called a *master gene* for eye development; that is, it can turn on the cascade of an estimated 2500 genes that guide development of the eye. The power of Pax-6 is shown by the formation of ectopic eyes on antennae and legs in *Drosophila* when the gene is improperly expressed. In the absence of Pax-6 expression (*eyeless* mutant), eyes do not form. In the *small eye* mutation, the

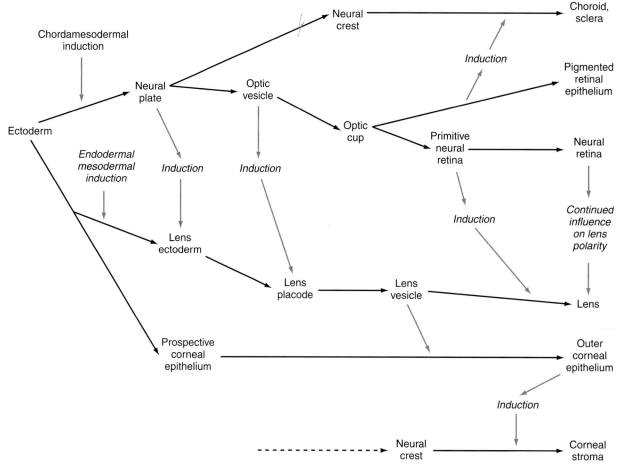

**FIGURE 13-3** Flow chart of major inductive events and tissue transformations in eye development. Inductive events are indicated by colored arrows.

mammalian equivalent of *eyeless*, the early optic vesicle forms, but, as previously noted, eye development does not progress because the surface ectoderm is unable to respond to the inductive signal emitted by the optic vesicle. The recent identification in humans of two genes (*Eya* [eyes absent] and *Six* [sine oculis]) that are activated by Pax-6 in *Drosophila* strongly suggests that despite major differences in the structure and development of the vertebrate and insect eye, the basic genetic apparatus has been conserved throughout phylogeny. In mice, **Eya-1** and **Eya-2** are expressed in the lens placodes and appear to be required for placodal induction and early differentiation, but in the absence of Pax-6 function, they are not expressed, and eye development fails to proceed.

As the process of lens induction occurs, the outer face of the optic vesicle begins to flatten and ultimately becomes concave. This results in the transformation of the optic vesicle to the **optic cup** (see Figure 13-2). Meanwhile, the induced lens ectoderm thickens and invaginates to form a **lens vesicle**, which detaches from the surface epithelium from which it originated (Figures 13-2 and 13-4). Then the lens vesicle takes over and

becomes the primary agent of a new inductive reaction by acting on the overlying surface ectoderm and causing it to begin corneal development (see Figure 13-3).

Formation of the optic cup is an asymmetrical process that occurs at the ventral margin of the optic vesicle rather than at its center. This results in the formation of a gap called the *choroid fissure*, which is continuous with a groove in the **optic stalk** (Figure 13-5). During much of early ocular development, the choroid fissure and optic groove form a channel through which the **hyaloid artery** passes into the posterior chamber of the eye. Differential expression of *Pax* genes determines which cells will become optic cup (future retina) and which will become optic stalk (future optic nerve). Through exposure to high concentrations of shh, the expression of **Pax-6** is inhibited and **Pax-2** is induced in the optic stalk, whereas a lower concentration of shh more distally permits the expression of Pax-6 in the optic vesicle, paving the way toward formation of the retina.

The optic stalk initially represents a narrow neck that connects the optic cup to the diencephalon, but as development progresses, it is invaded by neuronal processes

**FIGURE 13-4** Scanning electron micrograph of the optic cup *(left)* and lens vesicle *(center)* in the chick embryo. (Courtesy K. Tosney, Ann Arbor, Mich.)

emanating from the ganglion cells of the retina. Pax-2–expressing cells in the optic stalk provide guidance cues to outgrowing retinal axons that pass through the optic nerve and optic chiasm and enter the contralateral optic tract. After the neuronal processes have made their way to the appropriate regions of the brain, the optic stalk is properly known as the **optic nerve**.

Later in development, the choroid fissure closes, and no trace of it is seen in the normal iris. Nonclosure of the choroid fissure results in the anomaly of coloboma (see Figure 13-18, *B*). In certain forms of coloboma, especially those that are associated with anomalies of the kidneys,

mutations of *Pax-2* genes are seen. In *Pax-2* mutant mice, retinal axons do not cross the midline through the optic chiasm, but rather remain in the ipsilateral optic tract.

## Formation of the Lens

From the earliest stages, formation of the lens depends on genetic instructions provided by *Pax-6*. *Pax-6* expression is required for the surface ectoderm to respond to inductive signals from the underlying optic vesicle by activating and combining with another transcription factor, Sox-2. This leads to the thickening of the surface ectoderm to form the **lens placode** (see Figure 13-2, *D*). *Pax-6* expression continues as the lens placode invaginates to form the **lens vesicle**, which ultimately breaks off from the surface ectoderm. At this point *Pax-6* plays a new role in regulating the activity of the genes governing the formation of the lens crystallin proteins.

When it is breaking off from the surface ectoderm, the lens vesicle is roughly spherical and has a large central cavity (see Figure 13-2, *E*). At the end of the sixth week the cells at the inner pole of the lens vesicle begin to elongate in an early step toward their transformation into the long, transparent cells called **lens fibers** (Figure 13-6, *A*).

Differentiation of the lens is a very precise and well-orchestrated process involving several levels of organization. At the cellular level, relatively nonspecialized lens epithelial cells, under the influence of Sox and other proteins paired with an oncogene called **Maf**, undergo a profound transformation into transparent, elongated cells that contain large quantities of specialized **crystallin proteins**. At the tissue level the entire lens is responsive to signals from the retina and other structures of the eye so that its shape and overall organization are best adapted for the transmission of undistorted light rays from the corneal entrance to the light-receiving cells of the retina.

**FIGURE 13-5** Optic cup and stalk showing the choroid fissure containing the hyaloid artery.

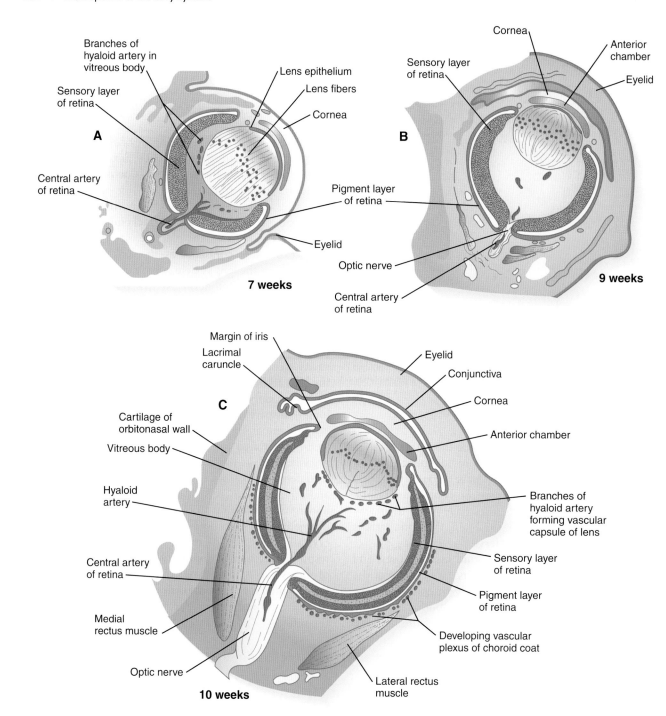

**FIGURE 13-6** Later stages of eye development drawn from coronal sections through heads of human embryos. **A,** At **7 weeks. B,** At **9 weeks. C,** At **10 weeks.** (Modified from Carlson B: *Patten's foundations of embryology,* ed 6, New York, 1996, McGraw-Hill.)

At the cellular level, cytodifferentiation of the lens consists of the transformation of mitotically active lens epithelial cells into elongated postmitotic lens fiber cells. Up to 90% of the soluble protein in these postmitotic cells consists of crystallin proteins. The mammalian lens contains three major crystallin proteins: $\alpha$, $\beta$, and $\gamma$.

The formation of crystallin-containing lens fibers begins with the elongation of epithelial cells from the inner pole of the lens vesicle (see Figure 13-2). These cells make up the fibers of the **lens nucleus** (Figure 13-7). The remainder of the lens fibers arise from the transformation of the cuboidal cells of the anterior lens epithelium. During embryonic life, mitotic activity is

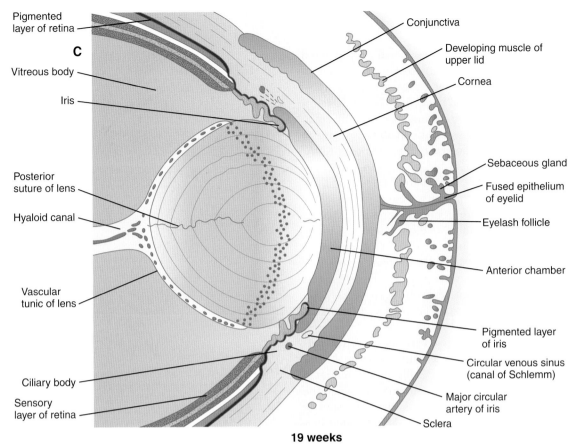

C

Pigmented layer of retina

Vitreous body

Iris

Posterior suture of lens

Hyaloid canal

Vascular tunic of lens

Ciliary body

Sensory layer of retina

Conjunctiva

Developing muscle of upper lid

Cornea

Sebaceous gland

Fused epithelium of eyelid

Eyelash follicle

Anterior chamber

Pigmented layer of iris

Circular venous sinus (canal of Schlemm)

Major circular artery of iris

Sclera

**19 weeks**

**FIGURE 13-6, CONT'D D,** At **19 weeks.** (Modified from Carlson B: *Patten's foundations of embryology,* ed 6, New York, 1996, McGraw-Hill.)

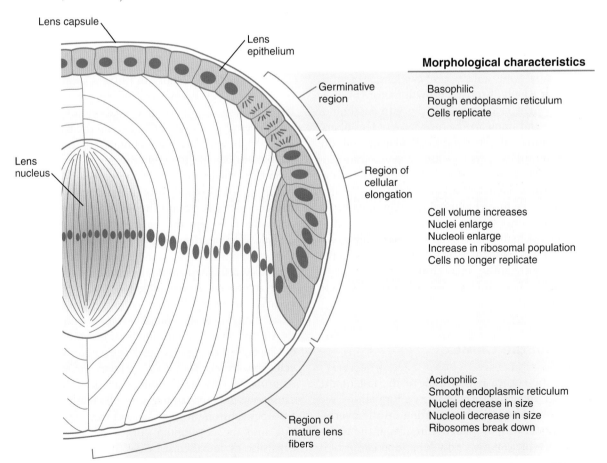

Lens capsule

Lens epithelium

Germinative region

Lens nucleus

Region of cellular elongation

Region of mature lens fibers

**Morphological characteristics**

Basophilic
Rough endoplasmic reticulum
Cells replicate

Cell volume increases
Nuclei enlarge
Nucleoli enlarge
Increase in ribosomal population
Cells no longer replicate

Acidophilic
Smooth endoplasmic reticulum
Nuclei decrease in size
Nucleoli decrease in size
Ribosomes break down

**FIGURE 13-7** Organization of the vertebrate lens. As the lens grows, epithelial cells from the germinative region stop dividing, elongate, and differentiate into lens fiber cells that produce lens crystallin proteins. (From Papaconstantinou J: *Science* 156:338–346, 1967.)

spread throughout the outer lens epithelial cells. Around the time of birth, mitotic activity ceases in the central region of this epithelium, leaving a germinative ring of mitotically active cells around the central region. Daughter cells from the germinative region move into the equatorial region of cellular elongation, where they cease to divide and take on the cytological characteristics of RNA-producing cells and begin to form crystallin messenger RNAs. These cells soon elongate tremendously, fill up with crystallins, and transform into secondary lens fibers that form concentric layers around the primary fibers of the lens nucleus. The midline region where secondary lens fibers from opposite points on the equator join is recognized as the anterior and posterior **lens suture** (see Figure 13-6, *D*). With this arrangement, the lens fibers toward the periphery are successively younger. As long as the lens grows, new secondary fibers move in from the equator onto the outer cortex of the lens.

The crystallin proteins show a very characteristic pattern and sequence of appearance, with the α-crystallins appearing first in the morphologically undifferentiated epithelial cells. Synthesis of β-crystallins is seen when the lens fibers begin to elongate, whereas the expression of γ-crystallins is restricted to terminally differentiated lens fiber cells. Each of the crystallin protein families contains several members. They show different patterns of activation (some members of a family being coordinately activated) and different patterns of accumulation. These facilitate the optical clearing of the lens to allow the efficient transmission of light.

Throughout much of its life the lens is under the influence of the retina. After induction of the lens, secretions of the retina, of which **fibroblast growth factor (FGF)** is a major component, accumulate in the vitreous humor behind the lens and stimulate the formation of lens fibers. A striking example of the continued influence of the retina on lens morphology is seen after a developing lens is rotated so that its outer pole faces the retina. Very rapidly, under the influence of retinal secretions, the low epithelial cells of the former outer pole begin to elongate and form an additional set of lens fibers (Figure 13-8). A new lens epithelium forms on the corneal side of the rotated lens. Such structural adaptations are striking evidence of a mechanism that ensures correct alignment between the lens and the rest of the visual system throughout development.

## Formation of the Cornea

Formation of the cornea is the result of the last of the series of major inductive events in eye formation (see Figure 13-3), with the lens vesicle acting on the overlying surface ectoderm. This induction results in the transformation of a typical surface ectoderm, consisting of a basal layer of cuboidal cells and a superficial periderm,

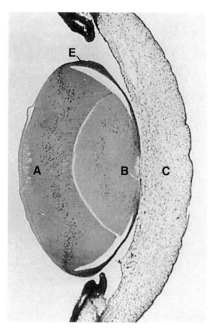

**FIGURE 13-8** Section through the lens of an 11-day-old chick embryo. At 5 days the lens was surgically reversed so that the anterior epithelial cells *(E)* faced the vitreous body and retina. The formerly low epithelial cells elongated to form new lens fibers *(A)*. Because of the reversal of the polarity of the equatorial zone of the lens, new epithelial cells were added over the original mass of lens fibers *(B)* onto the corneal face of the reversed lens. *C*, Cornea. (From Coulombre JL et al: *Science* 142:1489–1490, 1963.)

to a transparent, multilayered structure with a complex extracellular matrix and cellular contributions from several sources.

The inductive influence of the lens stimulates a change in the basal ectodermal cells. They increase in height, largely as a result of the elaboration of secretory organelles (e.g., Golgi apparatus) on the basal ends of the cells. As these changes are completed, the cells begin to secrete epithelially derived collagen types I, II, and IX to form the **primary stroma** of the cornea (Figure 13-9).

Using the primary stroma as a basis for migration, neural crest cells around the lip of the optic cup migrate centrally between the primary stroma and the lens capsule. Although mesenchymal in morphology during their migration, these cells become transformed into a cuboidal epithelium called the **corneal endothelium** once their migration is completed. At this point the early cornea consists of (1) an outer epithelium, (2) a still acellular primary stroma, and (3) an inner endothelium.

After the corneal endothelium has formed a continuous layer, its cells synthesize large amounts of **hyaluronic acid** and secrete it into the primary stroma. Because of its pronounced water-binding capacities, hyaluronic acid causes the primary stroma to swell greatly. This provides a proper substrate for the second wave of cellular migration into the developing cornea (Figure 13-10). These cells, also of neural crest origin, are fibroblastic in nature. They migrate and proliferate in the hyaluronate-rich

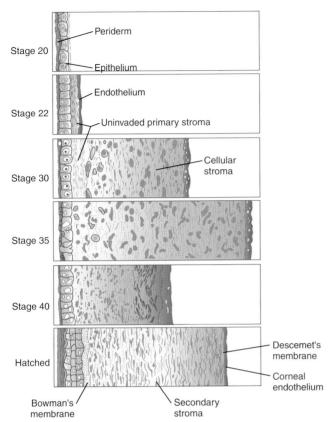

Stage 20 — Periderm, Epithelium

Stage 22 — Endothelium, Uninvaded primary stroma

Stage 30 — Cellular stroma

Stage 35

Stage 40

Hatched — Descemet's membrane, Corneal endothelium

Bowman's membrane, Secondary stroma

**FIGURE 13-9** Stages (Hamburger-Hamilton) in the formation of the cornea in the chick embryo. (Based on studies by Hay ED, Revel JP: *Monogr Devel Biol* 1:1–144, 1969.)

spaces between layers of collagen in the primary corneal stroma. The migratory phase of cellular seeding of the primary corneal stroma ceases when these cells begin to produce large amounts of **hyaluronidase**, which breaks down much of the hyaluronic acid in the primary stroma. In other parts of the embryo (e.g., limb bud), there is also a close correlation between high amounts of hyaluronic acid and cellular migration and a cessation of migration with its removal. With the removal of hyaluronic acid, the cornea decreases in thickness. Once the migratory fibroblasts have settled, the primary corneal stroma is considered to have been transformed into the **secondary stroma.**

The fibroblasts of the secondary stroma contribute to its organization by secreting coarse collagen fibers to the stromal matrix. Nevertheless, prominent layers of acellular matrix continue to be secreted by both epithelial and endothelial cells of the cornea. These secretions provide the remaining layers that constitute the mature cornea. Listed from outside in, they are (1) the outer epithelium, (2) **Bowman's membrane**, (3) the secondary stroma, (4) **Descemet's membrane**, and (5) the corneal endothelium (see Figure 13-9).

The final developmental changes in the cornea involve the formation of a transparent pathway free from optical distortion, through which light can enter the eye. A major change is a great increase in transparency, from about 40% to 100% transmission of light. This is accomplished by removing much of the water from the secondary stroma. The initial removal of water occurs with the degradation of much of the water-binding hyaluronic acid. The second phase of dehydration is mediated by **thyroxine**, which is secreted into the blood by the maturing thyroid gland. Thyroxine acts on the corneal endothelium by causing it to pump sodium from the secondary stroma into the anterior chamber of the eye. Water molecules follow the sodium ions, thus effectively completing the dehydration of the corneal stroma. The role of the thyroid gland in this process was demonstrated in two ways. When relatively mature thyroid glands were transplanted onto the extraembryonic membranes of young chick embryos, allowing thyroid hormone to gain access to the embryonic circulation via the blood vessels supplying the membrane (**chorioallantoic membrane**), premature dehydration of the cornea took place. Conversely, the application of thyroid inhibitors retarded the clearing of the cornea.

The other late event in the cornea is a pronounced change in its radius of curvature in relation to that of the eyeball as a whole. This morphogenetic change, which involves a number of mechanical events, including intraocular fluid pressure, allows the cornea to work with the lens in bringing light rays into focus on the retina. If irregularities develop in the curvature of the cornea during its final morphogenesis, the individual develops **astigmatism**, which causes distortions in the visual image.

## Retina and Other Derivatives of the Optic Cup

While the lens and cornea are taking shape, profound changes are also occurring in the optic cup (see Figure 13-2). The inner layer of the optic cup thickens, and the epithelial cells begin a long process of differentiation into neurons and light receptor cells of the **neural retina**. The outer layer of the optic cup remains relatively thin and ultimately becomes transformed into the **pigment layer of the retina** (see Figure 13-6). At the same time, the outer lips of the optic cup undergo a quite different transformation into the iris and ciliary body, which are involved in controlling the amount of light that enters the eye and the curvature of the lens, respectively.

The neural retina is a multilayered structure; its embryonic development can be appreciated only after its adult organization is understood (Figure 13-11). When seen in cross section under a microscope, the neural retina consists of alternating light- and dense-staining strips that correspond to layers rich in nuclei or cell processes, respectively. The direct sensory pathway in the neural retina is a chain of three neurons that traverse the thick-

**FIGURE 13-10** Major events in corneal morphogenesis in the chick embryo. (Based on Toole BP, Trelstad RL: *Dev Biol* 26:28–35, 1971; and on studies by Hay ED, Revel JP: *Monogr Devel Biol* 1:1–144, 1969.)

ness of the retina. The first element of the chain is the light receptor cell, either a **rod** or a **cone**. A light ray that enters the eye passes through the entire thickness of the neural retina until it impinges on the outer segment of a rod or cone cell (photoreceptor) in the extreme outer layer of the retina. The nucleus of the stimulated rod and cone cell is located in the **outer nuclear layer**. The photoreceptor cell sends a process toward the **outer plexiform layer**, where it synapses with a process from a bipolar cell located in the **inner nuclear layer**. The other process from the bipolar neuron leads into the **internal plexiform layer** and synapses with the third neuron in the chain, the **ganglion cell**. The bodies of the ganglion cells, which are located in the **ganglion cell layer**, send out long processes that course through the innermost **nerve fiber layer** toward their exit site from the eye, the optic nerve, through which they reach the brain.

If all light signals were processed only through the simple three-link series of neurons in the retina, visual acuity would be much less than it actually is. Many levels of integration have occurred by the time a visual pattern

is stored in the visual cortex of the brain. The first is in the neural retina. At synaptic sites in both the inner and outer plexiform layers of the retina, other cells such as **horizontal** and **amacrine cells** (see Figure 13-11) are involved in the horizontal redistribution of the simple visual signal. This facilitates the integration of components of a visual pattern. Another prominent cell type in the retina is the **Müller glial cell**, which sends processes to almost all layers of the retina and appears to play a role similar to that of astrocytes in the central nervous system.

### Neural retina

From the original columnar epithelium of the inner sensory layer of the optic cup (see Figure 13-6), the primordium of the neural retina takes on the form of a mitotically active, thickened pseudostratified columnar epithelium organized in a manner similar to that of the early neural tube. During the early stages of development of the retina, its polarity becomes fixed according to the

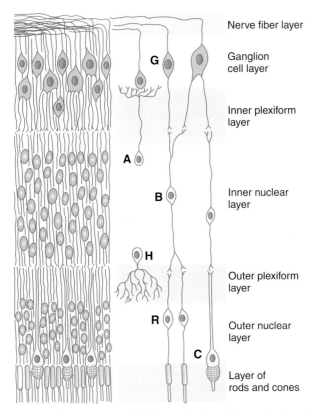

Nerve fiber layer

Ganglion cell layer

Inner plexiform layer

Inner nuclear layer

Outer plexiform layer

Outer nuclear layer

Layer of rods and cones

**FIGURE 13-11** Tissue and cellular organization of the neural retina of a human fetus. *A,* Amacrine cell; *B,* bipolar cell; *C,* cone; *G,* ganglion cell; *H,* horizontal cell; *R,* rod.

same axial sequence as that seen in the limbs (see Chapter 10). The nasotemporal (anteroposterior) axis is fixed first; this is followed by fixation of the dorsoventral axis. Finally, radial polarity is established.

To process distinct visual signals, the retina must develop according to a well-defined pattern, and that pattern must in turn be carried on to the brain so that distinct visual images will be produced. Despite its cuplike shape, patterning in the retina is often described in a two-dimensional manner, with dorsoventral and nasotemporal gradients serving as the basis for retinal pattern formation and differentiation.

Dorsoventral patterning is initiated through the presence of bone morphogenetic protein-4 (**BMP-4**) dorsally and ***shh*** ventrally (Figure 13-12, *A*). The presence of shh ventrally stimulates the production of **Otx-2** in the outer layer of the optic vesicle and its differentiation into the pigment layer of the retina. Within the inner layer of the optic vesicle, shh and a protein, **ventroptin,** both antagonists of BMP-4, stimulate the expression of the transcription factors **Vax-2** and **Pax-2** in the ventral retina. In the dorsal part of the future retina, BMP-4 signals the expression of **Tbx-5,** the transcription factor that also specifies the formation of the forelimb (see page 216). Although many molecules are unequally distributed along the two axes of the retina, opposing gradients of specific ephrins and their receptors are heavily involved

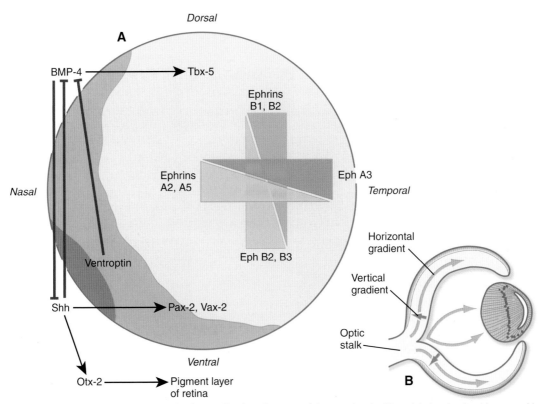

**FIGURE 13-12 A,** Molecular basis for the specification of pattern of the neural retina. The original molecular drivers are shh ventrally and BMP-4 dorsally. The molecular interactions indicated by the arrows are supplemented by dorsoventral and nasotemporal gradients of ephrins and their receptors. **B,** Horizontal and vertical gradients in the differentiation of the layers of the neural retina.

in the characterization of the retinal axes (see Figure 13-12, *A*).

As the number of cells in the early retina increases, the differentiation of cell types begins. There are two major gradients of differentiation in the retina. The first proceeds roughly vertically from the inner to the outer layers of the retina. The second moves horizontally from the center toward the periphery of the retina (Figure 13-12, *B*).

Very recent evidence obtained on fish retinas suggests that the horizontal gradient of neurogenesis may be driven by an initial point source of shh in a manner similar to a more well-understood process that occurs in *Drosophila*. Differentiation in the horizontal gradient begins with the appearance of ganglion cells and the early definition of the ganglion cell layer (Figure 13-13). As the ganglion cells differentiate, the surrounding cells are prevented from premature differentiation by the activity of the **Notch** gene. A major function of *Notch* is to maintain populations of cells in the nondifferentiated state until the appropriate local cues for their further differentiation appear. With the later differentiation of the horizontal and amacrine cells, the inner and outer nuclear layers take shape. As the cells within the nuclear layers send out processes, the inner and outer plexiform layers become better defined. The bipolar neurons and cone cells differentiate last, thus completing the first gradient.

The horizontal gradient of differentiation of the neural retina is based on the outward spread of the first vertical gradient from the center to the periphery of the retina.

The retina cannot grow from within. Thus during the phase of growth in the human eye (or throughout life in the case of continuously growing animals such as fish), developmentally immature retinal precursor cells along the edge of the retina undergo mitosis as an ever-expanding concentric ring on the periphery of the retina. Just inside the ring of mitosis, cellular differentiation takes place in a manner corresponding roughly to that of the vertical gradient.

Cell lineage experiments involving the use of retroviral or other tracers (such as horseradish peroxidase) introduced into neuronal precursors in the early retina have revealed two significant cellular features of retinal differentiation. First, progeny of a single labeled cell are distributed in a remarkably straight radial pattern following the vertical axis of retinal differentiation. There seems to be little lateral mixing among columns of retinal cells (Figure 13-14). The second cellular feature of retinal differentiation is that a single labeled precursor cell can give rise to more than one type of differentiated retinal cell.

A later stage in retinal differentiation is the growth of axons from the ganglion cells along the innermost layer of the retina towards and into the optic stalk. Once the axons reach the optic stalk, they grow into it, following cues provided by Pax-2–expressing cells. As the axons reach the area of the optic chiasm, they undergo a segregation so that the axons that arise from the temporal half of the retina remain on the same side and those from the nasal half of the retina decussate through the optic

**FIGURE 13-13** Progressive development of retinal layers in the chick embryo. At the far left, the ganglion cell layer begins to take shape from the broad neuroblast layer *(N)*. With time, further layers take shape until all layers of the retina are represented *(far right)*. (From Sheffield JB, Fischman DA: *Z Zellforsch Mikrosk Anat* 104(3):405–418, 1970.)

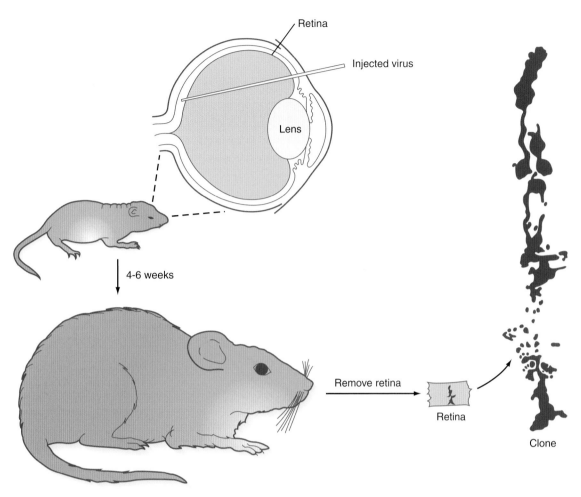

**FIGURE 13-14** Experiment illustrating the origins and lineages of retinal cells in the rat. *Top,* Injection of a retroviral vector that includes the gene for β-galactosidase into the space between the neural and pigmented retinal layers. About 4 to 6 weeks later, the retinas were removed, fixed, and histochemically reacted for β-galactosidase activity. The drawing at the right illustrates a vertical clone of cells derived from a virally infected precursor cell. Several cell types (rods, a bipolar cell, and a Müller glial cell) constituted this clone. (Modified from Turner DL, Cepko CL: *Nature* 328:131–136, 1987.)

chiasm over to the other side. The choice of pathways involves precise local signaling, with **netrin 1** serving as a growth cone attractor and **shh** playing a new role as a repulsive signal to axonal outgrowth. During this phase of retinal axonal outgrowth, the precise retinal map is maintained in the organization of the optic nerve, and it is ultimately passed on to the visual centers of the brain.

### Iris and Ciliary Body

At the lip of the optic cup where the developing neural and pigment retinas meet, differentiation of the **iris** and **ciliary body** occurs. Rather than being sensory in function, these structures are involved in modulating the amount and character of light that ultimately impinges on the retina. The iris partially encircles the outer part of the lens, and through contraction or relaxation, it controls the amount of light passing through the lens. The iris contains an inner unpigmented epithelial layer and an outer pigmented layer, which are continuous with the neural and pigmented layers of the retina, respectively (Figure 13-15). The **stroma of the iris**, which is superficial to the outer pigmented layer of the iris, is of neural crest origin and secondarily migrates into the iris. Within the stroma of the iris lie the primordia of the **sphincter pupillae** and **dilator pupillae** muscles. These muscles are unusual because they are of neurectodermal origin; they seem to arise from the anterior epithelial layer of the iris.

Between the iris and neural retina lies the ciliary body, a muscle-containing structure that is connected to the lens by radial sets of fibers called the **suspensory ligament of the lens**. By contractions of the ciliary musculature acting through the suspensory ligament, the ciliary body modulates the shape of the lens in focusing light rays on the retina. Normal development of the ciliary body depends on an appropriate amount of intraocular fluid pressure. If some of the fluid of the developing eye is shunted off, a defective ciliary body results.

**FIGURE 13-15** Two stages (earlier stage at left) in the development of the iris and ciliary body, including the sphincter and dilator pupillae muscles.

Eye color results from levels and distribution of pigmentation in the iris. The bluish color of the iris in most newborns is caused by the intrinsic pigmentation of the outer pigmented layer of the iris. Pigment cells also appear in the iridial stroma in front of the pigmented epithelium. The greater the density of pigment cells in this area, the browner the eye color. Definitive pigmentation of the eye gradually develops over the first 6 to 10 months of postnatal life.

## Vitreous Body and Hyaloid Artery System

During early development of the retina, a loose mesenchyme invades the cavity of the optic cup and forms a loose fibrillar mesh along with a gelatinous substance that fills the space between the neural retina and lens. This material is called the **vitreous body.**

During much of embryonic development the vitreous body is supplied by the hyaloid artery and its branches (Figure 13-16). The hyaloid artery enters the eyeball through the choroid fissure of the optic stalk (see Figure 13-5), passes through the retina and vitreous body, and terminates in branches to the posterior wall of the lens. As development progresses, the portions of the hyaloid artery (as well as its branches supplying the lens) in the vitreous body regress through apoptosis of their endothelial cells, leaving a **hyaloid canal.** The more proximal part of the hyaloid arterial system persists as the **central artery of the retina** and its branches.

## Choroid Coat and Sclera

Outside the optic cup lies a layer of mesenchymal cells, largely of neural crest origin. Reacting to an inductive influence from the pigmented epithelium of the retina, these cells differentiate into structures that provide vascular and mechanical support for the eye. The innermost cells of this layer differentiate into a highly vascular tunic called the **choroid coat** (see Figure 13-6, C) and the outermost cells form a white, densely collagenous covering known as the **sclera.** The opaque sclera, which serves as a tough outer coating of the eye, is continuous with the cornea. The extraocular muscles,

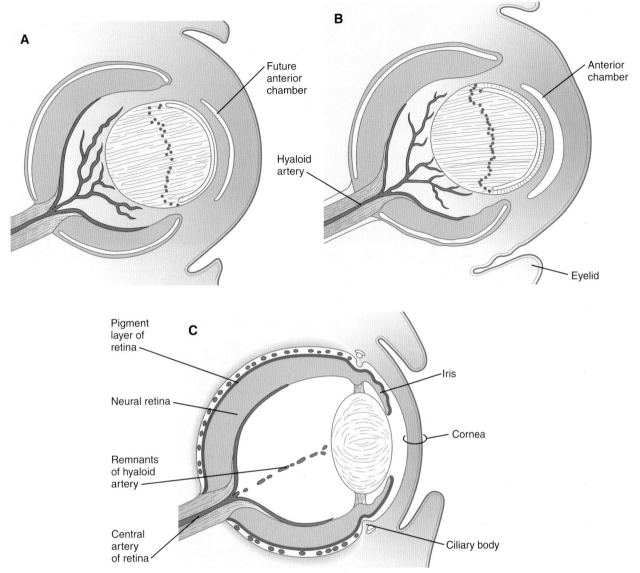

**FIGURE 13-16** Stages in development and regression of the hyaloid artery in the embryonic eye.

which provide gross movements to the eyeball, attach to the sclera.

## Eyelids and Lacrimal Glands

The eyelids first become apparent during the seventh week as folds of skin that grow over the cornea (Figures 13-6 and 13-17, *A*). Once their formation has commenced, the eyelids rapidly grow over the eye until they meet and fuse with one another by the end of the ninth week (Figures 13-17, *B* and 18-4). The temporary fusion involves only the epithelial layers of the eyelids, resulting in a persisting epithelial lamina between them. Before the eyelids reopen, eyelashes and the small glands that lie along the margins of the lids begin to differentiate from the common epithelial lamina. Although signs of loosen-

ing of the epithelial union of the lids can be seen in the sixth month, reopening of the eyelids normally does not occur until well into the seventh month of pregnancy.

The space between the front of the eyeball and the eyelids is known as the **conjunctival sac**. Multiple epithelial buds grow from the lateral surface ectoderm at about the time when the eyelids fuse. These buds differentiate into the lacrimal glands, which produce a watery secretion that bathes the outer surface of the cornea when mature. This secretion ultimately passes into the nasal chamber by way of the **nasolacrimal duct** (see Chapter 14). The lacrimal glands are not fully mature at birth, and newborns typically do not produce tears when crying. The glands begin to function in lacrimation at about 6 weeks.

Despite the many types of malformations of the eye and visual system, the incidence of most individual types of defects is uncommon. Examples of a few of the

**FIGURE 13-17 A,** Head of a human embryo approximately **47 days old.** Upper and lower eyelids have begun to form. The external ear is still low set and incompletely formed. **B,** A **5½-month-old** (200 mm crown-rump length) human embryo. The upper and lower eyelids are fused and the external ear is better formed. Note the receding chin. (**A** From Streeter G: *Carnegie contributions to embryology*, No. 230, 165-196, 1951; **B** EH 1196 from the Patten Embryological Collection at the University of Michigan, courtesy A. Burdi, Ann Arbor, Mich.)

many ocular malformations are given in Clinical Correlation 13-1.

## EAR

The ear is a complex structure consisting of three major subdivisions: the external, middle, and internal ear. The **external ear** consists of the **pinna** (auricle), the **external auditory meatus** (external ear canal), and the outer layers of the **tympanic membrane** (eardrum) and functions principally as a sound-collecting apparatus. The middle ear acts as a transmitting device. This function is served by the chain of three middle ear ossicles, which connect the inner side of the tympanic membrane to the oval window of the inner ear. Other components of the middle ear are the middle ear cavity (**tympanic cavity**), the **auditory tube** (eustachian tube), the middle ear musculature, and the inner layer of the tympanic membrane. The inner ear contains the primary sensory apparatus, which is involved with both hearing and balance. These functions are served by the **cochlea** and **vestibular apparatus**, respectively.

From an embryological standpoint the ear has a dual origin. The inner ear arises from a thickened ectodermal placode at the level of the rhombencephalon. The structures of the middle and external ear are derivatives of the first and second pharyngeal arches and the intervening first pharyngeal cleft and pharyngeal pouch.

### Development of the Inner Ear

Development of the ear begins with preliminary inductions of the surface ectoderm, first by the notochord

(chordamesoderm) and then by the paraxial mesoderm (Figure 13-19). These inductions prepare the ectoderm for a third induction, in which the rhombencephalon induces the adjacent surface ectoderm to thicken and form the **otic placode** (Figure 13-20). Recent evidence suggests that **FGF-19,** produced in the paraxial mesoderm, induces the expression of **Wnt-8c** in the rhombencephalic neuroepithelium, which in turn stimulates the secretion of FGF-3. Late in the fourth week, possibly under the influence of **FGF-3** secreted by the adjacent rhombencephalon, the otic placode invaginates and then separates from the surface ectoderm to form the **otic vesicle,** or otocyst. Even at the earliest stages of development of the otocyst, the localized expression of certain molecules presages the formation of specific morphological derivatives of the otocyst.

The otic vesicle soon begins to elongate, forming a dorsal vestibular region and a ventral cochlear region (Figure 13-21, *A*). The paired box gene, *Pax-2,* is heavily involved in early development of the otic vesicle. In the absence of Pax-2 function, neither the cochlea nor the spiral ganglion form. Quite early, the **endolymphatic duct** arises as a short, fingerlike projection from the dorsomedial surface of the otocyst (Figure 13-21, *B*). FGF-3, secreted by rhombomeres 5 and 6, appears to be necessary for normal development of the endolymphatic duct. At about 5 weeks, the appearance of two ridges in the vestibular portion of the otocyst foreshadows the formation of two of the **semicircular ducts** (Figure 13-21, *C*). As the ridges expand laterally, their opposing epithelial walls approximate each other, forming a **fusion plate.** Programmed cell death in the central area of epithelial fusion or epithelial cell migration away from this area converts the flangelike structures to canals by setting up

## Congenital Malformations of the Eye

### ANOPHTHALMOS AND MICROPHTHALMOS

Anophthalmos, the absence of an eye, is very rare and can normally be attributed to lack of formation of the optic vesicle. Since this structure acts as the inductive trigger for much of subsequent eye development, many local inductive interactions involved in the formation of eye structures fail to occur. **Microphthalmos,** which can range from an eyeball that is slightly smaller than normal to one that is almost vestigial, can be associated with genetic defects (e.g., aniridia) or various other causes, including intrauterine infections (Figure 13-18, A).

### COLOBOMA OF THE IRIS

Nonclosure of the choroid fissure of the iris during the sixth or seventh week results in its persistence as a defect called **coloboma iridis** (Figure 13-18, B). The location of colobomas of the iris (typically at the 5 o'clock position in the right eye and the 7 o'clock position in the left) marks the position of the embryonic choroid fissure.

### CONGENITAL CATARACT

Cataract is a condition characterized by opacity of the lens of the eye. Not so much a structural malformation as a dysplasia, congenital cataracts first came into prominence as one of the triad of defects resulting from exposure of the embryo to the rubella virus.

**FIGURE 13-18 A,** Microphthalmos of the right eye. **B,** Congenital coloboma of the iris. The fissure is in the region of closure of the choroid fissure. (**A** from Smith B: *Ophthalmic plastic and reconstructive surgery,* vol 2, St Louis, 1987, Mosby. **B** from Newell F: *Ophthalmology: principles and concepts,* St Louis, 1986, Mosby.)

a zone of resorption (Figure 13-21, C). The epithelial precursors of the semicircular canals express the homeobox transcription factor gene *Nkx 5-1,* which is important for the development of the dorsal vestibular portion of the inner ear. Other transcription factors play a role in the formation of individual semicircular canals. In the absence of *Otx-1* the lateral semicircular canal fails to form, and the homeobox transcription factor *Dlx-5* must be expressed for the anterior and posterior canals to develop. Thus the development of the two main parts of the inner ear is under separate genetic control: Pax-2 for the auditory portion (cochlea) and Nkx5 for the vestibular portion (semicircular canals). The cochlear part of the otocyst begins to elongate in a spiral, having attained one complete revolution at 8 weeks and two revolutions by 10 weeks (Figure 13-21, C through F). The last half turn of the cochlear spiral (a total of $2\frac{1}{2}$ turns) is not completed until 25 weeks.

The inner ear (membranous labyrinth) is encased in a capsule of skeletal tissue that begins as a condensation of mesenchyme around the developing otocyst at 6 weeks' gestation. The process of encasement of the otocyst begins with an induction of the surrounding mesenchyme by the epithelium of the otocyst (see Figure 13-19). This induction stimulates the mesenchymal cells, mainly of mesodermal origin, to form a cartilaginous matrix (starting at about 8 weeks). The capsular cartilage then serves as a template for the later formation of the true bony labyrinth. The conversion from the cartilaginous to the bony labyrinth occurs between 16 and 23 weeks' gestation.

The sensory neurons that make up the eighth cranial nerve (specifically the **statoacoustic ganglion**) arise from cells that migrate out from a portion of the medial wall of the otocyst (see Figure 13-20). The cochlear part (**spiral ganglion**) of the eighth nerve fans out in close association with the sensory cells (collectively known as the **organ of**

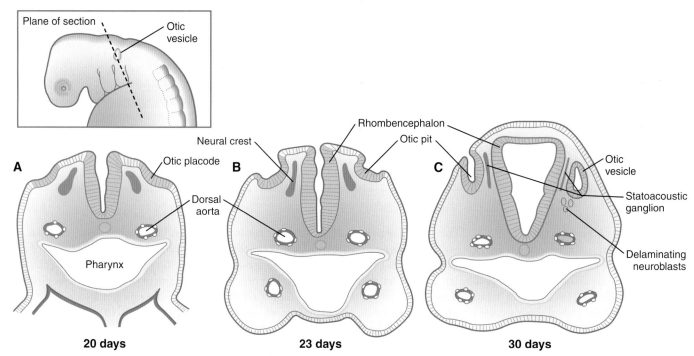

**FIGURE 13-19** Flow chart of major inductive events and tissue transformations in the developing ear. Colored arrows refer to inductive events. (Based on McPhee JR, van de Water TR. In Jahn AF, Santos-Sacchi J, eds: *Physiology of the ear*, New York, 1988, Raven, pp 221–242.)

**FIGURE 13-20** Formation of the otic vesicles from thickened otic placodes.

Corti) that develop within the cochlea. Neural crest cells invade the developing statoacoustic ganglion and ultimately form the satellite and supporting cells within it. The sensory cells of the organ of Corti are also derived from the epithelium of the otocyst. They undergo a very complex pattern of differentiation (Figure 13-22). The generation of sensory neuroblast precursors in the inner ear appears to use the **Notch pathway** to control the pro-

portion of epithelial cells that differentiate into neuroblasts vs. supporting cells in a manner similar to that described for the differentiation of ganglion cells in the early retina (see p. 302). As in other sensory systems, highly regulated developmental controls ensure precise matching between sensory cells designed to receive sound waves at different frequencies or gravitational information and the neurons that transmit the signals to the brain.

**FIGURE 13-21** Development of the human inner ear. **A,** At **28 days. B,** At **33 days. C,** At **38 days. D,** At **41 days. E,** At **50 days. F,** At **56 days,** lateral view. **G,** At **56 days,** medial view. **H,** Central reference drawing at **56 days.** (From Carlson B: *Patten's foundations of embryology,* ed 6, New York, 1996, McGraw-Hill.)

## Development of the Middle Ear

Formation of the middle ear is intimately associated with developmental changes in the first and second pharyngeal arches (see Chapter 14). Both the **middle ear cavity** and the **auditory tube** arise from an expansion of the first pharyngeal pouch called the **tubotympanic sulcus** (Figure 13-23). Such an origin ensures that the entire middle ear cavity and auditory tube are lined with an endodermally derived epithelium.

By the end of the second month of pregnancy, the blind end of the tubotympanic sulcus (pharyngeal pouch 1) approaches the innermost portion of the first pharyngeal cleft. Nonetheless, these two structures are still

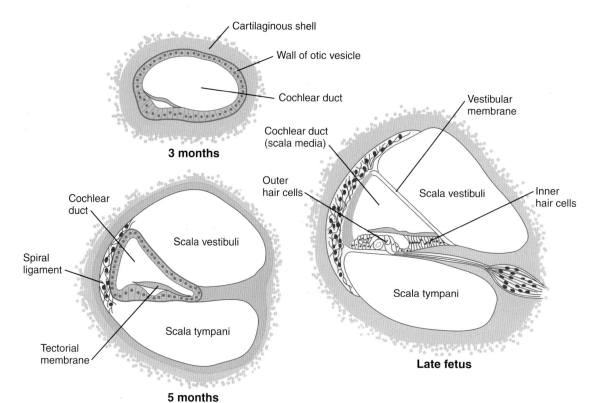

**FIGURE 13-22** Cross sections through the developing organ of Corti.

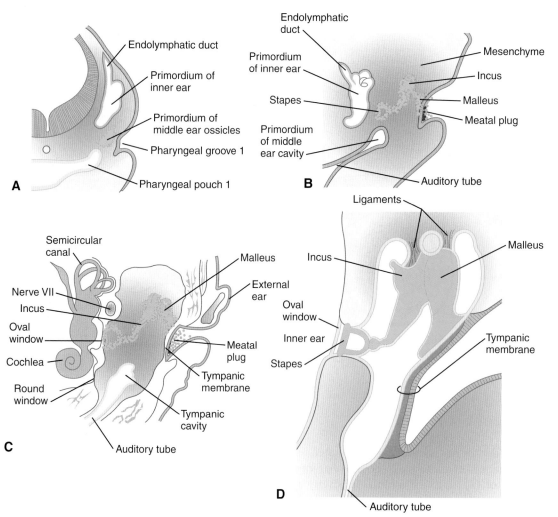

**FIGURE 13-23** Stages in development of the middle ear.

separated by a mass of mesenchyme. Later the endodermal epithelium of the tubotympanic sulcus becomes more closely apposed to the ectoderm lining the first pharyngeal cleft, but they are always separated by a thin layer of mesoderm. This complex, containing tissue from all three germ layers, becomes the **tympanic membrane** (eardrum). During fetal life a prominent ring-shaped, neural crest–derived bone, called the **tympanic ring**, supports the tympanic membrane. Experiments have shown that the tympanic ring is actively involved in morphogenesis of the tympanic membrane. Later the tympanic ring becomes absorbed into the temporal bone.

Just dorsal to the end of the tubotympanic sulcus, a conspicuous condensation of mesenchyme of neural crest origin appears at 6 weeks and gradually takes on the form of the middle ear ossicles. These ossicles, which lie in a bed of very loose embryonic connective tissue, extend from the inner layer of the tympanic membrane to the oval window of the inner ear. Although the middle ear cavity is surrounded by the developing temporal bone, the future middle ear cavity remains filled with loose mesenchyme until late in pregnancy. During the eighth and ninth month, programmed cell death and other resorptive processes gradually clear the middle ear cavity, leaving the auditory ossicles suspended within it. Even at the time of birth, remains of the middle ear connective tissue may dampen the free movement of the auditory ossicles. Free movement of the auditory ossicles is acquired within 2 months after birth. Coincident with the removal of the connective tissue of the middle ear cavity is the expansion of the endodermal epithelium of the tubotympanic sulcus, which ultimately lines the entire middle ear cavity.

The middle ear ossicles themselves have a dual origin. According to comparative anatomical evidence, the **malleus** and **incus** arise from neural crest–derived mesenchyme of the first pharyngeal arch, whereas the **stapes** originates from second-arch mesenchyme (Figure 13-24).

Two middle ear muscles help modulate the transmission of auditory stimuli through the middle ear. The **tensor tympani muscle**, which is attached to the malleus, is derived from first arch mesoderm and is correspondingly innervated by the trigeminal nerve (V). The **stapedius muscle** is associated with the stapes, is of

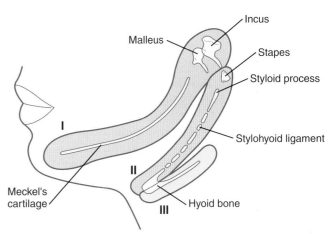

**FIGURE 13-24** According to the traditional theory of the formation of the middle ear ossicles, the malleus and incus are derived from arch I and the stapes from arch II.

second arch origin, and is innervated by the facial nerve (VII), which supplies derivatives of that arch.

## Development of the External Ear

The external ear (pinna) is derived from mesenchymal tissue of the first and second pharyngeal arches that flank the first (hyomandibular) pharyngeal cleft. During the second month, three nodular masses of mesenchyme (**auricular hillocks**) take shape along each side of the first pharyngeal cleft (Figure 13-25). The auricular hillocks enlarge asymmetrically and ultimately coalesce to form a recognizable external ear. During its formation, the pinna shifts from the base of the neck to its normal adult location on the side of the head. Because of its intimate association with the pharyngeal arches and its complex origin, the external ear is a sensitive indicator of abnormal development in the pharyngeal region. Other anomalies of the first and second arches are often attended by misshapen or abnormally located external ears.

The external auditory meatus takes shape during the end of the second month by an inward expansion of

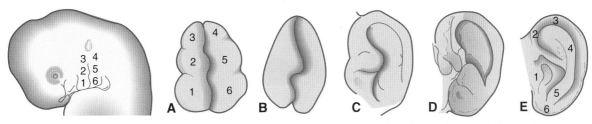

**FIGURE 13-25** Stages in development of the external ear. Components derived from the mandibular arch (I) are unshaded; those derived from the hyoid arch (II) are shaded.

the first pharyngeal cleft. Early in the third month the ectodermal epithelium of the forming meatus proliferates, forming a solid mass of epithelial cells called the **meatal plug** (see Figure 13-23). Late during the fetal period (at 28 weeks), a channel within the meatal plug extends the existing external auditory meatus to the level of the tympanic membrane.

The external ear and external auditory meatus are very sensitive to drugs. Exposure to agents such as streptomycin, thalidomide, and salicylates during the first trimester can cause agenesis or atresia of both of these structures. Congenital malformations of the ear are discussed in Clinical Correlation 13-2.

## SUMMARY

◯ The eye begins as an outpocketing (optic groove) of the lateral wall of the diencephalon. The optic grooves enlarge to form the optic vesicles, which induce the

---

### CLINICAL CORRELATION 13-2

## Congenital Malformations of the Ear

The ear is subject to a wide variety of genetically based defects, ranging from those that affect the function of specific hair cells in the inner ear to those that produce gross malformations of the middle and external ear. Defects of the middle and external ear are often associated with genetic conditions that affect broader areas of cranial tissues or regions. Therefore many malformations involving the first or second pharyngeal arches are also accompanied by malformations of the ear and reduced acuity of hearing.

### CONGENITAL DEAFNESS

Many disturbances of development of the ear can lead to hearing impairments, which affect one in every 1000 newborns. Conditions such as **rubella** can lead to maldevelopment of the organ of Corti, causing inner ear deafness. Abnormalities of the middle ear ossicles or ligaments, which can be associated with anomalies of the first and second arches, can interfere with transmission, resulting in middle ear deafness. Agenesis or major

atresias of the external ear can cause deafness by interfering with the primary collection of sound waves.

The very recent surge of molecular studies on the development of the inner ear has identified in both mice and humans a variety of mutants of the inner ear that could lead to deficits in hearing, equilibrium, or both. Mutants, such as those of Pax-3 causing variants of the Waardenburg's syndrome (see p. 288), can affect development at levels from gross morphogenesis to specific cellular defects in the cochleosaccular complex.

### AURICULAR ANOMALIES

Because of the multiple origins of its components, there is great variety in the normal form of the pinna. Variations include obvious malformations such as **auricular appendages,** or **sinuses** (Figure 13-26). Many malformations of the external ears are not functionally important but are associated with other developmental anomalies such as malformations of the kidneys and pharyngeal arches.

**FIGURE 13-26 A,** Auricular anomalies and tags associated with the mandibular arch (I) component of the external ear. **B,** Anotia. The external ear is represented only by a couple of small tags. (Courtesy M Barr, Ann Arbor, Mich.)

overlying ectoderm to form the lens primordium. The optic stalk, which connects the optic cup to the diencephalon, forms a groove containing the hyaloid artery, which supplies the developing eye. The paired box gene *Pax-6* acts as a master control gene for eye development.

◯ Under the influence of Pax-6, the lens forms from an ectodermal thickening that invaginates to form a lens vesicle. The cells of the inner wall of the lens vesicle elongate and synthesize lens-specific crystallin proteins. In the growing lens the inner epithelium forms a spherical mass of banana-shaped lens fibers (epithelial cells). The anterior lens epithelium consists of cuboidal epithelial cells. The overall polarity of the lens is under the influence of the retina.

◯ The cornea is formed through induction of the surface ectoderm by the lens. After induction, the basal ectodermal cells secrete an extracellular matrix that serves as a substrate for the migration of neural crest cells forming the corneal endothelial layer. The corneal endothelial cells secrete large amounts of hyaluronic acid into the early cornea. This permits the migration of a second wave of neural crest cells into the cornea. These fibroblast-like cells secrete collagen fibers into the coarse corneal stroma matrix. Under the influence of thyroxine, water is removed from the corneal matrix, and it becomes transparent.

◯ The neural retina differentiates from the inner layer of the optic cup. The outer layer forms the pigment layer of the retina. The neural retina is a complex multilayered structure with three layers of neurons connected by cellular processes. Cellular differentiation in the neural retina follows both vertical and horizontal gradients. Under the influence of Pax-2, cell processes grow from retinal neurons through the optic stalk to make connections with optic centers within the brain.

◯ The iris and ciliary body form from the outer edge of the optic cup. Sphincter and dilator pupillae muscles form within the iris. Eye color is related to the levels and distribution of pigmentation within the iris. Outside the optic cup, mesenchyme differentiates into a vascular

choroid coat and a tough collagenous sclera. Eyelids begin as folds of skin that grow over the cornea and then fuse, closing off the eyes. The eyelids reopen late in the seventh month.

◯ The developing eyes are sensitive to a number of teratogens and intrauterine infections. Exposure to these can cause microphthalmia or congenital cataracts. Nonclosure of the choroid fissure results in coloboma.

◯ The inner ear arises by an induction of the surface ectoderm by the developing hindbrain. Steps in its formation include ectodermal thickening (placode), invagination to form an otic vesicle, and later, growth and morphogenesis into auditory (cochlea) and vestibular (semicircular canals) portions. Normal development of the cochlea depends on the proper expression of Pax-2, whereas Nkx5 is required for the formation of the semicircular canals.

◯ Development of the middle ear is associated with the first pharyngeal cleft and the arches on either side. Middle ear ossicles and associated muscles take shape within the middle ear cavity.

◯ The external ear arises from six modular masses of mesenchyme that take shape in the pharyngeal arch tissue surrounding the first pharyngeal cleft.

◯ Congenital deafness can occur after a number of intrauterine disturbances such as a rubella infection. Structural anomalies of the external ear are common.

## Review Questions

1. **Neural crest–derived cells constitute a significant component of which tissue of the eye?**
   A. Neural retina
   B. Lens
   C. Optic nerve
   D. Cornea
   E. None of the above

2. **The otic placode arises through an inductive message given off by the:**
   A. Telencephalon
   B. Rhombencephalon
   C. Infundibulum
   D. Diencephalon
   E. Mesencephalon

3. **What molecule plays a role in guidance of advancing retinal axons through the optic nerve?**
   A. Pax-2
   B. FGF-3
   C. Bone morphogenetic protein-4
   D. Pax-6
   E. Bone morphogenetic protein-7

### CLINICAL VIGNETTE

A pediatrician is asked to examine a young boy who has arrived from a country with poor access to medical care. The boy has low-set, misshapen ears, an underslung lower jaw, and a severe hearing deficit. The boy's teeth are also poorly aligned.

What is the common denominator for this set of conditions?

The doctor orders an imaging study of the boy's kidneys and urinary tract. Why does she do that?

4. Surface ectoderm is induced to become corneal epithelium by an inductive event originating in the:
   A. Optic cup
   B. Chordamesoderm
   C. Optic vesicle
   D. Lens vesicle
   E. Neural retina

5. The second pharyngeal arch contributes to the:
   A. Cochlea, ear lobe
   B. Auditory tube, incus
   C. Stapes, ear lobe
   D. Auditory tube, stapes
   E. Otic vesicle, stapes

6. During a routine physical examination, an infant was found to have a small segment missing from the lower part of one iris. What is the diagnosis, what is the basis for the condition, and why might the infant be sensitive to bright light?

7. Why does a person sometimes get a runny nose while crying?

8. What extracellular matrix molecule is often associated with migrations of mesenchymal cells, and where does such an event occur in the developing eye?

9. Why is the hearing of a newborn often not as acute as it is a few months later?

10. Why are malformations or hypoplasia of the lower jaw commonly associated with abnormalities in the shape or position of the ears?

## REFERENCES

Alvarez G, Schwarz M, Gruss P: Pax-2 in the chiasm, *Cell Tissue Res* 290:197–200, 1997.

Anniko M: Embryonic development of vestibular sense organs and their innervation. In Romand R, ed: *Development of auditory and vestibular systems*, New York, 1983, Academic, pp 375–423.

Anson BJ, Hanson JS, Richany SF: Early embryology of auditory ossicles and associated structures in relation to certain anomalies observed clinically, *Ann Otol Rhinol Laryngol* 69:427–447, 1960.

Ashery-Padan R and others: Pax6 activity in the lens primordium is required for lens formation and for correct placement of a single retina in the eye, *Genes Devel* 14:2701–2711, 2000.

Baker CVH, Bronner-Fraser M: Vertebrate cranial placodes I. Embryonic induction, *Devel Biol* 232:1–61, 2001.

Barishak YR: *Embryology of the eye and its adnexae*, Basel, Switzerland, 1992, Karger.

Cantos R and others: Patterning of the mammalian cochlea, *Proc Natl Acad Sci USA* 97:11707–11713, 2000.

Carlson B: *Patten's foundations of embryology*, ed 6, New York, 1996, McGraw-Hill.

Chalupa LM, ed: Development and organization of the retina: cellular, molecular and functional perspectives, *Seminars Cell Devel Biol* 9:239–318, 1998.

Corwin J, ed: Developmental biology of the ear, *Semin Cell Dev Biol* 8:215–284, 1997.

Coulombre AJ, Coulombre JL: The role of intraocular pressure in the development of the chick eye. III. Ciliary body, *Am J Ophthalmol* 44:85–92, 1957.

Cvekl A, Piatigorsky J: Lens development and crystallin gene expression: many roles for Pax-6, *BioEssays* 18:621–630, 1996.

Deeison M, Le Roux I, Lewis J: Notch signaling in the development of the inner ear: lessons from *Drosophila*, *Proc Natl Acad Sci* USA 97:11692–11699, 2000.

Fekete DM: Cell fate specification in the inner ear, *Curr Opin Neurobiol* 6:533–541, 1996.

Fekete DM and others: Involvement of programmed cell death in morphogenesis of the vertebrate inner ear, *Development* 124:2451–2461, 1997.

Fini ME, Strissel KJ, West-Mays JA: Perspectives on eye development, *Dev Genet* 20:175–185, 1997.

Fritsch B, Barald KF, Lomax MI: Early embryology of the vertebrate ear. In Rubel EW, Popper AN, Fay RR, eds: *Development of the auditory system*, New York, 1997, Springer, pp 80–145.

Graw J: Genetic aspects of embryonic eye development in vertebrates, *Dev Genet* 18:181–197, 1996.

Hadrys T and others: Nkx5-1 controls semicircular canal formation in the mouse inner ear, *Development* 125:33–39, 1998.

Hay ED: Development of the vertebrate cornea, *Int Rev Cytol* 63:263–322, 1980.

Hyatt GA, Dowling JE: Retinoic acid: a key molecule for eye and photoreceptor development, *Invest Ophthalmol Vis Sci* 38:1471–1475, 1997.

Jakobiec FA, ed: *Ocular anatomy, embryology and teratology*, Philadelphia, 1982, Harper & Row.

Kiernan AE, Steel KP, Fekete DM: Development of the mouse inner ear. In Rossant J, Tam PPL, eds: *Mouse development: patterning, morphogenesis, and organogenesis*, San Diego, 2002, Academic, pp 539–566.

Kondoh H: Development of the eye. In Rossant J, Tam PPL, eds: *Mouse development: patterning, morphogenesis, and organogenesis*, San Diego, 2002, Academic, pp 519–539.

Kraus P, Lufkin T: Mammalian *Dlx* homeobox gene control of craniofacial and inner ear morphogenesis, *J Cell Biochem Suppl* 32/33:133–140, 1999.

Ladher RK and others: Identification of synergistic signals initiating inner ear development, *Science* 290:1965–1967, 2000.

Lang RA: Apoptosis in mammalian eye development: lens morphogenesis, vascular regression and immune privilege, *Cell Death Differen* 4:12–20, 1997.

Lewis WH: Experimental studies on the development of the eye in amphibia. I. On the origin of the lens, *Am J Anat* 3:505–536, 1904.

MacDonald R, Wilson SW: Pax proteins and eye development, *Curr Opin Neurobiol* 6:49–56, 1996.

Mallo M: Embryological and genetic aspects of middle ear development, *Int J Dev Biol* 42:11–22, 1998.

Mann I: *The development of the human eye*, ed 3, New York, 1964, Grune & Stratton.

McKay IJ, Lewis J, Lumsden A: The role of FGF-3 in early inner ear development: an analysis in normal and kreisler mutant mice, *Dev Biol* 174:370–378, 1996.

McPhee JR, van de Water TR: Structural and functional development of the ear. In Jahn AF, Santos-Sacchi J, eds: *Physiology of the ear*, New York, 1988, Raven, pp 221–242.

Mui SH and others: The homeodomain protein Vax2 patterns the dorsoventral and nasotemporal axes of the eye, *Development* 129:797–804, 2002.

Neumann CJ, Nuesslein-Volhard C: Patterning of the zebrafish retina by a wave of sonic hedgehog activity, *Science* 289:2137–2139, 2000.

Nishimura Y, Kumoi T: The embryologic development of the human external auditory meatus, *Acta Otolaryngol* 112:496–503, 1992.

Noden DM, van de Water TR: The developing ear: tissue origins and interactions. In Ruben RW and others, eds: *The biology of change in otolaryngology*, Amsterdam, 1986, Elsevier Science, pp 15–46.

Noden DM, van de Water TR: Genetic analysis of mammalian ear development, *Trends Neurosci* 15:235–237, 1992.

O'Rahilly R: The timing and sequence of events in the development of the human eye and ear during the embryonic period proper, *Anat Embryol* 168:87–99, 1983.

Otteson DC and others: Pax2 expression and retinal morphogenesis in the normal and Krd mouse, *Dev Biol* 193:209–224, 1998.

Piatigorsky J: Lens differentiation in vertebrates, *Differentiation* 19:134–153, 1981.

Pichaud F, Desplan C: Pax genes and eye organogenesis, *Curr Opin Genet Devel* 12:430–434, 2002.

Represa J, Frenz DA, van de Water TR: Genetic patterning of embryonic inner ear development, *Acta Otolaryngol* 120:5–10, 2000.

Rubel EW: Ontogeny of auditory system function, *Annu Rev Physiol* 46: 213–229, 1984.

Sakuta H and others: Ventroptin: a BMP-4 antagonist expressed in a double-gradient pattern in the retina, *Science* 293:111–115, 2001.

Spemann H: *Embryonic development and induction*, New Haven, Conn, 1938, Yale University.

Stark MR and others: Neural tube–ectoderm interactions are required for trigeminal placode formation, *Development* 124:4287–4295, 1997.

Streeter GC: Development of the auricle in the human embryo, *Contr Embryol Carnegie Inst* 14:111–138, 1922.

Toole BP, Trelstad RL: Hyaluronate production and removal during corneal development in the chick, *Dev Biol* 26:28–35, 1971.

Torres M, Gomez-Pardo E, Gruss P: Pax2 contributes to inner ear patterning and optic nerve trajectory, *Development* 122:3381–3391, 1996.

Traboulsi EI: Developmental genes and ocular malformation syndromes, *Am J Ophthalmol* 115:105–107, 1993.

Trousse F and others: Control of retinal ganglion cell axon growth: a new role for sonic hedgehog, *Development* 128:3927–3936, 2001.

Vendrell V and others: Induction of inner ear fate by FGF3, *Development* 127:2011–2019, 2000.

Wride MA: Cellular and molecular features of lens differentiation: a review of recent advances, *Differentiation* 61:77–93, 1996.

Zhang X-M, Yang X-J: Temporal and spatial effects of sonic hedgehog signaling in chick eye morphogenesis, *Devel Biol* 233:271–290, 2001.

Ziman MR and others: *Pax* genes in development and maturation of the visual system: implications for optic nerve regeneration, *Histol Histopathol* 16:239–249, 2001.

# CHAPTER 14

# Head and Neck

Among the earliest vertebrates the cranial region consisted of two principal components: (1) a **chondrocranium** associated with the brain and the major sense organs (nose, eye, ear) and (2) a **viscerocranium**, a series of branchial (pharyngeal) arches associated with the oral region and the pharynx (Figure 14-1, *A*). As vertebrates became more complex, the contributions of the neural crest to the head became much more prominent, and the face and many dermal (intramembranously formed) bones of the skull (**dermocranium**) were added. With the early evolution of the face, the most anterior of the branchial arches underwent a transformation to form the upper and lower jaws as well as two of the middle ear bones, the malleus and the incus. Along with an increase in complexity of the face (Figure 14-1, *B*) came a corresponding increase in complexity of the forebrain (the telencephalon and diencephalon). From both structural and molecular aspects, the rostral (anteriormost) part of the head shows distinctly different characteristics from the pharyngeal region, as follows:

1. The pharyngeal region and hindbrain are highly segmented (see Figure 14-3), whereas segmentation is less evident in the forebrain and rostral part of the head.

2. Structural segmentation in the pharyngeal region is associated with complex segmental patterns of gene expression (see Figure 11-11).

3. Formation of the forebrain and associated structures of the rostral part of the head depends on the actions of specific genes (e.g., *Lim-1* [see Figure 5-11], *Emx-1*, *Emx-2*, *Otx-1*, and *Otx-2*) and inductive signaling by the prechordal mesoderm or anterior visceral endoderm.

4. Much of the connective tissue and skeleton of the rostral (phylogenetically newer) part of the head is derived from the neural crest. The anterior end of the notochord, terminating at the hypophysis, constitutes the boundary between the mesodermally derived chondrocranium and the more rostral neural crest–derived chondrocranium. Neural crest cells are also prominent contributors to the ventral part of the pharyngeal region.

In previous chapters the development of certain components of the head (e.g., the nervous system, neural crest, bones of the skull) has been detailed. The first part of this chapter provides an integrated view of early craniofacial development to show how the major components are interrelated. The remainder of the chapter concentrates on the development of the face, pharynx, and pharyngeal arch system. Clinical Correlations 14-1 and 14-2 present malformations associated with the head and neck. These are located later in the chapter.

## EARLY DEVELOPMENT OF HEAD AND NECK

Development of the head and neck begins early in embryonic life and continues until the cessation of postnatal growth in the late teens. Cephalization begins with the

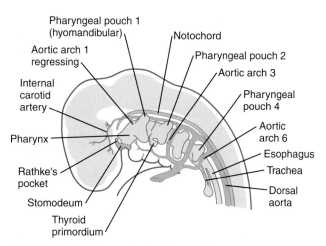

**FIGURE 14-1** Organization of the major components of the vertebrate skull. **A,** Skull of a primitive aquatic vertebrate, showing the chondrocranium *(green)*, the viscerocranium *(orange)*, and the dermocranium *(brown)*. **B,** Human fetal head, showing the distribution of the same components of the cranial skeleton.

**FIGURE 14-2** Basic organization of the pharyngeal region of the human embryo at the end of the **first month.**

rapid expansion of the rostral end of the neural plate. Very early the future brain is the dominant component of the craniofacial region. Beneath the brain, the face, which does not take shape until later in embryogenesis, is represented by the **stomodeum** (Figure 14-2). In the early embryo the stomodeum is sealed off from the primitive gut by the **oropharyngeal membrane**, which breaks down by the end of the first embryonic month (see Figure 6-21). Surrounding the stomodeum are several tissue prominences that constitute the building blocks of the face (see Figure 14-5). In keeping with its origin from the anterior neural ridge and its later serving as the tissue of origin of Rathke's pouch, the ectoderm of the oropharyngeal membrane is first characterized by its expression of the homeodomain transcription factor Pitx-2. In the rostral midline is the frontonasal prominence, which is populated by mesenchymal cells derived from forebrain and some midbrain neural crest. On either side of the frontonasal prominence, ectodermal nasal placodes, which arose from the anterior neural ridge (see page 108), develop into horseshoe-shaped structures, each consisting of a nasomedial process, also derived from forebrain neural crest, and a nasolateral process, derived from midbrain neural crest. Farther caudally, the stomodeum is bounded by maxillary and mandibular processes, which are also filled with neural crest–derived mesenchyme.

The future cervical region is dominated by the pharyngeal apparatus, consisting of a series of pharyngeal pouches, arches, and clefts. Many components of the face, ears, and glands of the head and neck arise from the pharyngeal region. Also prominent are the paired ectodermal placodes (see Figure 13-1), which form much of the sensory tissue of the cranial region.

## Tissue Components and Segmentation of the Early Craniofacial Region

The early craniofacial region consists of a massive neural tube beneath which lie the notochord and a ventrally situated pharynx (see Figure 14-2). The pharynx is surrounded by a series of pharyngeal arches. Many of the tissue components of the head and neck are organized segmentally. Figure 14-3 illustrates the segmentation of the tissue components of the head. As discussed in earlier chapters, distinct patterns of expression of certain homeobox-containing genes are associated with morphological segmentation in some cranial tissues, particularly the central nervous system (see Figure 11-11). The chain of events between segmental patterns of gene expression and the appearance of morphological segmentation in parts of the cranial region remains incompletely understood.

## Early Cellular Migrations and Tissue Displacements in the Craniofacial Region

Early craniofacial development is characterized by a number of massive migrations and displacements of cells and tissues. The neural crest is the first tissue to exhibit such migratory behavior, with cells migrating from the nervous system even before closure of the cranial neural tube (see Chapter 12). Initially, segmental groups of neural crest cells are segregated, especially in the pharyngeal region (see Figure 14-3). However, these populations of cells become confluent during their migrations through the pharyngeal arches.

The early cranial mesoderm consists mainly of the **paraxial** and **prechordal mesoderm** (see Figure 14-3). Mesenchymal cells originating in the paraxial mesoderm (somitomeres) form the connective tissue and skeletal elements of the caudal part of the cranium and the dorsal part of the neck. Somitomere-derived myogenic cells from paraxial mesoderm undergo extensive migrations to form the bulk of the muscles of the cranial region. Like their counterparts in the trunk and limbs, these myogenic cells become integrated with local connective tissue to form muscles. Another similarity with the trunk musculature is that morphogenetic control appears to reside within the connective tissue elements of the muscles rather than in the myogenic cells themselves. In the face and ventral pharynx, this connective tissue is of neural crest origin.

The prechordal mesoderm, which emits important forebrain inductive signals in the early embryo, is a transient mass of cells located in the midline, rostral to the tip of the notochord. Although the fate of these cells is controversial, some investigators feel that myoblasts contributing to the extraocular muscles take origin from these cells. On their way to the eye, cells of the prechordal mesoderm may pass through the rostralmost somites. Other investigators feel that the extraocular muscles have a purely somitomeric origin.

The **lateral mesoderm** is not well defined in the cranial region. Transplantation experiments have shown that it gives rise to endothelial and smooth muscle cells and at least in birds, to some portions of the laryngeal cartilages.

Another set of tissue displacements of importance in the cranial region is the joining of cells derived from the ectodermal placodes with those of the neural crest to form parts of sense organs and ganglia of certain cranial nerves (see Figure 13-1).

## FUNDAMENTAL ORGANIZATION OF PHARYNGEAL REGION

Because many components of the face are derived from the pharyngeal region, an understanding of the basic organization of this region is important. In the 1-month-old embryo the pharyngeal part of the foregut contains four lateral pairs of endodermally lined outpocketings called **pharyngeal pouches** and an unpaired ventral midline diverticulum, the **thyroid primordium** (Figure 14-4). If the contours of the ectodermal covering over the pharyngeal region are followed, bilateral pairs of inpocketings called **pharyngeal grooves** that almost make contact with the lateralmost extent of the pharyngeal pouches are seen (Figure 14-4, C).

Alternating with the pharyngeal grooves and pouches are paired masses of mesenchyme called **pharyngeal (branchial) arches**. Central to each pharyngeal arch is a prominent artery called an **aortic arch**, which extends

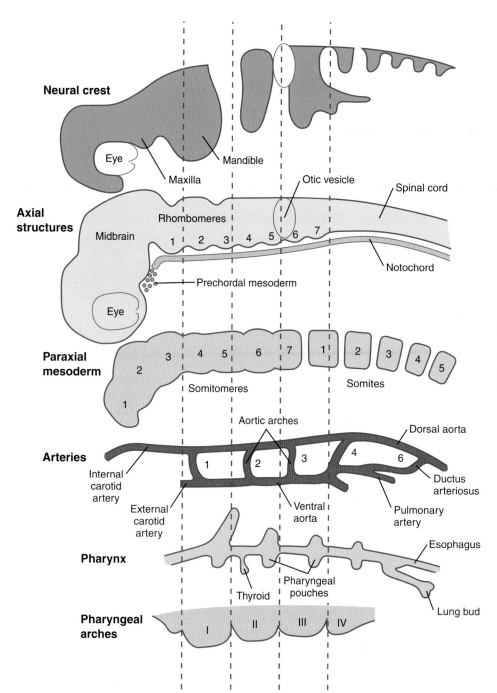

**FIGURE 14-3** Lateral view of the organization of the head and pharynx of a **30-day-old** human embryo, with individual tissue components separated but in register through the dashed lines. (Based on Noden DM: *Brain Behav Evol* 38:190–225, 1991.)

from the ventral to the dorsal aorta (see Chapter 17 and Figure 14-2). The mesenchyme of the pharyngeal arches is of dual origin. The mesenchyme of the incipient musculature originates from mesoderm, specifically the somitomeres. Much of the remaining pharyngeal arch mesenchyme, especially that of the ventral part, is derived from the neural crest, whereas mesoderm makes varying contributions to the dorsal pharyngeal arch mesenchyme. The early formation of the pharyngeal arches is closely associated with the spread of expression of products of the *HOXB* gene family from the rhombomeres of the

neural tube to the pharyngeal arch mesenchyme and ultimately the overlying ectoderm (see Figure 12-9).

The pharyngeal arches are evolutionarily complex structures, and the arches or their components give rise to a wide variety of structures in the head and neck. Both experimental and molecular research have shown control mechanisms operating along both the anteroposterior and proximodistal axes during the formation and development of the pharyngeal arches. Recent evidence suggests that the pharyngeal endoderm induces arch formation.

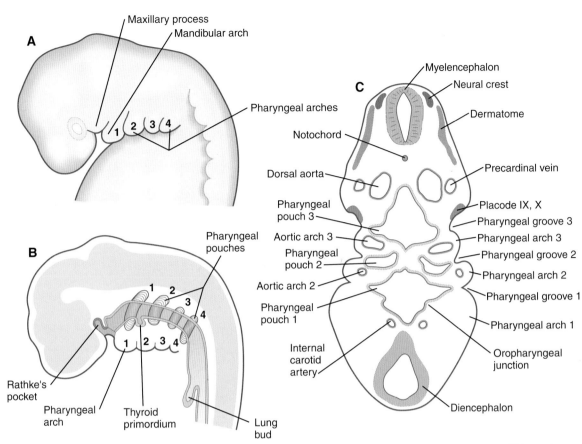

**FIGURE 14-4 A** and **B,** Superficial and sagittal views of the head and pharynx of a human embryo during the **fifth week. C,** Cross section through the pharyngeal region of a human embryo of the same age. Because of the strong C curvature of the head and neck of the embryo, a single section passes through the levels of both the forebrain *(bottom)* and hindbrain *(top).*

# DEVELOPMENT OF FACIAL REGION

## Formation of the Face and Jaws

Development of the face and jaws is a complex three-dimensional process involving the patterning, outgrowth, fusion, and molding of a variety of tissue masses. The forebrain acts as both a mechanical substrate and a signaling center for early facial development, and the stomodeum serves as a morphological point of reference. The lower face (maxillary region and lower jaw) is phylogenetically derived from a greatly expanded first pharyngeal arch. Much of the mesenchyme of the face is neural crest, originating from the forebrain to the first two rhombomeres. Each of the tissue components of the early face is the product of a unique set of morphogenetic determinants and growth signals, and there is increasing evidence that specific sets of molecular signals control their development along both the proximodistal and rostrocaudal axes. At a higher level, the building blocks of the face relate to one another in highly specific ways, and clues to their origins and relationships can be derived by examination of their blood supply. Disturbances at this

level regularly result in the production of craniofacial anomalies, and an understanding of the fundamental elements of facial morphogenesis is crucial to rational surgical approaches to these malformations.

Structures of the face and jaws originate from several primordia that surround the stomodeal depression of the 4- to 5-week-old human embryo (Figure 14-5). These primordia consist of an unpaired **frontonasal prominence;** paired **nasomedial** and **nasolateral processes,** which are components of the horseshoe-shaped olfactory (nasal) primordia; and paired **maxillary processes** and **mandibular prominences,** both components of the first pharyngeal arches. The upper jaw contains a mixed population of neural crest cells derived from the forebrain and midbrain, whereas the lower jaw contains mesenchymal cells derived from midbrain and hindbrain (rhombomeres 1 and 2) neural crest. The specific morphology of the facial skeletal elements, whether cartilage or membranous bones, is determined by yet undefined signaling between the pharyngeal endoderm and the neural crest precursors of the facial bones.

The frontonasal process is a prominent structure in the earliest phases of facial development, and its formation is the result of an exquisitely sensitive signaling system that

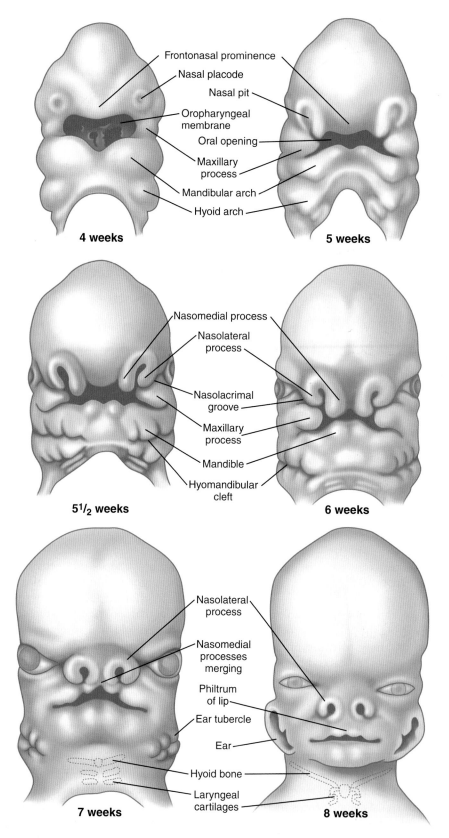

**FIGURE 14-5** Frontal and lateral views of heads of human embryos from **4** to **8 weeks** of age.

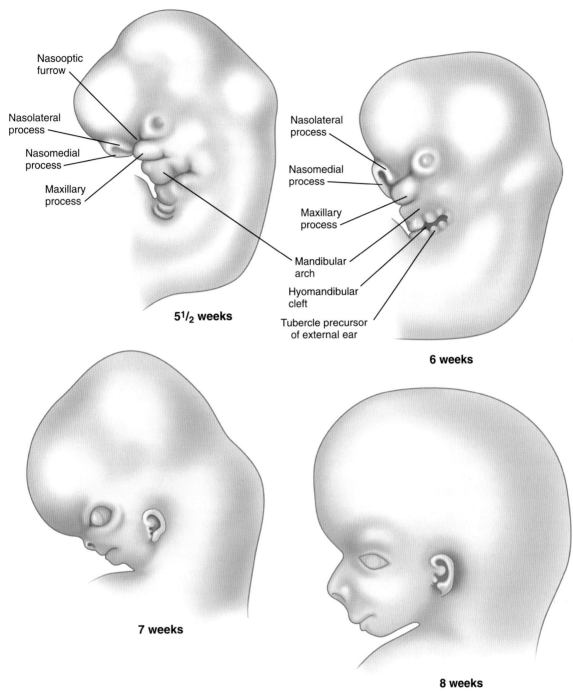

Nasooptic
furrow

Nasolateral
process

Nasomedial
process

Maxillary
process

**5¹/₂ weeks**

Nasolateral
process

Nasomedial
process

Maxillary
process

Mandibular
arch

Hyomandibular
cleft

Tubercle precursor
of external ear

**6 weeks**

**7 weeks**

**8 weeks**

**FIGURE 14-5, CONT'D**.

begins with the synthesis of **retinoic acid** in a localized region of ectoderm opposite the forebrain. The retinoic acid, possibly through the mediation of the most rostral wave of neural crest cells, maintains the signaling of fibroblast growth factor-8 (**FGF-8**) and **sonic hedgehog** (shh) in both anterior forebrain and the overlying frontonasal ectoderm. These two signaling molecules stimulate cell proliferation in the neural crest mesenchyme of the frontonasal process. In the absence of such signaling,

cell death in the region increases and cell proliferation decreases, resulting in a variety of midfacial defects (see Clinical Correlation 14-1). Retinoic acid is unusual in that both deficiencies and excess amounts can cause very similar defects. From 4 to 5 weeks the frontonasal process is a dominant structure of the early face (see Figure 14-5), but with subsequent growth of the maxillary process and the nasomedial and nasolateral processes, it recedes from the oral region.

The maxillary and mandibular processes are derivatives of the first pharyngeal arch. It has been suggested that the growth of the maxillary process from the first arch is the result of the establishment of a secondary signaling center, possibly involving FGF-8, in that part of the arch. As with the limb buds, outgrowth of the frontonasal prominence and the maxillary and mandibular processes depends upon mesenchymal-ectodermal interactions. In contrast to the limb, however, the signaling system (FGF and shh) is concentrated in the apical ectoderm of these processes, where it may act as a morphogenetic organizer and a stimulus for mesenchymal outgrowth of the facial primordia. The homeobox-containing gene **Msx-1** is expressed in the rapidly proliferating mesenchyme at the tips of the facial primordia. The parallel with expression of *Msx-1* in the progress zone of the limb (see page 216) suggests that similar mechanisms operate in both outgrowing limb and facial primordia. *Hox* genes are not expressed in the first pharyngeal arch, in contrast to the more posterior arches. Instead, expression of the transcription factor **Otx-2** characterizes precursors of the first arch. Specific combinations of subtypes of **bone morphogenetic proteins** (BMPs) and retinoic acid appear to determine the initial identity of the facial processes. In fact, inactivation of BMPs and the addition of retinoic acid can transform a maxillary process into a frontonasal process in avian embryos.

Despite the relatively featureless appearance of the early mandibular process (first pharyngeal arch), both mediolateral (oral-aboral) and proximodistal axes are tightly specified. This recognition has considerable clinical significance, because increasing numbers of genetic mutants are recognized to affect only certain regions of the arch, for example, the absence of distal (adult midline) vs. proximal structures. The medial (oral) region of the mandibular process, which appears to be the driver of mandibular growth, responds to local epithelial signals (possibly FGF-2 and FGF-4) by stimulating proliferation of the underlying mesenchyme through the mediation of Msx-1, much like the progress zone of the limb bud. In contrast growth of the lateral region depends upon FGF-8 signaling to the proliferating mesenchyme. Mandibular growth may be regulated through apoptosis mediated by BMP-4 and BMP-7, produced in the lateral region of the mandibular process.

Proximodistal organization of the arch is reflected by nested expression patterns of the transcription factor **Dlx** (the mammalian equivalent of *distalless* in *Drosophila*) along the arch. The paralogues Dlx-3 and Dlx-7 are expressed most distally; expression of Dlx-5 and Dlx-6 extends more proximally; and Dlx-1 and Dlx-2 expression extends most proximally. In mice, only Dlx-1 and Dlx-2 are expressed in the maxillary process. Although mutants of individual *Dlx* genes produce minor abnormalities, mice in which both *Dlx-5* and *Dlx-6* have been knocked out develop with a homeotic transformation of the distal lower jaws into upper jaws. It appears that *Dlx-5* and *Dlx-6* are selector genes that control the rostrocaudal identity of the distal segments of the first pharyngeal arch.

Through differential growth between 4 and 8 weeks (see Figure 14-5), the nasomedial and maxillary processes become relatively more prominent and ultimately fuse to form the upper lip and jaw (Figure 14-6). As this is occurring, the frontonasal prominence, which was a prominent tissue bordering the stomodeal area in the 4- and 5-week-old embryo, is displaced without contributing significantly to the upper jaw as the two nasomedial processes merge. The merged nasomedial processes form the **intermaxillary segment**, which is a precursor for (1) the **philtrum** of the lip, (2) the **premaxillary component** of the upper jaw, and (3) the **primary palate**.

Between the maxillary process and the nasal primordium (nasolateral process) is a **nasolacrimal groove** (nasooptic furrow) that extends to the developing eye (see Figure 14-5). The ectoderm of the floor of the nasolacrimal groove thickens to form a solid epithelial cord, which detaches from the groove. The epithelial cord then undergoes canalization and forms the **nasolacrimal duct** and near the eye, the **lacrimal sac**. The nasolacrimal duct extends from the medial corner of the eye to the nasal cavity (inferior meatus) and in postnatal life acts as a drain for lacrimal fluid. This connection explains why people can get a runny nose when crying. Meanwhile, the expanding nasomedial process fuses with the maxillary process, and over the region of the nasolacrimal groove, the nasolateral process merges with the superficial region of the maxillary process. The region of fusion of the nasomedial and maxillary processes is marked by an epithelial seam, called the **nasal fin**. Mesenchyme soon penetrates the nasal fin, resulting in a continuous union between the nasomedial and maxillary processes.

The lower jaw is formed in a simpler manner. The bilateral mandibular prominences enlarge, and their medial components merge in the midline, forming the point of the lower jaw. The midline dimple that is seen in the lower jaw of some individuals is a reflection of variation in the degree of merging of the mandibular prominences. A prominent cartilaginous rod called **Meckel's cartilage** differentiates within the lower jaw (see Figure 14-22, *D*). Derived from neural crest cells of the first pharyngeal arch, Meckel's cartilage forms the basis around which membrane bone (which forms the definitive skeleton of the lower jaw) is laid down. Experimental evidence indicates that the rodlike shape of Meckel's cartilage is related to the inhibition of further chondrogenesis by the surrounding ectoderm. If the ectoderm is removed around Meckel's cartilage, large masses of cartilage form instead of a rod. These properties are similar to the inhibitory interactions between ectoderm and chondrogenesis in the limb bud.

Shortly after the basic facial structures take shape, they are invaded by mesodermal cells associated with the first

**FIGURE 14-6 A,** Scanning electron micrograph showing the general facial features of an **8-week-old** human embryo. **B,** Higher magnification of the ear, which is located in the neck in **A.** (From Jirásek JE: *Atlas of human prenatal morphogenesis,* Amsterdam, 1983, Martinus Nijhoff.)

and second pharyngeal arches. These cells form the muscles of mastication (first arch derivatives, which are innervated by cranial nerve V) and the muscles of facial expression (second arch derivatives, which are innervated by cranial nerve VII).

Although the basic structure of the face is established between the fourth and eighth weeks, changes in the proportionality of the various regions continue until well after birth. In particular, the midface remains underdeveloped during embryogenesis and even early postnatal life.

## Temporomandibular Joint and Its Relationship to the Jaw Joint of Lower Vertebrates

Of considerable clinical importance and evolutionary interest is the **temporomandibular joint (TMJ)**, which represents the hinge between the mandibular condyle and the squamous part of the temporal bone. The TMJ, which phylogenetically appeared with the evolution of mammals, is a complex synovial joint surrounded by a capsule and containing an **articular disc** between the two bones. It is formed relatively late during development,

first appearing as mesenchymal condensations associated with the temporal bone and mandibular condyle during the seventh week of development. The articular disc and capsule begin to take shape a week later, with the actual joint cavity forming between weeks 9 and 11.

In lower vertebrates, the jaw opens and closes on a hinge between cartilaginous portions of the mandibular process—the **articular bone** in the lower jaw and the **quadrate bone** in the upper jaw, both derivatives of Meckel's cartilage. During phylogenesis, the distal membranous bone (the **dentary bone**) associated with Meckel's cartilage increased in prominence as the jaw musculature became more massive. The dentary bone of contemporary mammals and humans constitutes the vast majority of the lower jaw, and Meckel's cartilage is only seen as a prominent cartilaginous rod within the forming jaw complex during the late embryonic stage of development.

In mammals, over many millions of years, the original jaw-opening joint became less prominent and was incorporated into the middle ear as the malleus (derivative of articular bone of the lower jaw) and the incus (derivative of the ancestral quadrate bone in the skull). The incus connects with the stapes (a derivative of the second pharyngeal arch). The **tympanic ring**, a neural crest–derived

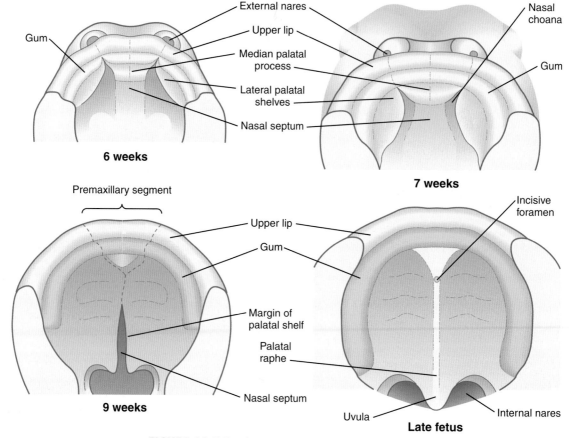

FIGURE 14-7 Development of the palate as seen from below.

bone that surrounds and supports the tympanic membrane, is derived from the **angular bone**, one of the first arch membrane bones that overlies the proximal part of Meckel's cartilage.

## Formation of Palate

The early embryo possesses a common oronasal cavity, but in humans the **palate** forms between the sixth and tenth weeks to separate the oral from the nasal cavity. The palate is derived from three primordia: an unpaired **median palatine process** and a pair of **lateral palatine processes** (Figure 14-7).

The median palatine process is an ingrowth from the newly merged nasomedial processes. As it grows, the median palatine process forms a triangular bony structure called the **primary palate**. In postnatal life the skeletal component of the primary palate is referred to as the **premaxillary component of the maxilla**. The four upper incisor teeth arise from this structure (Figure 14-8).

Formation of the palate involves (1) growth of the palatal shelves, (2) their elevation, (3) their fusion, and (4) removal of the epithelial seam at the site of fusion. The lateral palatine processes, which are the precursors

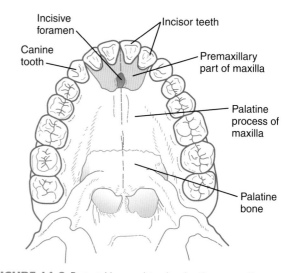

FIGURE 14-8 Postnatal bony palate, showing the premaxillary segment.

of the **secondary palate**, first appear as outgrowths of the maxillary processes during the sixth week. At first they grow downward on either side of the tongue (Figure 14-9). Like other facial primordia, outgrowth of the palatal shelves involves ectodermal-mesenchymal inter-

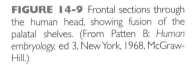

FIGURE 14-9 Frontal sections through the human head, showing fusion of the palatal shelves. (From Patten B: *Human embryology*, ed 3, New York, 1968, McGraw-Hill.)

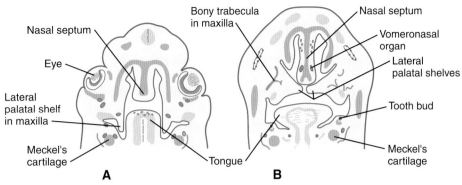

actions and specific growth factors. The action of Msx-1 in the palatal shelf mesenchyme stimulates a downstream cascade of BMP-4 signaling in the mesenchyme, leading to shh signaling in the apical ectoderm. The shh, in turn, induces BMP-2 signaling in the underlying mesenchyme, and the combination of BMP-2– and BMP-4–stimulates mesenchymal proliferation and outgrowth of the palatal shelf. During the seventh weeks, the lateral palatine processes (**palatal shelves**) dramatically dislodge from their positions alongside the tongue and become oriented perpendicularly to the maxillary processes. The apices of these processes meet in the midline and begin to fuse.

Despite many years of investigation, the mechanism underlying the elevation of the palatine shelves remains obscure. Swelling of the extracellular matrix of the palatal shelves appears to impart a resiliency that allows them to approximate one another shortly after their becoming dislodged from along the tongue. Recent research suggests that the period of rapid closure of the palatal shelves is accomplished by the flowing of the internal tissues rather than by a reaction that approximates the closure of swinging doors.

Another structure involved in formation of the palate is the **nasal septum** (see Figures 14-7 and 14-9). This midline structure, which is a downgrowth from the frontonasal prominence, reaches the level of the palatal shelves when the latter fuse to form the definitive secondary palate. Rostrally, the nasal septum is continuous with the primary palate.

At the gross level, the palatal shelves fuse in the midline, but rostrally they also join the primary palate. The midline point of the fusion of the primary palate with the two palatal shelves is marked by the **incisive foramen** (see Figure 14-8).

Because of its clinical importance, fusion of the palatal shelves has been investigated intensively. When the palatal shelves first make midline contact, each is covered throughout by a homogeneous epithelium. During the process of fusion, however, the midline epithelial seam disappears. The epithelium on the nasal surface of the palate differentiates into a ciliated columnar type, whereas the epithelium takes on a stratified squamous form on the oral surface of the palate. Significant developmental questions include the following:

1. What causes the disappearance of the midline epithelial seam?
2. What signals result in the diverse pathways of differentiation of the epithelium on either side of the palate?

The disappearance of the midline epithelial seam after the approximation of the palatal shelves involves several fundamental developmental processes (Figure 14-10). Some of the epithelial cells at the fusion seam undergo apoptosis and disappear. Others may migrate out from the plane of fusion and become inserted into the epithelial lining of the oral cavity. Still other epithelial cells undergo a morphological transformation into mesenchymal cells through the action of **transforming growth factor-β3** (TGF-β3). TGF-β3 is expressed by the ectodermal cells of the distal rim of the palatal shelves just prior to fusion and loses prominence shortly thereafter. In TGF-β3 mutant mice the lateral palatal shelves approximate in the midline, but the epithelial seam fails to disappear, and the mice develop isolated cleft palate.

Experiments involving the in vitro culture of a single palatal shelf of a number of species have shown clearly

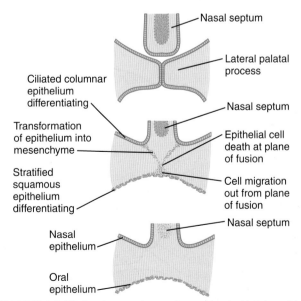

FIGURE 14-10 Developmental processes associated with fusion of the palatal shelves and the nasal septum.

that all aspects of epithelial differentiation (cell death in the midline and different pathways of differentiation on the oral and nasal surfaces) can occur in the absence of contact with the opposite palatal shelf. These different pathways of differentiation are not intrinsic to the regional epithelia but are mediated by the underlying neural crest–derived mesenchyme. The mechanism underlying this regional specification of the epithelium remains little understood. According to one model, the underlying mesenchyme produces growth factors that influence the production and regional distribution of extracellular matrix molecules (e.g., type IX collagen). The way these events are received and interpreted by the epithelial cells is unknown.

## Formation of the Nose and Olfactory Apparatus

The human olfactory apparatus first becomes visible at the end of the first month as a pair of thickened ectodermal **nasal placodes** located on the frontal aspect of the head (Figure 14-11, *A*). Like the formation of the lens placodes, the formation of the nasal placodes requires the expression of **Pax-6**. In the absence of Pax-6 expression, neither the nasal nor the lens placodes form. The nasal placodes originate from the anterolateral edge of the neural plate before its closure.

Soon after their formation, the nasal placodes form a surface depression (the **nasal pits**) surrounded by horseshoe-shaped elevations of mesenchymal tissue with the open ends facing the future mouth (see Figure 14-5). The two limbs of the mesenchymal elevations are the **nasomedial** and **nasolateral processes.** As the nasal primordia merge toward the midline during the sixth and seventh weeks, the nasomedial processes form the tip and crest of the nose along with part of the nasal septum, and the nasolateral processes form the wings (**alae**) of the nose. The receding frontonasal process contributes to part of the bridge of the nose.

Meanwhile, the nasal pits continue to deepen toward the oral cavity and form substantial cavities themselves (see Figure 14-11). By 6½ weeks only a thin **oronasal membrane** separates the oral from the nasal cavities. The

**FIGURE 14-11** Sagittal sections through embryonic heads with special emphasis on development of the nasal chambers. **A,** At **5 weeks. B,** At **6 weeks. C,** At **6½ weeks. D,** At **7 weeks. E,** At **12 weeks.**

oronasal membrane soon breaks down, making the nasal cavities continuous with the oral cavity through openings behind the primary palate called **nasal choanae**. With the fusion of the lateral palatal shelves, the nasal cavity is considerably lengthened and ultimately communicates with the upper pharynx.

Like the other major sensory organs of the head, the epithelium of each nasal pit induces the surrounding neural crest mesenchyme to form a cartilaginous capsule around it. In a three-dimensionally complex manner, the medial parts of the nasal capsules combine with more centrally derived deep neural crest mesenchyme to form the midline nasal septum and ethmoid bones. The lateral region of the nasal capsule forms the nasal bones. During the third month, shelflike structures called **nasal conchae** form from the ethmoid bones on the lateral wall of the nasal cavity. These structures increase the surface area available for conditioning the air within the nasal cavity. Late in fetal life and for several years after birth the paranasal sinuses form as outgrowths from the walls of the nasal cavities. The size and shape of these structures have a significant impact on the form of the face during its postnatal growth period.

At 6 to 7 weeks, a pair of epithelial ingrowths can be seen in each side of the nasal septum near the palate. Developing as invaginations from the medial portion of the nasal placode, these diverticula, known as **vomeronasal organs** (see Figure 14-9, *B*), reach a maximum size of about 6 to 8 mm at around the sixth fetal month and then begin to regress, leaving small cystic structures. In most mammals and many other vertebrates the vomeronasal organs, which are lined with a modified olfactory epithelium, remain prominent and appear to be involved in the olfaction of food in the mouth or sexual olfactory stimuli (e.g., pheromones).

The dorsalmost epithelium of the nasal pits undergoes differentiation as a highly specialized olfactory epithelium (see Figure 14-11). Beginning in the embryonic period and throughout life, the olfactory epithelium is able to form primitive sensory bipolar neurons, which send axonal projections toward the olfactory bulb of the brain. Preceding axonal ingrowth, some cells break free from this epithelium and migrate toward the brain. Some of these cells may synthesize a substrate for the ingrowth of the olfactory axons. Other cells migrating from the olfactory placode (specifically, the vomeronasal primordium) synthesize **luteinizing hormone–releasing hormone** and migrate to the hypothalamus, the site of synthesis and release of this hormone in the adult. The embryonic origin of these cells in the olfactory placode helps to understand the basis for **Kallman syndrome,** which is characterized by anosmia and hypogonadotropic hypogonadism. Cells of the olfactory placode also form supporting (sustentacular) cells and glandular cells in the olfactory region of the nose. Physiological evidence demonstrates that the olfactory epithelium is

capable of some function in late fetal life but that full olfactory function is not attained until after birth.

## Formation of the Salivary Glands

Starting in the sixth week the **salivary glands** originate as solid, ridgelike thickenings of the oral epithelium (Figure 14-12). Extensive epithelial shifts in the oral cavity make it difficult to determine the germ layer origins of the salivary gland epithelium. The parotid glands are probably derived from ectoderm, whereas the submandibular and sublingual glands are thought to be derived from endoderm.

As with other glandular structures associated with the digestive tract, the development of salivary glands depends on a continuing series of epitheliomesenchymal interactions. The basal lamina that surrounds the early epithelial lobular ingrowths differs in composition depending on the growth potential of the region. Around the stalk and in clefts, the basal lamina contains types I and IV collagen and a basement membrane-1 (BM-1) proteoglycan. These components are not found in the regions of the lobules that undergo further growth. Under the influence of the surrounding mesenchyme, the basal lamina in growing regions loses the collagens and proteoglycans that are associated with stable structures (e.g., stalks, clefts). In addition to alterations in the basal lamina, branching is associated with the local contraction of ordered microfilaments within the apices of epithelial cells at the branch points. Continued growth at the tips of lobules of the glands is supported by high levels of mitotic activity of the epithelium and the deposition of newly synthesized glycosaminoglycans in the area. The structural and functional differentiation of the epithelium of the salivary gland continues throughout fetal life.

## Formation of the Teeth

A tooth is a highly specialized extracellular matrix consisting of two principal components—enamel and dentin—each secreted by a different embryonic epithelium. Tooth development is a highly orchestrated process involving intimate interactions between the epithelia that produce the dentin and enamel. Extending a common theme of development into the macroscopic dimension, teeth undergo an **isoform transition**, with the postnatal replacement of the deciduous teeth by their permanent adult counterparts.

### Patterning of the Dentition

Each human tooth has a distinctive morphology, and each type of tooth forms in a characteristic location. For many years virtually nothing was known about the patterning

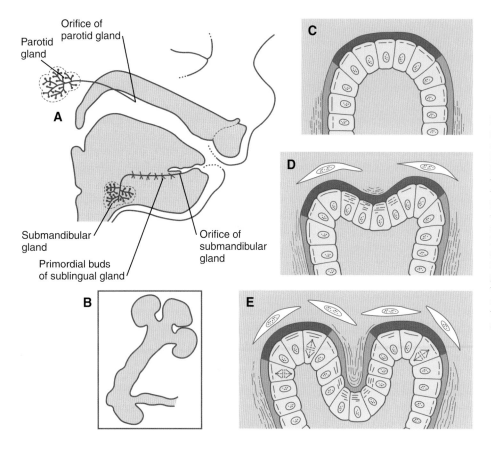

**FIGURE 14-12** Development of the salivary glands. **A,** Salivary gland development in an **11-week-old** human embryo. **B,** Development of salivary gland epithelium in vitro. **C,** Accumulation of newly synthesized glycosaminoglycans *(dark green)* in the basal lamina at the end of a primary lobule. **D,** Early cleft formation is associated with the contraction of bundles of microfilaments in the apices of the epithelial cells lining the cleft. Collagen fibers *(wavy lines)* are lined up lateral to the lobule and in the newly forming cleft. **E,** As the cleft deepens, glycosaminoglycan synthesis is reduced in the cleft, and collagen deposition continues. (**C** through **E** show the relationship between disposition of the extracellular matrix and lobulaton of the glandular primordium.)

of the dentition, but analysis of certain types of genetically modified mice has provided some of the first concrete clues to the molecular basis of dental patterning. The homeobox-containing genes *Dlx-1* and *Dlx-2* are expressed in the maxillary arch and in the proximal part of the mandibular arch. When both of these genes are knocked out in mice, the upper jaw develops without molar teeth, although molars develop in the lower jaws. The incisor teeth in both jaws develop normally. Another homeobox-containing gene, *Barx-1*, is induced by FGF-8 in proximal ectoderm of the mandibular process, and it may compensate in the formation of molar teeth for the absence of Dlx-1 and Dlx-2 in the lower jaw. **Msx-1** and **Msx-2** may be involved in patterning the incisor teeth, but the evidence is less clear.

Not only the location, but the type of tooth is under tight developmental control. The difference in morphology between an incisor tooth, possessing a single cusp, and a molar tooth, which contains several cusps, is related to the number of enamel knots (see below) that the developing tooth contains. This also appears to be under molecular control. A striking example is the conversion of incisor teeth to molars in mice. In the distal part of the mandibular arch, ectodermal BMP-4 signals normally repress the expression of Barx-1, but when BMP-4 signaling is inhibited by the implantation of noggin beads, Barx-1 expression is induced in the dental mesenchyme

and the developing incisor teeth are transformed into molars.

### Stages of Tooth Development

Tooth development begins with the migration of neural crest cells into the regions of the upper and lower jaws. The overlying oral ectoderm then thickens into **C**-shaped bands (**dental laminae**) in the upper and lower jaws. The appearance of the dental laminae during the sixth week is the first manifestation of a series of ectodermal-mesenchymal interactions that continues until tooth formation is virtually completed.

Although each tooth has a specific time sequence and morphology of development, certain general developmental stages are common to all teeth (Figure 14-13). As the dental lamina grows into the neural crest mesenchyme, epithelial primordia of the individual teeth begin to take shape as **tooth buds**. In keeping with their interactive mode of development, the tooth buds are associated with condensations of mesenchymal cells. The tooth bud soon expands, passing through a mushroom-shaped **cap stage** before entering the **bell stage** (see Figure 14-13, *D*).

By the bell stage the tooth primordium already has a complex structure, even though it has not formed any components of the definitive tooth. The epithelial com-

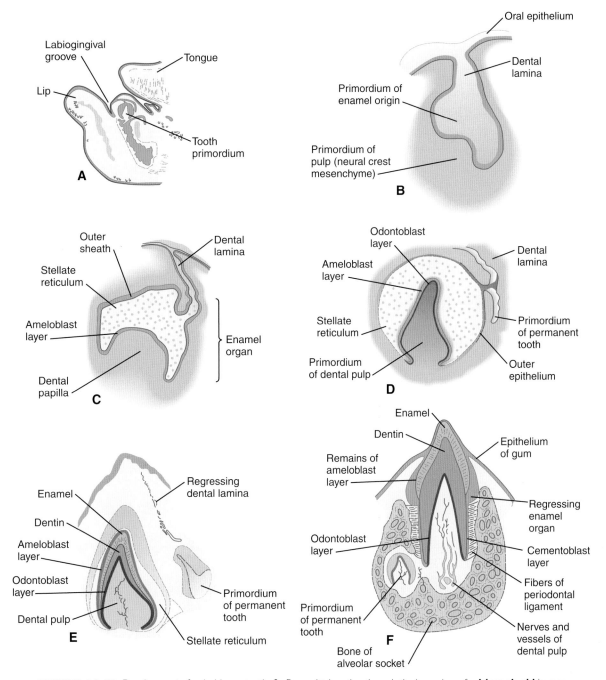

**FIGURE 14-13** Development of a deciduous tooth. **A,** Parasagittal section through the lower jaw of a **14-week-old** human embryo showing the relative location of the tooth primordium. **B,** Tooth primordium in the bud stage in a **9-week-old** embryo. **C,** Tooth primordium at the cap stage in an **11-week-old** embryo, showing the enamel organ. **D,** Central incisor primordium at the bell stage in a **14-week-old** embryo before deposition of enamel or dentin. **E,** Unerupted incisor tooth in a term fetus. **F,** Partially erupted incisor tooth showing the primordium of a permanent tooth near one of its roots. (After Patten B: *Human embryology*, ed 3, New York, 1968, McGraw-Hill.)

ponent, called the **enamel organ**, is still connected to the oral epithelium by an irregular stalk of dental lamina, which soon begins to degenerate. The enamel organ consists of an **outer sheath** of epithelium, a mesenchyme-like **stellate reticulum**, and an inner epithelial **ameloblast layer**. Ameloblasts are the cells that begin to secrete the enamel of the tooth. Within the concave surface

of the enamel organ is a condensation of neural crest mesenchyme called the **dental papilla**. Cells of the dental papilla opposite the ameloblast layer become transformed into columnar epithelial cells called **odontoblasts** (Figure 14-14). These cells secrete the dentin of the tooth. Attached to the dental lamina close to the enamel organ is a small bud of the permanent tooth (see Figure 14-13,

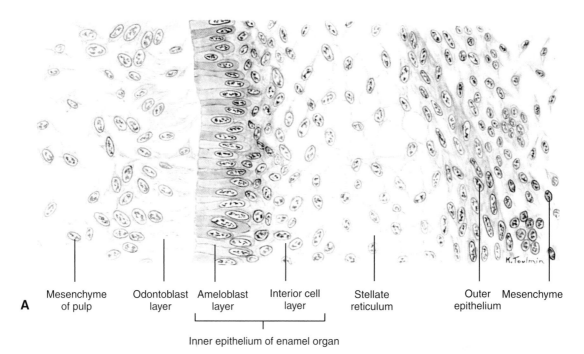

**A**    Mesenchyme of pulp    Odontoblast layer    Ameloblast layer    Interior cell layer    Stellate reticulum    Outer epithelium    Mesenchyme

Inner epithelium of enamel organ

**B**    Blood vessel in pulp    Odontoblast    Dentinal fiber    Thomes' process    Ameloblast layer    Outer epithelium of enamel organ

Dentine    Enamel    Blood vessel in mesenchyme

**FIGURE 14-14** Pig embryos showing the cellular configuration of the enamel organ and adjacent pulp of forming teeth before and after the beginning of deposition of enamel and dentin. **A,** Stage equivalent to a **4-month-old** human embryo. **B,** Stage equivalent to a **5-month-old** human embryo. (After Patten B: *Human embryology*, ed 3, New York, 1968, McGraw-Hill.)

*E and F).* Although delayed, it goes through the same developmental stages as the deciduous tooth.

Late in the bell stage the odontoblasts and ameloblasts begin to secrete precursors of dentin and enamel, beginning first at the future apex of the tooth. Over several months the definitive form of the tooth takes shape (see Figure 14-13). Meanwhile, a condensation of mesenchy-mal cells forms around the developing tooth. Cells of this structure, called the **dental sac,** produce specialized extracellular matrix components (**cementum** and the **periodontal ligament**) that provide the tooth a firm attachment to the jaw. While these events are occurring, the tooth elongates and begins to erupt through the gums (**gingiva**).

## Tissue Interactions in Tooth Development

Teeth are formed by a series of inductive interactions. Tissue recombination experiments have shown that the thickened ectoderm of the dental lamina initiates tooth formation. Early in development dental ectoderm can induce nondental cranial neural crest mesenchyme to participate in the formation of a tooth, but predental neural crest mesenchyme cannot induce nondental ectoderm to form a tooth. Recent research suggests that the transcription factor **Lef-1** (lymphoid enhancer factor-1) may stimulate the predental surface ectoderm to secrete **FGF-8**, which in turn induces the underlying mesenchyme to express **Pax-9** (Figure 14-15). In the absence of Pax-9 expression, tooth development does not proceed past the bud stage. **BMP-2** and **BMP-4**, also produced by the surface ectoderm, inhibit the action of FGF-8, and it has been suggested that such inhibition is the basis for the non–tooth forming spaces between the developing teeth, although how the specific pattern is set up remains unknown. Another characteristic transcription factor induced in the mesenchyme beneath the thickened dental lamina is Msx-1.

Slightly later in dental development BMP-4, instead of functioning as an inhibitor, acts along with FGF-8 and shh to stimulate the mesenchyme of the tooth bud to express a variety of characteristic molecules, including the transcription factors **Msx-1**, **Msx-2**, and **EGR-1** (early growth response-1); the extracellular matrix molecules **tenascin** and **syndecan**; and **BMP-4**. If the overlying ectoderm is separated from the neural crest mesenchyme, the predental mesenchyme does not develop into a dental papilla and a tooth does not form. The role of BMP-4 as an inducer was demonstrated by adding a small bead soaked in BMP-4 to a small mass of cultured predental neural crest mesenchyme (see Figure 14-15, B). Under the influence of the BMP-4 released from the bead, the mesenchyme began to express Msx-1, Msx-2, Egr-1, and BMP-4. The mesenchyme did not, however, produce tenascin or syndecan, showing that other signals in addition to BMP-4 are required to achieve the full inductive response.

With the initial induction of the dental mesenchyme, that tissue itself becomes the next prime mover in tooth development. Inductive signals emanating from the dental mesenchyme next act on the ectoderm of the dental ledge, now in the late bud to early cap stage. Recombination experiments have shown that the dental mesenchyme determines the specific form of the tooth. When molar mesenchyme is combined in vitro with incisor epithelium, a molar tooth takes shape, whereas combining incisor mesenchyme with molar epithelium results in the formation of an incisor.

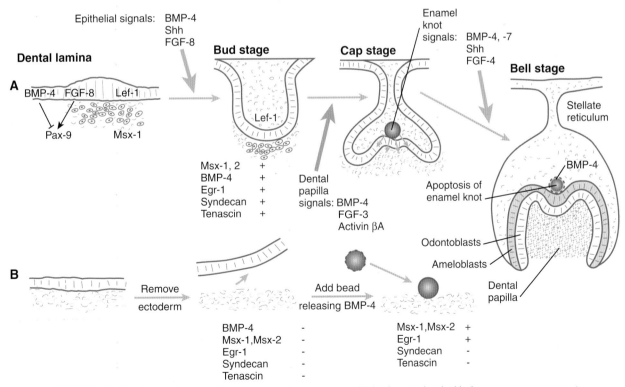

**FIGURE 14-15 A,** Inductive interactions during tooth development. Molecules associated with the green arrow represent components of the signal from dental lamina ectoderm to underlying neural crest mesenchyme; molecules associated with the violet arrow are signals from the dental papilla to the overlying ectoderm; molecules associated with the pink arrow are signals from the enamel knot to dental papilla. **B,** In vitro experiment showing that a bead releasing BMP-4 can induce dental mesenchyme to express specific markers (Msx-1, Msx-2, and Egr-1).

Under the inductive influence of the dental mesenchyme, now called the **dental papilla**, a small group of ectodermal cells at the tip of the dental papilla cease dividing. This mass of cells, called the **enamel knot** (Figure 14-16), serves as a signaling center that regulates the shape of the developing tooth. Through the production of several signaling molecules, including **shh, FGF-4, and BMP-2, BMP-4, and BMP-7**, the enamel knot stimulates the proliferation of cells in the dental cap down and away from itself. By serving as a fixed point in this process, the enamel knot determines the site of the tip of a cusp in the developing tooth. In the case of molar teeth, which have multiple cusps, secondary enamel knots form—one for each cusp. Ultimately, the cells of the enamel knot undergo apoptosis, possibly under the influence of BMP-4, which stimulates cell death in several other developmental systems. The appearance of apoptosis terminates the inductive signaling from this structure.

### Formation of Dentin and Enamel

Late in their differentiation, odontoblasts withdraw from the cell cycle, elongate, and start secreting **predentin** from their apical surfaces, which face the enamel organ. The production of predentin signals a shift in the patterns of synthesis from type III collagen and fibronectin to type I collagen and other molecules (e.g., **dentin phosphoprotein, dentin osteocalcin**) that characterize the dentin matrix. The first dentin is laid against the inner surface of the enamel organ at the apex of the tooth (see Figure 14-14, *B*). With the secretion of additional dentin, the accumulated material pushes the odontoblastic epithelium from the odontoblast-ameloblast interface.

Terminal differentiation of the ameloblasts occurs after the odontoblasts begin to secrete predentin. In response to inductive signals from the odontoblasts, the ameloblasts withdraw from the cell cycle and begin a new pattern of synthesis, producing two classes of proteins: **amelogenins** and **enamelins**. About 5% of enamel consists of organic matrix, and amelogenins account for about 90% of this, with enamelins constituting most of the remainder. Enamelins are secreted before the amelogenins, and they may serve as nuclei for the formation of crystals of **hydroxyapatite**, the dominant inorganic component of enamel.

The amelogenin genes are located on the X and Y chromosomes in humans. Enamel genes have been highly conserved during vertebrate phylogeny. It has been suggested that in early vertebrates, enamel once served as part of an electroreceptor apparatus.

### Tooth Eruption and Replacement

Each tooth has a specific time of eruption and replacement (Table 14-1). With the growth of the root, the enamel-covered crown pushes through the oral epithelium. The sequence of eruption begins with the central incisor teeth, usually a few months after birth, and continues generally stepwise until the last of the deciduous molars forms at the end of the second year. A total of 20 deciduous teeth are formed.

Meanwhile, the primordium of the permanent tooth is embedded in a cavity extending into the bone on the lingual side of the alveolar socket in which the tooth is embedded (see Figure 14-13, *F*). As the permanent tooth develops, its increasing size causes resorption of the root of the deciduous tooth. When a sufficient amount of the root is destroyed, the deciduous tooth falls out, leaving

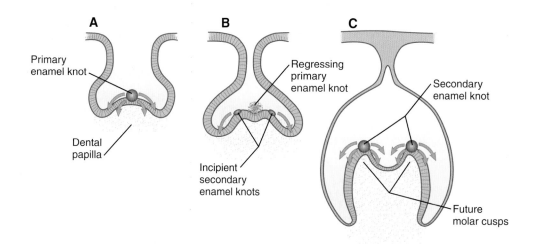

**FIGURE 14-16** The enamel knot as a signaling center in the developing molar tooth. **A,** The primary enamel knot induces proliferation on either side. **B,** Two secondary enamel knots form on each side of the regressing primary enamel knot. **C,** Under the influence of the secondary enamel knots, the future cusps of the molar begin to form.

**TABLE 14-1** *Usual Times of Eruption and Shedding of Deciduous and Permanent Teeth*

| Teeth | Eruption | Shedding |
|---|---|---|
| **DECIDUOUS** | | |
| Central incisors | 6–8 mo | 6–7 yr |
| Lateral incisors | 7–10 mo | 7–8 yr |
| Canines | 14–18 mo | 10–12 yr |
| First molars | 12–16 mo | 9–11 yr |
| Second molars | 20–24 mo | 10–12 yr |
| **PERMANENT** | | |
| Central incisors | 7–8 yr | |
| Lateral incisors | 8–9 yr | |
| Canines | 11–13 yr | |
| First premolars | 10–11 yr | |
| Second premolars | 11–12 yr | |
| First molars | 6–7 yr | |
| Second molars | 12–13 yr | |
| Third molars | 15–25 yr | |

room for the permanent tooth to take its place. The sequence of eruption of the permanent teeth is the same as that of the deciduous teeth, but an additional 12 permanent teeth (for a total of 32) are formed without deciduous counterparts.

The formation and eruption of teeth are important factors in midfacial growth, much of which occurs after birth. Tooth development and the corresponding growth of the jaw to accommodate the teeth, along with the development of the paranasal sinuses, account for much of the tissue mass of the midface.

## DEVELOPMENT OF PHARYNX AND ITS DERIVATIVES

Considering the complexity of the structural arrangements of the embryonic pharynx, it is not surprising that a wide variety of structures originate in the pharyngeal region. This provides many opportunities for abnormal development, discussed in Clinical Correlation 14-2 at the end of this section. This section details aspects of later development that lead to the formation of specific structures. Adult derivatives of the regions of the pharynx and pharyngeal arches are summarized in Figure 14-21.

## External Development of the Pharyngeal Region

Externally, the pharyngeal (branchial) region is characterized by four pharyngeal arches and grooves interposed between the arches (see Figure 14-4). These structures give rise to a diverse array of derivatives.

### Pharyngeal Arches

It is becoming increasingly apparent that development of the pharyngeal arches is under complex genetic control. Although there is an underlying unity in the tissue organization of the arches, each arch has a specific morphological identity. Molecular signals from the ectoderm of the pharyngeal clefts and possibly from the endoderm of the pharyngeal grooves play an important role in determining anteroposterior characteristics of the arches, and nested sets of homeobox-containing genes, such as *Dlx*, control development along the proximodistal axis. Formation of the first arch is independent of retinoic acid, but in the absence of retinoic acid, the second and fourth pharyngeal arches do not form properly.

In addition to being packed with mesenchyme (mainly of neural crest origin except for the premuscle mesoderm, which migrates from the somitomeres), each pharyngeal arch is associated with a major artery (aortic arch) and a cranial nerve (see Figure 14-21). Each also contains a central rod of precartilaginous mesenchyme, which is transformed into characteristic adult skeletal derivatives. Understanding the relationship between the pharyngeal arches and their innervation and vascular supply is very important, since tissues often maintain their relationship with their original nerve as they migrate out or become displaced from their site of origin in the pharyngeal arch system.

The **first pharyngeal arch** (mandibular) contributes mainly to structures of the face (both mandibular and maxillary portions) and ear (see Figure 14-21). Its central cartilaginous rod, Meckel's cartilage, is a prominent component of the embryonic lower jaw until it is surrounded by locally formed intramembranous bone, which forms the definitive jaw. During later development the distal part of Meckel's cartilage undergoes resorption because of extensive apoptosis of the chondrocytes. More dorsally, Meckel's cartilage forms the **sphenomandibular ligament,** the **anterior ligament of the malleus,** and the **malleus** (Figure 14-22). In addition, the **incus** arises from a primordium of the **quadrate cartilage.** The first arch musculature is associated with the masticatory apparatus, the pharynx, and the middle ear. A common feature of these muscles is their innervation by the trigeminal nerve (V).

The molecular basis for development of the first pharyngeal arch is quite different from that of the other arches, starting with the origin of the neural crest that

### CLEFT LIP AND PALATE

Cleft lip and cleft palate are relatively common malformations, with an incidence of approximately 1 in 1000 and 1 in 2500 births, respectively. Numerous combinations and degrees of severity exist, ranging from a unilateral cleft lip to a bilateral cleft lip associated with a fully cleft palate.

Structurally, **cleft lip** results from the lack of fusion of the maxillary and nasomedial processes. In the most complete form of the defect, the entire premaxillary segment is separated from both maxillae, resulting in bilateral clefts that run through the lip and the upper jaw between the lateral incisors and the canine teeth (Figure 14-17). The point of convergence of the two clefts is the incisive foramen (see Figure 14-8). The premaxillary segment commonly protrudes past the normal facial contours when viewed from the side. The mechanism frequently underlying cleft lip is hypoplasia of the maxillary process, preventing contact between the maxillary and nasomedial processes from being established.

**Cleft palate** results from incomplete or absent fusion of the palatal shelves (Figures 14-17, B, and 14-18). The extent of palatal clefting ranges from involvement of the entire length of the palate to something as minor as a bifid uvula. As with cleft lip, cleft palate is usually multifactorial. Some chromosomal syndromes (such as trisomy 13) are characterized by a high incidence of clefts. In other cases, cleft lip and palate can be linked to the action of a chemical teratogen (e.g., anticonvulsant medications).

Experiments on mice have shown that the incidence of cleft palate after exposure to a dose of cortisone is strongly related to the genetic background of the mouse. In humans, mutations of *Msx-1* are strongly associated with non syndromic cleft palate. The higher incidence of cleft palate in females may be related to the palatal shelves in females fusing about a week later than they do in males, thus prolonging the susceptible period.

### OBLIQUE FACIAL CLEFT

This rare defect results when the nasolateral process fails to fuse with the maxillary process, usually resulting from hypoplasia of one of the tissue masses (Figure 14-19, A). It frequently manifests as an epithelially lined fissure running from the upper lip to the medial corner of the eye.

### MACROSTOMIA (LATERAL FACIAL CLEFT)

An even rarer condition called **macrostomia** (Figure 14-19, B) results from hypoplasia or poor merging of the maxillary and mandibular processes. As the name implies, this condition manifests as a very large mouth on one or both sides. In severe cases the cleft can reach almost to the ears.

### MEDIAN CLEFT LIP

Another rare anomaly, **median cleft lip**, results from incomplete merging of the two nasomedial processes (Figure 14-19, C).

**A**                                                                  **B**

**FIGURE 14-17 A,** Front and lateral views of an infant with bilateral cleft lip and palate. On the lateral view, note how the premaxillary segment is tipped outward. **B,** Unilateral cleft lip and complete cleft palate. Note the duplicated uvula at the back of the oral cavity. (Courtesy A. Burdi, Ann Arbor, Mich.)

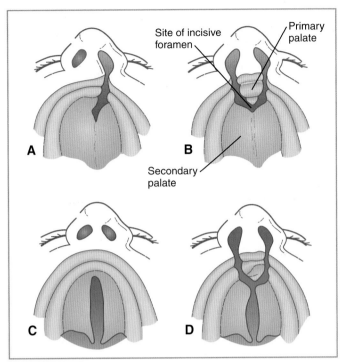

**FIGURE 14-18** Common varieties of cleft lip and palate. **A,** Unilateral cleft passing through the lip and between the premaxilla (primary palate) and secondary palate. **B,** Bilateral cleft lip and palate similar to that seen in the patient in Figure 14-17, A. **C,** Midline palatal cleft. **D,** Bilateral cleft lip and palate continuous with a midline cleft of the secondary palate.

**FIGURE 14-19** Varieties of facial clefts. **A,** Oblique facial cleft combined with a cleft lip. **B,** Macrostomia. **C,** Medial cleft lip with a partial nasal cleft.

## HOLOPROSENCEPHALY

Holoprosencephaly includes a broad spectrum of defects, all based on defective formation of the forebrain (prosencephalon) and structures whose normal formation depends on influences from the forebrain. The defect arises in early pregnancy when the forebrain is taking shape, and the brain defects usually involve archencephalic structures (e.g., the olfactory system). Because of the influence of the brain on surrounding structures, especially the cranial base, primary defects of the forebrain often manifest externally as facial malformations, typically a reduction in tissue of the frontonasal process.

In extreme cases, holoprosencephaly can take the form of cyclopia (see Figure 8-16), in which the near absence

*Continued*

FIGURE 14-20 Varying degrees of frontonasal dysplasia. (Courtesy A. Burdi, Ann Arbor, Mich.)

of upper and midfacial tissue results in a convergence and fusion of the optic primordia. Reduction defects of the nose can also be components of this condition. The nose can be either absent or represented by a tubular **proboscis** (or two such structures), sometimes even located above the eye (see Figure 8-16). Midline defects of the upper lip can also be attributed to holoprosencephaly (see Figure 14-19, C).

Some cases of holoprosencephaly (e.g., **Meckel's syndrome**, which includes midline cleft lip, olfactory bulb absence or hypoplasia, and nasal abnormalities) can be attributed to genetic causes. Meckel's syndrome is an autosomal recessive condition. Recent research has shown that several types of hereditary holoprosencephaly result from mutations of the **sonic hedgehog** gene, which normally induces the formation of a number of midline structures in the forebrain. In their absence, normally bilateral primordia, such as the optic fields, fuse, resulting in varying degrees of cyclopia. Exposure to an excess of retinoic acid, which causes misregulation of genes in the sonic hedgehog pathway, also causes holoprosencephaly in laboratory animals and possibly in humans as well. Most cases of holoprosencephaly appear to be multifactorial, although maternal consumption of alcohol during the first month of pregnancy is suspected to be a leading cause of this condition. As many as 1% to 2% of infants born to diabetic mothers develop some degree of holoprosencephaly. Trisomies of chromosomes 13 and 18 are commonly associated with holoprosencephaly.

## FRONTONASAL DYSPLASIA

Frontonasal dysplasia encompasses various nasal malformations that result from an excess of tissue in the frontonasal process. The spectrum of anomalies usually includes a broad nasal bridge and **hypertelorism** (an excessive distance between the eyes). In very severe cases the two external nares are separated, often by several centimeters, and a median cleft lip can also occur (Figure 14-20).

## ABNORMALITIES OF THE TEETH

A wide variety of conditions affect the teeth. Some are abnormalities of pattern, which could be a reflection of abnormal morphogenetic instructions of the early neural crest or secondary to growth defects of the jaw. Abnormal morphogenesis of individual teeth is common, with frequent variations including extra or distorted roots, enamel "pearls" (small masses of enamel) along the tooth, and abnormally shaped crowns. At a different level are **amelogenesis imperfecta** and **dentinogenesis imperfecta.** These rare genetic conditions are characterized by a defect in expression of one or more matrix proteins of the enamel or dentin. Progress is being made in identifying the specific genes that are defective in these conditions. For example, a single point mutation in Msx-1 has been found in individuals who lack all permanent second premolars and third molars. Knockouts of many of the genes that are important in early tooth development result in deficient or absent tooth formation.

## Pharyngeal arch structures

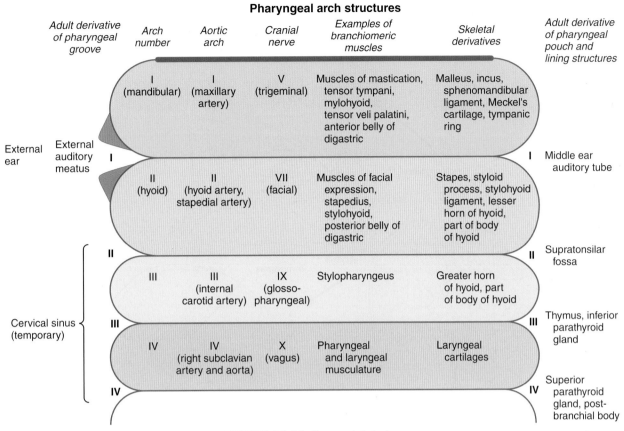

| Adult derivative of pharyngeal groove | Arch number | Aortic arch | Cranial nerve | Examples of branchiomeric muscles | Skeletal derivatives | Adult derivative of pharyngeal pouch and lining structures |
|---|---|---|---|---|---|---|
| External ear — External auditory meatus | I (mandibular) | I (maxillary artery) | V (trigeminal) | Muscles of mastication, tensor tympani, mylohyoid, tensor veli palatini, anterior belly of digastric | Malleus, incus, sphenomandibular ligament, Meckel's cartilage, tympanic ring | I — Middle ear auditory tube |
| | II (hyoid) | II (hyoid artery, stapedial artery) | VII (facial) | Muscles of facial expression, stapedius, stylohyoid, posterior belly of digastric | Stapes, styloid process, stylohyoid ligament, lesser horn of hyoid, part of body of hyoid | II — Supratonsilar fossa |
| Cervical sinus (temporary) | III | III (internal carotid artery) | IX (glosso-pharyngeal) | Stylopharyngeus | Greater horn of hyoid, part of body of hyoid | III — Thymus, inferior parathyroid gland |
| | IV | IV (right subclavian artery and aorta) | X (vagus) | Pharyngeal and laryngeal musculature | Laryngeal cartilages | IV — Superior parathyroid gland, post-branchial body |

**FIGURE 14-21** Pharyngeal derivatives.

populates it. The neural crest cells that populate the first arch are derived from rhombomeres 1 and 2 and midbrain, which are anterior to the expression domain of the *Hox* genes. Cellular precursors of the first arch mesenchyme are instead associated with the expression of Otx-2. The role of signaling molecules and transcription factors, such as Dlx and Msx, has been discussed earlier (see page 324).

The **second pharyngeal arch** (hyoid) also forms a string of skeletal structures from the body of the hyoid bone to the **stapes** of the middle ear. Although much of the second arch mesoderm migrates to the face to form the **muscles of facial expression**, additional muscles become associated with other second arch skeletal derivatives, a good example being the **stapedius muscle**, which is associated with the stapes bone. These second arch muscles are innervated by the facial nerve (VII).

Patterning of the second pharyngeal arch is strongly influenced by the homeobox gene *Hoxa-2*. When this gene is knocked out in mice, skeletal derivatives of the second arch fail to form. Interestingly, the second arch in such mutant animals contains mirror image duplicates of many of the proximal bones of the first arch skeleton. This may be a result of the response of the mutant second arch mesenchyme to an ectodermal signal from the first pharyngeal cleft that plays a role in patterning the first

arch. The formation of mirror image first arch structures is analogous to the formation of mirror image supernumerary limbs after transplantation of the zone of polarizing activity in the limb bud (see page 215). The fact that only proximal structures were affected reflects the different genetic control of proximal and distal segments of the arches.

The **third** and **fourth pharyngeal arches** are otherwise unnamed. The third arch gives rise to structures related to the hyoid bone and upper pharynx. The third arch skeleton becomes the greater horn of the hyoid bone. The one muscular derivative (stylopharyngeus) of the third arch is innervated by the glossopharyngeal nerve (IX). The fourth arch gives rise to certain muscles and cartilages of the larynx and lower pharynx. The muscles are innervated by the vagus nerve (X), which also grows into the thoracic and abdominal cavities.

### Pharyngeal Grooves

The first pharyngeal groove is the only one that persists as a recognizable adult structure: the **external auditory meatus**. Grooves II and III become covered by the enlarged external portion of the second arch (a phylogenetic homologue of the operculum [gill cover] of fish). The enlargement of the second arch is caused by the

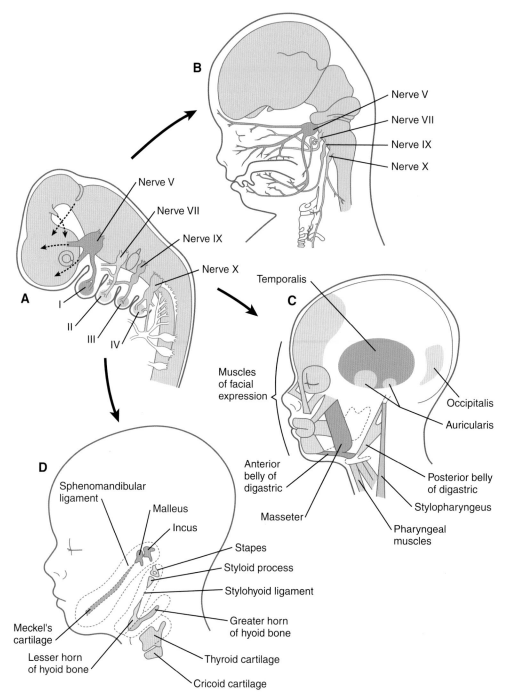

**FIGURE 14-22** Pharyngeal arch system **(A)** and adult derivatives of the neural **(B)**, muscular **(C)**, and skeletal **(D)** components of the arches.

presence of a signaling center in the ectoderm at its tip; such a signaling center is not present in arches 3 or 4. As in the facial primordia, this signaling center produces sonic hedgehog, FGF-8, and BMP-7, which stimulate growth of the underlying mesenchyme. During the period of their overshadowing by the hyoid (second) arch, grooves II and III are collectively known as the **cervical sinus** (Figure 14-23). As development progresses, the posterior ectoderm of the second arch fuses with ectoderm of a swelling (cardiac swelling) just posterior to the fourth arch, causing the cervical sinus to disappear and the external contours of the neck to become smooth.

## Pharynx and Pharyngeal Pouches

The embryonic pharynx is directly converted to the smooth-walled pharynx of the adult. Of greater develop-

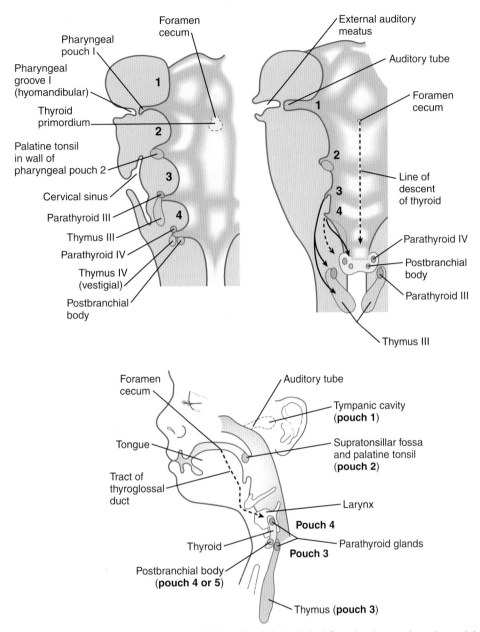

**FIGURE 14-23** Embryonic origins and pathways of primordia of glands derived from the pharyngeal pouches and the floor of the pharynx.

mental interest is the fate of the pharyngeal pouches and their lining epithelium.

As with their corresponding first pharyngeal clefts, the **first pharyngeal pouches** become intimately involved in the formation of the ear. The end of each pouch expands to become the **tympanic cavity** of the middle ear, and the remainder becomes the **auditory (eustachian) tube,** which connects the middle ear with the pharynx (see Figure 13-23).

The **second pharyngeal pouches** become shallower and less conspicuous as development progresses. Late in the fetal period, patches of lymphoid tissue form aggregations in the walls to create the **palatine (faucial) tonsils.**

The pouches themselves are represented only as the **supratonsillar fossae.**

The **third pharyngeal pouch** is a more complex structure, consisting of a solid, dorsal epithelial mass and a hollow, elongated ventral portion (see Figure 14-23). By the fifth week of gestation, cells identifiable as **parathyroid** tissue can be recognized in the endoderm of the solid dorsal mass. The ventral elongation of the third pouch differentiates into the epithelial portion of the **thymus gland.** The primordia of both the thymus and the parathyroid glands lose their connection with the third pharyngeal pouch and migrate caudally from their site of origin. Although the parathyroid III primordia initially comigrate with the thymic primordia, they ultimately continue to migrate toward the midline. There they join with the thyroid gland, passing the parathyroid primordia of the fourth pouch to form the **inferior parathyroid glands**. The third pharyngeal pouch disappears.

The **fourth pharyngeal pouch** is organized somewhat like the third, with a solid, bulbous, dorsal parathyroid IV primordium. It also contains a small ventral epithelial outpocketing, which contributes a minor component to the thymus in some species. In humans the thymic component of the fourth pouch is vestigial. At the ventralmost part of each fourth pouch is another structure called the **postbranchial (ultimobranchial) body** (see Figure 14-23).

Uncertainty surrounds the cellular origins and composition of the postbranchial bodies. Although according to one view the postbranchial bodies arise purely from pharyngeal endoderm, recent data suggest that neural crest cells migrate into the postbranchial bodies and ultimately become the secretory component of these structures.

As with their counterparts from the third pouch, the parathyroid IV primordia lose their connection with the fourth pouch and migrate toward the thyroid gland as the **superior parathyroid glands**. The postbranchial bodies also migrate toward the thyroid, where they become incorporated as **parafollicular** or **C cells**. The parafollicular cells, which are of neural crest origin, produce the polypeptide hormone **calcitonin**, which acts to reduce the concentration of calcium in the blood. The parathyroid glands produce **parathyroid hormone**, which causes an increase in blood calcium levels.

### Midline Structures Arising from the Pharynx

An unpaired primordium of the **thyroid gland** appears in the ventral midline of the pharynx between the first and second pouches (see Figure 14-23). Starting during the fourth week as an endodermal thickening just caudal to the median tongue bud (tuberculum impar), the thyroid primordium soon elongates to form a prominent downgrowth called the **thyroid diverticulum**. Caudal extension of the thyroid diverticulum continues during pharyngeal development. During its caudal migration, the tip of the thyroid diverticulum expands and bifurcates to form the thyroid gland itself, which consists of two main lobes connected by an isthmus. For some time the gland remains connected to its original site of origin by a narrow **thyroglossal duct**. By about the seventh week, when the thyroid has reached its final location at the level of the second and third tracheal cartilages, the thyroglossal duct has largely regressed. Nevertheless, in almost half the population the distal portion of the thyroglossal duct persists as the **pyramidal lobe of the thyroid**. The original site of the thyroid primordium persists as the **foramen cecum**, a small blind pit at the base of the tongue.

The thyroid gland undergoes histodifferentiation and begins functioning relatively early in embryonic development. By the tenth week of gestation, follicles containing some colloid material are evident, and a few weeks thereafter the gland begins to synthesize noniodinated **thyroglobulin**. Secretion of **triiodothyronine**, one of the forms of thyroid hormone, is detectable by late in the fourth month.

### Thymus and Lymphoid Organs

The paired endodermal thymic primordia begin to migrate from their third pharyngeal pouch origins during the sixth week. Their path of migration takes them through a substrate of mesenchymal cells until they reach the area of the future mediastinum behind the sternum. By the end of their migration, the two closely apposed thymic lobes are still epithelial structures. Soon, however, they become invested with a capsule of neural crest–derived connective tissue, which also forms septa among the endodermal epithelial cords. In the absence of neural crest the thymus fails to develop. Thus an interaction between the neural crest and endodermal components of the thymic primordia conditions the latter for subsequent differentiation of thymic structure and function.

At about 9 to 10 weeks' gestation, blood-borne thymocyte precursors (**prothymocytes**), which originate in the hematopoietic tissue, begin to invade the epithelial thymus, presumably in response to the secretion of peptides by the thymus. Just before the prothymocytes invade the thymus, the thymic epithelium begins to express the transcription factor **WHN**, which is necessary for colonization of the thymic epithelium by the prothrombocytes. In homozygous *whn* mutants the absence of such colonization results in the absence of functional T cells, leaving the individual severely immunocompromised and unable to reject foreign cells and tissue. Within the thymus the prothymocytes force apart the epithelial cells, causing them to form a spongy **epithelial reticulum**. Responding to signals from the thymic epithelium, the prothymocytes proliferate and redistribute, forming the cortical and medullary regions of the thymus. By 14 to 15 weeks, blood vessels grow into the thymus, and a week later, some epithelial cells aggregate into small, spherical **Hassal's corpuscles**. At this point the overall organization of the thymus is the same as that of adults. Functionally, the action of various **thymic hormones** causes the thymus to condition or instruct the prothymocytes migrating into it to become competent members of the **T lymphocyte** family. The T lymphocytes leave the thymus and populate other lymphoid organs (e.g., lymph nodes, spleen) as fully functional immune cells.

The T lymphocytes are principally involved in **cellular immune responses**. Another population of lymphocytes that also originates in the bone marrow is instructed to become **B lymphocytes**, which are the mediators of **humoral immune responses**. B lymphocyte precursors (**pro B cells**) must also undergo conditioning to become fully functional, but their conditioning does not occur in the thymus. In birds, the pro B cells pass through a cloacal lymphoid organ known as the **bursa of Fabricius**, where conditioning occurs. Humans do not possess a bursa, but its functional equivalent, although still not

defined, is assumed to exist. B lymphocyte conditioning is thought to occur in the bone marrow; in early embryos, conditioning possibly occurs in the liver.

The thymus and the bursa or mammalian equivalent are commonly referred to as **central lymphoid organs**. The lymphoid structures that are seeded by B and T lymphocytes are called **peripheral lymphoid organs**. (Figure 14-24 shows the development and function of the lymphoid system.)

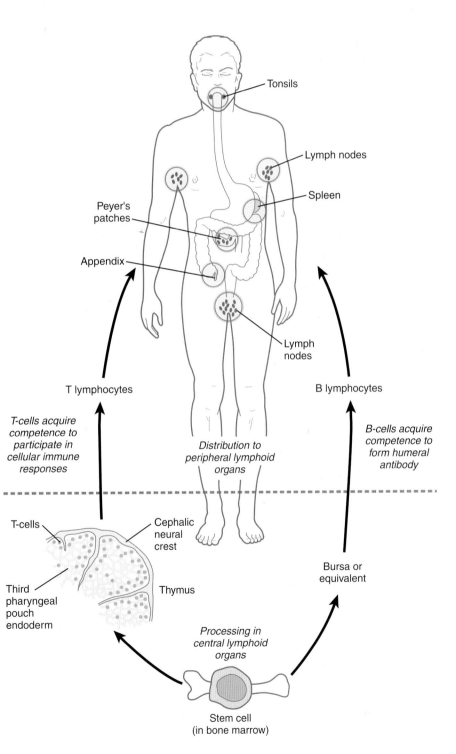

**FIGURE 14-24** Embryonic development of the lymphoid system.

### Formation of the Tongue

The tongue begins to take shape from a series of ventral swellings in the floor of the pharynx about the same time as the palate forms in the mouth. Major shifts in the positions of tissues of the tongue occur, making the characteristics of the adult form difficult to comprehend without knowledge of the basic elements of its embryonic development.

In 5-week-old embryos the tongue is represented by a pair of **lateral lingual swellings** in the ventral regions of the first pharyngeal arches and two median unpaired swellings. The **tuberculum impar** is located between the first and second arches, and the **copula** (yoke) unites the second and third arches (Figure 14-25, *A* and *B*). The foramen cecum, which marks the original location of the thyroid primordium, serves as a convenient landmark delineating the border between the original tuberculum impar and the copula. Caudal to the copula is another swelling that represents the **epiglottis**.

Growth of the body of the tongue is accomplished by a great expansion of the lateral lingual swellings, with a minor contribution by the tuberculum impar (Figure 14-25, *C* and *D*). The root of the tongue is derived from the copula along with additional ventromedial tissue between the third and fourth pharyngeal arches.

The dorsal surface of the tongue is covered with a large number of papillae. Development of the **filiform papillae**, which constitute the bulk of the papillae, follows a developmental course that is remarkably similar to that of hair follicles. The ectoderm, which surrounds a mesenchymal core, expresses Hoxc-13, as well as the signaling factors

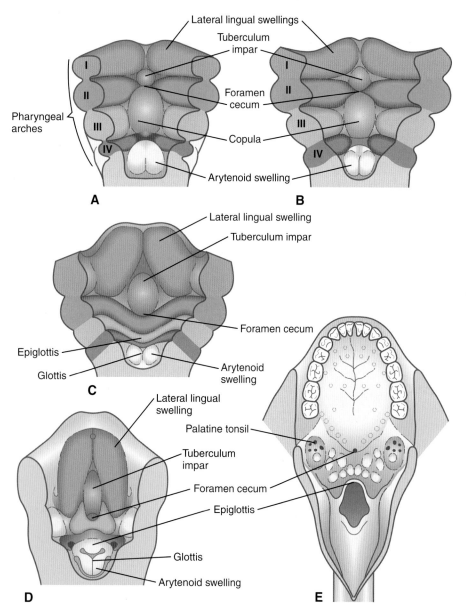

**FIGURE 14-25** Development of the tongue as seen from above. **A,** At **4 weeks. B,** Late in the **fifth week. C,** Early in the **sixth week. D,** Middle of the **seventh week. E,** Adult.

sonic hedgehog, BMP-2 and BMP-4, and FGF-8. These molecular components characterize the inductive signaling system in almost all ectodermal derivatives, including hairs, feathers, and teeth.

Corresponding to its innervation by the hypoglossal nerve (XII), the musculature of the tongue migrates from a considerable distance (the **occipital [postotic] myotomes**). Like their counterparts in the limb, the myoblasts express Pax-3 during their migration to the tongue. The general sensory innervation of the tongue accurately reflects the pharyngeal arch origins of the epithelium. Thus the lingual epithelium over the body of the tongue is innervated by the trigeminal nerve (V) in keeping with the first arch origins of the lateral lingual swellings. Correspondingly, the root of the tongue is innervated by the glossopharyngeal nerve (IX—third arch) and vagus nerve (X—fourth arch). The epithelium of the second arch is overgrown by that of the third arch; therefore there is no general sensory innervation of the tongue by the seventh nerve.

The seventh (facial) and ninth nerves innervate the taste buds. The contribution of the seventh nerve is facilitated by its chorda tympani branch, which joins with the lingual branch of the trigeminal nerve and thus has access to the body of the tongue. Taste buds appear during the seventh week of gestation. In contrast to an earlier hypothesis that they are induced by fibers of the visceral afferent nerves VII and IX, which innervate taste buds postnatally, recent evidence suggests that taste bud formation is nerve independent. An intrinsic signaling mechanism within the endodermal lingual epithelium, possibly mediated by a mechanism involving shh, Gli-1, and patched, appears to be the basis for the initial formation of taste buds. Once formed, taste buds become strongly dependent upon innervation for their maintenance. Considerable evidence indicates that the fetus is able to taste, and it has been postulated that the fetus uses the taste function to monitor its intraamniotic environment.

## CLINICAL VIGNETTE

A nervous-looking 23-year-old woman complains to her physician of feeling too hot, losing too much weight, and sweating more than she had previously. On physical examination, her skin is warm and fine in texture, she has a fine tremor of her fingers, and her eyes bulge slightly. As part of the diagnostic follow-up, she is given a dose of radioactive iodine; then scanning is performed to localize the iodine. The scans show that most of the radioactive iodine is localized to a small mass of tissue at the base of the tongue. A neoplastic growth in the tissue mass is diagnosed, but the location of the mass is attributed to a congenital malformation.

Explain the embryological basis for the location of the neoplastic growth.

## SUMMARY

○ The early craniofacial region arises from the rostral portions of the neural tube, the notochord, and the pharynx, which is surrounded by a series of paired aortic arches. Between the aortic arches and the overlying ectoderm are large masses of neural crest and mesodermally derived mesenchyme. A number of these components show evidence of anatomical segmentation or segmental patterns of gene expression.

○ Massive migrations of segmental groups of neural crest cells provide the mesenchyme for much of the facial region. The musculature of the craniofacial region is derived from somitomeric mesoderm or the occipital somites. The connective tissue component of the facial musculature is of neural crest origin.

○ The pharyngeal (branchial) region is organized around paired mesenchymal pharyngeal arches, which alternate with endodermally lined pharyngeal pouches and ectodermally lined pharyngeal grooves.

○ The face and lower jaw arise from an unpaired frontonasal prominence and paired nasomedial, maxillary, and mandibular processes. Through differential growth and fusion, the nasomedial processes form the upper jaw and lip, and the frontonasal prominence forms the upper part of the face. The expanding mandibular processes merge to form the lower jaw and lip. A nasolacrimal groove between the nasolateral and maxillary processes ultimately becomes canalized to form the nasolacrimal duct, which connects the orbit to the nasal cavity.

○ The palate arises from the fusion of an unpaired median palatine process and paired lateral palatine processes. The former forms the primary palate, and the latter forms the secondary palate. Fusion of the lateral palatal shelves involves removal of the midline epithelial seam by a combination of apoptosis, migration, and transformation of epithelial cells into mesenchyme.

○ The olfactory apparatus begins as a pair of thickened ectodermal nasal placodes. As these sink to form nasal pits, they are surrounded by horseshoe-shaped nasomedial and nasolateral processes. The former form the bridge and septum of the nose, and the nasolateral processes form the alae of the nose. The deepening nasal pits break into the oral cavity, and only later are the nasal cavities separated from the oral cavity by the palate.

○ The salivary glands arise as epithelial outgrowths of the oral epithelium. Through a series of continuing interactions with the surrounding mesenchyme, the expanding glandular epithelium branches and differentiates.

○ Teeth form from interactions between oral ectoderm (dental lamina) and neural crest mesenchyme. A

## SYNDROMES INVOLVING THE FIRST PHARYNGEAL ARCH

Several syndromes involve hypoplasia of the mandible and other structures arising from the first pharyngeal arch. A variety of mechanisms can account for them. Certainly, a number have a genetic basis, and others result from exposure to environmental teratogens. The numerous studies on genetically manipulated mice are beginning to produce malformations that may have human counterparts. With the fine balance of signaling molecules and transcription factors that are involved in the development of the pharyngeal arches, it is not surprising that disturbances in the function of single genes, whether through mutation or the action of teratogens, can result in a visible morphological anomaly. For example, hypoplasia of the lower face has been associated with the ingestion of isotretinoin (a vitamin A derivative used for the treatment of acne) during early pregnancy.

The **Pierre Robin syndrome** involves extreme **micrognathia** (small mandible), cleft palate, and associated defects of the ear. An imbalance often exists between the size of the tongue and the very hypoplastic jaw, which can lead to respiratory distress caused by mechanical interference of the pharyngeal airway by the relatively large tongue. Although many cases of Pierre Robin syndrome are sporadic, others appear to have a genetic basis.

**Treacher Collins syndrome (mandibulofacial dysostosis)** is typically inherited as an autosomal dominant condition. The responsible gene, called *Treacle*, has recently been identified. It includes a wide variety of anomalies, not all of which are found in the same patient. Common components of the syndrome include hypoplasia of the mandible and facial bones, malformations of the external and middle ears, high or cleft palate, faulty den-

tition, and coloboma-type defects of the lower eyelid (Figure 14-26).

The most extreme form of first arch hypoplasia is **agnathia**, in which the lower jaw basically fails to form (Figure 14-27). In severe agnathia the external ears remain in the ventral cervical region and may even join in the ventral midline.

## LATERAL CYSTS, SINUSES, AND FISTULAS

Structural malformations such as lateral cysts, sinuses, and fistulas can be related directly to the abnormal persistence of pharyngeal grooves, pharyngeal pouches, or both. A **cyst** is a completely enclosed, epithelially lined cavity that may be derived from the persistence of part of a pharyngeal pouch, a pharyngeal groove, or a cervical sinus. A **sinus** is closed on one end and open to the outside or to the pharynx. A **fistula** (Latin for "pipe") is an epithelially lined tube that is open at both ends—in this case to the outside and to the pharynx.

The postnatal location of these structures accurately marks the location of their embryonic precursors. External openings of fistulas are typically found anterior to the sternocleidomastoid muscle in the neck (Figure 14-28). Fistulas from remnants of pharyngeal grooves II or III may result from incomplete closure of the cervical sinus by tissue of the hyoid arch. Although present from birth, cervical cysts are often not manifested until after puberty. At that time they expand because of increased amounts of secretions by the epithelium that lines the inner surface of the cyst, corresponding to maturational changes in the normal epidermis.

**Preauricular sinuses** or **fistulas**, which are found in a triangular region in front of the ear, are also common. These structures are assumed to represent persistent clefts between preauricular hillocks on the first and second arches.

**FIGURE 14-26** Siblings with Treacher Collins syndrome. (Courtesy A. Burdi, Ann Arbor, Mich.)

**FIGURE 14-27** Agnathia. **A,** Ventral view of the upturned face of an infant. **B,** Lateral view of the face of a fetus with agnathia. Note the cervical location of the external ears. (Courtesy M. Barr, Ann Arbor, Mich.)

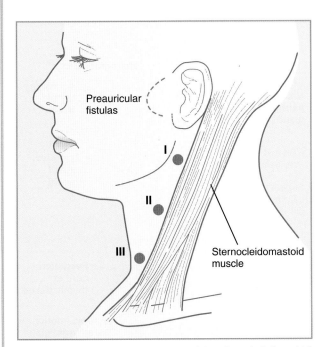

**FIGURE 14-28** Common locations of lateral cervical (branchial) cysts and sinuses *(red circles)* and preauricular fistulas. The roman numerals refer to the cervical cleft origin of the cysts.

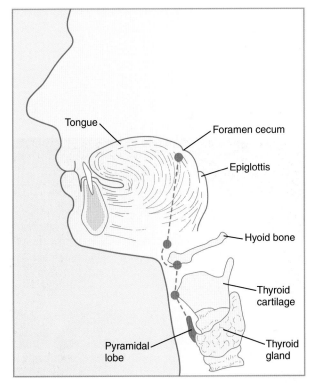

**FIGURE 14-29** Common locations *(red circles)* of thyroglossal duct remnants.

True fistulas (**cervicoaural fistulas**) represent persisting ventral portions of the first pharyngeal groove. These extend from a pharyngeal opening to somewhere along the auditory tube or even the external auditory meatus.

## THYROGLOSSAL DUCT REMNANTS

Various abnormal structures can persist along the pathway of the thyroglossal duct. **Ectopic thyroid tissue**

can be found anywhere along the pathway of migration of the thyroid primordium from the foramen cecum in the tongue to the isthmus of the normal thyroid gland (Figure 14-29). This fact must be considered in the clinical diagnosis or surgical treatment of carcinomas and other conditions affecting thyroid tissue. Less common are midline cysts or sinuses involving the former thyroglossal duct (Figure 14-30). Because of their location, they can usually be easily distinguished from their lateral cervical counterparts.

## MALFORMATIONS OF THE TONGUE

The most common malformation of the tongue is **ankyloglossia** (tongue-tie). This condition is caused by less-than-normal regression of the **frenulum**, the thin midline tissue that connects the ventral surface of the tongue to the floor of the mouth. Less common malformations of the tongue are **macroglossia** and **microglossia**, which are characterized by hyperplasia and hypoplasia of lingual tissue, respectively.

## ECTOPIC PARATHYROID OR THYMIC TISSUE

Because of their extensive migrations during early embryogenesis, parathyroid glands and components of

the thymus gland are often found in abnormal sites (Figure 14-31). Typically, this displacement is not accompanied by functional abnormalities, but awareness of the possibility of ectopic tissue or even supernumerary parathyroid glands is important for the surgeon.

## DIGEORGE SYNDROME

DiGeorge syndrome is a cranial neural crest deficiency and is manifest by immunological defects and hypoparathyroidism (see Box 12-1). The underlying pathological condition is failure of differentiation of the thymus and parathyroid glands. Associated anomalies are malformations of first arch structures and defects of the outflow tract of the heart, which contains an important cranial neural crest contribution as well. Hoxa-3 mutant mice exhibit many of the characteristics of the human DiGeorge syndrome.

FIGURE 14-30 Individual with a thyroglossal duct sinus in the ventral midline of the neck. (Courtesy A. Burdi, Ann Arbor, Mich.)

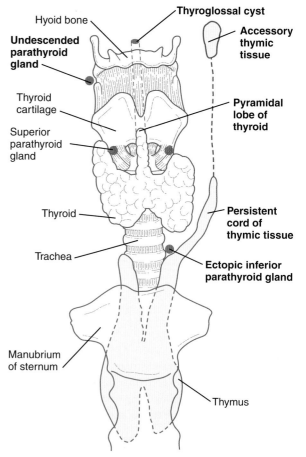

FIGURE 14-31 Locations where abnormally positioned pharyngeal glands or portions of glands can be found.

developing tooth is first a tooth bud, which then passes through a cap and bell stage. Late in the bell stage, ectodermal cells (ameloblasts) of the epithelial enamel organ begin to form enamel, and the neural crest–derived epithelium (odontoblasts) begins to secrete dentin. Precursors of the permanent teeth form dental primordia along the more advanced primary teeth.

◯ Malformations of the face are relatively common. Many, such as cleft lip and cleft palate, represent the persistence of the structural arrangements that are normal for earlier embryonic stages. Others, such as holoprosencephaly and hypertelorism, result from growth disturbances in the frontonasal process. Most facial malformations appear to be multifactorial in origin, involving both genetic susceptibility and environmental causes.

◯ Components of the pharynx (pharyngeal grooves, pharyngeal arches, and pharyngeal pouches) give rise to a wide variety of structures. The first arch gives rise to the upper and lower jaws and associated structures. The first groove and pouch, along with associated mesenchyme from the first and second arches, form the many structures of the external and middle ear. The second, third, and fourth pharyngeal grooves become obliterated and form the outer surface of the neck, and the components of the second through fourth arches form the pharyngeal skeleton and much of the musculature and connective tissue of the pharyngeal part of the neck. The endoderm of the third and fourth pouches forms the thymus and parathyroid glands. The thyroid gland arises from an unpaired ventral endodermal outgrowth of the upper pharynx.

◯ The tongue originates from multiple ventral swellings in the floor of the pharynx. The bulk of the tongue comes from the paired lateral lingual swellings in the region of the first pharyngeal arches. The unpaired tuberculum impar and copula also contribute to the formation of the tongue. The tongue musculature, along with the hypoglossal nerve (cranial nerve XII), which supplies the muscles, arises from the occipital somites. General sensory innervation of the tongue (from cranial nerves V, IX, and X) corresponds with the embryological origin of the innervated part of the tongue. Cranial nerves VII and IX innervate the taste buds on the tongue.

◯ Many malformations of the lower face and jaw are related to hypoplasia of the first pharyngeal arches. Cysts, sinuses, and fistulas of the neck are commonly caused by abnormal persistence of pharyngeal grooves or pouches. Ectopic glandular tissue (thyroid, thymus, or parathyroid) is explained by the persistence of tissue rests along the pathway of migration of the glands. Certain syndromes (e.g., DiGeorge syndrome), which seemingly affect disparate organs, can be attributed to neural crest defects.

## Review Questions

1. The facial (VII) nerve supplies muscles derived from which pharyngeal arch?
   A. First
   B. Second
   C. Third
   D. Fourth
   E. Sixth

2. Cleft lip results from lack of fusion of the:
   A. Nasomedial and nasolateral processes
   B. Nasomedial and maxillary processes
   C. Nasolateral and maxillary processes
   D. Nasolateral and mandibular processes
   E. Nasomedial and mandibular processes

3. In cases of holoprosencephaly, defects of facial structures are typically secondary to defects of the:
   A. Pharynx
   B. Oral cavity
   C. Forebrain
   D. Eyes
   E. Hindbrain

4. Meckel's cartilage is a prominent structure in the early formation of the:
   A. Upper jaw
   B. Hard palate
   C. Nasal septum
   D. Soft palate
   E. Lower jaw

5. An early induction in tooth development consists of the ectoderm of the dental epithelium acting on the underlying neural crest mesenchyme. Which of the following molecules is an important mediator of the inductive stimulus?
   A. BMP-4
   B. Tenascin
   C. Hoxb-13
   D. Msx-1
   E. Syndecan

6. A 15-year-old boy with mild acne developed a tender boil along the anterior border of the sternocleidomastoid muscle. What embryological condition would be included in a differential diagnosis?

7. The physician of the 15-year-old boy determined that the boy had a congenital cyst that needed to be removed surgically. What should the surgeon consider during removal of the cyst?

8. Why does a person sometimes get a runny nose when crying?

9. A woman who took an anticonvulsant drug during the tenth week of pregnancy gave birth to an infant with bilateral cleft lip and cleft palate. She sued the physician, blaming the facial malformations on the drug, and you are called in as an expert witness for the defense. What would be the basis for your case?

10. A woman who averaged three mixed drinks a day during pregnancy gave birth to an infant who was mildly retarded and who had a small notch in an upturned upper lip and a reduced olfactory sensitivity. What is the basis for this constellation of defects?

## REFERENCES

Barlow LA: A taste for development, *Neuron* 22:209–212, 1999.

Belloni E and others: Identification of sonic hedgehog as a candidate gene responsible for holoprosencephaly, *Nature Genet* 14:353–356, 1996.

Brickell P, Thorogood P: Retinoic acid and retinoic acid receptors in craniofacial development, *Semin Cell Dev Biol* 8:437–443, 1997.

Burdi AR: Sexual differences in closure of the human palatal shelves, *Cleft Palate J* 6:1–7, 1969.

Carstens MH: Development of the facial midline, *J Craniofacial Surg* 13:129–187, 2002.

Cohen MM, Shiota K: Teratogenesis of holoprosencephaly, *Am J Med Genet* 109:1–15, 2002.

Couly G and others: Interactions between Hox-negative cephalic neural crest cells and the foregut endoderm in patterning the facial skeleton in the vertebrate head, *Development* 129:1061–1082, 2002.

Dassule HR and others: Sonic hedgehog regulates growth and morphogenesis of the tooth, *Development* 127:4775–4785, 2000.

Depew MJ, Tucker AS, Sharpe PT: Craniofacial development. In Rossant J, Tam PPL, eds: *Mouse Development*, San Diego, 2002, Academic Press, pp 421–498.

Depew MJ, Lufkin T, Rubenstein JLR: Specification of jaw subdivisions by *Dlx* genes, *Science* 298:381–385, 2002.

Dixon MJ: Treacher Collins syndrome: an example of a craniofacial development defect, *Semin Dev Biol* 5:283–291, 1994.

Francis-West P and others: Signalling interactions during facial development, *Mech Devel* 75:3–28, 1998.

Gans C, Northcutt RG: Neural crest and the origin of vertebrates: a new head, *Science* 220:268–274, 1983.

Gendron-Maguire M and others: Hoxa-2 mutant mice exhibit homeotic transformation of skeletal elements derived from cranial neural crest, *Cell* 75:1317–1331, 1993.

Grindley JC, Davidson DR, Hill RE: The role of Pax-6 in eye and nasal development, *Development* 121:1433–1442, 1995.

Grobstein C: Epithelio-mesenchymal specificity in the morphogenesis of mouse submandibular rudiments in vitro, *J Exp Zool* 124:383–413, 1953.

Hanken J, Hall BK, eds: *The skull*, vol 1, *Development*, Chicago, 1993, University of Chicago Press.

Helms JA and others: Sonic hedgehog participates in craniofacial morphogenesis and is down-regulated by teratogenic doses of retinoic acid, *Dev Biol* 187:25–35, 1997.

Hieda Y, Nakanishi Y: Epithelial morphogenesis in mouse embryonic submandibular gland: its relationship to the tissue organization of epithelium and mesenchyme, *Dev Growth Differentiation* 39:1–8, 1997.

Hu P, Helms JA: The role of sonic hedgehog in normal and abnormal craniofacial morphogenesis, *Development* 126:4873–4884, 1999.

Jirásek JE: *Atlas of human prenatal morphogenesis*, Amsterdam, 1983, Martinus Nijhoff.

Kramer PR, Wray S: Midline nasal tissue influences nestin expression in nasal-placode-derived luteinizing hormone-releasing hormone neurons during development, *Devel Biol* 227:343–357, 2000.

Kraus P, Lufkin T: Mammalian *Dlx* homeobox gene control of craniofacial and inner ear morphogenesis, *J Cell Biochem Suppl* 32/33:133–140, 1999.

Kumoi T, Nishimura Y, Shiota K: The embryonic development of the human anterior nasal aperture, *Acta Otolaryngol* 113:93–97, 1993.

Kuratani S, Matsuo I, Aizawa S: Developmental patterning and evolution of the mammalian viscerocranium: genetic insights into comparative morphology, *Dev Dynam* 209:139–155, 1997.

Lee S-H and others: Noggin and retinoic acid transform the identity of avian facial prominences, *Nature* 414:909–912, 2001.

Lidral AC, Reising BC: The role of Msx1 in human tooth agenesis, *J Dent Res* 81:274–278, 2002.

Manley NR, Capecchi MR: The role of Hoxa-3 in mouse thymus and thyroid development, *Development* 121:1989–2003, 1995.

Matsuo I and others: Mouse Otx2 functions in the formation and patterning of rostral head, *Genes Dev* 9:2646–2658, 1995.

Mazzola RF: Congenital malformations in the frontonasal area: their pathogenesis and classification, *Clin Plast Surg* 3:573–609, 1976.

Merida-Velasco JR and others: Development of the human temporomandibular joint, *Anat Rec* 255:20–33, 1999.

Mina M and others: Experimental analysis of *Msx-1* and *Msx-2* gene expression during chick mandibular morphogenesis, *Dev Dynam* 202:195–214, 1995.

Mina M and others: Region- and stage-specific effects of FGFs and BMPs in chick mandibular morphogenesis, *Devel Dyn* 223:333–352, 2002.

Mombaerts P, ed: Development of the olfactory system, *Semin Cell Dev Biol* 8:151–213, 1997.

Muenke M, Cohen MM: Genetic approaches to understanding brain development: holoprosencephaly as a model, *Mental Retard Devel Disabil Res Rev* 6:15–21, 2000.

Nehls M and others: Two genetically separable steps in the differentiation of thymic epithelium, *Science* 272:886–889, 1996.

Neubuser A and others: Antagonistic interactions between FGF and BMP signaling pathways: a mechanism for positioning the sites of tooth formation, *Cell* 90:247–255, 1997.

Noden DM: Cell movements and control of patterned tissue assembly during craniofacial development, *J Craniofac Genet Dev Biol* 11:192–213, 1991.

Noden DM: Vertebrate craniofacial development: the relation between ontogenetic process and morphological outcome, *Brain Behav Evol* 38:190–225, 1991.

Osumi-Yamashita N: Retinoic acid and mammalian craniofacial morphogenesis, *J Biosci* 21:313–327, 1996.

Richman JM and others: Effect of fibroblast growth factors on outgrowth of facial mesenchyme, *Development* 189:135–147, 1997.

Rijli FM and others: A homeotic transformation is generated in the rostral branchial region of the head by disruption of *Hoxa-2*, which acts as a selector gene, *Cell* 75:1333–1349, 1993.

Ruch JV, Lesot H, Begue-Kirn C: Odontoblast differentiation, *Int J Dev Biol* 39:51–68, 1995.

Salzer GM, Zenker W: Das juxtaorale Organ, *Bibl Anat* 3:1–113, 1962.

Schneider RA and others: Local retinoid signaling coordinates forebrain and facial morphogenesis by maintaining FGF8 and SHH, *Development* 128:2755–2767, 2002.

Smith KK, Schneider RA: Have gene knockouts caused evolutionary reversals in the mammalian first arch? *BioEssays* 20:245–255, 1998.

Smith TD, Bhatnagar KP: The human vomeronasal organ. Part II: Prenatal development, *J Anat* 197:421–436, 2000.

Sperber GH: *Craniofacial embryology*, ed 4, London, 1989, Butterworth.

Stock DW, Weiss KM, Zhao Z: Patterning of the mammalian dentition in development and evolution, *BioEssays* 19:481–490, 1997.

Stricker M and others, eds: *Craniofacial malformations*, Edinburgh, 1990, Churchill Livingstone.

Ten Berge D and others: *Prx1* and *Prx2* are upstream regulators of sonic hedgehog and control cell proliferation during mandibular arch morphogenesis, *Development* 128:2929–2938, 2001.

Thesleff I and others: Molecular mechanisms of cell and tissue interactions during early tooth development, *Anat Rec* 245:151–161, 1996.

Thesleff I, Jernvall J: The enamel knot: A putative signaling center regulating tooth development, *Cold Spring Harbor Symp Quant Biol* 62:257–267, 1997.

Thesleff I, Mikkola M: The role of growth factors in tooth development, *Internat Rev Cytol* 217:93–135, 2002.

Thesleff I, Sharpe P: Signalling networks regulating dental development, *Mech Devel* 67:111–123, 1997.

Thorogood P, Tickle C, eds: Craniofacial development, *Development* 103(suppl):1–257, 1988.

Tolarova MM, Cervenka J: Classification and birth prevalence of orofacial clefts, *Am J Med Genet* 75:126–137, 1998.

Tucker AS and others: Fgf-8 determines rostral-caudal polarity in the first branchial arch, *Development* 126:51–61, 1998.

Tucker AS, Matthews KL, Sharpe PT: Transformation of tooth type induced by inhibition of BMP signaling, *Science* 282:1136–1138, 1998.

Tucker AS, Sharpe PT: Molecular genetics of tooth morphogenesis and patterning: the right shape in the right place, *J Dent Res* 78:826–834, 1999.

Wendling O and others: Retinoid signaling is essential for patterning the endoderm of the third and fourth pharyngeal arches, *Development* 127:1553–1562, 2000.

Whiting J: Craniofacial abnormalities induced by the ectopic expression of homeobox genes, *Mutation Res* 396:97–112, 1997.

Xu P-X and others: *Eya1* is required for the morphogenesis of mammalian thymus, parathyroid and thyroid, *Development* 129:3033–3044, 2002.

Young DL: Genetic and teratogenic approaches to craniofacial development, *Crit Rev Oral Biol Med* 11(3):304–317, 2000.

Zeichner-David M and others: Control of ameloblast differentiation, *Int J Dev Biol* 39:69–92, 1995.

Zhang Z and others: Rescue of cleft palate in *Msx1*-deficient mice by transgenic *Bmp4* reveals a network of BMP and Shh signaling in the regulation of mammalian palatogenesis, *Development* 129:4135–4146, 2002.

Zimmerman EF, ed: Palate development: normal and abnormal, cellular and molecular aspects, *Curr Top Dev Biol* 19:1–243, 1984.

# CHAPTER 15

# Digestive and Respiratory Systems and Body Cavities

The initial formation of the digestive system by the lateral folding of the endodermal germ layer into a tube is described in Chapter 6. From its beginnings as a simple tubular gut, development of the digestive system proceeds on several levels. These include molecular patterning, elongation and morphogenesis of the digestive tube itself, inductions and tissue interactions leading to the formation of the digestive glands, and the biochemical maturation of the secretory and absorptive epithelia associated with the digestive tract. Clinical Correlations 15-1 to 15-3 discuss malformations associated with the digestive system.

Formation of the respiratory system begins with a very unimposing ventral outpocketing of the foregut. Soon, however, this outpocketing embarks on a unique course of development while still following some of the basic patterns of epithelial-mesenchymal interactions characteristic of other gut-associated glands. Initially, both the digestive and respiratory systems form in a common body cavity, but functional considerations later necessitate the division of this primitive body cavity. Clinical Correlation 15-4 presents malformations associated with the respiratory system. Clinical Correlation 15-5 discusses malformations related to other body cavities.

## DIGESTIVE SYSTEM

Chapter 6 describes the formation of the primitive endodermal digestive tube, which is bounded at its cephalic end by the **oropharyngeal membrane** and at its caudal

end by the **cloacal plate** (see Figure 6-18). Because of its intimate relationship with the yolk sac through the **yolk stalk,** the gut can be divided into a **foregut,** an open-bottomed **midgut,** and a **hindgut.**

Like the nervous system, patterning of the regions of the digestive system is based upon the orderly expression of groups of homeobox-containing genes (Figure 15-1). Mice bearing mutant copies of some of these genes develop several of the common structural malformations of the digestive tract that occur in humans. Development of the gut tube proper involves continuous elongation, herniation past the body wall, and rotation and folding for efficient packing into the body cavity, as well as histogenesis and later functional maturation.

As early as the end of the first month, small endodermal diverticula, which represent primordia of the major digestive glands, can be identified (Figure 15-2). (Development of the pharynx and its glandular derivatives is discussed in Chapter 14.) The digestive glands and respiratory structures grow in complex branching patterns, resembling fractals, as the result of continuous epithelial-mesenchymal interactions. These interactions also occur in the developing digestive tube itself, with specific regional mesenchymal influences determining the character of the epithelium lining that part of the digestive tract.

### Formation of the Esophagus

Just caudal to the most posterior pharyngeal pouches of the 4-week-old embryo the pharynx becomes abruptly

**FIGURE 15-1** *Hox* gene expression along the developing digestive tract. Expression along the gut endoderm *(right)* and in the gut-associated mesoderm *(left)*. The circles represent areas where sphincters are located.

narrowed, and a small ventral outgrowth (lung bud) appears (see Figure 6-18). The region of foregut just caudal to the lung bud is the **esophagus**. This segment is initially very short, with the stomach seeming to reach almost to the pharynx. In the second month of development, during which the gut elongates considerably, the esophagus assumes nearly postnatal proportions in relation to the location of the stomach.

Although the esophagus grossly resembles a simple tube, it undergoes a series of striking differentiative changes at the tissue level. In its earliest stages the endodermal lining epithelium of the esophagus is stratified columnar. By the eighth week the epithelium has partially occluded the lumen of the esophagus, and large vacuoles appear (Figure 15-3). In succeeding weeks the vacuoles coalesce, and the esophageal lumen recanalizes but with a multilayered ciliated epithelium. During the fourth month, this epithelium finally becomes replaced with the stratified squamous epithelium that characterizes the mature esophagus.

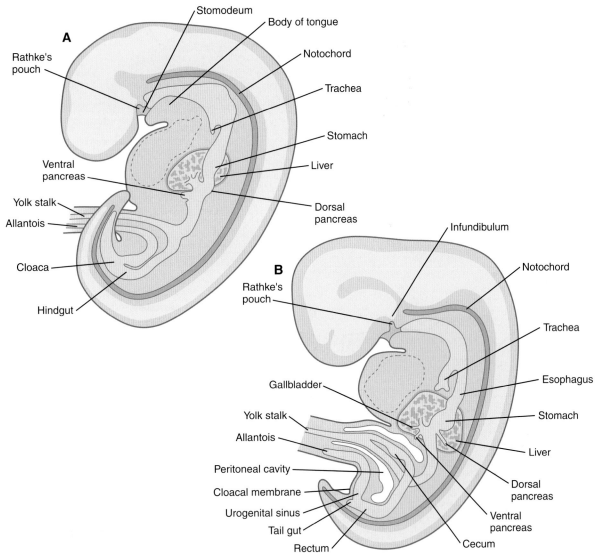

**FIGURE 15-2** Early stages in the formation of the digestive tract as seen in sagittal section. **A,** Early in the **fifth week. B,** Early in the **sixth week.**

Deeper in the esophageal wall, layers of muscle also differentiate in response to inductive signals from the gut endoderm. Very early (5 weeks' gestation) the primordium of the inner circular muscular layer of esophagus is recognizable, and by 8 weeks the outer longitudinal layer of muscle begins to take shape. The esophageal wall contains both smooth and skeletal muscle. The smooth muscle cells differentiate from the local splanchnic mesoderm associated with the gut. Experiments on mouse embryos have shown that the skeletal muscle cells in the esophageal wall arise by the direct transformation of existing smooth muscle cells into skeletal muscle.* This

conversion of phenotype is mediated by the expression of the myogenic regulatory factor, **myf-5** (see. p. 200) in the outer smooth muscle of the upper esophagus. All esophageal musculature is innervated by the vagus nerve (X).

The cross-sectional structure of the esophagus, like that of the rest of the gut, is organized into discrete layers. The innermost layer (**mucosa**) consists of the epithelium, derived from endoderm, and an underlying layer of connective tissue, the **lamina propria** (Figure 15-3, *C, D*). A thick layer of loose connective tissue (**submucosa**) separates the mucosa from the outer layers of muscle (usually smooth muscle, with the exception of the upper esophagus). This radial organization is regulated by the epithelial expression of **sonic hedgehog** (shh), acting through its receptor, **patched,** and bone morphogenetic protein-4 (**BMP-4**) in the underlying mesenchyme, but

* The direct transformation of one differentiated cell type to another is called **transdifferentiation**. Transdifferentiation is rare in vertebrates, occurring in processes such as regeneration of the lens from the dorsal iris or neural retina from pigmented retina in amphibians.

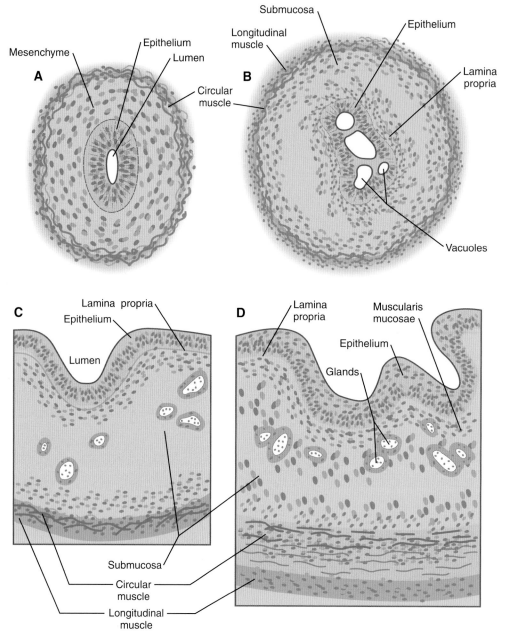

**FIGURE 15-3** Stages in the histogenesis of the esophagus. **A,** At **7 weeks. B,** At **8 weeks. C,** At **12 weeks. D,** At **34 weeks.**

the mechanism remains unclear. The net effect is the lack of differentiation of smooth muscle and enteric neurons in the mesenchyme close to the epithelium (the submucosa). Farther from the source of the endodermal shh, smooth muscle can differentiate in the outer wall of the intestine.

## Formation of the Stomach

Very early in the formation of the digestive tract the **stomach** is recognizable as a dilated region with a shape

remarkably similar to that of the adult stomach (see Figure 15-2). The early stomach is suspended from the dorsal body wall by a portion of the dorsal mesentery called the **dorsal mesogastrium**. It is connected to the ventral body wall by a ventral mesentery that also encloses the developing liver (Figure 15-4).

When the stomach first appears, its concave border faces ventrally, and its convex border faces dorsally. Two concomitant positional shifts bring the stomach to its adult configuration. The first is an approximately 90-degree rotation about its craniocaudal axis so that its originally dorsal convex border faces left and its ventral

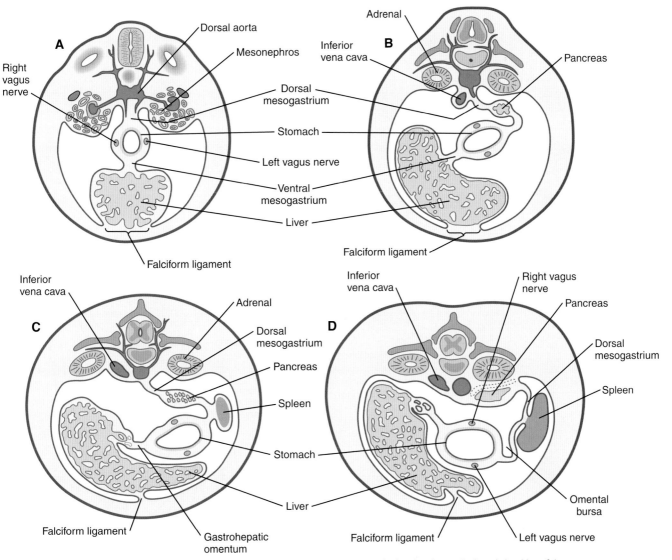

**FIGURE 15-4** Cross sections through the level of the developing stomach, showing changes in the relationships of the mesenteries as the stomach rotates.

concave border faces right. The other positional shift consists of a minor tipping of the caudal (pyloric) end of the stomach in a cranial direction so that the long axis of the stomach is positioned somewhat diagonally across the body (Figure 15-5).

During rotation of the stomach, the dorsal mesogastrium is carried with it, leading to the formation of a pouchlike structure called the **omental bursa** (*bursa* comes from a Latin word meaning "sac" or "pouch"). Both the spleen and the tail of the pancreas are embedded in the dorsal mesogastrium (see Figure 15-4).

The development of the **spleen** is very poorly understood. It is first recognizable in the dorsal mesogastrium at four weeks, and its normal left-sided location is determined early by the mechanisms that dictate heart asymmetry. In fact, the homeobox gene, *Nkx 2*, which is an important determinant of early heart development, is

a marker of splenic precursor cells. The spleen does not appear in mutants of the homeobox genes, *Barx-1* and *Hox-11*. The early splenic primordium consists of a condensation of mesenchyme covered by overlying mesothelium of the dorsal mesogastrium, both of which contribute to the stroma of the spleen. Later the splenic primordium becomes infiltrated with lymphoid cells, and by the fourth month the complex vascular structure of the red pulp begins to take shape. From the third to fifth months the spleen is an important site of embryonic hematopoiesis.

As the stomach rotates, the dorsal mesogastrium and the omental bursa that it encloses enlarge dramatically. Soon, part of the dorsal mesogastrium, which becomes the **greater omentum**, overhangs the transverse colon and portions of the small intestines as a large, double flap of fatty tissue (Figure 15-6). The two sides of the greater

**FIGURE 15-5** Stages in the development and rotation of the gut. **A,** At **5 weeks. B,** At **6 weeks. C,** At **11 weeks. D,** At **12 weeks. E,** Fetal period. Areas between the green lines represent the midgut, which is supplied by the superior mesenteric artery.

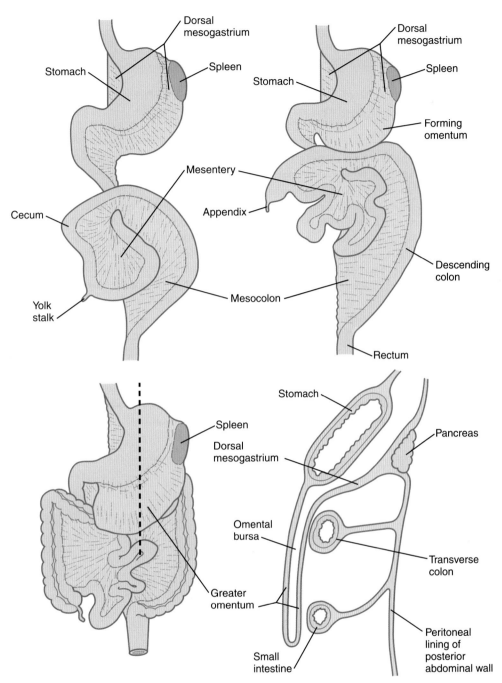

**FIGURE 15-6** Stages in the rotation of the stomach and intestines and development of the greater omentum. A section through the level of the dashed line *(lower left)* is shown *(lower right)*.

omentum ultimately fuse, obliterating the omental bursa within the greater omentum. The rapidly enlarging liver occupies an increasingly large portion of the ventral mesentery.

At the histological level the **gastric mucosa** begins to take shape late in the second month with the appearance of folds (**rugae**) and the first **gastric pits**. During the early fetal period, the individual cell types that characterize the gastric mucosa begin to differentiate. Biochemical and cytochemical studies have shown the gradual functional differentiation of specific cell types during the late fetal period. In most mammals, including humans, cells of the gastric mucosa begin to secrete hydrochloric acid shortly before birth.

The caudal end of the stomach is physiologically separated from the small intestine by the muscular **pyloric sphincter**. Formation of the pyloric sphincter is directed by the transcription factor **Nkx 2.5**, whose expression in the area of pyloric mesoderm is stimulated by BMP-4 signals. In addition, several *Hox* genes are needed to make

## Malformations of the Esophagus and Stomach

### ESOPHAGUS

The most common anomalies of the esophagus are associated with abnormalities of the developing respiratory tract (see p. 381). Other rather rare anomalies are **stenosis** and **atresia** of the esophagus. Stenosis is usually attributed to abnormal recanalization of the esophagus after epithelial occlusion of its lumen. Atresia of the esophagus is most commonly associated with abnormal development of the respiratory tract. In both of these conditions, impaired swallowing by the fetus can lead to an excessive accumulation of amniotic fluid (**polyhydramnios**). Just after birth a newborn with these anomalies commonly has difficulty swallowing milk, and regurgitation and choking while drinking are indications for examination of the patency of the esophagus.

### STOMACH

#### Pyloric Stenosis

Pyloric stenosis, which appears to be more physiological than anatomical, consists of hypertrophy of the circular layer of smooth muscle that surrounds the pyloric (outlet) end of the stomach. The hypertrophy causes a narrowing (stenosis) of the pyloric opening and impedes the passage of food. Several hours after a meal the infant violently vomits (**projectile vomiting**) the contents of that meal. The enlarged pyloric end of the stomach can often be palpated on physical examination. Although pyloric stenosis is commonly treated by a simple surgical incision through the layer of circular smooth muscle of the pylorus, the hypertrophy sometimes diminishes untreated by several weeks after birth. The pathogenesis of this defect remains unknown, but it seems to have a genetic basis. Pyloric stenosis is more common in males than in females, and the incidence has been reported as from 1 in 200 to 1 in 1000 infants.

#### Heterotopic Gastric Mucosa

Heterotopic gastric mucosa has been found in a variety of otherwise normal organs (Figure 15-7). This condition is often of clinical significance because if the heterotopic mucosa secretes hydrochloric acid, ulcers can form in unexpected locations.

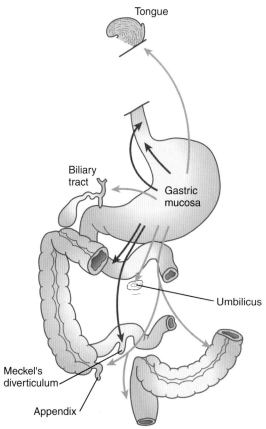

**FIGURE 15-7** Locations of heterotopic gastric tissue. The red arrows point to the most frequently occurring sites. The pink arrows indicate less common sites of occurrence. (Based on Gray SW, Skandalakis JE: *Embryology for surgeons*, Philadelphia, 1972, WB Saunders.)

each of the three major sphincters (pyloric, ileocecal, and anal) in the digestive tract.

## Formation of the Intestines

The intestines are formed from the posterior part of the foregut, the midgut, and the hindgut (Table 15-1). Table 15-2 summarizes the chronology of major stages in the development of the digestive tract. Two points of reference are useful in understanding the gross transformation of the primitive gut tube from a relatively straight cylinder to the complex folded arrangement characteristic of the adult intestinal tract. The first is the yolk stalk, which extends from the floor of the midgut to the yolk sac. In the adult the site of attachment of the yolk stalk is on the small intestine about 2 feet cranial to the junction between small and large intestine (**ileocecal junction**). On the dorsal side of the primitive gut an unpaired ventral branch of the aorta, the **superior mesenteric artery**, and its branches feed the midgut (see Figure 15-5). The superior mesenteric artery itself serves as a pivot point about which later rotation of the gut occurs.

As early as the fifth week, rapid growth of the gut tube causes it to buckle out in a hairpinlike loop. The major change that causes the intestines to assume their adult positions is a counterclockwise rotation of the caudal limb of the intestinal loop (with the yolk stalk attachment and superior mesenteric artery as reference points) around the cephalic limb from its ventral aspect. The main consequence of this rotation is to bring the future colon across

**TABLE 15-1** *Derivatives of Regions of the Primitive Gut*

| Blood supply | Adult derivatives |
|---|---|
| **FOREGUT** | |
| Celiac artery (lower esophagus to duodenum) | Pharynx<br>Esophagus<br>Stomach<br>Upper duodenum<br>Glands of pharyngeal pouches, respiratory tract, liver and gallbladder, pancreas |
| **MIDGUT** | |
| Superior mesenteric artery | Lower duodenum<br>Jejunum and ileum<br>Cecum and vermiform appendix<br>Ascending colon<br>Cranial half of transverse colon |
| **HINDGUT** | |
| Inferior mesenteric artery | Caudal half of transverse colon<br>Descending colon<br>Rectum<br>Superior part of anal canal |

**TABLE 15-2** *Timelines in Development of the Digestive System*

| Normal time | Developmental events |
|---|---|
| 3 weeks | Tubular gut begins to form; early induction of major digestive glands |
| 4 weeks | Most of gut tubular; primordia of liver, dorsal and ventral pancreas, and trachea visible; rupture of oropharyngeal membrane |
| 5 weeks | Expansion and early rotation of stomach; intestinal loop begins to form; cecum and bile duct evident |
| 6 weeks | Rotation of stomach completed, prominent intestinal loop; allantois and appendix appear; urorectal septum begins to subdivide cloaca into rectum and urogenital sinus |
| 7 weeks | Herniation of intestinal loop; rapid growth of liver; fusion of dorsal and ventral pancreas; cloacal septation complete |
| 8 weeks | Counterclockwise rotation of herniated intestinal loop; recanalization of intestine; early penetration of parasympathetic neuronal precursors from cranial neural crest into gut |
| 9 weeks | Return of herniated gut into the body cavity; differentiation of epithelial types in intestinal lining |
| 11 weeks | Villi appear in small intestine; differentiation of goblet cells. |
| 16 weeks | Villi line entire intestine (including colon) |
| 20 weeks | Peyer's patches seen in small intestine |

the small intestine so that it can readily assume its C-shaped position along the ventral abdominal wall (see Figure 15-5). Behind the colon the small intestine undergoes a great elongation and becomes packed in its characteristic position in the abdominal cavity.

The rotation and other positional changes of the gut occur partly because the length of the gut increases more than the length of the embryo. From almost the first stages the volume of the expanded gut tract is greater than the body cavity can accommodate. Consequently, the developing intestines herniate into the body stalk (the umbilical cord after further development) (Figure 15-8). Intestinal herniation begins as early as the sixth or seventh week of embryogenesis. By the ninth week the abdominal cavity has enlarged sufficiently to accommodate the intestinal tract, and the herniated intestinal loops begin to move through the intestinal ring back into the abdominal cavity. Coils of small intestine return first. As they do, they force the distal part of the colon, which was

**Week 6**

**Week 8**

**Week 9**

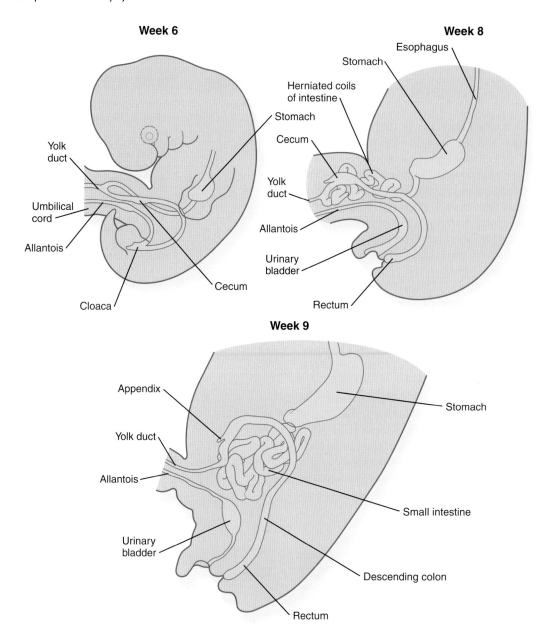

**FIGURE 15-8** Stages of herniation of the intestines into the body stalk and their return.

never herniated, to the left side of the peritoneal cavity, thus establishing the definitive position of the descending colon. After the small intestine has taken its intraabdominal position, the herniated proximal part of the colon also returns, with its cecal end swinging to the right and downward (see Figure 15-5).

During these coilings, herniations, and return movements, the intestines are suspended from the dorsal body wall by a mesentery (Figure 15-9). As the intestines assume their definitive positions within the body cavity, their mesenteries follow. Parts of the mesentery associated with the duodenum and colon (**mesoduodenum and mesocolon**) fuse with the peritoneal lining of the dorsal body wall.

Starting in the sixth week the primordium of the **cecum** becomes apparent as a swelling in the caudal limb of the midgut (see Figure 15-5). In succeeding weeks the cecal enlargement becomes so prominent that the distal small intestine enters the colon at a right angle. The sphincterlike boundary at the cecum between the small and large intestines, like that in other regions of the gut, is regulated by a sequence of *Hox* gene expression. In mice, deletion of *Hoxd-4*, *Hoxd-8* to *Hoxd-11*, and *Hoxd-13* results in the absence of this region.

The tip of the cecum elongates, but its diameter does not increase in proportion to the rest of the cecum. This wormlike appendage is aptly called the **vermiform appendix**.

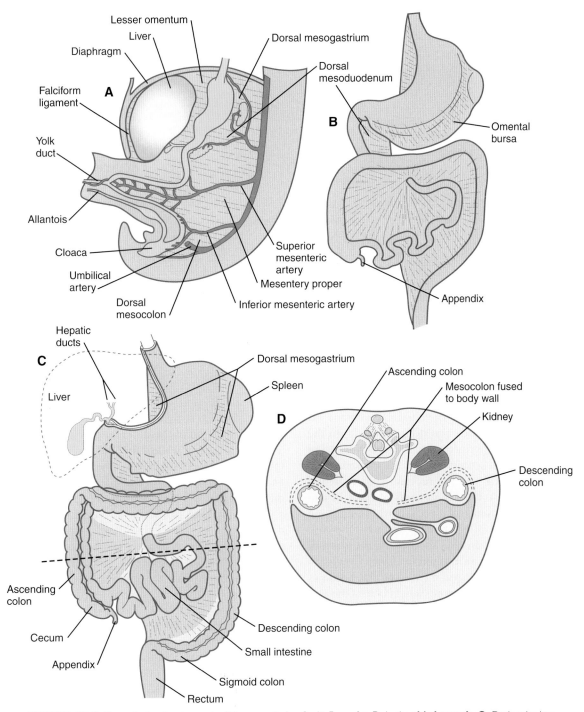

**FIGURE 15-9** Stages in the development of the mesenteries. **A,** At **5 weeks. B,** In the **third month. C,** During the late fetal period. **D,** Cross section through the dashed line in **C.** In **C,** the shaded areas represent regions where the mesentery is fused to the dorsal body wall.

## Partitioning of the Cloaca

In the early embryo the caudal end of the hindgut terminates in the endodermally lined **cloaca**, which in lower vertebrates serves as a common termination for the digestive and urogenital systems. The cloaca also includes the base of the allantois, which later expands as a common urogenital sinus (see Chapter 16). A **cloacal (proctodeal) membrane** consisting of apposed layers of ectoderm and endoderm acts as a barrier between the cloaca and an ectodermal depression known as the **proctodeum** (Figure 15-10). A shelf of mesodermal tissue called the **urorectal septum** is situated between the hindgut and the base of the allantois. During the sixth and seventh weeks, the

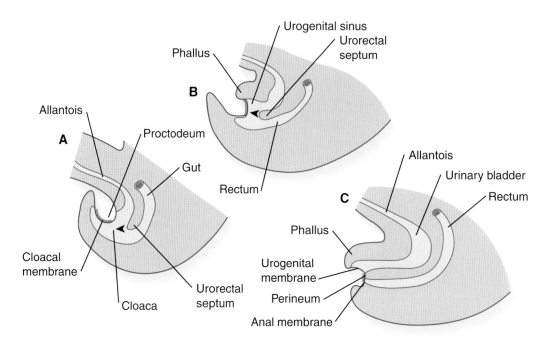

**FIGURE 15-10** Stages in the subdivision of the common cloaca by the urorectal septum. **A,** In the **fifth week. B,** In the **sixth week. C,** In the **eighth week.** The arrowheads indicate the direction of growth of the urorectal septum.

urorectal septum grows toward the cloacal membrane. At the same time, lateral mesodermal ridges extend into the cloaca. The combined ingrowth of the lateral ridges and growth of the urorectal septum toward the cloacal membrane divide the cloaca into the **rectum** and **urogenital sinus** (Figure 15-10, *B*). Double mutants of *Hoxa-13* and *Hoxd-13* result in the absence of cloacal partitioning along with hypodevelopment of the phallus (genital tubercle). In addition, they result in the absence of the smooth muscle component of the anal sphincter. Once the cloaca becomes partitioned, the cloacal membrane also becomes subdivided into an **anal membrane,** which blocks the end of the hindgut, and a **urogenital membrane,** which seals the urogenital sinus from the exterior. By the end of the eighth week the anal membrane ruptures and affords free access between the hindgut and the exterior of the body. The area where the urorectal septum and lateral mesodermal folds fuse with the cloacal membrane becomes the **perineal body,** which represents the partition between the digestive and urogenital systems.

### Histogenesis of the Intestinal Tract

Shortly after its initial formation the intestinal tract consists of a simple layer of columnar endodermal epithelium surrounded by a layer of splanchnopleural mesoderm. Three major phases are involved in the histogenesis of the intestinal epithelium: (1) an early phase of epithelial proliferation and morphogenesis, (2) an intermediate period of cellular differentiation in which the distinctive cell types characteristic of the intestinal epithelium

appear, and (3) a final phase of biochemical and functional maturation of the different types of epithelial cells. The mesenchymal wall of the intestine also differentiates into several layers of highly innervated smooth muscle and connective tissue. An overall craniocaudal gradient of differentiation is present within the developing intestine.

The endoderm of the early foregut is capable of producing cell types other than those of the gut tube itself, such as liver cells. A two-phase series of inhibitory influences from the gut mesoderm restricts the overlying endoderm to forming only the appropriate epithelial cell types through the activity of the transcription factors hepatic nuclear factor-3 (**HNF-3**) and **GATA-4,** which are essential for formation of anterior regions of endoderm.

Early in the second month the epithelium of the small intestine begins a phase of rapid proliferation that results in the epithelium temporarily occluding the lumen by 6 to 7 weeks' gestation. Within a couple of weeks, recanalization of the intestinal lumen has occurred. At about this time, small, cracklike secondary lumina appear beneath the surface of the multilayered epithelium, and aggregates of mesoderm push into the epithelium. A combination of coalescence of the secondary lumina with continued mesenchymal upgrowth beneath the epithelium results in the formation of numerous fingerlike **intestinal villi,** which greatly increase the absorptive surface of the intestinal surface. By this time the epithelium has transformed from a stratified into a simple columnar type.

With the formation of villi, pitlike **intestinal crypts** also form at the base of the villi. The crypts contain **epithelial stem cells,** which have a high rate of mitosis and serve as the source of epithelial cells for the entire intestinal surface (Figure 15-11). Experimental studies suggest that there are four to six stem cells per crypt. When a stem cell divides, one of the progeny retains stem cell qualities, and the other continues to proliferate as it migrates up the villus. Over 4 to 7 days, this cell continues to divide for approximately five more generations. As these descendents of the original stem cell move up the intestinal villus, they differentiate into four different mature cell types (see Figure 15-11). When they reach the tip of the villus, these cells die and are shed into the intestinal lumen. Human intestinal epithelial cells develop the intrinsic capacity for **apoptosis** by 18 to 20 weeks gestation.

By the end of the second trimester of pregnancy, all cell types found in the adult intestinal lining have differentiated, but many of these cells do not possess adult functional patterns. A number of specific biochemical patterns of differentiation are present as early as 12 weeks' gestation and mature during the fetal period. For example, **lactase**, an enzyme that breaks down the disaccharide **lactose** (milk sugar), is one of the digestive enzymes synthesized in the fetal period in anticipation of the early postnatal period during which the newborn subsists principally on the mother's milk. Further biochemical differentiation of the intestine occurs after birth, often in response to specific dietary patterns.

Histodifferentiation of the intestinal tract is not an isolated property of the individual tissue components of the intestinal wall. During the early embryonic period and sometimes into postnatal life the epithelial and mesodermal components of the intestinal wall communicate by inductive interactions. Interspecies recombination experiments show that the gut mesoderm exerts a regional influence on intestinal epithelial differentiation (e.g., whether the epithelium differentiates into a duodenal or colonic phenotype). Once regional determination is set, however, the controls for biochemical differentiation of the epithelium are inherent. This pattern of inductive influence and the epithelial reaction are very similar to those outlined earlier for dermal-epidermal interactions in the developing skin (see Chapter 9).

Final enzymatic differentiation of intestinal absorptive cells is strongly influenced by glucocorticoids, and the underlying mesoderm appears to mediate this hormonal effect. In a converse inductive influence the intestinal endoderm, through the action of shh signaling, induces the differentiation of smooth muscle from mesenchymal cells in the wall of the intestine.

Although the intestine develops many functional capabilities during the fetal period, no major digestive function occurs until feeding begins after birth. The intestines of the fetus contain a greenish material called **meconium** (see Figure 18-9), which is a mixture of lanugo hairs and vernix caseosa sloughed from the skin, desquamated cells from the gut, bile secretion, and other materials swallowed with the amniotic fluid.

## Formation of Enteric Ganglia

As was outlined in Chapter 12, the **enteric ganglia** of the gut are derived from neural crest. Pax-3–expressing

**FIGURE 15-11** Differentiation of intestinal epithelial cells from stem cells located in the crypts. The time scale shows the typical course of migration of daughter cells starting with their generation from the stem cell population to their being shed from the villus into the intestinal lumen.

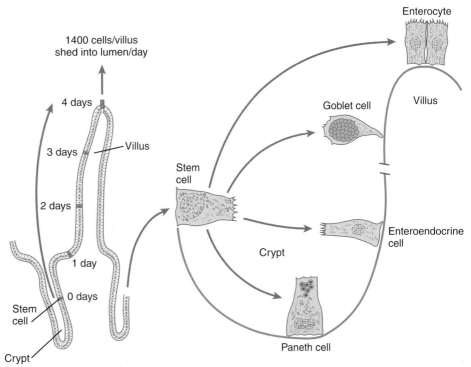

## Malformations of the Intestinal Tract

### DUODENAL STENOSIS AND ATRESIA

Duodenal stenosis and atresia typically result from absent or incomplete recanalization of the duodenal lumen after it is plugged by endothelium. These malformations are rare.

### VITELLINE DUCT REMNANTS

The most common family of anomalies of the intestinal tract is some form of persistence of the **vitelline (yolk) duct**. The most common member of this family is **Meckel's diverticulum**, which is present in 2% to 4% of the population. A typical Meckel's diverticulum is a blind pouch a few centimeters long located on the antimesenteric border of the ileum about 50 cm cranial from the ileocecal junction (Figure 15-12, *A* and *E*). This structure represents the persistent proximal portion of the yolk stalk. Simple Meckel's diverticula are often asymptomatic, but they occasionally become inflamed or contain ectopic tissue (e.g., gastric, pancreatic, or even endometrial tissue), which can cause ulceration. It has been suggested that in the absence of intestinal mesodermal restriction (the wall of a Meckel's diverticulum is derived from the yolk duct) of the endoderm lining a Meckel's diverticulum, the endoderm retains the developmental capability to form a variety of types of cellular phenotypes derived from endoderm.

In some cases a ligament connects a Meckel's diverticulum to the umbilicus (Figure 15-12, *B*), or a simple vitelline ligament that may have an associated persisting **vitelline artery** can connect the intestine to the umbilicus. Occasionally the intestine rotates about such a ligament, causing a condition known as **volvulus** (Figure 15-12, *D*). This can lead to strangulation of the bowel.

A persistent vitelline duct can take the form of a **vitelline fistula** (Figure 15-12, *C*), which constitutes a direct connection between the intestinal lumen and the outside of the body via the umbilicus. Rarely, a **vitelline duct cyst** is present along the length of a vitelline ligament.

### OMPHALOCELE

**Omphalocele** represents the failure of return of the intestinal loops into the body cavity during the tenth week. The primary defect in omphalocoele is most likely a reduced prominence of the lateral body wall that does not provide sufficient space for the complete return of the intestines to the body cavity. After birth, the intestinal loops can be easily seen within an almost transparent sac consisting of amnion on the outside and peritoneal membrane on the inside (Figure 15-13). The incidence of omphalocele is approximately 1 in 3500 births, but half of the infants with this condition are stillborn.

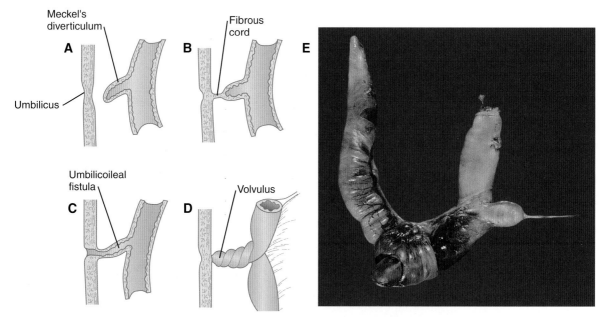

**FIGURE 15-12** Varieties of vitelline duct remnants. **A,** Meckel's diverticulum. **B,** Fibrous cord connecting a Meckel's diverticulum to the umbilicus. **C,** Umbilicoileal (vitelline) fistula. **D,** Volvulus caused by rotation of the intestine around a vitelline duct remnant. **E,** Meckel's diverticulum protruding at the right from a segment of ileum. The bowel below the diverticulum is reddish because of an associated intussusception just below the Meckel's diverticulum (Photo 2681 from the Arey-DaPeña Pediatric Pathology Photographic Collection, Human Development Anatomy Center, National Museum of Health and Medicine, Armed Forces Institute of Pathology, Washington, DC.)

## CONGENITAL UMBILICAL HERNIA

In congenital umbilical hernia, which is especially common in premature infants, the intestines return normally into the body cavity, but the musculature (rectus abdominis) of the ventral abdominal wall fails to close the umbilical ring, allowing a varying amount of omentum or bowel to protrude through the umbilicus. In contrast to omphalocele, the protruding tissue in an umbilical hernia is covered by skin rather than amniotic membrane.

Both omphalocele and congenital umbilical hernia are associated with closure defects in the ventral abdominal wall. If these defects are large, they may be accompanied by massive protrusion of abdominal contents or with other closure defects such as exstrophy of the bladder (see Chapter 16).

## ABNORMAL ROTATION OF THE GUT

Sometimes the intestines undergo no or abnormal rotation as they return to the abdominal cavity. This can result in a wide spectrum of anatomical anomalies (Figure 15-14). In most cases these are asymptomatic, but occasionally, they can lead to volvulus or another form of strangulation of the gut. The major rotation of the gut occurs after smooth muscle has formed in the intestinal walls. Mice mutant for both *sonic hedgehog* and *Indian hedgehog* have greatly reduced smooth muscle in the gut wall and frequently exhibit malrotation of the intestines.

## INTESTINAL DUPLICATIONS, DIVERTICULA, AND ATRESIA

As with the esophagus and duodenum, the remainder of the intestinal tract is susceptible to various anomalies that seem to be based on incomplete recanalization of the lumen after the stage of temporary blocking of the lumen by epithelium during the first trimester. Some of the variants of these conditions are shown in Figure 15-15.

## AGANGLIONIC MEGACOLON (HIRSCHSPRUNG'S DISEASE)

The basis of aganglionic megacolon, which is manifested by great dilatation of certain segments of the colon, is the absence of parasympathetic ganglia in the affected walls of the colon. Hirschsprung's disease appears to be truly multifactorial, with both dominant and recessive mutations resulting in the condition. Many patients with Hirschsprung's disease do not express the *c-RET* onco-

**FIGURE 15-13** Omphalocele in a stillborn. Loops of small intestine can be clearly seen through the nearly transparent amniotic membrane that covers the omphalocele. (Courtesy M. Barr, Ann Arbor, Mich.)

*Continued*

## Malformations of the Intestinal Tract (Continued)

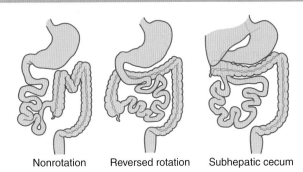

Nonrotation　　　Reversed rotation　　　Subhepatic cecum

**FIGURE 15-14** Types of abnormal rotations of the gut.

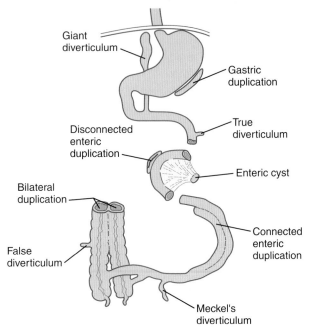

**FIGURE 15-15** Types of diverticula and duplications that can occur in the digestive tract. (Based on Gray SW, Skandalakis JE: *Embryology for surgeons*, Philadelphia, 1972, WB Saunders.)

gene. C-RET, along with a co-receptor Gfra-1, is a receptor for glia-derived neurotrophic factor (GDNF). This gene is activated by the combination of Pax-3 with SOX-10, both of which are necessary for the formation of enteric ganglia. Similarly, mutations of SOX-10, which probably interferes with Pax-3 function, can result in a combined Waardenburg-Hirschsprung syndrome. Mutants of *Ret, Gfra-1,* and *GDNF* interfere with the migration of vagal neural crest cells into the gut. Known mutations presently account for only about half of the cases of Hirschsprung's disease. Other mutations underlying aganglionic megacolon could involve defects in the migration or proliferation of neural crest precursor cells. Death of precursor cells before or after they reach their final destination in the hindgut could reduce the number of enteric ganglia. Or, the local environment could prevent the successful migration of neural crest cells into the colon. Evidence from mutant mice developing aganglionic segments of the bowel strongly suggests that the environment of the gut wall inhibits the migration of neural crest cells into the affected segment of gut. This was shown by experiments in which crest cells from mutant mice were capable of colonizing normal gut, but normal crest cells could not migrate into gut segments of mutant mice. The accumulation of laminin in the gut wall as the result of overproduction of **endothelin-3** serves as a stop signal for neural crest migration. The distal colon is the most affected region for aganglionosis, but in a small number of cases, aganglionic segments extend as far cranially as the ascending colon. Estimates of the frequency of megacolon vary widely—from 1 in 1000 to 1 in 30,000 births.

Recent experiments have shown that cells derived from the vagal neural crest exhibit much stronger migratory properties in the hindgut than do cells from the sacral crest. This has led to the suggestion that vagal crest cells be transplanted into aganglionic segments of the colon in an attempt to correct the deficit of enteric neurons in this area.

### IMPERFORATE ANUS

Imperforate anus includes a spectrum of anal defects that can range from a simple membrane covering the anal opening (persistence of the anal membrane) to atresia of varying lengths of the anal canal, rectum, or both structures. Grossly, all are characterized by the absence of an anal opening (Figure 15-16). Deletions of *Hoxa-13* and *Hoxd-13* in mice result in defects in morphogenesis of the anal sphincter, and mutants of *sonic hedgehog* and its downstream molecules *Gli-2* and *Gli-3* result in the colon ending in a blind sac, with no anus forming. Any examination of a newborn must include a determination of the presence of an anal opening. Of considerable importance when considering the surgical treatment of imperforate anus is the extent of the atretic segment. Treatment of a persistent anal membrane can be trivial, whereas more extensive defects, especially those involving the anal musculature, constitute very challenging surgical problems.

### HINDGUT FISTULAS

In many cases, anal atresia is accompanied by a fistula linking the patent portion of the hindgut to another structure in the region of the original urogenital sinus region. Common types of fistulas connect the hindgut with the vagina, the urethra, or the bladder, and others may lead to the surface in the perineal area (Figure 15-17).

**FIGURE 15-16** Anal atresia in a newborn. No trace of an anal opening is seen. (Courtesy M. Barr, Ann Arbor, Mich.)

**FIGURE 15-17** Varieties of hindgut fistulas and atresias. **A,** Persistent anal membrane. **B,** Anal atresia. **C,** Anoperineal fistula. **D,** Rectovaginal fistula. **E,** Rectourethral fistula. **F,** Rectovesical fistula.

cells from the vagal neural crest migrate into the foregut and then spread in a wavelike fashion throughout the entire length of the gut. Slightly later, cells from the sacral crest enter the hindgut and intermingle with cells derived from the vagal neural crest. The migratory properties of vagal crest cells are much more pronounced than those of cells from the sacral crest. Initially, the vagal crest cells migrate throughout the mesenchyme of the gut, but as the smooth muscle of the intestines begins to differentiate, the migrating vagal crest cells become preferentially distributed between the smooth muscle and the serosa, where the myenteric plexuses will form. During their migration through the gut, the population of neural crest cells undergoes a massive expansion until the number of enteric neurons ultimately exceeds the number of neurons present in the spinal cord. Glial cells also differentiate from neural crest precursors in the gut, but the environmental factors that contribute to the differentiation of neural crest cells in the gut wall remain poorly understood.

## Glands of the Digestive System

The glands of the digestive system arise through inductive processes between the early epithelial outgrowths and the surrounding mesenchyme. The various glandular epithelia have considerably different requirements in the types of mesenchyme that can support their development. For example, in tissue recombination experiments, pancreatic epithelium undergoes typical development when juxtaposed with mesenchyme from almost any

source. The development of salivary gland epithelium, on the other hand, is supported by mesenchyme from lung or accessory sexual glands but not by many other types of mesenchyme. Inductive support of hepatic (liver) epithelium follows a distinctive pattern. Normal epithelial development is supported by mesenchyme derived from lateral or intermediate mesoderm, but axial mesenchyme (either somitic or neural crest) fails to support hepatic differentiation. The inductive properties of certain glandular mesenchymes may be correlated with different modes of vascularization of these mesenchymes (see p. 435).

## *Formation of the Liver*

Early in the third week an endodermal hepatic diverticulum arises from the floor of the foregut and grows into the mesenchyme of the **septum transversum** (see Figure 6-18). The hepatic diverticulum is the manifestation of a series of inductive processes that have already begun to take place (Figure 15-18). Before the hepatic diverticulum becomes recognizable, an induction by hepatocardiac mesoderm, mediated by fibroblast growth factor (FGF) signaling (FGF-1, FGF-2, and FGF-8) and joined with BMP-2, BMP-4, and BMP-7 signaling from the septum transversum, specifies the ventral foregut endoderm to become a precursor of the hepatic epithelium by expressing several liver-specific genes. In the absence of FGF signaling the ventral foregut endoderm differentiates into ventral pancreatic tissue by a default mechanism. As the hepatic diverticulum takes shape, precursors of vascular endothelial cells grow into the same area. These cells

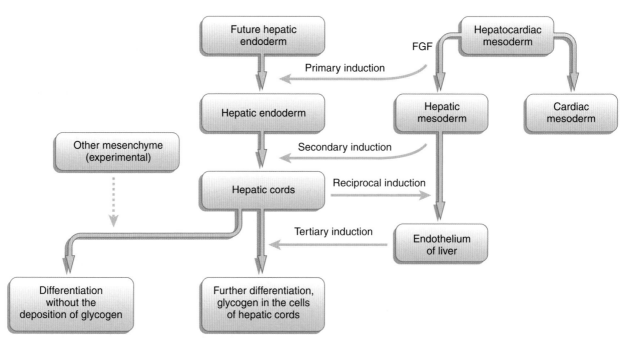

**FIGURE 15-18** Tissue interactions in the morphogenesis of the endodermal component of the liver.

appear to provide one or more factors that are necessary for further development of the hepatic endoderm.

The original hepatic diverticulum branches into many hepatic cords, which are closely associated with splanchnic mesoderm of the septum transversum. The mesoderm supports continued growth and proliferation of the hepatic endoderm. This occurs in part through the actions of **hepatic growth factor** (scatter factor), which is bound by the receptor molecule, c-**met,** located on the surface of the endodermal hepatocytes. A number of experimental studies have shown that mesoderm from either the splanchnopleural or somatopleural components of the lateral mesoderm can support further hepatic growth and differentiation, whereas paraxial mesoderm has only a limited capacity to support hepatic development.

In addition to cords of hepatic endoderm, a system of bile drainage ducts forms in the developing liver. Near the area where the hepatic ducts become confluent, a dilatation foreshadows the further development of the **gallbladder** (Figure 15-19). The hepatic cords form a series of loosely packed and highly irregular sheets that alternate with mesodermally lined **sinusoids,** through which blood percolates and exchanges nutrients with the **hepatocytes.** The developing liver is richly vascularized, with many major vessels passing through it in the embryonic period (see Figure 17-13).

The entire liver soon becomes too large to be contained in the septum transversum, and it protrudes into the ventral mesentery within the abdominal cavity. As it continues to expand, the rapidly growing liver remains covered by a glistening, translucent layer of mesenteric tissue that now serves as the connective tissue capsule of the liver. Between the liver and the ventral body wall is a thin, sickle-shaped piece of ventral mesentery: the **falciform ligament.** The ventral mesentery between

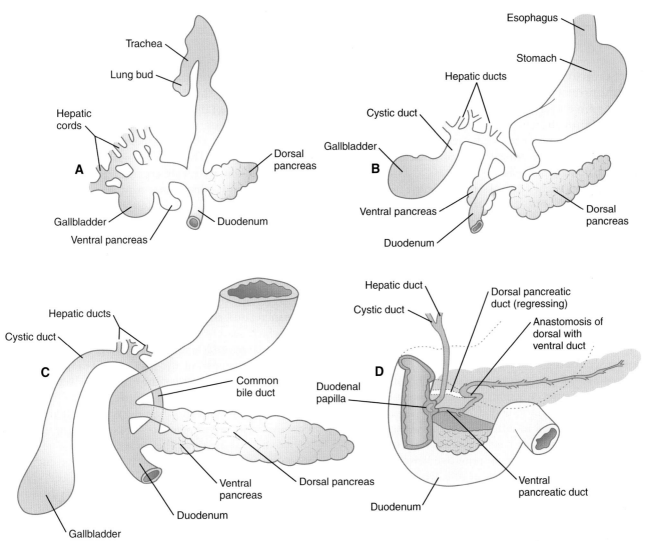

**FIGURE 15-19** Development of the hepatic and pancreatic primordia from the ventral aspect. **A,** In the **fifth week. B,** In the **sixth week. C,** In the **seventh week. D,** In the late fetus, showing fusion of the dorsal and ventral pancreatic ducts and regression of the distal portion of the dorsal duct.

the liver and the stomach is the **lesser omentum** (see Figure 15-4).

### Development of Hepatic Function

Development of the liver is not only a matter of increasing its mass and structural complexity. As the liver develops, its cells gradually acquire the capacity to perform the many biochemical functions characterizing the mature, functioning liver. One characteristic major function of the liver is to produce the plasma protein **serum albumin.** The messenger RNA for albumin has been detected in mammalian hepatocytes during the earliest stages of their ingrowth into the hepatic mesoderm, and it appears to depend on the earlier expression of the transcription factor HNF-3.

A major function of the adult liver is the synthesis and storage of **glycogen,** which serves as a carbohydrate reserve. As the fetal period progresses, the liver actively stores glycogen. This function is strongly stimulated by adrenocortical hormones and is indirectly stimulated by the anterior pituitary. Similarly, the fetal period includes the functional development of the system of enzymes involved in the synthesis of urea from nitrogenous metabolites. By birth, these have attained full functional capacity.

A major function of the embryonic liver is the production of blood cells. After yolk sac hematopoiesis, the liver is one of the chief sites of intraembryonic blood formation. Hematopoietic cells, seeding the liver from origins in other sites, appear in small clusters among the hepatic parenchymal cells.

At approximately 12 weeks' gestation the hepatocytes begin to produce **bile** largely through the breakdown of hemoglobin. The bile drains down the newly formed bile duct system and is stored in the gallbladder. As bile is released into the intestines, it stains the other intestinal contents a dark green, which is one of the characteristics of meconium.

### Formation of the Pancreas

The pancreas begins as separate dorsal and ventral primordia within the duodenal endoderm (see Figure 6-18, D). Interestingly, early development of each of these two primordia is under different molecular controls. As was seen previously, ventral endoderm of the hepatic diverticulum is patterned to differentiate into ventral pancreatic tissue by a default mechanism in areas where liver induction does not occur. In primitive vertebrates, pancreatic function is distributed in cells within the foregut rather than in a discrete gland, and some investigators have speculated that the ventral pancreatic bud represents the extension of this system, whereas the discrete dorsal pancreas is an evolutionary newcomer.

The dorsal pancreas is induced from the dorsal gut endoderm by **activin** and **FGF** signals emanating from the notochord, which early in development is directly opposed to the endoderm (Figure 15-20). Sonic hedgehog activity in the dorsal endoderm must be repressed or pancreatic differentiation will not occur. During the earliest stages of pancreatic bud formation the **pancreatic progenitor cells** express the transcription factors Pdx-1 and Hlxb-9. If Pdx-1 expression is eliminated by targeted mutagenesis, development of the pancreatic bud ceases. From this point, different environmental signals and intracellular responses result in the differentiation of two lineages of cells, the **pancreatic exocrine cells** and the **pancreatic endocrine cells** (see Figure 15-20).

During the phase of early growth, the dorsal pancreas becomes considerably larger than the ventral pancreas. At about the same time the duodenum rotates to the right and forms a **C**-shaped loop, carrying the ventral pancreas and common bile duct behind it and into the dorsal mesentery. The ventral pancreas soon makes contact and fuses with the dorsal pancreas.

Both the dorsal and the ventral pancreas possess a large duct. After fusion of the two pancreatic primordia, the main duct of the ventral pancreas makes an anastomotic connection with the duct of the dorsal pancreas. The portion of the dorsal pancreatic duct between the anastomotic connection and the duodenum normally regresses, leaving the main duct of the ventral pancreas (**duct of Wirsung**) the definitive outlet from the pancreas into the duodenum (see Figure 15-19).

The pancreas is a dual organ with both endocrine and exocrine functions. The exocrine portion consists of large numbers of **acini,** which are connected to a secretory duct system. The endocrine component consists of roughly a million richly vascularized **islets of Langerhans,** which are scattered among the acini.

In certain pancreatic progenitor cells, the action of the signaling molecules, **follistatin,** and several **FGFs** emanating from the surrounding mesoderm, in combination with the activation of the **Notch** receptor system (see page 76), results in the differentiation of many of the pancreatic cells along the exocrine pathway. These cells, which secrete digestive hormones such as **amylase** and **carboxypeptidase,** are ultimately responsible for the gross morphogenesis of the pancreas. During outgrowth of the pancreatic primordia, the exocrine cells take on the form of sequentially budding cords. From these cellular cords, both the acini and their ducts differentiate. Tissue recombination experiments, conducted both in vitro and in vivo, have shown that the presence of mesenchyme is necessary for the formation of acini but that ducts can form in the absence of mesenchyme if the endodermal precursor cells are exposed to a gel rich in basement membrane material. Although the presence of mesenchyme is required for the differentiation of acini, the mesenchyme need not be of pancreatic origin. In vitro, pancreatic endoderm combined with salivary gland mesoderm differentiates even better than that exposed to pan-

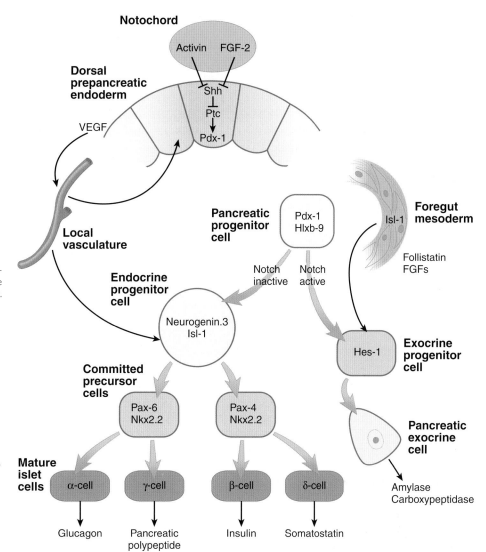

**Notochord**

Activin   FGF-2

**Dorsal prepancreatic endoderm**

VEGF

Shh
⊣
Ptc
↓
Pdx-1

**Local vasculature**

**Pancreatic progenitor cell**

Pdx-1
Hlxb-9

Notch inactive   Notch active

**Foregut mesoderm**

Isl-1

Follistatin
FGFs

**Endocrine progenitor cell**

Neurogenin.3
Isl-1

Hes-1   **Exocrine progenitor cell**

**Committed precursor cells**

Pax-6
Nkx2.2

Pax-4
Nkx2.2

**Pancreatic exocrine cell**

**Mature islet cells**

α-cell   γ-cell   β-cell   δ-cell

Amylase
Carboxypeptidase

Glucagon   Pancreatic polypeptide   Insulin   Somatostatin

**FIGURE 15-20** Molecular events underlying the differentiation of the endocrine and exocrine components of the pancreas.

creatic mesenchyme. This shows that in the case of the pancreas the inductive influence of the mesenchyme is permissive, rather than instructive.

Differentiation of the acini is divided into three phases (Figure 15-21). The first, called the **predifferentiated state,** occurs while the pancreatic primordia are first taking shape. A population of pancreatic progenitor cells that exhibits virtually undetectable levels of digestive enzyme activity is established. As the pancreatic buds begin to grow outward, the epithelium undergoes a transition into a second, **protodifferentiated state.** During this phase, the exocrine cells synthesize low levels of many hydrolytic enzymes that they will ultimately produce. After the main period of outgrowth, the pancreatic acinar cells pass through another transition before attaining a third, **differentiated state.** By this time, they have acquired an elaborate protein-synthesizing apparatus, and the inactive forms of the polypeptide digestive enzymes are stored in the cytoplasm as **zymogen granules.** Glucocorticoid hormones from the fetal adrenal

cortex stimulate increased production of a number of digestive enzymes.

Development of the islets of Langerhans follows a somewhat different course from that of the acini. They are formed from groups of epithelial cells that break away from the acinar epithelial cells during the second (protodifferentiated) phase of acinar cell development. In a pathway not involving activation of the Notch system, but requiring signals from the local vasculature, these cells enter the endocrine lineage as **endocrine precursor cells** (see Figure 15-20). Expressing the transcription factors **neurogenin-3** and **Isl-1,** the endocrine precursor cells give rise to two types of progeny (**committed precursor cells**), each of which is characterized by the expression of a different *Pax* gene. One, which differentiates at 8 to 9 weeks, gives rise to α- and γ-cells, which produce **glucagon** and **pancreatic polypeptide,** respectively. The other type, which differentiates later, gives rise to β- and δ-cells, which produce **insulin** and **somatostatin.** During the second phase of pancreatic differentiation (protodifferentiated state) the

**FIGURE 15-21** Stages of structural and functional differentiation of the pancreas. The green areas represent primitive islets. (Modified from Pictet R, Rutter W: *Handbook of physiology*, section 7: *Endocrinology*, vol 1, Washington, DC, 1972, American Physiological Society, pp 25–66.)

levels of glucagon synthesis considerably exceed those of insulin. By the third phase of pancreatic development, secretory granules are evident in the cytoplasm of most islet cells. Insulin and glucagon are present in the fetal circulation by the end of the fifth month of gestation.

## RESPIRATORY SYSTEM

The respiratory system is first seen during the fourth week as an inconspicuous midline **laryngotracheal groove** in the ventral midline at the posterior limit of the pharyngeal region. A principal mechanism underlying the early development of the **respiratory diverticulum** (future trachea) during the fifth week is the formation of a **tracheoesophageal septum** of splanchnic mesenchyme that is interposed between it and the esophagus (Figure 15-24, *A*). According to some authors, the trachea can be viewed as almost pinching off from the esophagus rather than growing out of it. Through a series of interactions with the surrounding mesoderm, the respiratory diverticulum elongates into a tracheal portion and begins to form the first of 23 sets of bifurcations (**lung buds**) that continue into postnatal life.

Many minor variations in the shape of the liver or bile ducts occur, but these normally have no functional significance. One of the most serious malformations involving the liver is **biliary atresia**. This can involve any level from the tiny bile canaliculi to the major bile-carrying ducts. The **Alagille syndrome**, which is characterized by biliary atresia and cardiac defects, is caused by mutations in **Jagged-1**, a ligand for the Notch receptor. Newborns with this condition typically develop severe **jaundice** shortly after birth. Some cases can be treated surgically; for others, a liver transplant is necessary.

On rare occasions a ring of pancreatic tissue completely encircles the duodenum, forming an **annular pancreas** (Figure 15-22). This can sometimes cause obstruction of the duodenum after birth. The cause of annular pancreas is not established, but a commonly accepted explanation is that outgrowths from a bifid

ventral pancreas may encircle the duodenum from both sides.

**Heterotopic pancreatic tissue** can occasionally be found along the digestive tract, and it occurs most frequently in the duodenum or mucosa of the stomach (Figure 15-23). About 6% of Meckel's diverticula contain heterotopic pancreatic tissue.

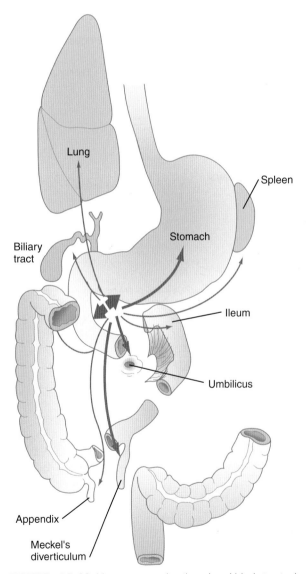

**FIGURE 15-23** Most common locations in which heterotopic pancreatic tissue can be found. The thickness of the arrows corresponds to the frequency of heterotopic tissue in that location. (Based on Gray SW, Skandalakis JE: *Embryology for surgeons*, Philadelphia, 1972, WB Saunders.)

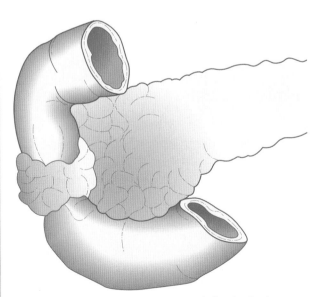

**FIGURE 15-22** Annular pancreas encircling the duodenum.

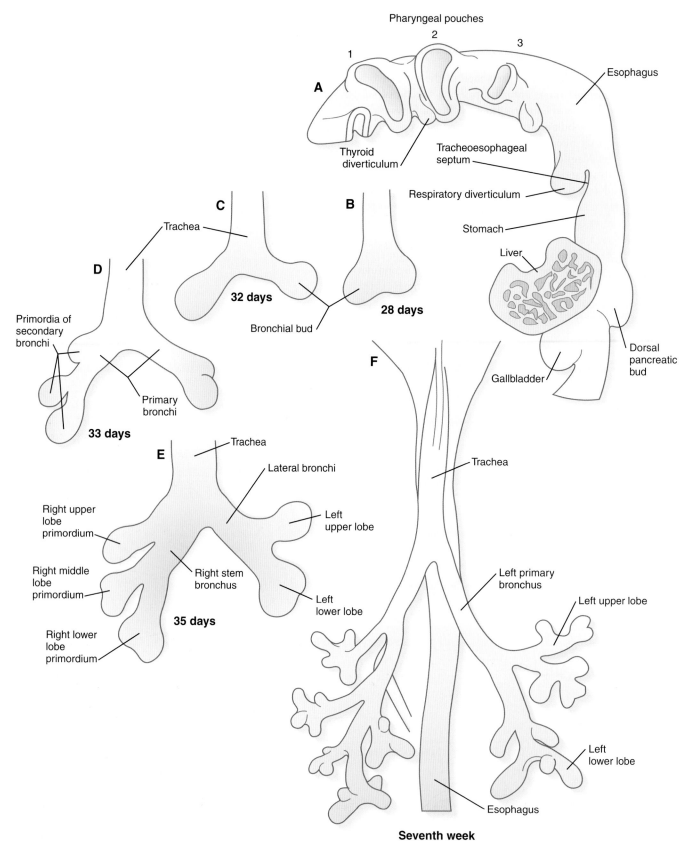

**FIGURE 15-24** Development of the major branching patterns of the lungs. **A,** Lateral view of the pharynx, showing the respiratory diverticulum in a **4-week-old** embryo. **B,** At **4 weeks. C,** At **32 days. D,** At **33 days. E,** At the end of the **fifth week. F,** Early in the **seventh week.**

## Formation of the Larynx

During the fourth and fifth weeks of gestation, a rapid proliferation of the fourth and sixth pharyngeal arch mesenchyme around the site of origin of the respiratory bud converts the opening slit from the esophagus into a T-shaped **glottis** bounded by two lateral **arytenoid swellings** and a cranial **epiglottis**. The mesenchyme surrounding the laryngeal orifice ultimately differentiates into the **thyroid, cricoid,** and **arytenoid cartilages,** which form the skeletal supports of the **larynx.** Like the esophagus, the lumen of the larynx undergoes a temporary epithelial occlusion. In the process of recanalization during the ninth and tenth weeks, a pair of lateral folds and recesses forms the structural basis for the **vocal cords** and adjacent **laryngeal ventricles.** The somitomere derived musculature of the larynx is innervated by branches of the vagus nerve (X), that associated with the fourth arch is innervated by the **superior laryngeal nerve,** and that of the sixth arch is innervated by the **recurrent laryngeal nerve.**

## Formation of the Trachea and Bronchial Tree

After the initial appearance of the respiratory diverticulum, a pair of bronchial buds appears at its end (Figure 15-24, *B*). The straight portion of the respiratory diverticulum is the primordium of the trachea. The bronchial buds, which ultimately become the primary bronchi, give rise to additional buds—three on the right and two on the left. These buds become the **secondary,** or **stem, bronchi,** and their numbers presage the formation of the three lobes of the right lung and the two lobes of the left (see Figure 15-24). From this point, each secondary bronchial bud undergoes a long series of branchings until a maximum 23 successive orders of branching have occurred. Morphogenesis of the lung continues after birth, and stabilization of the morphological pattern of the lungs does not occur until about 8 years of age. An array of *Hox* genes (*Hoxa-3* to *Hoxa-5* and *Hoxb-3* to *Hoxb-6*) is expressed early in the developing respiratory tract. Combinatorial patterns of expression of *Hox* genes may be involved in regional specification of the respiratory tract.

The mesoderm surrounding the endoderm controls the extent of branching within the respiratory tract. Numerous tissue recombination experiments have shown that the mesoderm surrounding the trachea inhibits branching, whereas that surrounding the bronchial buds promotes branching. If tracheal endoderm is combined with bronchial mesoderm, abnormal budding is induced. Conversely, tracheal mesoderm placed around bronchial endoderm inhibits bronchial budding. Mesoderm of certain other organs such as salivary glands can promote budding of the bronchial endoderm, but a pattern of branching characteristic of the mesoderm is induced. A mesoderm capable of promoting or sustaining budding must maintain a high rate of proliferation of the epithelial cells. Generally, the pattern of the epithelial organ is largely determined by the mesoderm. Structural and functional differentiation of the epithelium is a specific property of the epithelial cells, but the epithelial phenotype corresponds to the region dictated by the mesoderm.

The basic principles underlying pulmonary branching are similar to those operating in the development of the salivary glands and pancreas. At points of branching, epithelial cell proliferation is reduced, and the deposition of types I, III, and IV collagen; fibronectin; and proteoglycans stabilizes the morphology of the branching point and more proximal ductal regions. On the other hand, heightened epithelial cell proliferation characterizes the rapidly expanding portions of the epithelial buds (Figure 15-25).

The activities of many molecules contribute to lung morphogenesis. More than 50 genes are involved in morphogenesis of the tracheal system in *Drosophila,* which shows remarkable parallels to the mammalian respiratory system. A prime mover in generating branching is **FGF-10,** which is produced by the mesenchyme off the tip of a growing bud in the respiratory system. In FGF-10 knockout mice, budding of the developing lungs fails to occur. FGF-10 acts as a signaling center, stimulating cell proliferation in the epithelium at the tip of the bud and causing the epithelium to grow out toward the source of the FGF-10 (Figure 15-25, *A*). Apical epithelial proliferation is also promoted by the expression of the transcription factor **Nkx 2.1** in these cells.

Branching is initiated with the stimulation of secretion of **BMP-4** in the apical epithelial cells. This inhibits their proliferation. Simultaneously, **sonic hedgehog,** which is also produced by the epithelium, stimulates proliferation of the mesenchymal cells off the tip and inhibits the formation of FGF-10 (Figure 15-25, *B*). These mesenchymal cells begin to produce **transforming growth factor-β1** (TGF-β1), which in addition to inhibiting FGF-10 production along with shh, promotes the synthesis of extracellular matrix molecules just distal to the apical epithelial cells. These molecules, including **fibronectin** and **collagen types I, III,** and **IV,** stabilize the formerly growing epithelial tip.

While the cell proliferation in the epithelial tip is reduced and the cells become bound by newly secreted extracellular matrix molecules, FGF-10 is secreted by the mesenchyme lateral to the old apex, where the concentrations of shh and TGF-β1 are reduced below the inhibitory level (Figure 15-25, *C*). This sets up two new signaling centers on either side of the original one, and the cycle of apical epithelial proliferation begins anew. As the new apical growth centers mature, FGF-10 signaling is once again inhibited, and each of the two existing tips

**FIGURE 15-25** Molecular aspects of outgrowth and branching of the respiratory tree. **A,** The tip of an elongating respiratory duct. FGF-10 secretion in the mesenchyme stimulates the growth of the tip of the epithelial duct toward it. **B,** The prelude to branching. Inhibition of FGF-10 signaling at the tip of the duct leads to stabilization of that area. **C,** Cleft formation. Extracellular matrix molecules are deposited in the newly forming cleft, and two new centers of outgrowth, stimulated by FGF-10 signaling, indicate the start of branching. *BMP,* Bone morphogenetic protein; *FGF,* fibroblast growth factor; *Shh,* sonic hedgehog; *TGF,* transforming growth factor; *FGFR,* Fibroblast growth factor receptor; *, dividing cells.

will begin its own branching cycle. The concurrent presence of the epithelial cell–associated proteoglycan **syndecan** is important for maintaining the stability of epithelial sheets along the ducts. Interacting with the extracellular matrix protein **tenascin,** it is found along already formed ducts but not in areas where branching is occurring in terminal saccular regions of the developing airway (see Figure 15-25).

As with branching morphogenesis, the formation and maintenance of epithelially lined ducts involve special sets of molecular components. Hoxb-5 is expressed during the early development of smaller bronchioles (e.g., terminal bronchioles) but not in the components of the lung that will be involved in actual respiratory exchange (i.e., respiratory bronchioles, alveolar ducts, alveoli). The protein **epimorphin** is important in the later formation of epithelial tubes. Epimorphin is located in the mesenchyme and appears to provide a signal that allows overlying epithelial cells to establish proper polarity or cell arrangements. In the embryonic lung the developing epithelial ducts become disorganized and do not form lumens if epimorphin is blocked by specific antibodies.

## Stages in Lung Development

### Embryonic Stage (Weeks 4 to 7)

The embryonic stage includes the initial formation of the respiratory diverticulum up to the formation of all major bronchopulmonary segments. During this period, the developing lungs grow into and begin to fill the bilateral **pleural cavities**. These represent the major components of the thoracic body cavity above the pericardium (Figure 15-26).

### Pseudoglandular Stage (Weeks 8 to 16)

The pseudoglandular stage is the period of major formation and growth of the duct systems within the bronchopulmonary segments before their terminal portions form respiratory components. The histological structure of the lung resembles that of a gland (Figure 15-27), thus providing the basis for the designation of this stage. During this period, the pulmonary arterial system begins to form. The elongating vessels parallel the major developing ducts.

### Canalicular Stage (Weeks 17 to 26)

The canalicular stage is characterized by the formation of **respiratory bronchioles** as the result of budding of the terminal components of the system of bronchioles that formed during the pseudoglandular stage. The other major event during this stage is the intense ingrowth of blood vessels into the developing lungs and the close association of capillaries with the walls of the respiratory

bronchioles (see Figure 15-27). Occasionally a fetus born toward the end of this period can survive with intensive care, but respiratory immaturity is the principal reason for poor viability.

### Terminal Sac Stage (Weeks 26 to Birth)

During the terminal sac stage, the terminal air sacs (**alveoli**) bud off the respiratory bronchioles that largely formed during the canalicular stage. The epithelium lining the alveoli differentiates into two types of cells: **type I alveolar cells** (pneumocytes), across which gas exchange occurs after birth, and **type II alveolar (secretory epithelial) cells**. These latter cells form **pulmonary surfactant,** the material that spreads over the surface of the alveoli to reduce surface tension and facilitate expansion of the alveoli during breathing. Research involving specific markers of the epithelial cells has shown that the type II cells form first in the alveolar lining. After proliferation, some type II cells flatten, lose their characteristic secretory function, and undergo terminal differentiation into type I pneumocytes. Other type I cells may differentiate directly from a pool of epithelial precursor cells in the early alveolar lining. With increasing amounts of pulmonary surfactant being formed, the fetus has a correspondingly greater chance of survival if born prematurely. In the fetus the respiratory passageways in the lungs are filled with fluid (see Chapter 18). During the last 4 weeks of pregnancy, greatly increased formation of alveoli results in an exponential increase in the respiratory surface area of the lung. These weeks are sometimes referred to as the **alveolar period of lung development.**

### Postnatal Stage

At birth the mammalian lung is far from mature. An estimated 90% or more of the roughly 300 million alveoli found in the mature human lung are formed after birth. The major mechanism for this increase is the formation of secondary connective tissue septa that divide existing alveolar sacs. When they first appear, the secondary septa are relatively thick. In time, they transform into thinner mature septa capable of full respiratory exchange function.

## BODY CAVITIES

### Formation of the Common Coelom and Mesentery

As the lateral mesoderm of the early embryo splits and then folds laterally, the space between the somatic and splanchnic layers of mesoderm becomes the common

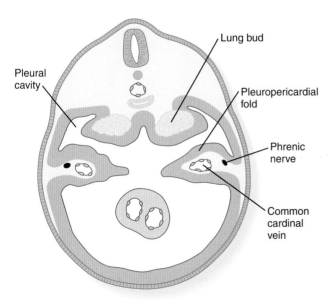

**FIGURE 15-26** Cross section through the thorax showing the lung buds growing into the pleural cavities. The pleuropericardial folds separate the future pleural from the pericardial cavities.

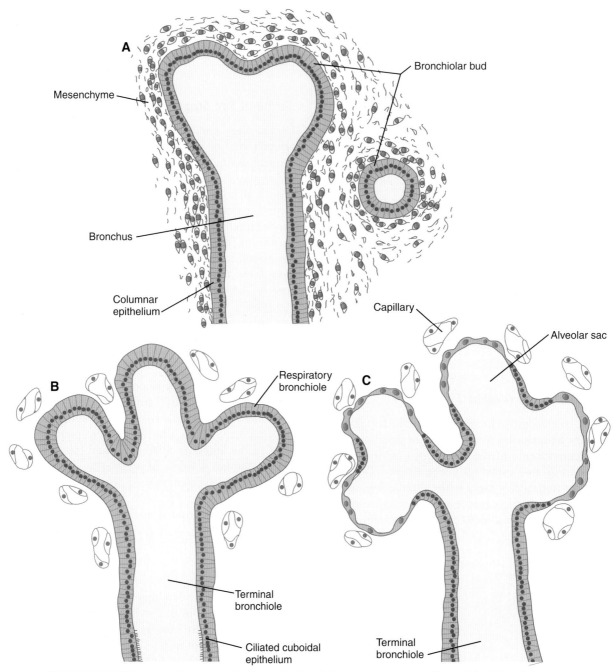

**FIGURE 15-27** Stages in histogenesis of the lungs. **A,** Pseudoglandular phase (up to **17 weeks**). **B,** Canalicular phase **(17** to **26 weeks). C,** Terminal sac phase (**26 weeks** to birth).

**intraembryonic coelom** (Figure 15-30) (see Chapter 6). The same folding process that results in the completion of the ventral body wall and the separation of the intraembryonic from the extraembryonic coelom also brings the two layers of splanchnic mesoderm around the newly formed gut as the **primary,** or **common, mesentery.** The primary mesentery suspends the gut from the dorsal body wall as the **dorsal mesentery** and attaches it to the ventral body wall as the **ventral mesentery.** This placement effectively divides the coelom into right and left components. Soon, however, most of the ventral mesentery breaks down and causes a confluence of the right and left halves of the coelom. In the region of the developing stomach and liver the ventral mesentery persists, forming the **ventral mesogastrium** and the falciform ligament of the liver (see Figure 15-4). Further cranially the tubular primordium of the heart is similarly supported by a **dorsal mesocardium** and briefly by a **ventral mesocardium,** which soon breaks down.

## TRACHEOESOPHAGEAL FISTULAS

The most common family of malformations of the respiratory tract is related to abnormal separation of the tracheal bud from the esophagus during early development of the respiratory system. Many common anatomical varieties of tracheoesophageal fistulas exist (Figure 15-28), but virtually all involve the stenosis or atresia of a segment of trachea or esophagus and an abnormal connection between them. These are manifested early after birth by the newborn's choking or regurgitation of milk when feeding.

Expression of a number of genes is important in the normal formation of a mesenchymal partition between the esophagus and the developing trachea. Mutants of the transcription factors, *Nkx2.1* and *Gli 2/3* and of the signaling molecule, *sonic hedgehog,* all result in the absence of septation between the trachea and esophagus. The genetic basis underlying specific variants of tracheoesophageal fistulas is less well understood.

## TRACHEAL OR PULMONARY AGENESIS

These rare malformations are incompatible with life. Tracheal agenesis appears to be due to defective septation between the esophagus and the respiratory diverticulum. Pulmonary agenesis is a primary consequence of a mutation of FGF-10, but it is likely that the same malformation can result from null mutations of other key molecules involved in early branching morphogenesis of the lung buds.

## GROSS MALFORMATIONS OF THE LUNGS

Because of their structural complexity, the lungs are subject to several structural variations or malformations (e.g., abnormal lobation). These are usually asymptomatic but can be foci of chronic respiratory infection. Recognition of the possibility of these variations from normal is important for the pulmonary surgeon.

## RESPIRATORY DISTRESS SYNDROME (HYALINE MEMBRANE DISEASE)

Respiratory distress syndrome is often manifested in infants born prematurely and is characterized by labored breathing. In infants who die of this condition, the lungs are underinflated, and the alveoli are partially filled with a proteinaceous fluid that forms a membrane over the respiratory surfaces (Figure 15-29). This is related to insufficiencies in the formation of surfactant by the type II alveolar cells.

## CONGENITAL CYSTS IN THE LUNG

Abnormal cystic structures can form in the lung or other parts of the respiratory tract. These can range from large single cysts to numerous small cysts located throughout the parenchyma of the lung. They may be associated with polycystic kidneys. If the cysts are numerous, they can cause respiratory distress.

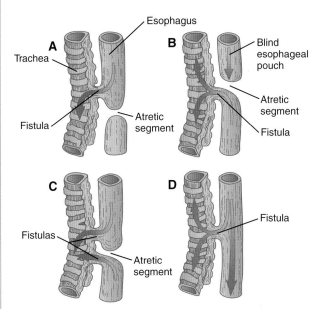

**FIGURE 15-28** Varieties of tracheoesophageal fistulas. **A,** Fistula above the atretic esophageal segment. **B,** Fistula below the atretic esophageal segment. **C,** Fistulas above and below the atretic esophageal segment. **D,** Fistula between the patent esophagus and the trachea.

**FIGURE 15-29** Photomicrograph from the lung of a newborn who died of hyaline membrane disease. The arrow points to the "membrane" that interferes with gas exchange. (Slide #427 from the Arey-DaPeña Pediatric Pathology Photographic Collection, Human Developmental Anatomy Center, National Museum of Health and Medicine, Armed Forces Institute of Pathology, Washington, DC.)

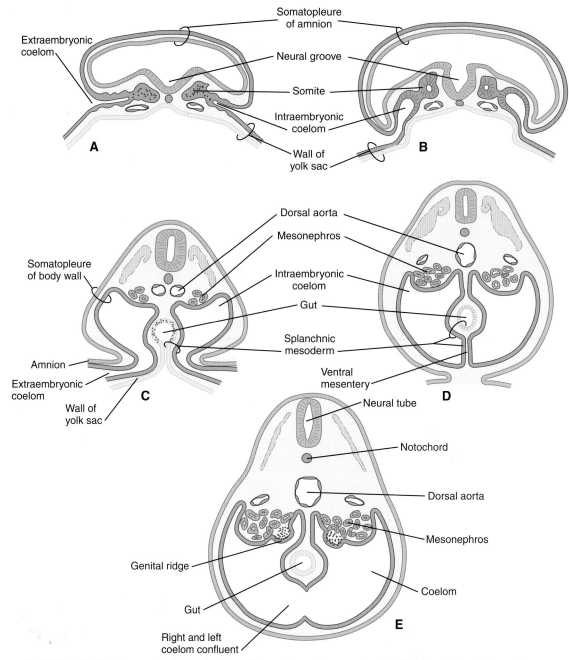

**FIGURE 15-30** Early stages in the development of the coelom and mesenteries. (Modified from Carlson B: *Patten's foundations of embryology,* ed 6, New York, 1996, McGraw-Hill.)

## Formation of the Septum Transversum and Pleural Canals

A major factor in division of the common coelom into thoracic and abdominal components is the **septum transversum**. This septum grows from the ventral body wall as a semicircular shelf, separating the heart from the developing liver (Figure 15-31). During its early development, a major portion of the liver is embedded in the septum transversum. Ultimately, the septum transversum

constitutes a significant component of the diaphragm (see p. 384).

The expanding septum transversum serves as a partial partition between the pericardial and peritoneal portions of the coelom. By the time the expanding edge of the septum transversum reaches the floor of the foregut, it has almost cut the common coelom into two parts. Two short channels located on either side of the foregut, however, connect the two major parts (Figure 15-32). Initially known as the **pleural (pericardioperitoneal) canals**, these

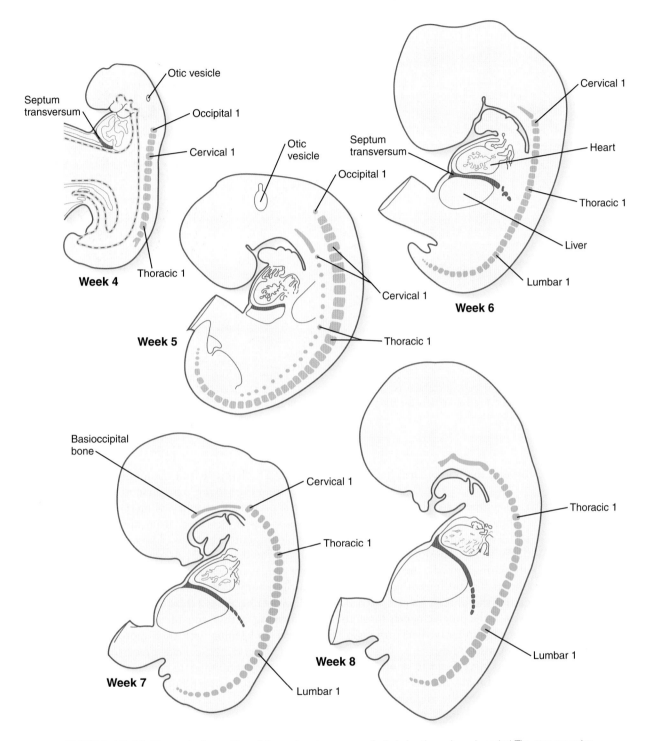

**FIGURE 15-31** Changes in the position of the septum transversum *(red)* during the embryonic period. The gray repeating structures are somites. The orange repeating structures are elements of the axial skeleton.

channels represent the spaces into which the developing lungs grow. The pleural canals enlarge greatly as the lungs increase in size and ultimately form the **pleural cavities**.

The pleural canals are partially delimited by two paired folds of tissue: the pleuropericardial and pleuroperitoneal folds. The **pleuropericardial folds** (see Figure 15-26) are ridges of tissue associated with the common cardinal

veins, which bulge into the dorsolateral wall of the coelom as they arch toward the midline of the thoracic portion of the coelom and enter the sinus venosus of the heart (Figure 15-33). Initially, the pleuropericardial folds are not large and cause only a narrowing at the junction of the pericardial cavity and pleural canals. However, as the lungs expand, the folds form prominent shelves that

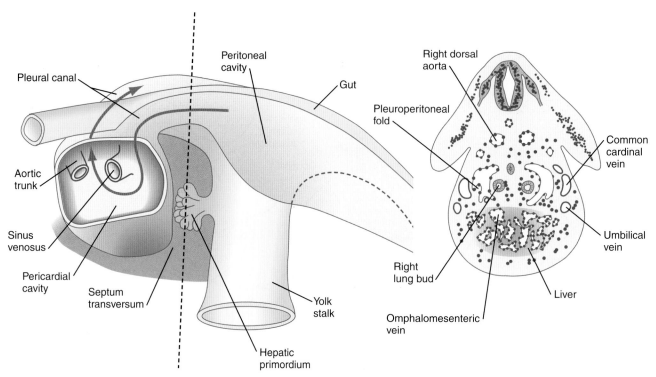

**FIGURE 15-32** Relationships among the pericardial cavity, pleural canals, and peritoneal cavity. The red arrow passes from the left pleural cavity into the pericardial cavity and then into the right pleural canal. The dashed line on the left represents the level of the cross section on the right.

meet at the midline, forming the fibrous (parietal) layer of the pericardium.

Associated with the pleuropericardial folds are the paired **phrenic nerves.** These arise from joined branches of cervical roots 3, 4, and 5 and supply the muscle fibers of the diaphragm. With the shifts in positions of various components of the body during growth, the diaphragm ultimately descends to the level of the lower thoracic vertebrae. As it does, it carries the phrenic nerves with it. Even in adults the pathway of the phrenic nerves through the fibrous pericardium is a reminder of their early association with the pleuropericardial folds.

At the caudal ends of the pleural canals, another pair of folds, the **pleuroperitoneal folds,** becomes prominent as the expanding lungs push into the mesoderm of the body wall. The pleuroperitoneal folds occupy successively greater portions of the pleural canal until they fuse with the septum transversum and the mesentery of the esophagus, effectively obliterating the pleural canal (Figure 15-34). All connections between the abdominal cavity and the thoracic cavity are thus eliminated.

## Formation of the Diaphragm

The **diaphragm,** which separates the thoracic from the abdominal cavity in adults, is a composite structure derived from several embryonic components (see Figure

15-34). The large ventral component of the diaphragm arises from the septum transversum, which fuses with the ventral part of the esophageal mesentery. Converging on the esophageal mesentery from the dorsolateral sides are the pleuroperitoneal folds. These components form the bulk of the diaphragm. As the lungs continue to grow, their caudal tips excavate additional space in the body wall. The body wall mesenchyme separated from the body wall proper becomes a third component of the diaphragm by forming a thin rim of tissue along its dorsolateral borders. In keeping with their motor innervation by the vagus (X) nerve, the cellular precursors of the diaphragmatic musculature migrate caudally into the body cavity from their site of origin in the occipital somites.

### CLINICAL VIGNETTE

A 14-year-old girl has been troubled for several years with moderately severe upper abdominal pains that recur on a fairly regular basis at roughly monthly intervals. After passing through several pediatric and medical clinics without obtaining relief, she is sent to a psychiatrist, who also cannot resolve her symptoms. Finally, an astute physician suspects that her symptoms might be caused by a congenital anomaly. Further testing and ultimately surgery proved this suspicion to be correct.

What was the diagnosis?

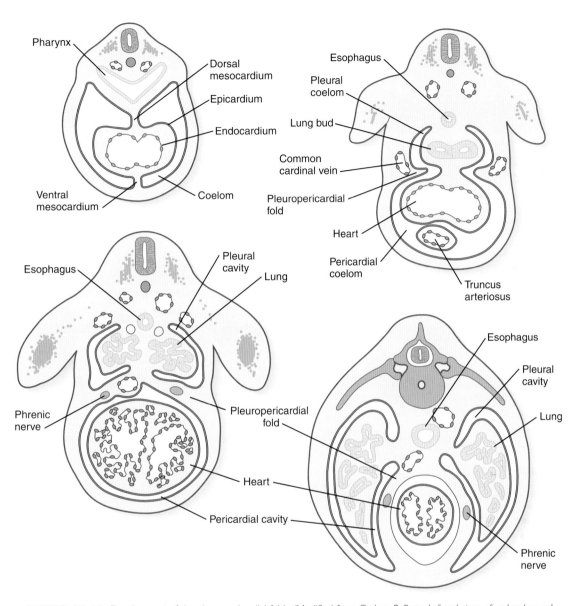

**FIGURE 15-33** Development of the pleuropericardial folds. (Modified from Carlson B: *Patten's foundations of embryology*, ed 6, New York, 1996, McGraw-Hill.)

## SUMMARY

◯ The digestive system arises from the primitive endodermally lined gut tube, which is bounded cranially by the oropharyngeal membrane and caudally by the cloacal membrane. The gut is divided into foregut, midgut, and hindgut segments, with the midgut opening into the yolk sac. Specification of the various regions of the gut tract depends upon a pattern set up by tightly regulated combinations of *Hox* genes. Development of virtually all parts of the gut depends on epithelial-mesenchymal interactions. Responding to such interactions, primordia of the respiratory system, the liver, the pancreas, and other digestive glands bud out from the original gut tube.

◯ The esophagus takes shape as a simple tubular structure between the pharynx and stomach. At one stage the epithelium occludes the lumen of the esophagus; the lumen later recanalizes. The developing stomach is suspended from a dorsal and ventral mesogastrium. Through two types of rotation, the stomach attains its adult position. Common malformations of the stomach are pyloric stenosis, which interferes with emptying of the stomach, and ectopic gastric mucosa, which can produce ulcers in unexpected locations.

◯ As they grow, the intestines form a hairpin loop that herniates into the body stalk. Further growth of the small intestine causes small intestinal loops to accumulate in the body stalk. While the intestines retract into the body

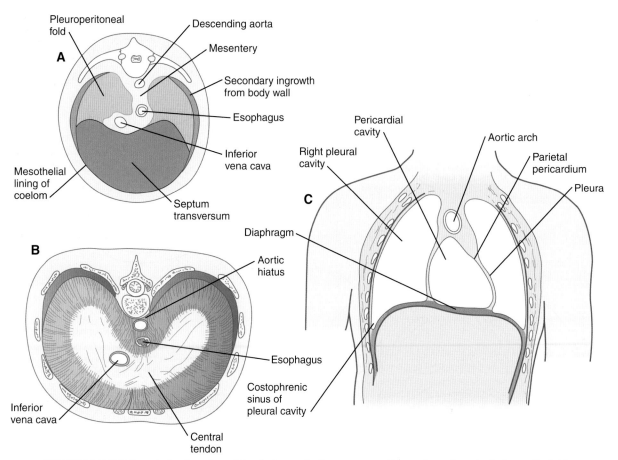

**FIGURE 15-34** Stages in the formation of the diaphragm. **A,** Components making up the embryonic diaphragm. **B,** Adult diaphragm as seen from the thoracic side. **C,** Frontal section showing relations of the diaphragm to the pleural and pericardial cavities.

cavity, they rotate around the superior mesenteric artery. This results in the characteristic positioning of the colon around the small intestine in the abdominal cavity. During these changes in position, parts of the dorsal mesentery fuse with the peritoneal lining of the dorsal body wall. In the posterior part of the gut the urorectal septum partitions the cloaca into the rectum and urogenital sinus.

◯ During its differentiation, the lining of the intestinal tract passes through phases of (1) epithelial proliferation, (2) cellular differentiation, and (3) biochemical and functional maturation. Like the esophagus, the small intestine goes through a period of occlusion of the lumen by the epithelium. At later stages, intestinal crypts located at the base of villi contain epithelial stem cells, which supply the entire intestinal epithelial surface with various epithelial cells.

◯ The intestinal tract is subject to a variety of malformations, including local stenosis, atresia, duplications, diverticula, and abnormal rotation. Incomplete resorption of the vitelline duct can give rise to Meckel's diverticulum, vitelline duct ligaments, cysts, or fistulas. Omphalo-

cele is the failure of the intestines to return to the body cavity from the body stalk. Aganglionic megacolon is caused by the failure of parasympathetic neurons to populate the distal part of the colon. Failure of the anal membrane to break down (imperforate anus) may be associated with fistulas connecting the digestive tract to various regions of the urogenital system.

◯ Digestive glands arise as epithelial diverticula from the gut. Their formation and further outgrowth are based on inductive interactions with the surrounding mesenchyme. The primordium of the liver arises in the septum transversum, but as it expands, it protrudes into the ventral mesentery. As it develops, the liver acquires the capacity to synthesize and secrete serum albumin and to store glycogen among other biochemical functions. The pancreas grows out as dorsal and ventral pancreatic buds that ultimately fuse to form a single pancreas. Within the pancreas the epithelium forms exocrine components, which secrete digestive enzymes, and endocrine components (islets of Langerhans), which secrete insulin and glucagon.

◯ The respiratory system arises as a ventral outgrowth from the gut just caudal to the pharynx. Through

## VENTRAL BODY WALL DEFECTS, ECTOPIA CORDIS, GASTROSCHISIS, AND OMPHALOCELE

The opposing sides of the body wall occasionally fail to fuse as the embryo assumes its cylindrical shape late in the first month. Several defective mechanisms such as hypoplasia of the tissues can account for these defects. A quantitatively minor defect in closure of the thoracic wall is manifested as **failure of sternal fusion** (Figure 15-35). If growth of the two sides of the thoracic wall is severely defective, the heart can form outside the thoracic cavity, resulting in **ectopia cordis** (Figure 15-36).

Closure defects of the ventral abdominal wall can lead to similar gross malformations. In many cases of omphalocele (see Figure 15-13), hypoplasia of the abdominal wall itself or deficiencies of abdominal musculature are evident. More serious cases involve evisceration of the abdominal contents through a fissure between the umbilicus and sternum (**gastroschisis**) (Figure 15-37). Caudal to

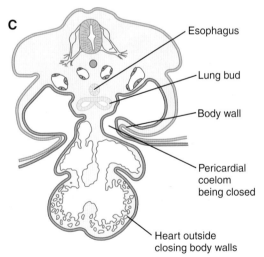

FIGURE 15-36 Ectopia cordis. **A,** Fetus with a major ventral abdominal wall defect that combines gastroschisis and ectopia cordis. **B** and **C,** Cross sections illustrating the inability of the folding sides of the body wall to encompass the developing heart, resulting in ectopia cordis. (Courtesy M. Barr, Ann Arbor, Mich.)

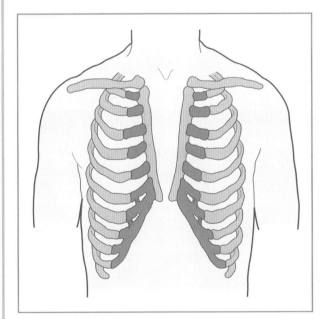

FIGURE 15-35 Failure of fusion of the paired components of the embryonic sternum.

*Continued*

the umbilicus, an associated closure defect of the urinary bladder (exstrophy of the bladder [see Figure 16-19]) is common.

### DIAPHRAGMATIC HERNIAS

Incomplete fusion or hypoplasia of one or more of the components of the diaphragm can lead to an open connection between the abdominal and thoracic cavities. If the defect is large enough, a variety of structures in the abdominal cavity (usually part of the stomach or intestines) can herniate into the thoracic cavity, or more rarely, thoracic structures can penetrate into the abdominal cavity. Minor cases of herniation can cause digestive symptoms. In the case of major defects, herniation of massive portions of the intestines can press against the heart or lungs and interfere with their function. Some common sites of defects in the diaphragm are shown in Figure 15-38.

FIGURE 15-37 Defective closure of the ventral abdominal wall cranial **(A)** and caudal **(B)** to the umbilicus. (Courtesy M. Barr, Ann Arbor, Mich.)

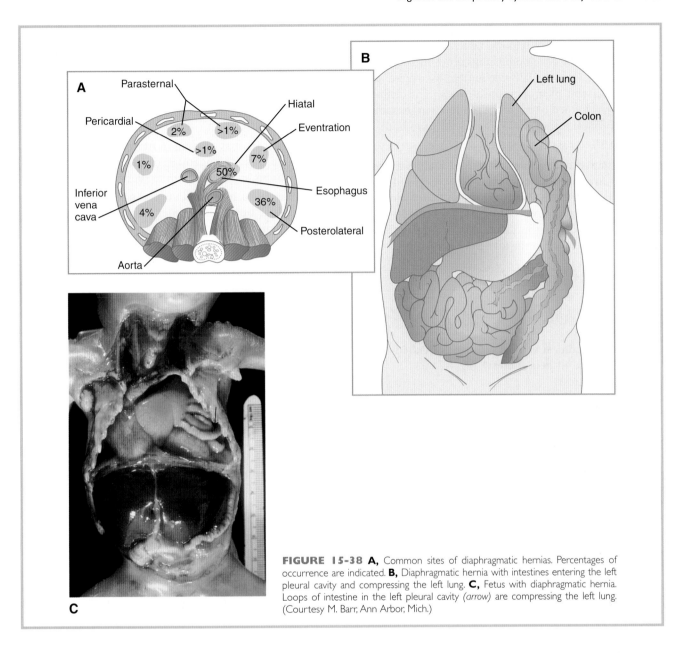

**FIGURE 15-38 A,** Common sites of diaphragmatic hernias. Percentages of occurrence are indicated. **B,** Diaphragmatic hernia with intestines entering the left pleural cavity and compressing the left lung. **C,** Fetus with diaphragmatic hernia. Loops of intestine in the left pleural cavity *(arrow)* are compressing the left lung. (Courtesy M. Barr, Ann Arbor, Mich.)

epithelial-mesenchymal interactions, the tip of the respiratory diverticulum undergoes up to 23 sets of dichotomous branchings. Other interactions with the surrounding mesenchyme stabilize the tubular parts of the respiratory tract by inhibiting branching. Lung development goes through several stages: (1) the embryonic stage, (2) the pseudo-glandular stage, (3) the canalicular stage, (4) the terminal sac stage, and (5) the postnatal stage.

◐ Important malformations of the respiratory tract include tracheoesophageal fistulas, which result in abnormal connections between the trachea and esophagus. Atresia of components of the respiratory system is rare,

but anatomical variations in the morphology of the lungs are common. Respiratory distress syndrome, commonly seen in premature infants, is related to insufficiencies in the formation of pulmonary surfactant by type II alveolar cells.

◐ In its most basic condition the intraembryonic coelom is separated into right and left components by the dorsal and ventral mesenteries, which suspend the gut. Except for the region of the stomach and liver, the ventral mesentery disappears. In the region of the heart the dorsal mesocardium persists, and the ventral mesocardium disappears.

○ The septum transversum divides the coelom into thoracic and abdominal regions, which are connected by pleural canals. The developing lungs grow into the pleural canals, which are partially delimited by paired pleuropericardial and pleuroperitoneal folds. The definitive diaphragm is formed from (1) the septum transversum, (2) pleuroperitoneal folds, and (3) ingrowths from body wall mesenchyme.

○ Quantitative deficiencies in ventral body wall tissue can result in abnormalities ranging from failure of sternal fusion to ectopia cordis in the thorax and omphalocele to gastroschisis and/or exstrophy of the bladder in the abdomen. Defects in the diaphragm are diaphragmatic hernias and can result in the intestines herniating into the thoracic cavity.

## Review Questions

1. Which condition is most closely associated with a disturbance of neural crest?
   A. Anal atresia
   B. Meckel's diverticulum
   C. Omphalocoele
   D. Volvulus
   E. Aganglionic megacolon

2. Meckel's diverticulum is most commonly located in the:
   A. Ileum
   B. Ascending colon
   C. Jejunum
   D. Transverse colon
   E. Duodenum

3. The primordium of which structure is located in the septum transversum?
   A. Dorsal pancreas
   B. Lung
   C. Liver
   D. Thymus
   E. Spleen

4. The yolk stalk is most closely associated with which artery?
   A. Celiac
   B. Umbilical
   C. Superior mesenteric
   D. Aorta
   E. Inferior mesenteric

5. The dorsal pancreatic bud is initially induced from the gut endoderm by the:
   A. Liver
   B. Notochord
   C. Lung bud
   D. Yolk sac
   E. None of the above

6. Splanchnic mesoderm acts as an inducer of all of the following tissues or organs except:
   A. Teeth
   B. Trachea
   C. Liver
   D. Lungs
   E. Pancreas

7. During its first feeding, a newborn begins to choke. What congenital anomalies should be included in the differential diagnosis?

8. A newborn took its first feeding of milk without incident but an hour later was crying in pain and vomited the milk with considerable force. Examination revealed a hard mass near the midline in the upper region of the abdomen. What was the diagnosis?

9. An infant was noted to extrude a small amount of mucus and fluid from the umbilicus when crying or straining. This should make the physician think of what congenital anomaly in the differential diagnosis?

10. A newborn was given a cursory physical examination and was taken home by the mother 1 day after delivery. Several days later the mother brought the child to the clinic. The newborn was in obvious severe discomfort with a swollen abdomen. Physical examination revealed that an important congenital anomaly had been overlooked at the original examination. What was that anomaly?

## REFERENCES

Alescio T, Cassini A: Induction in vitro of tracheal buds by pulmonary mesenchyme grafted on tracheal epithelium, *J Exp Zool* 150:83–94, 1962.

Avery ME, Wang N-S, Taeusch HW: The lung of the newborn infant, *Sci Am* 228:74–85, 1973.

Beck F, Tata F, Chawendsaksophak K: Homeobox genes and gut development, *BioEssays* 22:431–441, 2000.

Bellusci S and others: Fibroblast growth factor 10 (FGF10) and branching morphogenesis in the embryonic mouse lung, *Development* 124: 4867–4878, 1997.

Bossard P, Zaret KS: Repressive and restrictive mesodermal interactions with gut endoderm: possible relation to Meckel's diverticulum, *Development* 127:4915–4923, 2000.

Boyden EA: Development of the human lung, *Pract Pediatr* 4:1–17, 1975.

Burns AJ, Le Douarin NM: The sacral neural crest contributes neurons and glia to the post-umbilical gut: spatiotemporal analysis of the development of the enteric nervous system, *Development* 125:4335–4347, 1998.

Burri PH: Fetal and postnatal development of the lung, *Ann Rev Physiol* 46:617–628, 1984.

Cardoso WV: Molecular regulation of lung development, *Annu Rev Physiol* 63:471–494, 2001.

Colony PC: Successive phases of human fetal development. In Kretchmer N, Minkowski A, eds: *Nutritional adaptation of the gastrointestinal tract of the newborn*, New York, 1983, Raven, pp 3–28.

Duluc I and others: Fetal endoderm primarily holds the temporal and positional information required for mammalian intestinal development, *J Cell Biol* 126:211–221, 1994.

Gittes GK and others: Lineage-specific morphogenesis in the developing pancreas: role of mesenchymal factors, *Development* 122:439–447, 1996.

Godlewski G and others: Liver development in the rat and in man during the embryonic period (Carnegie stages 11–23), *Microsc Res Tech* 39: 314–327, 1997.

Grapin-Botton A, Melton DA: Endoderm development from patterning to organogenesis, *Trends Genet* 16:124–130, 2000.

Gray SW, Skandalakis JE: *Embryology for surgeons*, Philadelphia, 1972, WB Saunders.

Hirai Y and others: Epimorphin: a mesenchymal protein essential for epithelial morphogenesis, *Cell* 69:471–481, 1992.

Hogan BLM: Morphogenesis, *Cell* 96:225–233, 1999.

Hollinshead WH: Embryology and anatomy of the anal canal and rectum, *Dis Colon Rectum* 5:18–22, 1962.

Hollinshead WH: Embryology and surgical anatomy of the colon, *Dis Colon Rectum* 5:23–27, 1962.

Iwashita T and others: Hirschsprung disease is linked to defects in neural crest stem cell function, *Science* 301:972–976, 2003.

Jackson CM: On the developmental topography of the thoracic and abdominal viscera, *Anat Rec* 3:361–396, 1909.

Jacobs-Cohen RJ and others: Inability of neural crest cells to colonize the presumptive aganglionic bowel of ls/ls mutant mice: requirement for a permissive environment, *J Comp Neurol* 255:425–438, 1987.

Kablar B, Tajbakhsh S, Rudnicki MA: Transdifferentiation of esophageal smooth to skeletal muscle is myogenic bHLH factor–dependent, *Development* 127:1627–1639, 2000.

Kaplan F: Molecular determinants of fetal lung organogenesis, *Mol Genet Metabol* 71:321–341, 2000.

Kawazoe Y and others: Region-specific gastrointestinal *Hox* code during murine embryonal gut development, *Devel Growth Differen* 44:77–84, 2002.

Kedinger M and others: Epithelial-mesenchymal interactions in intestinal epithelial differentiation, *Scand J Gastroenterol* 23(suppl 151):62–69, 1988.

Kim SK, Hebrok M: Intercellular signals regulating pancreas development and function, *Genes Devel* 15:111–127, 2001.

Kim SK, Hebrok M, Melton DA: Notochord to endoderm signaling is required for pancreas development, *Development* 124:4243–4252, 1997.

Kondo T and others: Function of posterior *HoxD* genes in the morphogenesis of the anal sphincter, *Development* 122:2651–2659, 1996.

Lammert E, Cleaver O, Melton D: Induction of pancreatic differentiation by signals from blood vessels, *Science* 294:564–567, 2001.

Lang D and others: Pax3 is required for enteric ganglia formation and functions with Sox10 to modulate expression of c-ret, *J Clin Investig* 106:963–971, 2000.

Le Douarin NM: An experimental analysis of liver development, *Med Biol* 53:427–455, 1975.

Lewis FT: The form of the stomach in human embryos with notes upon the nomenclature of the stomach, *Am J Anat* 13:477–503, 1912.

Mall FP: Development of the human coelom, *J Morphol* 12:395–453, 1897.

Marshman E, Booth C, Potten CS: The intestinal epithelial stem cell, *BioEssays* 24:91–98, 2002.

Matsumoto K and others: Liver organogenesis promoted by endothelial cells prior to vascular function, *Science* 294:559–563, 2001.

McHugh KM: Molecular analysis of gastrointestinal smooth muscle development, *J Pediatr Gastroenterol Nutr* 23:379–394, 1996.

Mueller TS and others: Expression of avian Pax1 and Pax9 is intrinsically regulated in the pharyngeal endoderm, but depends on environmental influences in the paraxial mesoderm, *Dev Biol* 178:403–417, 1996.

O'Rahilly R: The timing and sequence of events in the development of the human digestive system and associated structures during the embryonic period proper, *Anat Embryol* 153:123–136, 1978.

O'Rahilly R, Boyden EA: The timing and sequence of events in the development of the human respiratory system during the embryonic period proper, *Z Anat Entwickl-Gesch* 141:237–250, 1973.

O'Rahilly R, Tucker JA: The early development of the larynx in staged human embryos, *Ann Otolaryngol Rhinol Laryngol* 82(suppl 7):1–27, 1973.

Park WY and others: FGF-10 is a chemotactic factor for distal epithelial buds during lung development, *Devel Biol* 201:125–134, 1998.

Patapoutian A, Wold BJ, Wagner RA: Evidence for developmentally programmed transdifferentiation in mouse esophageal muscle, *Science* 270:1818–1821, 1995.

Pepicelli CV, Lewis PM, McMahon AP: Sonic hedgehog regulates branching morphogenesis in the mammalian lung, *Curr Biol* 8:1083–1086, 1998.

Pictet R, Rutter WJ: Development of the embryonic endocrine pancreas. In *Handbook of physiology*, section 7: *Endocrinology*, vol 1, Washington, DC, 1972, American Physiological Society, pp 25–66.

Ponder BAJ and others: Derivations of mouse intestinal crypts from single progenitor cells, *Nature* 313:689–691, 1985.

Potten CS, Loeffler M: Stem cells: attributes, cycles, spirals, pitfalls and uncertainties—lessons for and from the crypt, *Development* 110: 1001–1020, 1990.

Ramalho-Santos M, Melton DA, McMahon AP: Hedgehog signals regulate multiple aspects of gastrointestinal development, *Development* 127:2763–2772, 2000.

Roberts DJ and others: Sonic hedgehog is an endodermal signal inducing *Bmp-4* and *Hox* genes during induction and regionalization of the chick hindgut, *Development* 121:3163–3174, 1995.

Roberts DJ: Molecular mechanisms of development of the gastrointestinal tract, *Devel Dyn* 219:109–120, 2000.

Scharfmann R: Control of early development of the pancreas in rodents and humans: implications of signals from the mesenchyme, *Diabetologia* 43:1083–1092, 2000.

Shiojiri N: Development and differentiation of bile ducts in the mammalian liver, *Microsc Res Tech* 39:328–335, 1997.

Simon-Assman P and others: Extracellular matrix components in intestinal development, *Experientia* 51:883–900, 1995.

Skandalakis LJ and others: Surgical embryology and anatomy of the pancreas, *Surg Clin North Am* 73:661–697, 1993.

Slack JMW: Developmental biology of the pancreas, *Development* 121:1569–1580, 1995.

Smith DM, Tabin CJ: BMP signalling specifies the pyloric sphincter, *Nature* 748–749, 1999.

Stephens FD: Embryology of the cloaca and embryogenesis of anorectal malformations, *Birth Defects Orig Artic Ser* 24:177–209, 1988.

Sukegawa A and others: The concentric structure of the developing gut is regulated by sonic hedgehog derived from endodermal epithelium, *Development* 127:1971–1980, 2000.

Teitleman G, Lee JK: Cell lineage analysis of pancreatic islet cell development: glucagon and insulin precursors arise from catecholaminergic precursors present in the pancreatic duct, *Dev Biol* 121:454–466, 1987.

Thompson ABR, Keelan M: The development of the small intestine, *Can J Physiol Pharmacol* 64:13–29, 1986.

Vachon PH and others: Early establishment of epithelial apoptosis in the developing human small intestine, *Int J Devel Biol* 44:891–898, 2000.

Van Veenendaal MB, Liem KD, Marres HAM: Congenital absence of the trachea *Eur J Pediatr* 159:8–13, 2000.

Volpe MAV and others: Hoxb-5 expression in the developing mouse lung suggests a role in branching morphogenesis and epithelial cell fate, *Histochem Cell Biol* 108:495–504, 1997.

Warot X and others: Gene dosage-dependent effects of the Hoxa-13 and Hoxd-13 mutations on morphogenesis of the terminal parts of the digestive and urogenital tracts, *Development* 124:4781–4791, 1997.

Wartiovaara K, Salo M, Sariola H: Hirschsprung's disease genes and the development of the enteric nervous system, *Ann Med* 30:66–74, 1998.

Wells LJ: Development of the human diaphragm and pleural sacs, *Carnegie Contr Embryol* 35:107–134, 1954.

Wells LJ, Boyden EA: The development of the human bronchopulmonary segments in human embryos of horizons XVII to XIX, *Am J Anat* 95:163–201, 1954.

Yasugi S, Mizuno T: Mesenchymal-epithelial interactions in the organogenesis of the digestive tract, *Zool Sci* 7:159–170, 1990.

Yokouchi Y, Sakiyama J-I, Kuroiwa A: Coordinated expression of Abd-B subfamily genes of the HoxA cluster in the developing digestive tract of chick embryo, *Dev Biol* 169:76–89, 1995.

Young HM, Newgreen D: Enteric neural crest–derived cells: origin, identification, migration, and differentiation, *Anat Rec* 262:1–15, 2001.

Zákány J, Duboule D: Hox genes and the making of sphincters, *Nature* 401:761–762, 1999.

Zaret KS: Liver specification and early morphogenesis, *Mech Devel* 92:83–88, 2000.

Zaret KS: Hepatocyte differentiation: from the endoderm and beyond, *Curr Opin Genet Devel* 11:568–574, 2001.

# CHAPTER 16

# Urogenital System

The urogenital system arises from the intermediate mesoderm of the early embryo (see Figure 6-6). Several major themes underlie the development of urinary and genital structures from this common precursor. The first is the interconnectedness of urinary and genital development, in which early components of one system are taken over by another during its later development. A second is the recapitulation during human ontogeny of kidney types (the equivalent of organ isoforms) that are terminal forms of the kidney in lower vertebrates. A third theme is the dependence of differentiation and maintenance of many structures in the urogenital system on epithelial-mesenchymal interactions. Finally, the sexual differentiation of many structures passes from an indifferent stage, in which male and female differences are not readily apparent, to a male or female pathway depending on the presence of specific promoting or inhibiting factors acting on the structure. Although phenotypic sex is genetically determined, genetic sex can be overridden by environmental factors, leading to a discordance between the two. Clinical Correlations 16-1 and 16-2 discuss abnormalities of the urinary and genital systems, respectively. These are found at the end of each section.

## URINARY SYSTEM

The urinary system begins to take shape before any gonadal development is evident. Embryogenesis of the kidney begins with the formation of an elongated pair of excretory organs similar in structure and function to the kidneys of lower vertebrates. These early forms of the kidney are later supplanted by the definitive metanephric kidneys, but as they regress, certain components are retained to be reused by other components of the urogenital system.

### Early Forms of the Kidney

The common representation of mammalian kidney development includes three successive phases beginning with the appearance of the **pronephros**, the developmental homologue of the type of kidney found in only the lowest vertebrates. In human embryos the first evidence of a urinary system consists of the appearance of a few segmentally arranged sets of epithelial cords that differentiate from the anterior intermediate mesoderm at about 22 days' gestation. These structures are more appropriately called **nephrotomes**. The nephrotomes connect laterally with a pair of **primary nephric (pronephric) ducts**, which grow toward the cloaca (Figure 16-1). Experimental evidence suggests that kidney development is initiated by a signal emanating from the paraxial mesoderm. The response to this signal is the expression of the transcription factors **Lim-1** and **Pax-2** in the intermediate mesoderm. Lim-1 is required for the aggregation of the mesenchymal cells of the intermediate mesoderm into the primary nephric ducts.

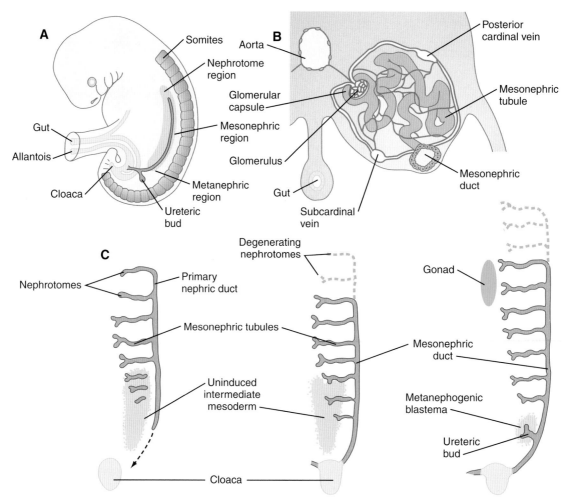

**FIGURE 16-1** Early stages in the establishment of the urinary system. **A,** Subdivision of the intermediate mesoderm into areas that will form nephrotomes, mesonephros, and metanephros. **B,** Cross section through mesonephros showing a well-developed mesonephric tubule and its associated vasculature. **C,** Caudal progression of formation of the mesonephros and degeneration of the most cranial segments of the primitive kidney.

As the primary nephric ducts extend caudally, they stimulate the intermediate mesoderm to form additional segmental sets of tubules. The conversion of the mesenchymal cells of the intermediate mesoderm into epithelial tubules depends upon the expression of Pax-2, and in the absence of this molecule further development of kidney tubules does not occur. These tubules are structurally equivalent to the **mesonephric tubules** of fishes and amphibians. A typical mesonephric unit consists of a vascular **glomerulus**, which is partially surrounded by an epithelial glomerular capsule. The glomerular capsule is continuous with a contorted mesonephric tubule, which is surrounded by a mesh of capillaries (see Figure 16-1, B). Each mesonephric tubule empties separately into the continuation of the primary nephric duct, which becomes known as the **mesonephric (wolffian) duct**.

The formation of pairs of mesonephric tubules occurs along a craniocaudal gradient. The first four to six pairs of mesonephric tubules (as well as the pronephric tubules)

appear to arise as outgrowths from the primary nephric ducts. Farther caudally, mesonephric tubules take shape separately in the intermediate mesoderm slightly behind the caudal extension of the mesonephric ducts. By the end of the fourth week of gestation the mesonephric ducts attach to the cloaca, and a continuous lumen is present throughout each. There is a difference in the developmental controls between the most cranial four to six pairs of mesonephric ducts and the remaining caudal ones. Knockouts for the *WT-1* (Wilms' tumor suppressor) gene result in the absence of posterior mesonephric tubules, whereas the cranial ones that bud off the pronephric duct form normally. As is the case in the formation of the metanephros (see later), *WT-1* appears to regulate the transformation from mesenchyme to epithelium during the early formation of renal (mesonephric) tubules. Very near its attachment site to the cloaca, the mesonephric duct develops an epithelial outgrowth called the **ureteric bud** (see Figure 16-1, A). Early in the fifth week the ureteric bud begins to grow into the most posterior region of the intermediate mesoderm. It then sets up a series of continuous inductive interactions leading to the formation of the definitive kidney, the **metanephros**.

Although there is evidence of urinary function in the mammalian mesonephric kidney, the physiology of the mesonephros has not been extensively investigated. Urine formation in the mesonephros begins with a filtrate of blood from the glomerulus into the glomerular capsule. This filtrate then flows into the tubular portion of the mesonephros, where the selective resorption of ions and other substances occurs. The return of resorbed materials to the blood is facilitated by the presence of a dense plexus of capillaries around the mesonephric tubules.

The structure of the human embryonic mesonephros is very similar to that of adult fishes and aquatic amphibians, and it functions principally to filter and remove body wastes. Because these species and the amniote embryo exist in an aquatic environment, there is little need to conserve water. Therefore the mesonephros does not develop a medullary region or an elaborate system for concentrating urine as the adult human kidney must.

The mesonephros is most prominent while the definitive metanephros is taking shape. Although it rapidly regresses as a urinary unit after the metanephric kidneys become functional, the mesonephric ducts and some of the mesonephric tubules persist in the male and become incorporated as integral components of the genital duct system (Figure 16-2).

## Metanephros

Development of the metanephros begins early in the fifth week, when the ureteric bud (**metanephric diverticulum**) grows into the posterior portion of the intermediate mesoderm. Mesenchymal cells of the intermediate mesoderm condense around the metanephric diverticulum to form the **metanephrogenic blastema** (see Figure 16-1, C). Outgrowth of the ureteric bud from the mesonephric duct is a response to the secretion of **glial cell line–derived neurotrophic factor** (**GDNF**) by the undifferentiated mesenchyme of the metanephrogenic blastema (Figure 16-3, A). This inductive signal is bound by **c-Ret**, a member of the tyrosine kinase receptor superfamily, which is located in the plasma membranes of the

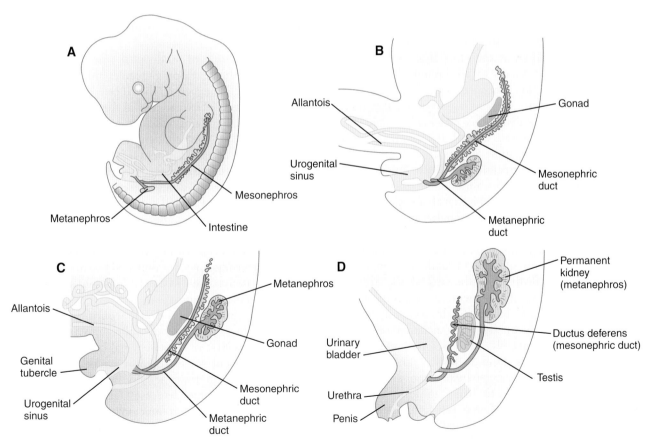

**FIGURE 16-2** Stages in the formation of the metanephros. **A,** At **6 weeks. B,** At **7 weeks. C,** At **8 weeks. D,** At **3 months** (male).

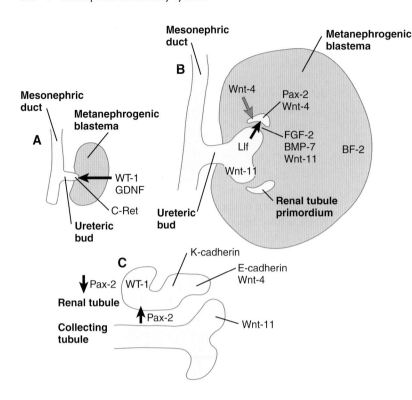

**FIGURE 16-3** Molecular basis for the early formation of the metanephros and ureter. **A,** Early induction of metanephros. **B,** Branching of ureteric bud. **C,** Early tubule formation. *BMP,* Bone morphogenetic protein; *FGF,* fibroblast growth factor; *GDNF,* glial cell line–derived neurotrophic factor.

epithelial cells of the early ureteric bud. The formation of GDNF in the metanephric mesenchyme is regulated by **WT-1**.

The morphological basis for the development of the metanephric kidney is the elongation and branching (up to 14 or 15 times) of the ureteric bud, which becomes the **collecting (metanephric) duct** system of the metanephros, and the formation of renal tubules from mesenchymal condensations (metanephrogenic blastema) located around the tips of the branches. The mechanism underlying these events is a series of reciprocal inductive interactions between the tips of the branches of the metanephric ducts and the surrounding metanephrogenic blastemal cells. Without the metanephric duct system, tubules do not form; conversely, the metanephrogenic mesoderm acts on the metanephric duct system, inducing its characteristic branching. Expression of **Wnt-11** and bone morphogenetic protein-7 (**BMP-7**) in the tips of the ureteric buds is important to the branching response to the mesenchymal inductive influences. In response to the GDNF inductive signal by the metanephric mesenchyme, the epithelial cells of the ureteric bud produce **fibroblast growth factor (FGF-2)**, **BMP-7**, and **leukemia inhibitory factor (LIF)**, which induce the surrounding metanephric mesenchyme to begin to form the epithelial precursors of renal tubules. Tubule formation also requires a sequential inductive signal, **Wnt-4**, which is produced by the metanephric mesenchyme itself. This early induction patterns the metanephric mesenchyme into a tubular epithelial domain, in which the cells express

Wnt-4 and Pax-2, and a stromal region, in which the mesenchymal cells express a winged helix transcription factor, **BF-2**, which may regulate stromal inductive signals.

The formation of individual functional tubules (**nephrons**) in the developing metanephros involves three mesodermal cell lineages: epithelial cells derived from the ureteric bud, mesenchymal cells of the metanephrogenic blastema, and ingrowing vascular endothelial cells. The earliest stage is the condensation of mesenchymal blastemal cells around the terminal bud of the ureteric bud (later to become the metanephric duct). The pre-induced mesenchyme contains several interstitial proteins, such as types I and III collagen and fibronectin. As the mesenchymal cells condense after local induction by the branching tips of the ureteric bud, these proteins are lost and are replaced with epithelial-type proteins (type IV collagen, syndecan-1, laminin, and heparin sulfate proteoglycan), which are ultimately localized to the basement membranes (Figure 16-4).

As the terminal bud of the metanephric duct branches, the surrounding mesenchyme splits into two parts. A single condensation of mesenchymal cells goes through a defined series of stages to form a renal tubule. After a growth phase, mitotic activity within the rounded blastemal mesenchyme decreases, and the primordium of the tubule assumes a comma shape (Figure 16-5, *A*). Within the comma a group of cells farthest from the end of the metanephric duct becomes polarized, forming a central lumen and a basal lamina on the outer surface. This marks the transformation of the induced mesenchy-

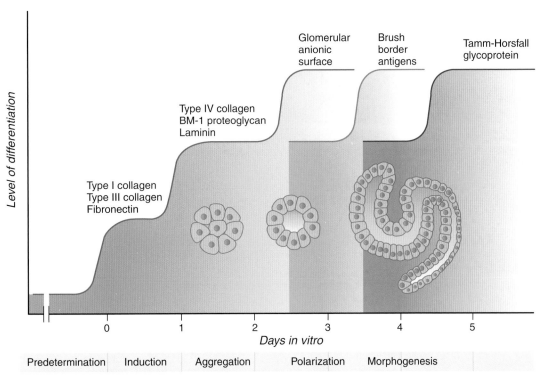

**FIGURE 16-4** Multiphasic determination and differentiation of mouse metanephric mesoderm in vitro. (Modified from Saxén L and others: *Biology of human growth*, New York, 1981, Raven.)

mal cells into an epithelium, specifically the specialized **podocytes**, which ultimately surround the vascular endothelium of the glomerulus.

A consequence of this epithelial transformation is the formation of a slit just beneath the transforming podocyte precursors in the tubular primordium (see Figure 16-5, *B*). Precursors of vascular endothelial cells grow into this slit, which ultimately forms the glomerulus. Induced metanephric mesenchyme stimulates the ingrowth of endothelial cells, possibly by the release of a factor similar to FGF. Uninduced mesenchyme does not possess this capability. The endothelial cells are connected with branches from the dorsal aorta, and they form a complex looping structure that ultimately becomes the renal glomerulus. Cells of the glomerular endothelium and the adjoining podocyte epithelium form a thick basement membrane between them. This basement membrane later serves as an important component of the renal filtration apparatus.

As the glomerular apparatus of the nephron takes shape, another slit forms in the comma-shaped tubular primordium, transforming it into an S-shaped structure (Figure 16-5, *C*). Cells in the rest of the tubule primordium also undergo an epithelial transformation to form the remainder of the renal tubule. This transformation involves the acquisition of polarity by the differentiating epithelial cells. It is correlated with the deposition of laminin in the extracellular matrix along the basal surface of the cells and the concentration of the integral

membrane glycoprotein **uvomorulin (E-cadherin)**, which seals the lateral borders of the cells (Figure 16-6). As the differentiating tubule assumes an **S** shape, differing patterns of gene expression are seen along its length. Near the future glomerular end, levels of Pax-2 expression fall as WT-1 becomes strongly expressed (see Figure 16-3). At the other end of the tubule (future distal convoluted tubule), Wnt-4 and E-cadherin remain prominent, whereas in the middle (future proximal convoluted tubule) K-cadherin is a prominent cellular marker. Many of the uninduced mesenchymal cells between tubules undergo apoptosis.

Differentiation of the renal tubule progresses from the glomerulus to the proximal and then distal convoluted tubule. During differentiation of the nephron, a portion of the tubule develops into an elongated hairpin loop that extends into the medulla of the kidney as the **loop of Henle**. During differentiation, the tubular epithelial cells develop molecular features characteristic of the mature kidney (e.g., brush border antigens or the Tamm-Horsfall glycoprotein [see Figure 16-4]).

Growth of the kidney involves the formation of approximately 15 successive generations of nephrons in its peripheral zone, with the outermost nephrons less mature than those farther inward. Development of the internal architecture of the kidney is very complex, involving the formation of highly ordered arcades of nephrons (Figure 16-7). Details are beyond the scope of this text.

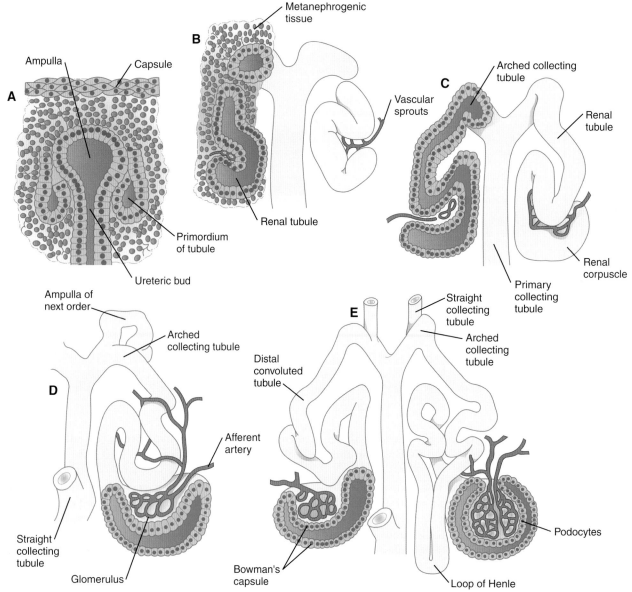

**FIGURE 16-5** Stages in the development of a metanephric tubule.

## Later Changes in Kidney Development

While the many sets of nephrons are differentiating, the kidney becomes progressively larger. The branched system of ducts also becomes much larger and more complex, forming the pelvis and system of **calyces** of the kidney (Figure 16-8). These structures collect the urine and funnel it into the ureters. During much of the fetal period, the kidneys are divided into grossly visible lobes. By birth the lobation is already much less evident, and it disappears during the neonatal period.

When they first take shape, the metanephric kidneys are located deep in the pelvic region. During the late embryonic and early fetal period, they undergo a pronounced shift in position that moves them into the abdominal region. This shift results partly from actual migration and partly from a marked expansion of the caudal region of the embryo. Two concurrent components to the migration occur. One is a caudocranial shift from the level of the fourth lumbar to the first lumbar or even twelfth thoracic vertebra (Figure 16-9). The other is a lateral displacement. These changes bring the kidneys into contact with the adrenal glands, which form a cap of glandular tissue on the cranial pole of each kidney. During their migration, the kidneys also undergo a 90-degree rotation, with the pelvis ultimately facing the midline. As they are migrating out of the pelvic cavity,

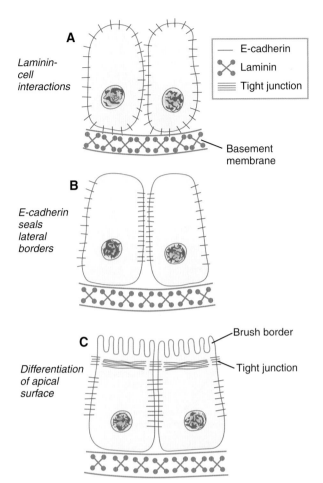

**FIGURE 16-6** Stages in the transformation of renal mesenchyme into epithelium, with emphasis on the role of laminin and E-cadherin (uvomorulin). **A,** Development of polarity is triggered by interactions between laminin and the cell surface, but E-cadherin is still distributed in a nonpolar manner. **B,** E-cadherin redistribution occurs, and E-cadherin interactions seal the lateral borders of the cells. **C,** Apical border of epithelial cells differentiates, as seen by formation of a brush border. (Based on Ekblom P: *FASEB J* 3:2141–2150, 1989.)

**FIGURE 16-7** Formation of arcades of nephrons in the developing human metanephros. **A,** Early stages. **B,** Arrangement of nephrons at the time of birth. (Based on Osathanondh V, Potter EL: *Arch Pathol* 76:271–302, 1963.)

## Formation of the Urinary Bladder

The division of the cloaca into the rectum and urogenital sinus region was introduced in Chapter 15 (see Figure 15-10). The urogenital sinus is continuous with the allantois, which has an expanded base continuous with the urogenital sinus and an attenuated tubular process that extends into the body stalk on the other end. The dilated base of the allantois continues to expand to form the **urinary bladder**, and its attenuated distal end solidifies into the cordlike urachus, which ultimately forms the median umbilical ligament leading from the bladder to the umbilical region (see Figure 16-18).

As the bladder grows, its expanding wall incorporates the mesonephric ducts and the ureteric buds (Figure 16-10). The result is that these structures open separately into the posterior wall of the bladder. Through a poorly defined mechanism possibly involving mechanical tension exerted by the migrating kidneys, the ends of the ureters open into the bladder laterally and cephalically to the mesonephric ducts. The region bounded by these structures is called the **trigone** of the bladder. At the entrance of the mesonephric ducts, the bladder becomes sharply attenuated. This region, originally part of the urogenital sinus, forms the **urethra**, which serves as the outlet of the bladder (see p. 419).

the kidneys slide over the large umbilical arteries, which branch from the caudal end of the aorta. All these changes take place behind the peritoneum, since the kidneys are retroperitoneal organs. During the early phases of migration of the metanephric kidneys, the mesonephric kidneys regress. The mesonephric ducts, however, are retained as they become closely associated with the developing gonads.

Although normally supplied by one large renal artery branching directly from the aorta, the adult kidney consists of five vascular lobes. The arteries feeding each of these lobes were originally segmental vessels that supplied the mesonephros and were taken over by the migrating metanephros. Their aortic origins are typically reduced to the single pair of renal arteries, but anatomical variations are common.

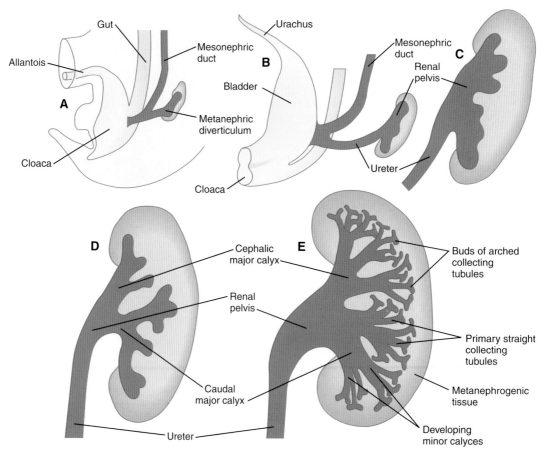

**FIGURE 16-8** Later changes in the development of the metanephros.

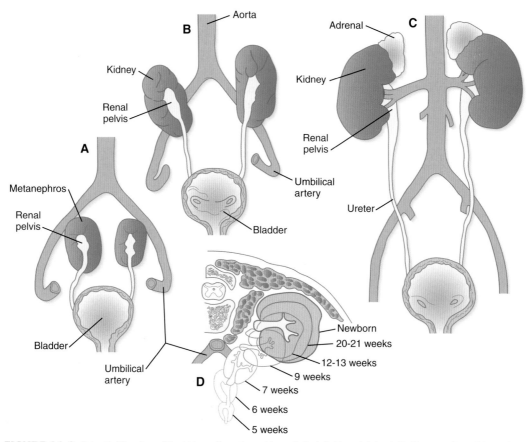

**FIGURE 16-9 A** to **C,** Migration of the kidneys from the pelvis to their definitive adult level. **D,** Cross section of the pathway of migration of the kidneys out of the pelvis.

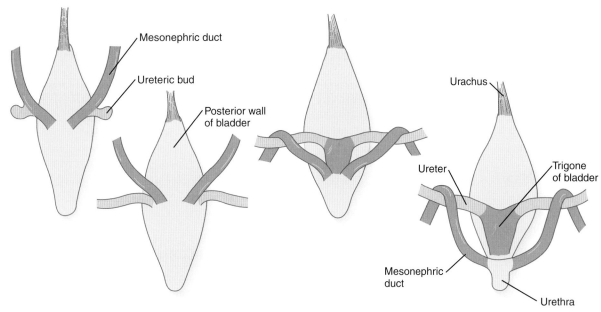

**FIGURE 16-10** Dorsal views of the developing urinary bladder showing changing relationships of the mesonephric ducts and the ureters as they approach and become incorporated into the bladder. In the two on the right, note the incorporation of portions of the walls of the mesonephric ducts into the trigone of the bladder.

## GENITAL SYSTEM

Development of the genital system is one phase in the overall sexual differentiation of an individual (Figure 16-20). Sexual determination begins at fertilization, when a Y chromosome or an additional X chromosome is joined to the X chromosome already in the egg. This phase represents the genetic determination of gender. Although the genetic gender of the embryo is fixed at fertilization, the gross phenotypic gender of the embryo is not manifested until the seventh week of development. Before that time, the principal morphological indicator of the embryo's gender is the presence or absence of the **sex chromatin (Barr body)** in the female. The Barr body is the result of inactivation of one of the X chromosomes. During this morphologically **indifferent stage** of sexual development, the gametes migrate into the gonadal primordia from the yolk sac.

The phenotypic differentiation of gender is traditionally considered to begin with the gonads* and progresses with gonadal influences on the sexual duct systems. Similar influences on the differentiation of the external genitalia and finally on the development of the secondary sexual characteristics (e.g., body configuration, breasts, hair patterns) complete the events that constitute the overall process of sexual differentiation. Sexual

differentiation of the brain, which has an influence on behavior, also occurs.

Under certain circumstances an individual's genetic gender can be overridden by environmental factors so that the genotypic and phenotypic sex do not correspond. An important general principle is that the development of phenotypic maleness requires the action of substances produced by the testis. In the absence of specific testicular influences or the ability to respond to them, a female phenotype results. The female phenotype is the baseline, or default, condition, which must be acted on by male influences to produce a male phenotype.

### Genetic Determination of Gender

Since 1923, scientists have recognized that the XX and XY chromosomal pairings represent the genetic basis for human femaleness and maleness. For many decades, they believed that the presence of two X chromosomes was the sex-determining factor, but in 1959, it was established that the differentiation between maleness and femaleness in humans depends on the presence of a Y chromosome. Nevertheless, the link between the Y chromosome and determination of the testis remained obscure. During recent decades, three candidates for the **testis-determining factor** have been proposed.

The first was the **H-Y antigen,** a minor histocompatibility antigen present on the cells of males but not females. The H-Y antigen has been mapped to the long arm of the human Y chromosome. It has been considered

* Recent research, however, has shown gender differences as early as the preimplantation embryo. The *Sry* genes (see later section) are already transcribed before implantation. In addition, the XY preimplantation embryo develops more rapidly than the XX embryo. Male and female preimplantation embryos are antigenically distinguishable. This suggests differences in gene expression.

## Congenital Anomalies of the Urinary System

Anomalies of the urinary system are relatively common (3% to 4% of live births). Many are asymptomatic, and others manifest only later in life. Figure 16-11 summarizes the locations of many of the more frequently encountered malformations of the urinary system.

### RENAL AGENESIS

**Renal agenesis** is the unilateral or bilateral absence of any trace of kidney tissue (Figure 16-12, *A*). Unilateral renal agenesis is seen in roughly 0.1% of adults, whereas bilateral renal agenesis occurs in 1 in 3000 to 4000 newborns. The ureter may be present. This anomaly is usually ascribed to a faulty inductive interaction between the ureteric bud and the metanephrogenic mesenchyme. Misexpression of molecules, such as Pax-2, WT-1, or Wnt-4, which are important in early metanephric development, is a likely cause of some cases of renal agenesis. Individuals with unilateral renal agenesis are often asymptomatic, but typically the single kidney undergoes **compensatory hypertrophy** to maintain a normal functional mass of renal tissue.

An infant born with bilateral renal agenesis dies within a few days after birth. Because of the lack of urine output,

reduction in the volume of amniotic fluid (**oligohydramnios**) during pregnancy is often an associated feature. Infants born with bilateral renal agenesis characteristically exhibit **Potter facies**, consisting of a flattened nose, wide interpupillary space, a receding chin, tapering fingers, and large, low-set ears (Figure 16-13). Potter facies is classified as a secondary disruption resulting from mechanical pressure of the uterus on the face of the fetus in the absence of the normal mechanical buffering of the amniotic fluid.

### RENAL HYPOPLASIA

An intermediate condition between renal agenesis and a normal kidney is **renal hypoplasia** (see Figure 16-12, *B*), in which one kidney or more rarely, both kidneys are substantially smaller than normal even though a certain degree of function may be retained. Although a specific cause for renal hypoplasia has not been identified, some cases may be related to deficiencies in growth factors or their receptors that are active during later critical phases of metanephrogenesis. As with renal agenesis, the normal counterpart to a hypoplastic kidney is likely to undergo compensatory hypertrophy.

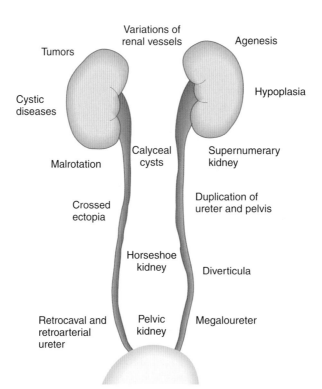

**FIGURE 16-11** Types and sites of anomalies of the kidneys and ureters. (Modified from Gray SW, Skandalakis JE: *Embryology for surgeons*, New York, 1972, WB Saunders.)

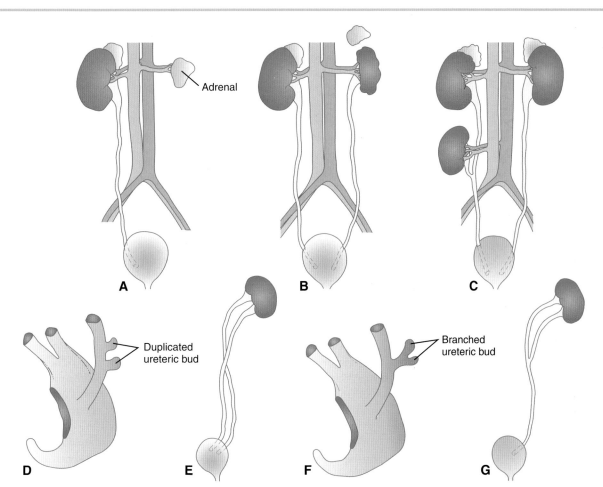

**FIGURE 16-12** Common renal anomalies. **A,** Unilateral renal agenesis. The ureter is also missing. **B,** Unilateral renal hypoplasia. **C,** Supernumerary kidney. **D** and **E,** Complete duplication of ureter, presumably arising from two separate ureteric buds. **F** and **G,** Partial duplication of ureter, presumably arising from a bifurcated ureteric bud.

**FIGURE 16-13 A,** Potter facies, which is characteristic of a fetus who has been exposed to oligohydramnios. Note the flattened nose and low-set ears. **B,** Potter hand with thickened, tapering fingers. (Courtesy M. Barr, Ann Arbor, Mich.)

*Continued*

## RENAL DUPLICATIONS

Renal duplications range from a simple duplication of the renal pelvis to a completely separate **supernumerary kidney.** Like hypoplastic kidneys, renal duplications may be asymptomatic, although the incidence of renal infections may be increased. Many variants of **duplications of the ureter** have also been described (see Figure 16-12). Duplication anomalies are commonly attributed to splitting or wide separation of branches of the ureteric bud.

## ANOMALIES OF RENAL MIGRATION AND ROTATION

The most common disturbance of renal migration leaves a kidney in the pelvic cavity (Figure 16-14, *A*). This is usually associated with malrotation of the kidney as well, so the hilus of the **pelvic kidney** faces anteriorly instead of toward the midline. Another category of migratory malformation is **crossed ectopia,** in which one kidney and its associated ureter are found on the same side of the body as the other kidney (Figure 16-14, *B*). In this condition the ectopic kidney may be fused with the normal kidney.

In the condition of **horseshoe kidney,** occurring in as many as 1 in 400 individuals, the kidneys are typically fused at their inferior poles (Figure 16-15). Horseshoe kidneys cannot migrate out of the pelvic cavity because the inferior mesenteric artery, coming off the aorta, blocks them. In most cases, horseshoe kidneys are asymptomatic, but occasionally pain or obstruction of the

ureters may occur. This condition may be associated with anomalies of other internal organs. Pelvic kidneys are subject to an increased incidence of infections and obstructions of the ureters.

## ANOMALIES OF THE RENAL ARTERIES

Instead of a single renal artery branching off each side of the aorta, duplications or major extrarenal branches of the renal artery are common. Because of the appropriation of segmental arterial branches to the mesonephros by the metanephros, consolidation of the major external arterial supply to the kidney occasionally does not occur.

## POLYCYSTIC DISEASE OF THE KIDNEY

**Congenital polycystic disease of the kidney,** an autosomal recessive condition in infants, is typically manifest by the presence of large numbers of cysts of different sizes within the parenchyma of the kidney (Figure 16-16). Neither the origin nor the pathogenesis of this condition has been definitively ascertained. According to one theory, it is caused by the lack of connection between the tubular part of the nephron and the collecting duct system. The cysts have also been attributed to dilatations of the collecting duct system. An autosomal dominant form of human polycystic disease results from mutations in two genes encoding transcription factors, **ADPKD-1** and **ADPKD-2 (autosomal dominant polycystic kidney disease),** which produce the proteins **polycystin-1** and **polycystin-2.** These proteins may normally function in the development of apical and basolateral polarity of the

Pelvic kidney

A    B

**FIGURE 16-14** Migration defects of the kidney. **A,** Pelvic kidney. **B,** Crossed ectopia. The right kidney has crossed the left ureter and has migrated only part of the normal distance.

FIGURE 16–15 Stages in the formation of a horseshoe kidney. **A** to **C,** As the kidneys migrate out of the pelvis, their caudal poles touch and fuse. **D,** Pelvic kidney in an adult. Note the lack of rotation of the kidneys so that the ureters face ventrally instead of medially. **E,** Horseshoe kidney. (**E,** Photo 914E from the Arey-DaPeña Pediatric Pathology Photographic Collection, Human Developmental Anatomy Center, National Museum of Health and Medicine, Armed Forces Institute of Pathology, Washington, DC.)

FIGURE 16–16 Polycystic kidneys. (Courtesy M. Barr, Ann Arbor, Mich.)

*Continued*

tubule epithelial cells. Cysts of other organs, especially the liver and pancreas, are frequently associated with polycystic kidneys.

### ECTOPIC URETERAL ORIFICES

Ureters may open into a variety of ectopic sites (Figure 16-17). Because of the continuous supply of urine flowing through them, these sites are symptomatic and usually relatively easy to diagnose. Their embryogenesis is commonly attributed to ectopic origins of the ureteric buds in the early embryo.

### CYSTS, SINUSES, AND FISTULAS OF THE URACHUS

If parts of the lumen of the allantois fail to become obliterated, **urachal cysts, sinuses,** or **fistulas** can form (Figure 16-18). In the case of a urachal fistula, urine seeps from the umbilicus. Urachal sinuses or cysts may swell in later life if they are not evident in the infant.

### EXSTROPHY OF THE BLADDER

**Exstrophy of the bladder** is a major defect in which the urinary bladder opens broadly onto the abdominal wall (Figure 16-19). Rather than being a primary defect of the urinary system, it is most commonly attributed to an insufficiency of mesodermal tissue of the ventral abdominal wall. Although initially the ventral body wall may be closed with ectoderm, it breaks down in the absence of mesoderm, and degeneration of the anterior wall of the bladder typically follows. In males, exstrophy of the bladder commonly involves the phallus, and a condition called **epispadias** results (see p. 424).

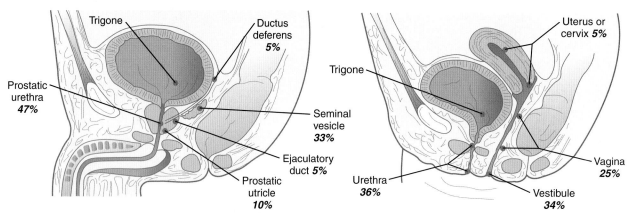

**FIGURE 16-17** Common sites of ectopic ureteral orifices. (Modified from Gray SW, Skandalakis JE: *Embryology for surgeons,* Philadelphia, 1972, WB Saunders.)

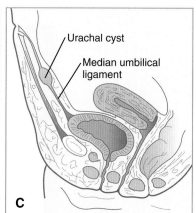

**FIGURE 16-18** Anomalies of the urachus. **A,** Urachal fistula. **B,** Urachal sinus. **C,** Urachal cyst.

**FIGURE 16-19** Exstrophy of the bladder in a male infant, showing protrusion of the posterior wall of the bladder through a defect in the lower abdominal wall. At the base of the open bladder is an abnormal, partially bifid penis with an open urethra (not seen) on its dorsal surface. A wide, shallow scrotum is separated from the penis. (From Crowley LV: *An introduction to clinical embryology,* St Louis, 1974, Mosby.)

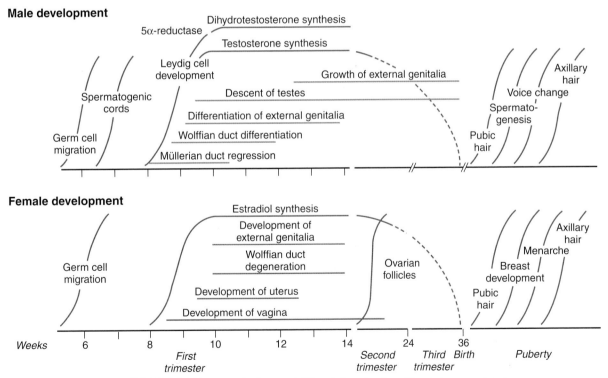

**FIGURE 16-20** Major events in the sexual differentiation of male and female human embryos.

to be the product of the mammalian testis-determining gene. However, a strain of mice (*Sxr*) was found to produce males in the absence of the H-Y antigen. *Sxr* mice were found to have a transposition of a region of the Y chromosome onto the X chromosome, but the locus coding for the H-Y antigen was not included. In addition, certain phenotypic human males with an XX genotype were shown to be missing the genetic material for the H-Y antigen.

The next candidate was a locus on the short arm of the Y chromosome called the *zinc finger Y (ZFY)* gene. With DNA hybridization techniques, this gene has been found in both XX male humans and in mice in which small pieces of the X and Y chromosomes were swapped during crossing-over in meiosis. Conversely, this gene was missing in some rare XY human females. However, certain XX males were found to lack the gene, and other rare cases of anomalies of sexual differentiation did not show a correspondence between sexual phenotype and the expected presence or absence of the ZFY gene.

The most recent candidate for the testis-determining gene is one called *Sry*, a member of the *Sox* family of transcription factors and probably an evolutionary derivative of *Sox-3*; it is also located within a 35-kilobase region on the short arm of the Y chromosome (Figure 16-21). The *Sry* gene encodes a 223-amino acid nonhistone protein belonging to a family of proteins that contain a highly conserved 79-amino acid DNA-binding region called a **high mobility group box**. After the gene was cloned, it was detected in many cases of gender reversal, including XX males with no *ZFY* genes. The *SRY* gene on the human Y chromosome is located near the homologous region, making it susceptible to translocation to the X chromosome.

The *Sry* gene is also absent in a strain of XY mice that are phenotypically female. Further experimental evidence consists of producing transgenic mice with the insertion of a 14-kilobase fragment of the Y chromosome containing the *Sry* gene. Many of the transgenic XX mice developed into phenotypic males with normal testes and male behavior. In situ hybridization studies in mice have shown that expression of the *Sry* gene product occurs in male gonadal tissue at the time of sex determination, but it is not expressed in the gonads of female embryos.

## Migration of Germ Cells into the Gonads

The early appearance of primordial germ cells in the lining of the yolk sac and their migration to the gonads in human embryos is briefly described in Chapter 1. Descriptive and experimental studies have shown that primordial germ cells in the mouse can first be demonstrated in the epiblast, where their formation is dependent upon **BMP-4** expression by the extraembryonic ectoderm. These cells pass through the early primitive streak and are next located as a small cluster of cells in the extraembryonic mesoderm near the base of the allantois. They then become associated with the endoderm of the posterior wall of the yolk sac (see Figure 1-1).

In human embryos the primordial germ cells migrate from the posterior wall of the yolk sac along the wall of the hindgut and through the dorsal mesentery until they reach the region of the newly appearing **genital ridges**. Experimental evidence suggests that the initial stages of migration of primordial germ cells at some distance from the gonads are accomplished by active ameboid

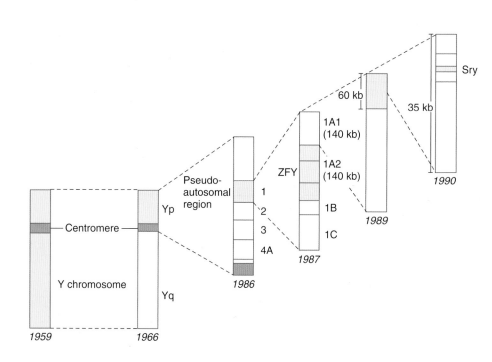

**FIGURE 16-21** A history in the progress of localization of the sex-determining gene on the Y chromosome. (Modified from Sultan C and others: *Horm Res* 36:1–3, 1991.)

movement of the cells in response to a permissive extracellular matrix substrate. Tissue displacements through differential growth of the posterior region of the embryo may also contribute. During their migration, many primordial germ cells are linked to one another through long cytoplasmic processes. How these interconnections control either migration or settling down in the gonads remains to be determined. Migrating germ cells proliferate in response to mitogenic factors such as *LIF* and **Steel factor**. Primordial germ cells express the transcription factor **Oct-4**, which is involved in the maintenance of their totipotent state much as this same gene maintains the undifferentiated condition of blastomeres of cleaving embryos (see p. 45).

As the germ cells approach the genital ridges late in the fifth week of development, they may be influenced by chemotactic factors secreted by the newly forming gonads. Such influences have been demonstrated by grafting embryonic tissues (e.g., hindgut, which contains dispersed germ cells) into the body cavity of a host embryo. The primordial germ cells of the graft typically concentrate on the side of the graft nearest the genital ridges of the host or sometimes migrate into the genital ridges from the graft. Approximately 1000 to 2000 primordial germ cells enter the genital ridges. Once the primordial germ cells have penetrated the genital ridges, their migratory behavior ceases.

Some primordial germ cells follow inappropriate migratory pathways, leading them to settle into extragonadal sites. These cells normally start to develop as oogonia, regardless of genotype; they then degenerate. In rare instances, however, they persist in ectopic sites, such as the mediastinum, and ultimately may give rise to **teratomas** (see Chapter 1).

## Establishment of Gonadal Gender

### Origin of the Gonads

The gonads arise from an elongated region of steroidogenic mesoderm along the ventromedial border of the mesonephros. Cells in the cranial part of this region condense to form the **adrenocortical primordia**, and those of the caudal part become the **genital ridges**, which are identifiable midway through the fifth week. The early genital ridges consist of two major populations of cells: one derived from the **coelomic epithelium** and the other arising from the **mesonephric ridge**.

One of the earliest genes required for development of the gonads is *WT-1*, which is expressed throughout the intermediate mesoderm and, as was seen earlier (page 394), is important in early kidney formation (see Figure 16-3). **Steroidogenic factor-1 (SF-1)** is expressed in the early indifferent gonad, as well as in the developing adrenal cortex. SF-1 appears to be involved in the somatic

cells of the early gonad, rather than the primordial germ cells. In keeping with its association with endocrine organs, SF-1 is also expressed in cells of the pituitary and hypothalamus. The other major gene involved in the earliest phase of gonadal development is *Lim-1*. As was noted earlier in this text (see Figure 5-11), the absence of *Lim-1* expression results in the lack of formation of the anterior head; in addition, neither kidneys nor gonads form.

### Differentiation of the Testes

When the genital ridges first appear, those of males and females are morphologically indistinguishable (indifferent stage). The general principle underlying gonadal differentiation is that under the influence of the *Sry* gene (testis-determining factor) on the Y chromosome, the indifferent gonad differentiates into a testis (Figure 16-22). In the absence of expression of products of this gene, the gonad later differentiates into an ovary.

In males, transcripts of the *Sry* gene are detected only in the genital ridge just at the onset of differentiation of the testis. Neither expression of the *Sry* gene nor later differentiation of the testis depends on the presence of germ cells. The sex-determining genes act on the somatic portion of the testis and not on the germ cells. The emerging picture is that *Sry* acts as a trigger for testis formation. It triggers testis formation by inhibiting the function of **Dax-1**, a member of a nuclear hormone receptor family. Dax-1, which is X-linked, is expressed in the early indifferent gonad at the same time as Sry. Unrestrained, Dax-1 functions as an inhibitor of testis formation, but the trigger function of Sry appears to be to inhibit Dax-1 inhibition, therefore allowing the male gonad to develop as a testis (Figure 16-23). This sequence is reminiscent of neural induction, in which inhibitors (noggin and chordin) inhibit an inhibitor (BMP-4) of neural plate formation in the dorsal ectoderm (see Figure 5-10).

Timing is important in differentiation of the testis. The testis develops more rapidly than the ovary. Precursors of the Sertoli cells must be prepared to receive the genetic signals (Sox-9) for testicular differentiation by a certain time. If not, the primordial germ cells begin to undergo meiosis and the gonad differentiates into an ovary. Early differentiation of the testis also appears to depend on a signal from the mesonephros, possibly WT-1. In the absence of the mesonephros, internal structures (testis cords) differentiate poorly.

The morphology of early gonadal differentiation has been controversial, with several scenarios of cell lineage and interactions being proposed. According to recent morphological evidence, the genital ridges first appear midway in the fifth week through the proliferation of **coelomic epithelial cells** along the medial border of the mesonephros (see Figure 16-23). Later in the fifth week the primordial germ cells enter the early genital ridge, and the coelomic epithelium sends short epithelial pillars

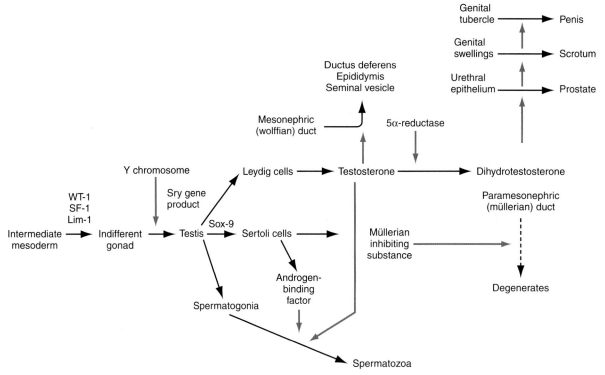

**FIGURE 16-22** Differentiation of the male phenotype.

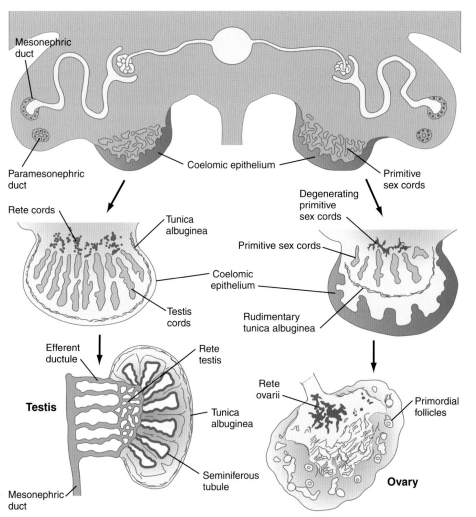

**FIGURE 16-23** Morphology of gonadal differentiation.

toward the interior of the gonad. Early in the sixth week, under the influence of the transcription factor **Sox-9**, a set of **primitive sex cords** takes shape in the genital ridge, and the primordial germ cells migrate into the primitive sex cords. The male gonad appears to give off a chemoattractive agent that stimulates the migration from the mesonephros of the myoid cells that surround the sex cords. In addition, endothelial cells and the myoepithelial cells that surround the vasculature migrate into the testis from the mesonephros. Ovarian tissue does not attract these cells.

Late in the sixth week the testis shows evidence of differentiation. The primitive sex cords enlarge and are better defined, and their cells are thought to represent the precursors of the Sertoli cells (Table 16-1). As the sex cords differentiate, they are separated from the surface epithelium (germinal epithelium) by a dense layer of connective tissue called the **tunica albuginea**. The deepest portions of the testicular sex cords are in contact with the fifth to twelfth sets of mesonephric nephrons. The outer portions of the testicular sex cords form the **seminiferous tubules**, and the inner portions become meshlike and ultimately form the **rete testis**. The rete testis ultimately joins the **efferent ductules**, which are derived from mesonephric tubules.

For the first 2 months of development, **Leydig cells** are not identifiable in the embryonic testis. These appear during the eighth week and soon begin to synthesize androgenic hormones (testosterone and androstenedione). This endocrine activity is important because differentiation of the male sexual duct system and the external genitalia depends on the sex hormones secreted by the fetal testis. Fetal Leydig cells secrete their hormonal products at just the period when differentiation of the hormonally sensitive genital ducts takes place (9 to 14 weeks). After weeks 17 and 18, the Leydig cells gradually involute and do not reappear until puberty, when they stimulate spermatogenesis. The fetal Leydig cells can be viewed as a cellular isoform that is later replaced by the definitive adult form of the cells. By 8 weeks the

---

**TABLE 16-1** *Functions of Sertoli Cells in Male Sexual Differentiation*

Induce migration of mesenchymal cells (future interstitial cells) from mesonephros into testis

Give off signals that inhibit the entry of male germ cells into meiosis

Emit signals that induce the differentiation of Leydig cells, which secrete testosterone

Secrete müllerian inhibiting substance

Secrete androgen-binding factor

---

embryonic Sertoli cells produce **müllerian inhibiting substance** (see p. 412), which also plays an important role in shaping the sexual duct system by causing involution of the precursors of the female genital ducts.

During the late embryonic and fetal periods and after birth, the primordial germ cells in the testis divide slowly by mitosis, but the fetal Sertoli cells are insensitive to androgens and fail to mature. Sertoli cells secrete a **meiosis-inhibiting factor**, but such a factor has not been isolated or characterized. The environment of the testis does not become favorable for meiosis and spermatogenesis until puberty.

## Differentiation of the Ovaries

In females, the expression of **Dax-1**, in the absence of the influence of Sry, suppresses the formation of testis structures and allows the gonads to develop as ovaries. In contrast to the testes, the presence of viable germ cells is essential for ovarian differentiation. If primordial germ cells fail to reach the genital ridges or if they are abnormal (e.g., XO) and degenerate, the gonad regresses, and **streak ovaries** (vestigial ovaries) result.

After the primordial germ cells have entered the future ovary, they remain concentrated in the outer cortical region or near the corticomedullary border. Like the testis, the ovary contains primitive sex cords in the medullary region, but these are not as well developed as those in the testis. The origin of the cells that form the ovarian follicles has not been established. Three sites of origin have been proposed for the follicular epithelial cells: (1) the coelomic epithelium (secondary sex cords), (2) the primitive sex cords of mesonephric origin, and (3) a combination of the two. The last possibility is in accordance with the presence of two distinct cell types—light and dark—within the early follicular epithelium.

The primary germ cells, now properly called **oogonia**, proliferate by mitosis from the time of their entry into the gonad until the start of the fourth month of gestation. At that time, some oogonia in the inner medullary region of the ovary enter prophase of the first meiotic division, possibly under the influence of a meiosis-stimulating factor emanating from the mesonephros. This influence may be associated with clumps of mesonephrically derived epithelia called the medullary **rete ovarii**. The meiotic oogonia, now called **oocytes**, become associated with follicular cells and form **primordial follicles** (see Figure 1-5). Meanwhile, the oogonia in the cortical region of the ovary continue to divide mitotically. The oogonia and early oocytes are connected by intercellular cytoplasmic bridges, which may play a role in synchronization of their development. By week 22, follicular development is well under way throughout the ovary. The oocytes continue in meiosis until they reach the diplotene stage of prophase of the first meiotic division. Meiosis is then arrested, and the oocytes remain in this stage until the block is removed. In the adult, this occurs in individual oocytes just days before ovulation. In premenopausal women, as many as 50 years may have elapsed since these oocytes entered the meiotic block in embryonic life.

In the fetal ovary an inconspicuous tunica albuginea forms at the corticomedullary junction. The cortex of the ovary is the dominant component, and it contains the majority of oocytes. The medulla fills with connective tissue and blood vessels that are derived from the mesonephros. The testis, on the other hand, is characterized by a dominance of the medullary component located inside a prominent tunica albuginea.

The developing ovary does not maintain a relationship with the mesonephros. Normally, the mesonephric tubules in the female embryo degenerate, leaving only a few remnants (Table 16-2).

**TABLE 16-2** *Homologies in the Male and Female Urogenital Systems*

| Indifferent structure | Male derivative | Female derivative |
|---|---|---|
| Genital ridge | Testis | Ovary |
| Primordial germ cells | Spermatozoa | Ova |
| Sex cords | Seminiferous tubules (Sertoli cells) | Follicular (granulosa) cells |
| Mesonephric tubules | Efferent ductules Paradidymis | Eoophoron Paroophoron |
| Mesonephric (wolffian) ducts | Appendix of epididymis Epididymal duct Ductus deferens Ejaculatory duct | Appendix of ovary Gartner's duct |
| Paramesonephric (müllerian) ducts | Appendix of testis Prostate utricle | Uterine tubes Uterus Upper vagina |
| Definitive urogenital sinus (lower part) | Penile urethra | Lower vagina Vaginal vestibule |
| Early urogenital sinus (upper part) | Urinary bladder Prostatic urethra | Urinary bladder Urethra |
| Genital tubercle | Penis | Clitoris |
| Genital folds | Floor of penile urethra | Labia minora |
| Genital swellings | Scrotum | Labia majora |

## SEXUAL DUCT SYSTEM

Like the gonads, the sexual ducts pass through an early indifferent stage. As the fetal testes begin to function in the male, their secretion products act on the indifferent ducts, causing some components of the duct system to develop further and others to regress. In females the absence of testicular secretory products results in the preservation of structures that regress and the regression of structures that persist in the male.

### Indifferent Sexual Duct System

The indifferent sexual duct system consists of the **mesonephric (wolffian) ducts** and the **paramesonephric (müllerian) ducts** (Figure 16-24). The paramesonephric ducts appear between 44 and 48 days of gestation as longitudinal invaginations of the surface epithelium along the mesonephric ridge lateral to the mesonephric ducts. The invaginations soon become epithelial cords, which grow caudally and terminate on the urogenital sinus between the ends of the mesonephric ducts without breaking into the sinus. These cords then develop a lumen in a craniocaudal direction. The cranial end of each paramesonephric duct opens into the coelomic cavity as a funnel-shaped structure. The fate of the indifferent genital ducts depends on the gender of the gonad.

### Sexual Duct System of Males

Development of the sexual duct system in the male depends on secretions from the testis. Under the influence of **müllerian inhibiting substance** (sometimes called antimüllerian hormone), a glycoprotein of the transforming growth factor-β family secreted by the Sertoli cells of the testes at 8 weeks' gestation, the paramesonephric ducts degenerate, leaving only remnants at their cranial and caudal ends (Figures 16-25 and 16-26 and Table 16-2). Müllerian inhibiting substance appears not to directly affect the epithelium of the paramesonephric ducts but rather the surrounding mesenchyme. These mesenchymal cells express a gene that encodes a serine/threonine kinase membrane-bound receptor, which binds the müllerian inhibiting substance. Under its influence, the surrounding mesenchymal cells instruct the epithelial cells of the müllerian duct to regress.

Under the influence of testosterone, which is secreted by the Leydig cells of the testes, the mesonephric ducts continue to develop even though the mesonephric kidneys are degenerating. The mesonephric ducts differentiate into the paired **ductus deferens**, which constitutes the path of sperm transport from the testis to the urethra. Portions of degenerating mesonephric tubules may persist near the testis as the **paradidymis**. *Hox* genes play a role

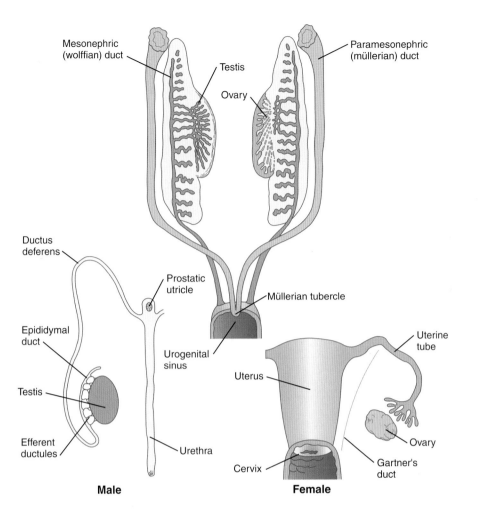

**FIGURE 16-24** Indifferent condition of the genital ducts in the embryo at approximately **6 weeks.**

Mesonephric (wolffian) duct
Paramesonephric (müllerian) duct
Testis
Ovary
Ductus deferens
Prostatic utricle
Müllerian tubercle
Epididymal duct
Urogenital sinus
Uterine tube
Uterus
Testis
Efferent ductules
Urethra
Ovary
Cervix
Gartner's duct

**Male**          **Female**

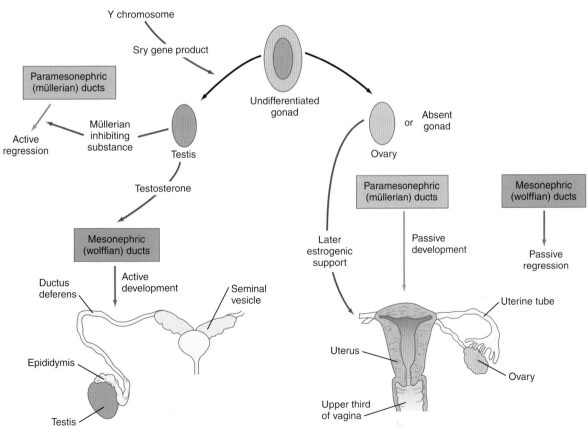

Y chromosome
Sry gene product
Paramesonephric (müllerian) ducts
Undifferentiated gonad
Absent gonad
Active regression
Müllerian inhibiting substance
Testis
Ovary
Paramesonephric (müllerian) ducts
Mesonephric (wolffian) ducts
Testosterone
Later estrogenic support
Passive development
Passive regression
Mesonephric (wolffian) ducts
Active development
Seminal vesicle
Ductus deferens
Uterine tube
Epididymis
Uterus
Ovary
Testis
Upper third of vagina

**FIGURE 16-25** Factors involved in sexual differentiation of the genital tract. (After Hutson JM and others. In Burger H, deKrester D, eds: *The testis,* ed 2, New York, 1989, Raven, pp 143–179.)

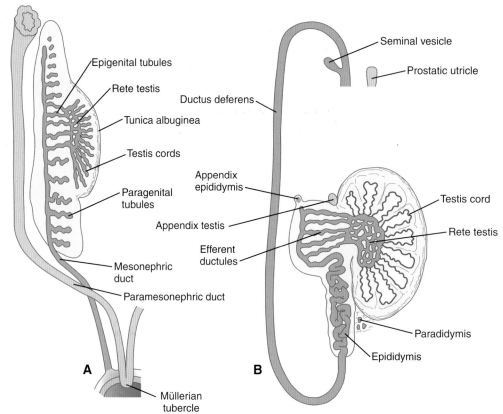

**FIGURE 16-26** Development of the male genital duct system. **A,** At the end of the **second month. B,** In the late fetus. (Modified from Sadler T: *Langman's medical embryology,* ed 6, Baltimore, 1990, Williams & Wilkins.)

in the specification of the various regions of the male reproductive tract. For example, **Hoxa-10** is expressed along the mesonephric duct from the caudal epididymis to the point where the ductus deferens inserts into the urethra. Mutants of both *Hoxa-10* and *Hoxa-11* exhibit a homeotic transformation, resulting in the partial transformation of ductus deferens to epididymis.

Associated with development of the male genital duct system (both the ductus deferens and the urethra) is the formation of the male accessory sex glands: the **seminal vesicles,** the **prostate,** and the **bulbourethral glands** (Figure 16-27). These glands arise as epithelial outgrowths from their associated duct systems (seminal vesicles from the ductus deferens and the others from the urogenital sinus, the precursor of the urethra), and their formation involves epithelial-mesenchymal interactions similar to those of other glands. In addition, these glands depend on androgenic stimulation for their development. Specifically, the mesenchymal cells develop androgen receptors and appear to be the primary targets of the circulating androgenic hormones. (At this stage the epithelial cells do not contain androgen receptors.) After stimulation by the androgens, the mesenchymal cells act on the associated epithelium through the local paracrine effects of growth factors, causing it to differentiate with gland-specific characteristics.

In the developing prostate, the urogenital mesenchyme induces epithelial outgrowths from the urogenital sinus endoderm just below the bladder. **Dihydrotestosterone** (see later), acting through receptors in the mesenchyme, and the resultant secretion of **FGF-10** and **TGF-β1** by the mesenchyme, regulates the production of **sonic hedgehog** (shh) in the epithelium of the urogenital sinus. In response to the shh signaling, the prostatic ducts begin to bud off the epithelium of the urogenital sinus. The extent of budding is regulated by the inhibitory action of **BMP-4,** which is most strongly expressed lateral to the area where the prostatic ducts begin to bud off. Underlying all of these molecular interactions is the action of the transcription factors, **Hoxa-13** and **Hoxd-13,** which appear to determine that the organ that will form in this site is, indeed, the prostate. Null mutants of these *Hox* genes show a reduced number of prostatic ducts. The developing prostatic epithelium also induces the surrounding mesenchyme to differentiate into smooth muscle cells.

Tissue recombination experiments in which glandular mesoderm from mice with **testicular feminization syndrome** (lack of testosterone receptors resulting in no response to testosterone) was combined with normal epithelium demonstrated that the mesodermal component of the glandular primordia is the hormonal target.

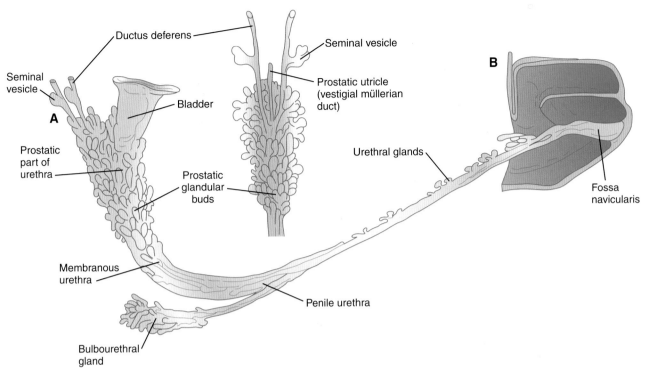

**FIGURE 16-27** Development of the male urethra and accessory sex glands in an embryo of approximately **16 weeks. A,** Lateral view. **B,** Dorsal view of prostatic region. (After Didusch. From Johnson FP: *J Urol* 4:447–502, 1920.)

Differentiation of the epithelium did not occur. In contrast, when normal glandular mesoderm was combined with epithelium from animals with testicular feminization syndrome, normal development took place.

In the embryo the tissues around the urogenital sinus synthesize an enzyme (**5α-reductase**) that converts testosterone to dihydrotestosterone. Through the action of appropriate receptors of either form of testosterone, critical tissues of the male reproductive tract are maintained and grow (Figure 16-28).

## Sexual Duct System of Females

If ovaries are present or if the gonads are absent or dysgenic, the sexual duct system differentiates into a female phenotype. In the absence of testosterone secreted by the testes, the mesonephric ducts regress, leaving only rudimentary structures (see Table 16-2). In contrast, the absence of müllerian inhibitory substance allows the paramesonephric (müllerian) ducts to continue to develop into the major structures of the female genital tract (Figure 16-29).

Early formation of the paramesonephric ducts is dependent upon Wnt signaling. In the absence of **Wnt-4**, the paramesonephric ducts fail to form. **Wnt-7a**, which is also involved in setting up the dorsoventral axis of the developing limb, is expressed in the epithelium throughout the entire paramesonephric ducts and is required for

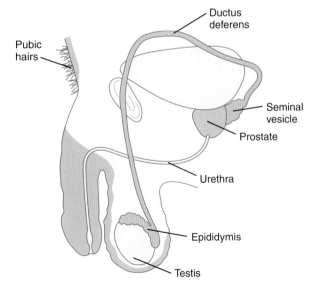

**FIGURE 16-28** Regions of the male reproductive tract sensitive to testosterone (*brown*) and dihydrotestosterone (*blue*).

their normal development. Later in development Wnt-7a expression becomes restricted to the uterine epithelium. In some manner, Wnt-7a seems to be involved in maintaining the expression of a sequence of *Hox* genes (**Hoxd-10** through **Hoxd-13**, as well as the Hoxa paralogues) that are spread along the female reproductive tract (Figure 16-30). For example, Hoxa-9 is expressed in the uterine

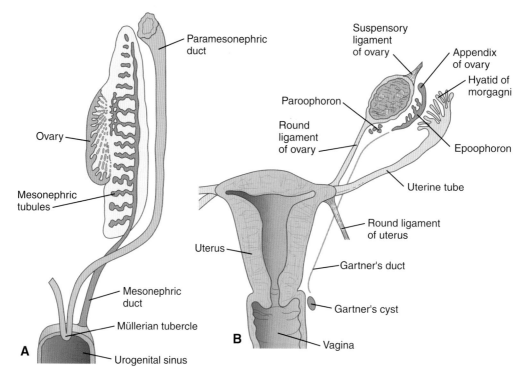

**FIGURE 16-29** Development of the female genital duct system. **A,** At the end of the second month. **B,** Mature condition. (Modified from Sadler T: *Langman's medical embryology*, ed 6, Baltimore, 1990, Williams & Wilkins.)

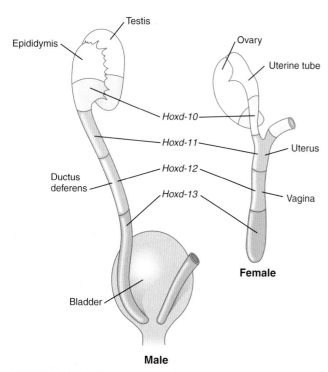

**FIGURE 16-30** Gradients of *Hoxd* gene expression in the male and female internal genitalia of mouse embryos. (Based on studies by Dolle and others [1991].)

tubes, Hoxa-10 in the uterus, Hoxa-11 in the uterus and cervix, and Hoxa-12 in the upper vagina. As is the case in the male reproductive tract, mutations of *Hox* genes result in homeotic transformations, for example, in the absence of Hoxa-10, the cranial part of the uterus becomes transformed into uterine tube. In contrast to other areas of the body, *Hox* gene expression throughout the female reproductive tract, at least in the mouse, continues into adult life. This may be related to the developmental plasticity required of the female reproductive tract throughout the reproductive cycle.

The cranial portions of the paramesonephric ducts become the **uterine tubes,** with the cranial openings into the coelomic cavity persisting as the fimbriated ends. Toward their caudal ends the paramesonephric ducts begin to approach the midline and cross the mesonephric ducts ventrally. This crossing and ultimate meeting in the midline are caused by the medial swinging of the entire urogenital ridge (Figure 16-31). The region of midline fusion of the paramesonephric ducts ultimately becomes the uterus, and the ridge tissue that is carried along with the paramesonephric ducts forms the **broad ligament of the uterus.**

The formation of the vagina remains poorly understood, and several explanations for its origin have been posited. According to one commonly held hypothesis, the fused paramesonephric ducts form the upper part of the vagina, and epithelial tissue from the **müllerian tubercle (uterovaginal plate)** hollows out to form the lower

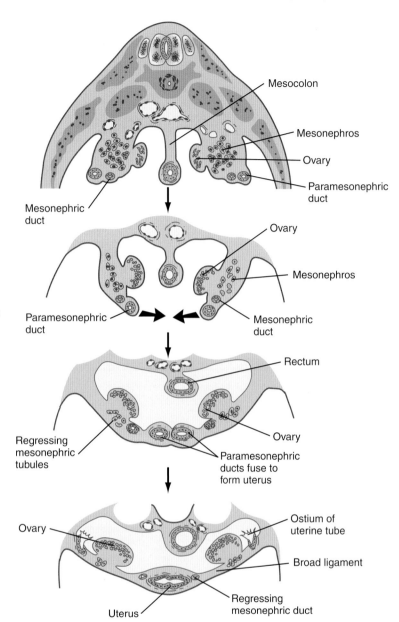

Mesocolon

Mesonephros

Ovary

Paramesonephric duct

Mesonephric duct

Ovary

Paramesonephric duct

Mesonephros

Mesonephric duct

Rectum

Regressing mesonephric tubules

Ovary

Paramesonephric ducts fuse to form uterus

Ovary

Ostium of uterine tube

Broad ligament

Regressing mesonephric duct

Uterus

**FIGURE 16-31** Formation of the broad ligament in the female embryo.

part (Figure 16-32). More recently, several investigators have suggested that the most caudal portions of the mesonephric ducts participate in the formation of the vagina either by directly contributing cells to its wall or by inductively acting on the paramesonephric tissue. Full development of the female reproductive tract depends on estrogenic hormones secreted by the fetal ovaries.

## Descent of the Gonads

### Descent of the Testes

The testes do not remain in their original site of development; they migrate from their intraabdominal location into the scrotum (Figure 16-33). Like the kidneys, the testes are retroperitoneal structures, and their descent occurs behind the peritoneal epithelium. Before their descent, the testes are anchored cranially to the **cranial suspensory ligament**, derived from the diaphragmatic ligament of the mesonephros, and caudally to the **inguinal (caudal) ligament of the mesonephros**, which in later development is called the **gubernaculum**.

Control of testicular descent occurs in three phases. The first is associated with the enlargement of the testes and the concomitant regression of the mesonephric kidneys. Under the influence of androgens, acting through androgen receptors in the cranial suspensory ligament, the ligament regresses, thus releasing the testis from its location near the diaphragm. This causes some caudal displacement of the testes. The second phase, commonly called **transabdominal descent**, brings the

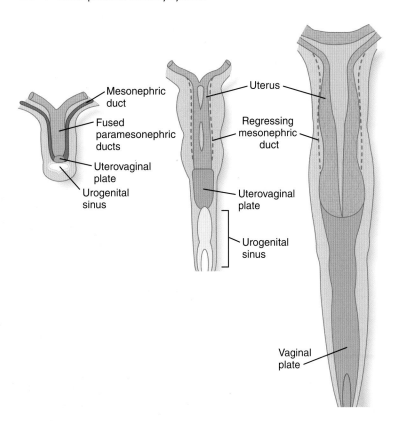

Mesonephric duct

Fused paramesonephric ducts

Uterovaginal plate

Urogenital sinus

Uterus

Regressing mesonephric duct

Uterovaginal plate

Urogenital sinus

Vaginal plate

**FIGURE 16-32** Development of the uterus and vagina. Contact between the fused müllerian ducts and urogenital sinus stimulates proliferation of the junctional endoderm to form the uterovaginal plate. Later canalization of the plate forms the lumen of the vagina.

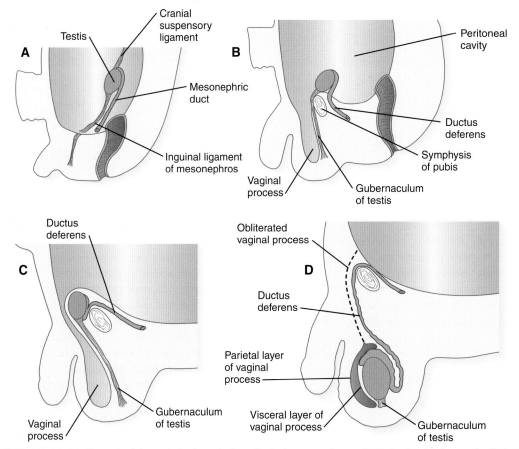

A

Testis

Cranial suspensory ligament

Mesonephric duct

Inguinal ligament of mesonephros

B

Peritoneal cavity

Ductus deferens

Symphysis of pubis

Vaginal process

Gubernaculum of testis

C

Ductus deferens

Vaginal process

Gubernaculum of testis

D

Obliterated vaginal process

Ductus deferens

Parietal layer of vaginal process

Visceral layer of vaginal process

Gubernaculum of testis

**FIGURE 16-33** Descent of the testis in the male fetus. **A,** In the **second month. B,** In the **third month. C,** In the **seventh month. D,** At term.

testes down to the level of the inguinal ring but not into the scrotum. This phase is dependent upon the activity of **Insl-3**, without which the testes remain high in the abdomen. The third phase, called **transinguinal descent**, brings the testes into the scrotum. This phase involves both the action of testosterone and the guidance of the **inguinal ligament of the mesonephros**, which in later development is called the **gubernaculum**. Whether the gubernaculum actively pulls the testis into the scrotum or just acts as a fixed point while the other tissues grow has not been resolved. Testicular descent begins during the seventh month and may not be completed until birth. As it descends into the scrotum, the testis slides behind an extension of the peritoneal cavity: the vaginal process (see Figure 16-33, C). Although this cavity largely closes off with maturation of the testis, it remains as a potential mechanical weak point. With straining, it can open and permit the herniation of intestine into the scrotum.

### Descent of the Ovaries

Although not as dramatically as the testes, the ovaries also undergo a distinct caudal shift in position. In conjunction with their growth and the crossing over of the para-mesonephric ducts, the ovaries move caudally and later-ally. Their position is stabilized by two ligaments, both of which are remnants of structures associated with the mesonephros. Cranially, the **diaphragmatic ligament of the mesonephros** becomes the **suspensory ligament of the ovary**. The superior portion of the inguinal ligament (called the **caudal gonadal ligament** by some authors) develops into the **round ligament of the ovary**, and the inferior portion of the inguinal ligament becomes the **round ligament of the uterus** (see Figure 16-29). The most caudal ends of the round ligaments of the uterus become embedded in the dense fascial connective tissue of the labia majora.

## EXTERNAL GENITALIA

### Indifferent Stage

The external genitalia are derived from a complex of mesodermal tissue located around the cloaca. A very early midline elevation called the **genital eminence** is situated just cephalic to the proctodeal depression. This structure soon develops into a prominent **genital tubercle** (Figure 16-34), which is flanked by a pair of **genital folds** extend-ing toward the proctodeum. Somewhat lateral to these are paired **genital swellings** (see Figure 16-36). When the original cloacal membrane breaks down during the eighth week, the urogenital sinus opens directly to the outside between the genital folds. An endodermal **urethral plate** lines much of the open urogenital sinus. These structures, which are virtually identical in male and female embryos

**FIGURE 16-34** Scanning electron micrograph of the inferior aspect of the indifferent external genitalia of a human embryo at the end of the eighth week of development. (From Jirásek JE: *Atlas of human prenatal morphogene-sis,* Amsterdam, 1983, Martinus Nijhoff.)

during the indifferent stage, form the basis for develop-ment of the external genitalia.

There are some interesting parallels between the development of the genital tubercle and the limb. Both utilize much the same cast of molecular players, starting with an underlying basis of *Hox* gene expression. Being at the terminal part of the urogenital system, the genital tubercle expresses the 5′ elements along the *Hox* gene clusters, specifically *Hoxa-13* and *Hoxd-13*. The early phase of outgrowth of the genital tubercle, which is the same in both male and female embryos, depends upon interacting signals of **shh** and **FGF-8** and **FGF-10**. Shh and FGF-8 are both expressed in the epithelium of the distal urethral plate, and FGF-10 is expressed in the distal mesenchyme of the genital tubercle. Small pieces of genital tubercle even exhibit polarizing activity when grafted into the anterior regions of the limb bud (see Chapter 10). BMP-4, a frequent mediator of programmed cell death in the embryo (e.g., in the interdigital spaces) is also present in the genital tubercle, but the effects of knockouts of BMP-4 are considerably less pronounced in the genital tubercle than in the developing limb. On the other hand, the genital tubercle fails to form in the absence of shh function, and the most distal part (glans) does not form in FGF-10 knockouts.

## External Genitalia of Males

Under the influence of dihydrotestosterone (see Figure 16-28), the genital tubercle in the male undergoes a second phase of elongation to form the penis, and the genital swellings enlarge to form scrotal pouches (see Figure 16-36, A). As this growth is occurring, the urethra takes shape. The male urethra forms in a proximodistal direction by the ventral folding and midline fusion of the genital folds. This results in the formation of a midline epithelial seam on the ventral face of the elongating genital tubercle (Figure 16-35, B). The midline seam undergoes remodeling by secondary canalization and detachment from the ventral surface epithelium to form the urethra proper (Figure 16-35, C). The mode of formation of the distal (glandular) portion of the male urethra has remained controversial for many years. According to one hypothesis, an ectodermal cordlike ingrowth from the tip of the glans meets the distally extending endodermal portion of the penile urethra. More recent research suggests that the entire length of the urethra is formed from the endodermal lining of the urogenital sinus and that the histological characteristic of the distal epithelial lining (a stratified squamous epithelium) can be accounted for by the specific inductive effect of the glandular mesenchyme acting upon the urethral epithelium. After the urethra has formed and has become detached from the ventral epithelial seam, the line of fusion of the urethral folds is marked by the persistence of a ventral **raphe**, which is continuous with the midline raphe that passes between the scrotal swellings.

## External Genitalia of Females

In females the pattern of external genitalia is similar to that of the indifferent stage (Figure 16-36, B). The genital tubercle becomes the **clitoris**, the genital folds become the **labia minora**, and the genital swellings develop into the **labia majora**. The urogenital sinus remains open as the vestibule, into which both the urethra and vagina open. The female **urethra**, developing from the more cranial part of the urogenital sinus, is equivalent to the prostatic urethra of the male, which has a similar origin.

## SUMMARY

◎ The urogenital system arises from the intermediate mesoderm. The urinary system arises before gonadal development begins.

◎ Kidney development begins with the formation of pairs of nephrotomes that connect with a pair of primary nephric ducts. Farther caudally to the nephrotomes, pairs of mesonephric tubules form in a craniocaudal sequence and connect to the primary nephric ducts, which become known as *mesonephric ducts*. In the caudal part of each mesonephric duct a ureteric bud grows out and induces the surrounding mesoderm to form the metanephros.

◎ Outgrowth of the ureteric bud is stimulated by GDNF, produced by the metanephrogenic mesenchyme. This inductive signal is bound by c-Ret on the ureteric bud. In turn, FGF-2, BMP-7, and LIF, secreted by the ureteric bud, stimulate the formation of renal tubules in the metanephrogenic mesenchyme.

◎ Within the developing metanephros, nephrons (functional units of the kidney) form from three sources: the metanephrogenic blastema, the metanephrogenic diverticulum, and ingrowing vascular endothelial cells. Nephrons continue to form throughout fetal life. The

---

**CLINICAL VIGNETTE**

A female athlete with amenorrhea is subjected to a routine sex chromatin test and is told that she cannot compete because she is a male.
  1. What was the appearance of the cells that were tested?
  2. What was the most likely basis for her female phenotype?
  3. What is the likely anatomy of her gonads and genital duct systems, and why?

---

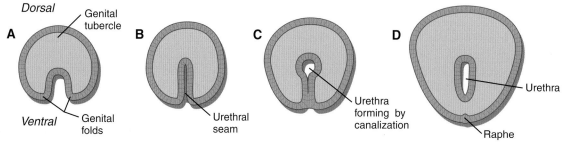

**FIGURE 16-35** Cross-sectional views through the developing penis, showing the mode of formation of the male penile urethra.

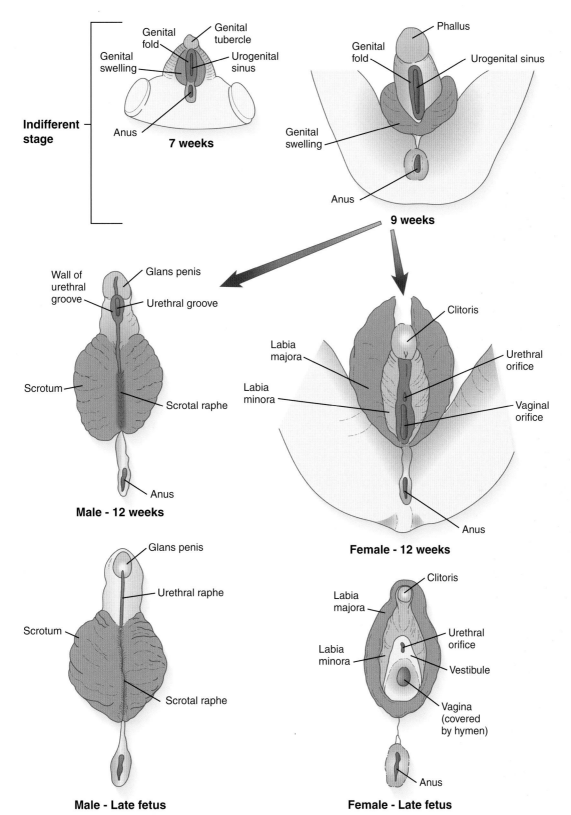

**FIGURE 16-36** Differentiation of the external genitalia of embryos.

## Malformations of the Genital System

### ABNORMALITIES OF SEXUAL DIFFERENTIATION

#### Turner's Syndrome (Gonadal Dysgenesis)

Turner's syndrome results from a chromosomal anomaly (45,XO) (see p. 157). Individuals with this syndrome possess primordial germ cells that degenerate shortly after reaching the gonads. Differentiation of the gonad fails to occur, leading to the formation of a **streak gonad**. In the absence of gonadal hormones the genitalia develop along female lines but remain infantile. The mesonephric duct system regresses for lack of androgenic hormonal stimulation.

#### True Hermaphroditism

Individuals with true hermaphroditism, which is an extremely rare condition, possess both testicular and ovarian tissue. In cases of genetic mosaicism, both an ovary and a testis may be present; in other cases, ovarian and testicular tissue are present in the same gonad (**ovotestis**). Most true hermaphrodites have a 46,XX chromosome constitution, and the external genitalia are basically female, although typically the clitoris is hypertrophied. Such individuals are usually reared as females.

#### Female Pseudohermaphroditism

Female pseudohermaphrodites are genetically female (46,XX) and are sex chromatin positive. The internal genitalia are typically female, but the external genitalia are masculinized, either from excessive production of androgenic hormones by the adrenal cortex (**congenital virilizing adrenal hyperplasia**) or from inappropriate hormonal treatment of pregnant women. The degree of external masculinization can vary from simple clitoral enlargement to partial fusion of the labia majora into a scrotumlike structure (see Figure 8-12).

#### Male Pseudohermaphroditism

Male pseudohermaphrodites are sex chromatin negative (46,XY). Because this condition commonly results from inadequate hormone production by the fetal testes, the phenotype can vary. It is often associated with hypoplasia of the phallus, and there may be varying degrees of persistence of paramesonephric duct structures.

#### Testicular Feminization (Androgen Insensitivity) Syndrome

Individuals with testicular feminization syndrome are genetic males (46,XY) and possess internal testes, but they typically have a normal female external phenotype and are raised as females (see Figure 9-12). Often, testicular feminization is not discovered until the person seeks treatment for amenorrhea or is tested for sex chromatin before athletic events. The testes typically produce testosterone, but because of a deficiency in receptors caused by a mutation on the X chromosome, the testosterone is unable to act on the appropriate tissues. Because müllerian inhibitory substance is produced by the testes, the uterus and upper part of the vagina are absent.

### VESTIGIAL STRUCTURES FROM THE EMBRYONIC GENITAL DUCTS

Vestigial structures are remnants from the regression of embryonic genital ducts, which is rarely complete. They are so common that they are not always considered to be malformations, although they can become cystic.

#### Mesonephric Duct Remnants

In males a persisting blind cranial end of the mesonephric duct can appear as the **appendix of the epididymis** (see Figure 16-26). Remnants of a few mesonephric tubules caudal to the efferent ductules occasionally appear as the **paradidymis**.

In females, the remains of the cranial parts of the mesonephros may persist as the **epoophoron**, or **paroophoron** (see Figure 16-29). The caudal part of the mesonephric ducts is often seen in histological sections along the uterus or upper vagina as **Gartner's ducts**. Portions of these duct remnants sometimes enlarge to form cysts.

#### Paramesonephric Duct Remnants

The cranial tip of the paramesonephric duct may remain as the small **appendix of the testis** (see Figure 16-26). The fused caudal ends of the paramesonephric ducts are commonly seen in the prostate gland as a small midline **prostatic utricle**, which represents the rudimentary uterine primordium. In newborn males the prostatic utricle is typically slightly enlarged because of the influence of maternal estrogenic hormones during pregnancy, but it regresses soon after birth. This structure can enlarge to form a uterus-like structure in some cases of male pseudohermaphroditism.

In females a small part of the cranial tip of the paramesonephric duct may persist at the fimbriated end of the uterine tube as the **hydatid of Morgagni** (see Figure 16-29).

### OTHER ABNORMALITIES OF THE GENITAL DUCT SYSTEM

#### Males

Abnormalities of the mesonephric duct system are relatively rare, but duplications or diverticula of the ductus deferens or urethra can occur. There is an interesting correlation of absent or rudimentary ductus deferens in males with cystic fibrosis. It may be the result of a defect in a gene situated along the gene causing the cystic fibrosis.

**Persistent müllerian duct syndrome,** characterized by the formation of a uterus and uterine tubes, has been described in a number of 46,XY phenotypic males. There is no single cause for this condition, and mutations of genes for both müllerian inhibiting substance and its receptor have been documented.

### Females

Malformations of the uterus or vagina are attributed to abnormalities of fusion or regression of the caudal ends of the paramesonephric ducts (Figure 16-37). Uterine anomalies range from a small septum extending from the dorsal wall of the uterus to complete duplication of the uterus and cervix. Numerous successful pregnancies have been recorded in women with uterine malformations. **Agenesis of the vagina** has been attributed to a failure of formation of the epithelial vaginal plate from the site of joining of the müllerian tubercle with the urogenital sinus.

## ABNORMALITIES OF TESTICULAR DESCENT

### Cryptorchidism

Undescended testes are common in premature males and are seen in about 3% of term males. Normally, the testes of these individuals descend into the scrotum within the first few months after birth. If they do not, the condition of **cryptorchidism** results. Descent of the testes requires the activity of **Insl-3** and androgens, but how disturbances in these molecules result in cryptorchidism remains obscure. Cryptorchidism results in sterility because spermatogenesis does not normally occur at the temperature of the body cavity. There is also a fiftyfold greater incidence of malignancy in undescended testes.

### Ectopic Testes

A testis occasionally migrates to some site other than the scrotum, including the thigh, perineum, and ventral abdominal wall. Because of the elevated temperature of the surrounding tissues, ectopic testes produce reduced numbers of viable spermatozoa.

### Congenital Inguinal Hernia

If the peritoneal canal that leads into the fetal scrotum fails to close, a condition called **persistent vaginal process** occurs. This space may become occupied by loops of bowel that herniate into the scrotum.

## MALFORMATIONS OF THE EXTERNAL GENITALIA

### Males

The most common malformation of the penis is **hypospadias,** in which the urethra opens onto the ventral surface

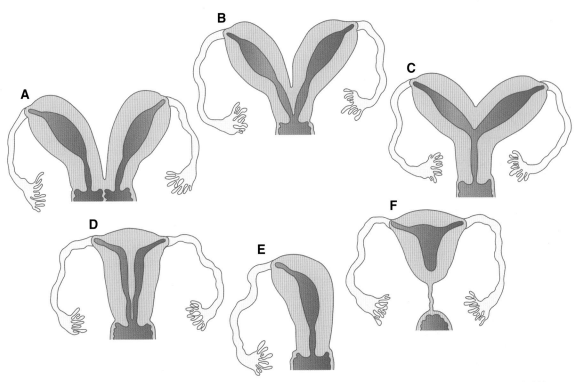

**FIGURE 16-37** Abnormalities of the uterus and vagina. **A,** Double uterus and double vagina. **B,** Double uterus and single vagina. **C,** Bicornuate uterus. **D,** Septate uterus. **E,** Unicornuate uterus. **F,** Atresia of the cervix.

*Continued*

of the penis rather than at the end of the glans (Figure 16-38). The degree of hypospadias can range from a mild ventral deviation of the urethral opening to an elongated opening representing an unfused portion of the urogenital sinus. In the more severe varieties the penis is often bowed ventrally (**chordee**).

Isolated **epispadias**, with the urethra opening on the dorsal surface of the penis, is very rare. A dorsal groove on the penis is commonly associated with exstrophy of the bladder (see Figure 16-19).

**Duplication of the penis** occurs most commonly in association with exstrophy of the bladder and appears to result from the early separation of the tissues destined to form the genital tubercle. Duplication of the penis very

rarely occurs separately from exstrophy of the bladder.

**Congenital absence of the penis** (or clitoris in the female) is rare. This condition is most likely results from mutations of the distalmost *Hox* genes, specifically, *Hoxa-13* or *Hoxd-13*.

### Females

Anomalies of the external genitalia in females can range from hormonally induced enlargement of the clitoris to duplications. Exposure to androgens may also masculinize the genital swellings, resulting in scrotalization of the labia majora (see Figure 8-12). Depending on the degree of severity, wrinkling of the skin and partial fusion may occur.

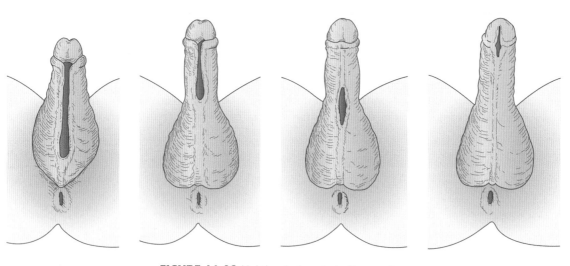

**FIGURE 16-38** Variations in the extent of hypospadias.

induction of nephrons involves reciprocal inductions between terminal branches of the collecting duct system (ureteric bud) and the metanephrogenic mesoderm. Many molecular interactions mediate these inductions.

◯ The kidneys arise in the pelvic basin, and during the late embryonic and early fetal period, they shift into the abdominal region, where they become associated with the adrenal glands. The urinary bladder arises from the base of the allantois.

◯ The urinary system is subject to various malformations. The most severe is renal agenesis, which is probably caused by faulty induction in the early embryo. Abnormal migration can result in pelvic kidneys, other ectopic kidneys, or horseshoe kidney. Polycystic disease of the

kidney is associated with cysts in other internal organs. Faulty closure of the allantois results in urachal cysts, sinuses, or fistulas.

◯ Sex determination begins at fertilization by the contribution of an X or a Y chromosome to the egg by the sperm. The early embryo is sexually indifferent. Through the action of the *Sry* gene, the indifferent gonad in the male develops into a testis. In the absence of this gene the gonad becomes an ovary.

◯ Gonadal differentiation begins after migration of the primordial germ cells into the indifferent gonads. Under the influence of the *Sry* gene product (testis-determining factor), the testis begins to differentiate. The presence of germ cells is not required for differentiation of testis cords. In the embryonic testis, Leydig cells secrete testosterone, and Sertoli cells produce müllerian inhibitory substance. In the absence of *Sry* expression, the gonad differentiates into an ovary and contains follicles. Ovarian follicular differentiation does not occur in the absence of germ cells.

○ The sexual duct system consists of the mesonephric (wolffian) and paramesonephric (müllerian) ducts. The duct system is originally indifferent. In the male, müllerian inhibitory substance causes regression of the paramesonephric duct system, and testosterone causes further development of the mesonephric duct system. In the female, the mesonephric ducts regress in the absence of testosterone, and the paramesonephric ducts persist in the absence of müllerian inhibitory substance.

○ In males the mesonephric ducts form the ductus deferens and give rise to the male accessory sex glands. In females the paramesonephric ducts form the uterine tubes, the uterus, and part of the vagina.

○ The testes descend from the abdominal cavity into the scrotum later in development. The ovaries also shift to a more caudal position. Faulty descent of the testes results in cryptorchidism and is associated with sterility and testicular tumors.

○ The external genitalia also begin in an indifferent condition. Basic components of the external genitalia are the genital tubercle, genital folds, and genital swellings. Under the influence of dihydrotestosterone the genital tubercle elongates into a phallus, and the genital folds fuse to form the penile urethra. The genital swellings form the scrotum. In the female the genital tubercle forms the clitoris, the genital folds form the labia minora, and the genital swellings form the labia majora.

○ If an individual possesses only one X chromosome (XO), Turner's syndrome results. Such individuals have a female phenotype with streak gonads. True hermaphroditism or pseudohermaphroditism can result from various causes. Testicular feminization is found in genetic males lacking testosterone receptors. Such individuals are phenotypic females. Major abnormalities of the sexual ducts are rare, but they can lead to duplications or the absence of the uterus in females.

## Review Questions

1. Which of the following does *not* connect directly with the primary nephric (mesonephric) duct?
   A. Metanephros
   B. Cloaca
   C. Nephrotomes
   D. Mesonephric tubules
   E. Ureteric bud

2. Which association is correct?
   A. Potter facies and hydramnios
   B. Urachal fistula and hydramnios
   C. Horseshoe kidney and superior mesenteric artery
   D. GDNF and metanephrogenic blastema
   E. Bilateral renal agenesis and compensatory hypertrophy

3. Which defect is strongly associated with oligohydramnios?
   A. Pelvic kidney
   B. Renal agenesis
   C. Horseshoe kidney
   D. Crossed ectopia
   E. Polycystic kidney

4. Which anomaly is most closely associated with exstrophy of the bladder?
   A. Epispadias
   B. Renal agenesis
   C. Anal atresia
   D. Pelvic kidney
   E. Ectopic ureteral orifice

5. The uterus arises from the
   A. Paramesonephric ducts
   B. Urogenital sinus
   C. Mesonephric tubules
   D. Pronephric ducts
   E. Mesonephric ducts

6. The floor of the penile urethra in the male is homologous to what structure in the female?
   A. Clitoris
   B. Trigone of the bladder
   C. Labia majora
   D. Labia minora
   E. Perineum

7. The metanephrogenic blastema is induced by the
   A. Pronephric duct
   B. Ureteric bud
   C. Mesonephric tubules
   D. Allantois
   E. Mesonephric duct

8. Drops of a yellowish fluid were observed around the umbilicus of a young infant. What is a likely diagnosis, and what is the embryological basis?

9. A woman who gained relatively little weight during pregnancy gives birth to an infant with large, low-set ears; a flattened nose; and a wide interpupillary space. Within hours after birth the infant is obviously in great distress and dies after 2 days. What is the diagnosis?

10. A seemingly normal woman experiences pelvic pain during the later stages of pregnancy. An ultrasound examination reveals that she has a bicornuate uterus. What is the embryological basis for this condition?

# REFERENCES

Acien P: Embryological observations on the female genital tract, *Hum Reprod* 7:437–445, 1992.

Baskin LS and others: Urethral seam formation and hypospadias, *Cell Tiss Res* 305:379–387, 2001.

Belville C, Josso N, Picard J-Y: Persistence of Müllerian derivatives in males, *Am J Med Genet* 89:218–223, 1999.

Behringer RR: The müllerian inhibitor and mammalian sexual development, *Phil Trans R Soc Lond B* 350:285–289, 1995.

Buehr M: The primordial germ cells of mammals: some current perspectives, *Exp Cell Res* 232:194–207, 1997.

Byskov AG: Differentiation of mammalian embryonic gonad, *Physiol Rev* 66:71–117, 1986.

Capel B: The role of Sry in cellular events underlying mammalian sex determination, *Curr Top Dev Biol* 32:1–37, 1996.

Carroll T and others: Molecular regulation of pronephric development, *Curr Top Devel Biol* 44:67–100, 1999.

Cunha GR and others: The endocrinology and developmental biology of the prostate, *Endocr Rev* 8:338–363, 1987.

Cunha G and others: Growth factors as mediators of stromal-epithelial interactions in steroid hormone target organs. In Dickson RB, Salomon DS, eds: *Hormones and Growth Factors in Development and Neoplasia*, New York, 1998, Wiley-Liss, pp 207–228.

Dollé P and others: Hox-4 genes and the morphogenesis of mammalian genitalia, *Genes Dev* 5:1767–1776, 1991.

Dressler GR: Development of the excretory system. In Rossant J, Tam PPL, eds: *Mouse Development*, San Diego, 2002, Academic Press, pp 395–420.

Eccles MR and others: *Pax* genes in development and disease: the role of *Pax2* in urogenital tract development, *Int J Dev Biol* 46:535–544, 2002.

Ekblom P: Developmentally regulated conversion of mesenchyme to epithelium, *FASEB J* 3:2141–2150, 1989.

Erickson RP: Does sex determination start at conception? *BioEssays* 19:1027–1032, 1997.

Ginsburg M, Snow MHL, McLaren A: Primordial germ cells in the mouse embryo during gastrulation, *Development* 110:521–528, 1990.

Godin I, Wylie C, Heasman J: Genital ridges exert long-range effects on mouse primordial germ cell numbers and direction of migration in culture, *Development* 108:357–363, 1990.

Gougeon A: Initiation of ovarian follicular growth: few facts and many hypotheses. In Filicori M, Flamigni C, eds: *The ovary: regulation, dysfunction and treatment*, Amsterdam, 1996, Elsevier Science, pp 3–12.

Greenfield A, Koopman P: SRY and mammalian sex determination, *Curr Top Dev Biol* 34:1–23, 1996.

Haraguchi R and others: Unique functions of sonic hedgehog signaling during external genitalia development, *Development* 128:4241–4250, 2001.

Hiort O, Holterhus P-M: The molecular basis of male sexual differentiation, *Eur J Endocrinol* 142:101–10, 2000.

Huhtaniemi I, Pelliniemi LJ: Fetal Leydig cells: cellular origin, morphology, life span, and special functional features, *Proc Soc Exp Biol Med* 201:125–140, 1992.

Hutson JM and others: Müllerian inhibiting substance. In Burger H, de Krester D, eds: *The testis*, ed 2, New York, 1989, Raven, pp 143–179.

Josso N, Picard J-Y: Anti-müllerian hormone, *Physiol Rev* 66:1038–1090, 1986.

Koopman P: Gonad development: signals for sex, *Curr Biol* 11:R481–R483, 2001.

Kuure S, Vuolteenaho R, Vainio S: Kidney morphogenesis: cellular and molecular regulation, *Mech Devel* 92:31–45, 2000.

Lamm MLG and others: Mesenchymal factor bone morphogenetic protein 4 restricts ductal budding and branching morphogenesis in the developing prostate, *Devel Biol* 232:301–314, 2001.

Lamm MLG and others: Sonic hedgehog activates mesenchymal Gli1 expression during prostate ductal bud formation, *Devel Biol* 249:349–366, 2002.

Lawson KA and others: BMP4 is required for the generation of primordial germ cells in the mouse embryo, *Genes Devel* 13:424–436, 1999.

Lechner MS, Dressler GR: The molecular basis of embryonic kidney development, *Mech Dev* 62:105–120, 1997.

Levy JB, Husmann DA: The hormonal control of testicular descent, *J Androl* 16:459–463, 1995.

Ludwig KS: The development of the caudal ligaments of the mesonephros and of the gonads: a contribution to the development of the human gubernaculum (Hunteri), *Anat Embryol* 188:571–577, 1993.

Mackay S: Gonadal development in mammals at the cellular and molecular levels, *Internat Rev Cytol* 200:47–99, 2000.

Makabe S and others: Migration of germ cells, development of the ovary, and folliculogenesis. In Familiari G, Makabe S, Motta PM, eds: *Ultrastructure of the ovary*, Norwell, Mass, 1991, Kluwer Academic, pp 1–27.

Marshall Graves JA: The rise and fall of *SRY*, *Trends Genet* 18:259–264, 1999.

Martineau J and others: Male-specific cell migration into the developing gonad, *Curr Biol* 7:958–968, 1997.

Mauch TJ and others: Signals from trunk paraxial mesoderm induce pronephros formation in chick intermediate mesoderm, *Devel Biol* 220:62–75, 2000.

McElreavey K, Fellous M: Sex determination and the Y chromosome, *Am J Med Genet* 89:176–185, 1999.

Migeon CJ, Wisniewski AB: Human sex differentiation: From transcription factors to gender, *Horm Res* 53:111–119, 2000.

Miyamoto N and others: Defects of urogenital development in mice lacking Emx2, *Development* 124:1653–1664, 1997.

Muller J, Shakkebaek NE: The prenatal and postnatal development of the testis, *Bailliere Clin Endocrinol Metab* 6:251–271, 1992.

O'Rahilly RO, Muecke EC: The timing and sequence of events in the development of the human urinary system during the embryonic period proper, *Z Anat Entwickl-Gesch* 138:99–109, 1972.

Osathanondh V, Potter EL: Development of the human kidney as shown by microdissection. I. II. III. *Arch Pathol* 76:271–302, 1963.

Piscione TD, Rosenblum ND: The malformed kidney disruption of glomerular and tubular development, *Clin Genet* 56:341–356, 1999.

Plisov SY and others: TGFβ2, LIF and FGF2 cooperate to induce nephrogenesis, *Development* 128:1045–1057, 2001.

Podlasek C and others: Posterior Hox gene expression in developing genitalia, *Evol Devel* 4:142–163, 2002.

Ramkissoon Y, Goodfellow P: Early steps in mammalian sex determination, *Curr Opin Genet Dev* 6:316–321, 1996.

Reyes FI, Winter JSD, Faiman C: Endocrinology of the fetal testis. In Burger H, de Kretser D, eds: *The testis*, ed 2, New York, 1989, Raven, pp 119–142.

Ryan G and others: Repression of Pax-2 by WT1 during normal kidney development, *Development* 121:867–875, 1995.

Sainio K and others: Differential regulation of two sets of mesonephric tubules by WT-1, *Development* 124:1293–1299, 1997.

Sainio K and others: Glial-cell-line neurotrophic factor is required for bud initiation from ureteric epithelium, *Development* 124:4077–4087, 1997.

Sariola H: Mechanisms and regulation of the vascular growth during kidney differentiation. In Feinberg RN, Sherer GK, Auerbach R, eds: *The development of the vascular system*, Basel, Switzerland, 1991, S Karger, pp 69–80.

Sassoon D: Wnt genes and endocrine disruption of the female reproductive tract: a genetic approach, *Mol Cell Endocrinol* 158:1–5, 1999.

Satoh M: Histogenesis and organogenesis of the gonad in human embryos, *J Anat* 177:85–107, 1991.

Saxén L: *Organogenesis of the kidney*, Cambridge, England, 1987, Cambridge University Press.

Schafer AJ, Goodfellow PN: Sex determination in humans, *BioEssays* 18:955–963, 1996.

Sinclair AH and others: A gene from the human sex-determining region encodes a protein with homology to a conserved DNA binding motif, *Nature* 346:240–244, 1990.

Simpson JL: Genetics of the female reproductive tracts, *Am J Med Genet* 89:224–229, 1999.

Simpson JL, Rajkovic A: Ovarian differentiation and gonadal failure, *Am J Med Genet* 89:186–200, 1999.

Sultan C and others: Sry and male sex determination, *Horm Res* 36:1–3, 1991.

Swain A, Lovell-Badge R: Sex determination and differentiation. In Rossant J, Tam PPL: *Mouse Development*, San Diego, 2002, Academic Press, pp 371–393.

Taylor HS, Vanden Heuvel GB, Igarashi P: A conserved Hox axis in the mouse and human female reproductive system: late establishment and persistent adult expression of the Hoxa cluster genes, *Biol Reprod* 57: 1338–1345, 1997.

Vainio S, Mueller U: Inductive tissue interactions, cell signaling, and the control of kidney organogenesis, *Cell* 90:975–978, 1997.

Van der Werff JFA and others: Normal development of the male anterior urethra, *Teratology* 61:172–183, 2000.

Wartenberg H: Differentiation and development of the testes. In Burger H, de Kretser D, eds: *The testis*, New York, 1989, Raven, pp 67–118.

Wartenberg H: Ultrastructure of fetal ovary including oogenesis. In Van Blerkom J, Motta PM, eds: *Ultrastructure of human gametogenesis and early embryogenesis*, Norwell, Mass, 1989, Kluer Academic, pp 61–84.

Wool AS: A molecular and genetic view of human renal and urinary tract malformations, *Kidney Internat* 58:500–512, 2000.

Woolf AS: Multiple causes of human kidney malformations, *Arch Dis Childhood* 77:471–473, 1997.

Wylie C: Germ cells, *Cell* 96:165–174, 1999.

Zaontz MR, Packer MG: Abnormalities of the external genitalia, *Pediatr Clin North Amer* 44:1267–1297, 1997.

# CHAPTER 17

# Cardiovascular System

This chapter follows the development of the heart from a simple tubular structure to the four-chambered organ that can assume the full burden of maintaining an independent circulation at birth. Similarly, the pattern of blood vessels is traced from their first appearance to an integrated system that carries blood to all parts of the embryo and the placenta. (The early stages in the establishment of the heart and blood vessels are described in Chapter 6 [see Figures 6-12 to 6-17], and the general plan of the embryonic circulation is summarized in Figure 6-24.) Cellular aspects of blood formation are also briefly described. Clinical Correlations 17-1 and 17-2 at the end of the chapter discuss malformations of the heart and the blood vessels, respectively. Table 17-5, also at the end of the chapter, summarizes the time lines in cardiac development.

Functionally, the embryonic heart needs only to act like a simple pump that maintains the flow of blood through the body of the embryo and into the placenta, where fetal wastes are exchanged for oxygen and nutrients. An equally important function, however, is to anticipate the radical changes in the circulation that take place at birth as a consequence of the abrupt cutting off of the placental circulation and the initiation of breathing. To meet the complex requirements of the postnatal circulatory system, the embryonic heart must develop four chambers that can receive or pump the full flow of blood circulating throughout the body. The heart must also adapt to the condition of the fetal lungs, which are poorly developed and for much of the fetal period do not possess

a vasculature that can accommodate a large flow of blood. This physiological dilemma is resolved by the presence of two shunts that allow each chamber of the heart to handle large amounts of blood while sparing the underdeveloped pulmonary vascular channels.

Cardiac morphogenesis involves intrinsic cellular and molecular interactions, but these must occur against a background of ongoing mechanical function. Some of these mechanisms remain elusive, but others are becoming better defined through research on normal and abnormal cardiac development.

Development of the vasculature at the level of gross patterns of arteries and veins has been well understood for many years. Only recently have new cellular and molecular markers enabled investigators to outline the cellular origins and factors controlling differentiation of the arteries and veins in specific organs or regions of the body.

## DEVELOPMENT OF VASCULAR SYSTEM

Development of the vascular system begins in the wall of the yolk sac during the third week of gestation (18 days) with the formation of blood islands (see Figure 6-17). At this time the embryo has attained a size that is too large for the distribution of oxygen to all tissues by diffusion alone. This necessitates the very early development of both the heart and the vascular system. Because the tissues that normally produce blood cells in the adult have not yet begun to form, yolk sac hematopoiesis serves as a temporary adaptation for accommodating the immediate needs of the embryo.

The founder cells of the blood islands, called **hemangioblasts**, have a bipotential developmental capacity and can give rise to either endothelial cells or hematopoietic cells. Once a commitment toward one of these two lineages has been made, daughter cells of the hemangioblasts lose the capacity to form the other type of cell.

## Embryonic Hematopoiesis

Although blood cell formation (**hematopoiesis**) begins in the yolk sac, evidence from animal experimentation suggests that the yolk sac–derived cells are soon replaced by other blood cells that are independently derived from intraembryonic sites of hematopoiesis (Figure 17-1).

The blood islands contain pluripotential **hematopoietic stem cells**, which can give rise to most types of cells found in the embryonic blood. The erythrocytes produced in the yolk sac are large nucleated cells that enter the bloodstream just before the heart tube begins to beat at about 22 days' gestation. For the first 6 weeks the circulating erythrocytes are almost entirely yolk sac derived,

but during that time, preparations for the next stages of hematopoiesis are taking place.

Analysis of human embryos has shown that, starting at 28 days, definitive **intraembryonic hematopoiesis** begins in small clusters of cells (**paraaortic clusters**) in the splanchnopleuric mesoderm associated with the ventral wall of the dorsal aorta and shortly thereafter in the **aorta/genital ridge/mesonephros (AGM) region**. By 5 to 6 weeks, sites of hematopoiesis become prominent in the liver. In both the yolk sac and early sites of embryonic hematopoiesis the endothelial cells themselves briefly retain the capacity for producing blood-forming cells.

The erythrocytes produced by the liver are quite different from those derived from the yolk sac. Although still considerably larger-than-normal adult red blood cells, liver-derived erythrocytes are nonnucleated and contain different types of hemoglobin. By 6 to 8 weeks of gestation in humans, the liver replaces the yolk sac as the main source of blood cells. Although the liver continues to produce red blood cells until the early neonatal period, its contribution begins to decline in the sixth month of pregnancy. At this time the formation of blood cells shifts to the bone marrow, the definitive site of adult hematopoiesis. This shift is controlled by cortisol secreted by the fetal adrenal cortex. In the absence of cortisol, hematopoiesis remains confined to the liver. Before hematopoiesis becomes well established in the bone

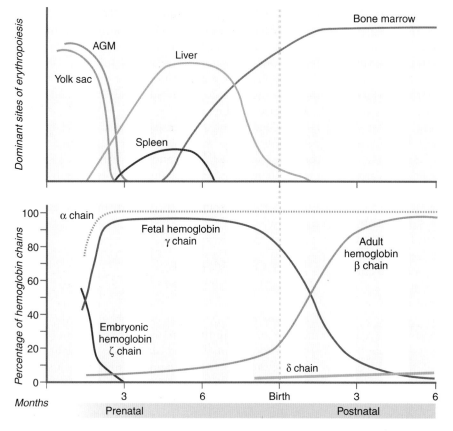

**FIGURE 17-1** Sites of hematopoiesis *(above)* and phases of hemoglobin synthesis *(below)* in the human embryo. The upper graph highlights the relative importance of the various sites of hematopoiesis. The lower graph shows the percentages of the various hemoglobin polypeptide chains present in the blood at any given time. The α chain is treated separately from the others. *AGM*, aorta, genital ridge, mesonephros region. (Based on Carlson B: *Patten's foundations of embryology*, ed 6, New York, 1996, McGraw-Hill).

marrow, small amounts of blood formation may also occur in the omentum and possibly the spleen.

## Cellular Aspects of Hematopoiesis

The first **hematopoietic stem cells** that arise in the embryo are truly pluripotential in that they can give rise to all the cell types found in the blood (Figure 17-2). These **pluripotent stem cells**, sometimes called **hemocytoblasts**, have great proliferative ability. They produce vast numbers of progeny, most of which are cells at the next stage of differentiation, but they also produce small numbers of their original stem cell type, which act as a reserve capable of replenishing individual lines of cells should the need arise. Very early in development, the line of active blood-forming cells subdivides into two separate lineages. **Lymphoid stem cells** ultimately form the two lines of lymphocytes: **B lymphocytes** (which are responsible for antibody production) and **T lymphocytes** (which are responsible for cellular immune reactions). **Myeloid stem cells** are precursors to the other lines of blood cells: erythrocytes, the granulocytes (neutrophils, eosinophils, and basophils), monocytes, and platelets. The second-generation stem cells (lymphoid and myeloid) are still pluripotent, although their develop-

mental potency is restricted, since neither can form the progeny of the other type.

Stemming from their behavior in certain experimental situations, the hematopoietic stem cells are often called **colony-forming units** (**CFUs**). The first-generation stem cell is called the *CFU-ML* because it can give rise to both myeloid and lymphoid lines of cells. Stem cells of the second generation are called *CFU-L* (*L,* lymphocytes) and *CFU-S* (*S,* spleen) (determined from experiments in which stem cell differentiation was studied in irradiated spleens). In all cases except one, the progeny of CFU-L and CFU-S are **committed stem cells,** which are capable of forming only one type of mature blood cell. For each lineage the forming cell types must pass through several stages of differentiation before they attain their mature phenotype.

What controls the diversification of stem cells into specific cell lines? Experiments begun in the 1970s provided evidence for the existence of specific **colony-stimulating factors** (**CSFs**) for each line of blood cell. CSFs are diffusible proteins that stimulate the proliferation of hematopoietic stem cells. Some CSFs act on a number of types of stem cells; others stimulate only one type. Although much remains to be learned about the sites of origin and modes of action of CSFs, many appear to be produced locally in stromal cells of the bone marrow,

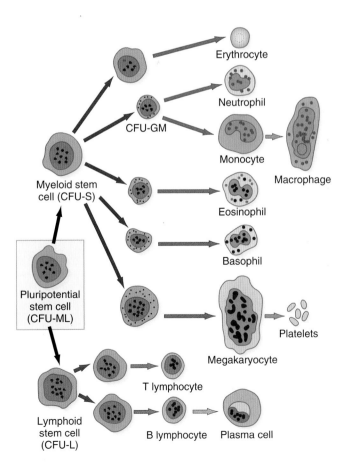

**FIGURE 17-2** Major cell lineages during hematopoiesis. Mature blood cells *(right). CFU,* colony-forming unit; *GM,* granulocyte and monocyte; *L,* lymphocyte; *ML,* myeloid and lymphoid; *S,* spleen.

and some may be stored on the local extracellular matrix. CSFs are bound by small numbers of surface receptors on their target stem cells. Functionally, CSFs represent mechanisms for stimulating the expansion of specific types of blood cells when the need arises. Recognition of the existence of CSFs has prompted considerable interest in their clinical application to conditions characterized by a deficiency of white blood cells (leukopenia).

Certain *Hox genes*, especially those of the *Hoxa* and *Hoxb* families, play an important role in some aspects of hematopoiesis. Exposure of bone marrow to antisense oligonucleotides against specific *Hox* genes results in the suppression of specific lines of differentiation of blood cells. Conversely, engineered overexpression of genes, such as *Hoxb-8, Hoxa-9,* and *Hoxa-10,* causes leukemia in mice. Evidence is increasing for the involvement of *Hox* genes in the pathogenesis of human leukemias. One important function of the *Hox* genes in hematopoiesis is the regulation of proliferation.

## Erythropoiesis

The erythrocyte lineage represents one line of descent from the CFU-S cells. Although the erythroid progenitor cells are restricted to forming only red blood cells, there are many generations of precursor cells (Figure 17-3). The earliest stages of erythropoiesis are recognized by the behavior of the precursor cells in culture rather than by morphological or biochemical differences. These are called **erythroid burst-forming units (BFU-E)** and **erythroid colony-forming units (CFU-E)**. Each responds to different stimulatory factors. The pluripotent CFU-S precursors (see Figure 17-2) respond to **interleukin-3,** a product of macrophages in adult bone marrow. A hormone designated as **burst-promoting activity (BPA)** stimulates mitosis of the BFU-E precursors (see Figure 17-3). A CFU-E cell, which has a lesser proliferative capacity than a BFU-E cell, requires the presence of **erythropoietin** as a stimulatory factor. Erythropoietin is a glycoprotein that stimulates the synthesis of the messenger RNA for globin and is first produced in the fetal liver. Later in development, synthesis shifts to the kidney, which remains the site of erythropoietin production in the adult. Under conditions of hypoxia (e.g., from blood loss or high altitudes) the production of erythropoietin by the kidneys increases, stimulating the production of more red blood cells to compensate for the increased need. In adult erythropoiesis the CFU-E stage seems to be the one most responsive to environmental influences. The placenta appears to be impervious to erythropoietin, thereby insulating the embryo from changes in erythropoietin levels of the mother as well as eliminating the influence of fetal erythropoietin on the blood-forming apparatus of the mother.

One or two generations after the CFU-E stage, successive generations of erythrocyte precursor cells can be

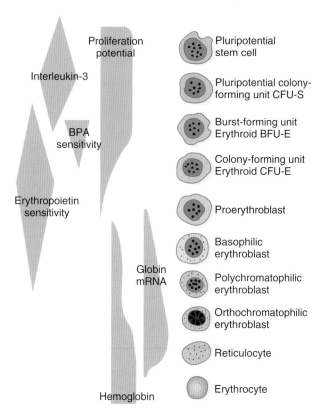

**FIGURE 17-3** *Right,* Morphological stages in the differentiation of a red blood cell from a pluripotential stem cell. *Left,* Molecular correlates of differentiation. The thickness of the tan background is proportional to the amount at the corresponding stages of erythropoiesis. *BFU,* burst-forming units; *BPA,* Burst-promoting activity; *CFU,* colony-forming unit; *E,* erythroid; *mRNA,* messenger ribonucleic acid; *S,* spleen.

recognized by their morphology. The first recognizable stage is the **proerythroblast** (Figure 17-4), a large, highly basophilic cell that has not yet produced sufficient hemoglobin to be detected by cytochemical analysis. Such a cell has a large nucleolus, much uncondensed nuclear chromatin, numerous ribosomes, and a high concentration of globin mRNAs. These are classic cytological characteristics of an undifferentiated cell.

Succeeding stages of erythroid differentiation (**basophilic, polychromatophilic,** and **orthochromatic erythroblasts**) are characterized by a progressive change in the balance between the accumulation of newly synthesized hemoglobin and the decline of first the RNA-producing machinery and later the protein-synthesizing apparatus. The overall size of the cell decreases, and the nucleus becomes increasingly **pycnotic** (smaller with more condensed chromatin) until it is finally extruded at the stage of the orthochromatic erythrocyte. After the loss of the nucleus and most cytoplasmic organelles, the immature red blood cell, which still contains a small number of polysomes, is a **reticulocyte.** Reticulocytes are released into the bloodstream, where they continue to produce small amounts of hemoglobin for 1 or 2 days.

The final stage of hematopoiesis is the mature **erythrocyte,** which is a terminally differentiated cell because

**FIGURE 17-4** Structural features of erythropoiesis. In successive stages, cytoplasmic basophilia decreases and the concentration of hemoglobin increases in the cells. The duration of stages is given in parentheses.

of the loss of its nucleus and most of its cytoplasmic organelles. Erythrocytes in embryos are larger than their adult counterparts and have a shorter life span (50 to 70 days in the fetus vs. 120 days in adults).

## Hemoglobin Synthesis and Its Control

Both the red blood cells and the hemoglobin within them undergo isoform transitions during embryonic development. The adult hemoglobin molecule is a complex composed of heme and four globin chains: two $\alpha$ and two $\beta$ chains. Both the $\alpha$ and $\beta$ subunits are products of genes located on chromosomes 16 and 11, respectively (Figure 17-5). Different isoforms of the subunits are encoded linearly on these chromosomes.

During the period of yolk sac hematopoiesis, embryonic globin isoforms are produced. The earliest embry-

**FIGURE 17-5** Organization of hemoglobin genes along chromosomes 11 and 16 and their sequential activation during embryonic development.

onic hemoglobin, sometimes called *Gower 1*, is composed of two $\zeta$ ($\alpha$-type) and two $\varepsilon$ ($\beta$-type) chains. After passing through a couple of transitional forms (Table 17-1), hemoglobin synthesis enters a fetal stage by 12 weeks, which corresponds to the shift in the site of erythropoiesis from the yolk sac to the liver. Fetal hemoglobin consists of two adult-type $\alpha$ chains, which form very early in embryogenesis, and two $\gamma$ chains, the major fetal isoform of the $\beta$ chain. Fetal hemoglobin is the predominant form during the remainder of pregnancy. The main adaptive value of the fetal isoform of hemoglobin is that it has a higher affinity for oxygen than the adult form. This is advantageous to the fetus, which depends on the oxygen concentration of the maternal blood. Starting at about 30 weeks' gestation, there is a gradual switch from the fetal to the adult type of hemoglobin, with $\alpha_2\beta_2$ being the predominant type. A minor but functionally similar variant is $\alpha_2\delta_2$.

**TABLE 17-1** *Developmental Isoforms of Human Hemoglobin*

| Developmental stage | Hemoglobin type | Globin-chain composition |
|---|---|---|
| Embryo | Gower 1 | $\zeta_2\varepsilon_2$ |
| Embryo | Gower 2 | $\alpha_2\varepsilon_2$ |
| Embryo | Portland | $\zeta_2\gamma_2$ |
| Embryo to fetus | Fetal | $\alpha_2\gamma_2$ |
| Fetus to adult | A (adult) | $\alpha_2\beta_2$ |
| Adult | $A_2$ | $\alpha_2\delta_2$ |
| Adult | Fetal | $\alpha_2\gamma_2$* |

Modified from Brown MS. In Stockman J, Pochedly C, eds: *Developmental and neonatal hematology*, New York, 1988, Raven.
* The fetal hemglobin expressed in adults differs from true fetal hemoglobin by an amino acid substitution at the 136 position of the $\gamma$ chain.

## Formation of Embryonic Blood Vessels

The early embryo is devoid of blood vessels. Although blood islands appear in the wall of the yolk sac and extraembryonic vascular channels form in association with them (see Figure 6-17), much of the vasculature of the embryonic body is derived from intraembryonic sources. During the early period of somite formation, networks of small vessels rapidly appear in many regions of the embryonic body.

The formation of blood vessels in the embryo consists of several phases (Figure 17-6). The first is the specification of a population of vascular precursors, called **angioblasts**. These cells then become organized into a **primary capillary plexus** through a process known as **vasculogenesis**. To keep pace with rapidly growing embryo,

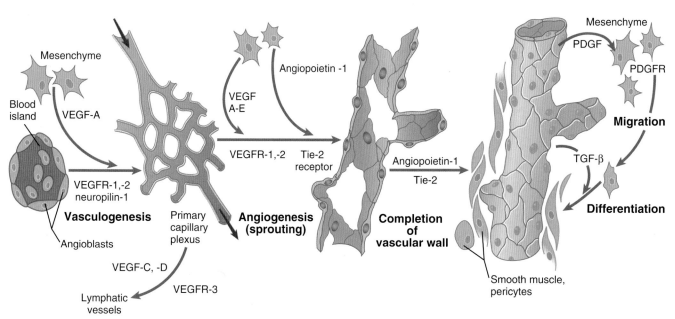

**FIGURE 17-6** Scheme illustrating vasculogenesis, angiogenesis, and assembly of the vascular wall. Angioblasts, initially expressing vascular endothelial growth factor receptor (VEGFR-2), are stimulated by VEGF-A, secreted by the surrounding mesenchyme, to form the primary capillary plexus by the process of vasculogenesis. Under additional stimulation by growth factors, competent endothelial cells of the primary capillary plexus form vascular sprouts in the earliest stages of angiogenesis. This is followed by the recruitment of surrounding mesenchymal cells to form the cellular elements of the vascular wall. Early in vasculogenesis, endothelial cells that express VEGFR-3 respond to VEGF stimulation by differentiating into the precursors of the lymphatic vessels. *PDGF*, platelet-derived growth factor; *PDGFR*, platelet-derived growth factor receptor.

the primary capillary plexus must rapidly undergo reorganization through the resorption of existing vessels and the sprouting of new branches to support the expanding vascular network. This latter process is called **angiogenesis**. Angiogenesis continues not only in the prenatal period, but throughout adult life, as tissues and organs continually adapt to changing conditions of life, whether normal or pathological.

Detailed descriptive studies and transplantation experiments involving intrinsic cellular labels or graft-specific monoclonal antibody labels have shown that **angioblasts** arise from most mesodermal tissues of the body except notochord and prechordal mesoderm (Table 17-2). Embryonic blood vessels form from angioblasts by three main mechanisms. Many of the larger blood vessels, such as the dorsal aortae, are formed by the coalescence of angioblasts in situ. Other equally large channels, such as the endocardium, are formed by angioblasts migrating into the region from other sites. Other vessels, especially the intersegmental vessels of the main body axis and vessels of the central nervous system, arise as vascular sprouts from existing larger vessels. Many of the angioblasts of the trunk are originally associated with the splanchnic mesoderm.

All stages in the formation of the vascular system occur in response to the influence of powerful growth factors and their receptors. The initial phase of recruitment of a population of angioblasts from the mesoderm is characterized

**TABLE 17-2** *Distribution of Endogenous Angioblasts in Embryonic Tissues*

| Tissues | Angioblasts |
| --- | --- |
| **CEPHALIC** | |
| Paraxial mesoderm | + |
| Lateral mesoderm | + |
| Prechordal mesoderm | − |
| Notochord | − |
| Brain | − |
| Neural crest | − |
| **TRUNK** | |
| Whole somites | + |
| Dorsal half somites | + |
| Segmental plate mesoderm | + |
| Lateral somatic mesoderm | + |
| Lateral splanchnic mesoderm | + |
| Spinal cord | − |

From Noden DM: *Ann NY Acad Sci* 588:236–249, 1990.

by the appearance of a transmembrane **vascular endothelial growth factor receptor (VEGFR-2)** on their surfaces (see Figure 17-6). Soon, in response to the production of **vascular endothelial growth factor (VEGF-A)** by the surrounding mesenchyme, the phase of vasculogenesis takes place, and the angioblasts form the cellular tubes that become the basis for the primary capillary plexus.

The formation of vascular endothelial sprouts, the cellular basis for angiogenesis, occurs against a background of VEGF/VEGFR-1 and -2 interactions, but with a new set of players added. A sprouting factor, **angiopoietin-1**, interacts with its receptor, **Tie-2**, on the endothelial cells at sites where endothelial sprouts will occur. The **Notch** signaling pathway is also strongly tied to the formation of vascular sprouts (a common denominator with other organ systems that display branching morphogenesis), but its connection to the angiopoietin-1/Tie-2 mechanism remains unclear.

The next step in building a blood vessel is formation of the vascular wall, which in the trunk and extremities is derived from local mesoderm that becomes associated with the endothelial lining of the vessel. In the head and many areas of the aortic arch system, mesenchyme derived from neural crest ectoderm is a major contributor to the connective tissue and smooth muscle of the vascular wall. The neural crest, however, does not give rise to endothelial cells.

Two-way molecular signaling is involved in building up the walls of blood vessels. In response to the angiopoietin-1/Tie-2 interaction that occurs during angiogenesis, the endothelial cells release their own signaling molecule, **platelet-derived growth factor (PDGF)**, which stimulates the migration of mesenchymal cells toward the vascular endothelium. The release of other growth factors (possibly transforming growth factor-β [TGF-β]) by the endothelial cells stimulates the differentiation of the mesenchymal cells into vascular smooth muscle or pericytes.

Recent research has shed considerable light on the differentiation of the arterial vs. venous system. In contrast to previous assumptions that physiological and local environmental factors determine whether a developing vessel will become an artery or a vein, it is now known that the arterial or venous identity of endothelial cells is established very early in their development—prior to angiogenesis and before the onset of circulation. Endothelial cells of developing arteries express the membrane-bound ligand **Ephrin-B2**, whereas those of developing veins express the receptor **Eph-B4** on their surface membranes. These characteristic phenotypes appear to be the result of earlier signaling by the Notch system. **Notch** and its ligands **Delta** and **Jagged** are expressed in arterial endothelium, and experimental evidence suggests that Notch signaling in developing arteries may act to suppress the venous identity of endothelial cells.

As with myoblasts, angioblasts appear to react to local environmental cues that determine the specific morphological pattern of a blood vessel. An unexpected recent finding is that in the skin, at least, the pattern of the peripheral innervation determines the pattern of the smaller arteries and that the effective patterning agent is the secretion of VEGF by the nerves. Tracing studies of transplanted angioblasts have shown that some can migrate long distances. Angioblasts that have migrated far from the place into which they were grafted become integrated into morphologically normal blood vessels in the areas where they settle.

Local factors also influence the initiation of vasculogenesis. In some organs (e.g., the liver) or parts of organs (e.g., the bronchi of the respiratory system), the blood vessels supplying the regions arise from local mesoderm, whereas other organs (e.g., the metanephric kidneys) or parts of organs (e.g., the alveoli of the lungs) are supplied by blood vessels that grow into the mesenchyme from other tissues. In the latter type of vascularization mecha-

nism, evidence is increasing that these organ primordia produce their own **angiogenesis factors** that stimulate the growth of vascular sprouts (by promoting mitosis of endothelial cells) into the glandular mesenchyme.

## Development of the Arteries

### Aortic Arches and Their Derivatives

The system of aortic arches in early human embryos is organized along the same principles as the system of arteries supplying blood to the gills of many aquatic lower vertebrates. Blood exits from a common ventricle in the heart into a ventral aortic root, from which it is distributed through the branchial arches by pairs of aortic arches (Figure 17-7, A). In gilled vertebrates the aortic arch arteries branch into capillary beds, where the

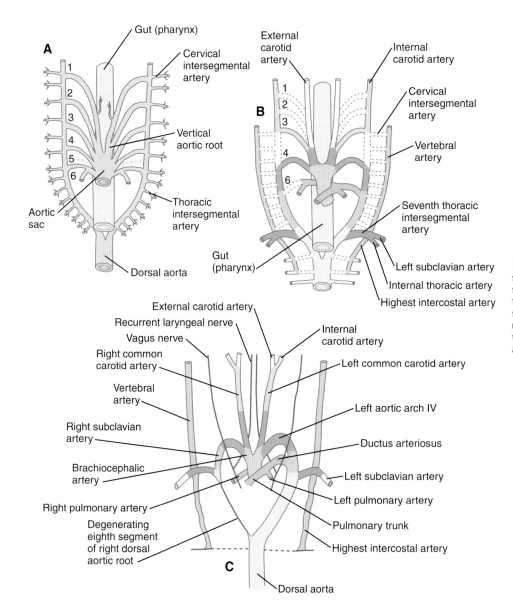

**FIGURE 17-7 A,** Schematic representation of the embryonic aortic arch system. **B** and **C,** Later steps in the transformation of the aortic arch system in the human. Disposition of the recurrent laryngeal nerve in relation to the right fourth and left sixth arch is also shown in **C.**

blood becomes reoxygenated as it passes through the gills. In mammalian embryos the aortic arches remain continuous vessels because gas exchange occurs in the placenta and not in the pharyngeal arches. The aortic arches empty into paired dorsal aortae where the blood enters the regular systemic circulation. In human embryos, all aortic arches are never present at the same time. Their formation and remodeling show a pronounced craniocaudal gradient. Blood from the outflow tract of the heart (the truncoconal region) flows into an **aortic sac**, which differs from the truncoconal region in the construction of its wall. The aortic arches branch off from the aortic sac.

The developmental anatomy of the aortic arch system well illustrates the principle of morphological adaptation of the vascular bed during different stages of embryogenesis (Table 17-3). Continued development of the cranial and cervical regions causes components of the first three arches and associated aortic roots to be remodeled into the carotid artery system (see Figure 17-7). With the

remodeling of the heart tube and the internal division of the outflow tract into aortic and pulmonary components, the fourth arches undergo an asymmetrical adaptation to the early asymmetry of the heart. The left fourth aortic arch is retained as a major channel (arch of the aorta), which carries the entire output from the left ventricle of the heart. The right fourth arch is incorporated into the right subclavian artery.

Embryology textbooks traditionally depict the aortic arch system as consisting of six pairs of vascular arches, but the fifth and sixth arches never appear as discrete vascular channels similar to the first through fourth arches. The fifth aortic arch, if it exists at all, is represented by no more than a few capillary loops. The sixth (**pulmonary arch**) arises as a capillary plexus associated with the early trachea and lung buds. The capillary plexus is supplied by ventral segmental arteries arising from the paired dorsal aortae in that region (Figure 17-8). The equivalent of the sixth arch is represented by a discrete distal segment (ventral segmental artery) connected to the dorsal aorta

**TABLE 17-3** *Adult Derivatives of the Aortic Arch System*

| | Right side | Left side |
|---|---|---|
| **AORTIC ARCHES** | | |
| 1 | Disappearance of most of structure | Disappearance of most of structure |
| | Part of maxillary artery | Part of maxillary artery |
| 2 | Disappearance of most of structure | Disappearance of most of structure |
| | Hyoid and stapedial arteries | Hyoid and stapedial arteries |
| 3 | Ventral part—common carotid artery | Ventral part—common carotid artery |
| | Dorsal part—internal carotid artery | Dorsal part—internal carotid artery |
| 4 | Proximal part of right subclavian artery | Part of arch of aorta |
| 5 | Rarely recognizable, even in early embryo | Rarely recognizable, even in early embryo |
| 6 (pulmonary) | Part of right pulmonary artery | Ductus arteriosus |
| | | Part of left pulmonary artery |
| **VENTRAL AORTIC ROOTS** | | |
| Cranial to third arch | External carotid artery | External carotid artery |
| Between third and fourth arches | Common carotid artery | Common carotid artery |
| Between fourth and sixth arches | Brachiocephalic artery | Ascending part of aorta |
| **DORSAL AORTIC ROOTS** | | |
| Cranial to third arch | Internal carotid artery | Internal carotid artery |
| Between third and fourth arches | Disappearance of structure | Disappearance of structure |
| Between fourth and sixth arches | Central part of right subclavian artery | Descending aorta |
| Caudal to sixth arch | Disappearance of structure | Descending aorta |

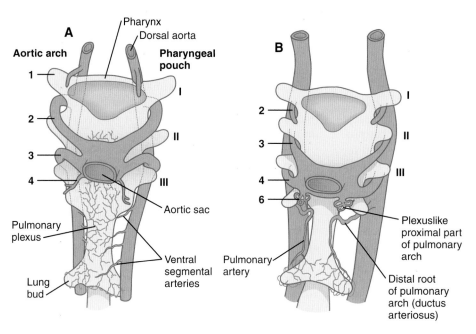

**FIGURE 17-8** Development of the pulmonary arch, showing the early pulmonary plexus in relation to several ventral segmental arteries associated with the early respiratory diverticulum **(A)** and their consolidation into discrete vessels that establish a connection with the bases of the fourth aortic arches **(B).** (Based on DeRuiter MC and others: *Anat Embryol* 179:309–325, 1989.)

and a plexuslike proximal segment that establishes a connection between the aortic sac at the base of the fourth arch and the distal segmental component. As the respiratory diverticulum and early lung buds elongate, parts of the pulmonary capillary network consolidate to form a pair of discrete **pulmonary arteries** that connect to the putative sixth arch. Although the term **sixth aortic arch** is frequently used in anatomical and clinical literature, **pulmonary arch** is a more appropriate term because it does not imply equivalence to the other aortic arches.

Like the fourth aortic arch, the pulmonary arch develops asymmetrically. On the left side it becomes a large channel. Its distal segment, which was derived from a ventral segmental artery, persists as a major channel (**ductus arteriosus**) that shunts blood from the left pulmonary artery to the aorta (see Figure 17-7, C). By this shunt the lungs are protected from a flow of blood that is greater than what their vasculature can handle during most of the intrauterine period. On the right side the distal segment of the pulmonary arch regresses, and the proximal segment (the base of the right pulmonary artery) branches off from the pulmonary trunk.

The asymmetry of the derivatives of the pulmonary arch accounts for the difference between the course of the right and left **recurrent laryngeal nerves**, which are branches of the vagus nerve (cranial nerve X). These nerves, which supply the larynx, hook around the pulmonary arches. As the heart descends into the thoracic cavity from the cervical region, the branch point from the vagus of each recurrent laryngeal nerve is correspondingly moved. On the left side the nerve is associated with the ductus arteriosus (see Figure 17-7, C), which persists throughout the fetal period, so it is pulled deep into the thoracic cavity. On the right side, however, with the

regression of much of the right pulmonary arch, the nerve moves to the level of the fourth arch, which constitutes an anatomical barrier. The positions of the right and left recurrent laryngeal nerves in the adult reflect this asymmetry, with the right nerve curving under the right subclavian artery (fourth arch) and the left nerve hooking around the **ligamentum arteriosum** (the adult derivative of the ductus arteriosus, the distal segment of the left pulmonary arch).

## Major Branches of the Aorta

In the early embryo, when the dorsal aortae are still paired vessels, three sets of arterial branches arise from them—**dorsal intersegmental, lateral segmental,** and **ventral segmental** (Figure 17-9). These branches undergo a variety of modifications in form before assuming their adult configurations (Table 17-4). The ventral segmental arteries arise as paired vessels that course over the dorsal and lateral walls of the gut and yolk sac. With the closure of the gut and the narrowing of the dorsal mesentery, certain branches fuse in the midline to form the celiac, superior, and inferior mesenteric arteries.

The **umbilical arteries** begin as pure ventral segmental branches supplying allantoic mesoderm, but their bases later connect with lumbar intersegmental vessels. The most proximal umbilical channels then regress, and the intersegmental branches become their main branches off the aorta. Like their subclavian counterparts in the arms, the initially small arterial branches (**iliac arteries**) supplying the leg buds appear as components of the dorsal intersegmental (lumbar) branches of the aorta. However, after the umbilical arteries incorporate the proximal segments of the intersegmental vessels, the iliac

**FIGURE 17-9** Types of segmental branches coming off the abdominal aorta at different stages of development.

| TABLE 17-4 *Major Arterial Branches of the Aorta* | |
| --- | --- |
| **Embryonic vessels** | **Adult derivatives** |
| **DORSAL INTERSEGMENTAL BRANCHES (PAIRED)** | |
| Cervical intersegmental (1–16) | Lateral branches joining to become vertebral arteries |
| Seventh intersegmentals | Subclavian arteries |
| Thoracic intersegmentals | Intercostal arteries |
| Lumbar intersegmentals | Iliac arteries |
| **LATERAL SEGMENTAL BRANCHES** | |
| Up to 20 pairs of vessels supplying the mesonephros | Adrenal arteries, renal arteries, gonadial (ovarian or spermatic) arteries |
| **VENTRAL SEGMENTAL BRANCHES*** | |
| Vitelline vessels | Celiac artery, superior and inferior mesenteric arteries |
| Allantoic vessels | Umbilical arteries |

* Originally paired in areas where the embryonic aorta itself consists of paired components.

arteries appear to arise as branches off the umbilical arteries.

## Arteries of the Head

The arteries supplying the head arise from two sources. Ventrally, the aortic arch system (first to third arches and corresponding roots) gives rise to the arteries supplying the face (**external carotid arteries**) and the frontal part of the base of the brain (**internal carotid arteries**) (see Figure 17-7).

At the level of the spinal cord, the **vertebral arteries**, which form through connections of lateral branches of dorsal intersegmental arteries, grow toward the brain. Soon they veer toward the midline and fuse, forming the unpaired **basilar artery** (Figure 17-10). This artery runs along the ventral surface of the brainstem, supplying it with a series of paired arteries. As the basilar artery approaches the level of the diencephalon and the internal carotid arteries, sets of branches from each of these major vessels grow out and fuse, forming **posterior communicating arteries**, which join the circulations of the basilar and internal carotid arteries. Two other small branches off the internal carotid system fuse in the midline to complete a vascular ring

Middle cerebral artery

Ophthalmic artery

Posterior communicating artery

Internal carotid artery

Basilar artery

External carotid artery

Vertebral artery

Common carotid artery

Ventral aortic root

Dorsal aortic root

**3 1/2 weeks**

**5 weeks**

Anterior cerebral artery

Anterior communicating artery

Middle cerebral artery

Internal carotid artery

Posterior communicating artery

Posterior cerebral artery

Superior cerebellar artery

Pontine artery

Anteror inferior cerebellar artery

Posterior inferior cerebellar artery

**7-8 weeks**

Vertebral artery

**Adult**

**FIGURE 17-10** Stages in the development of the major arteries supplying the brain.

(**circle of Willis**), which underlies the base of the diencephalon and encircles the optic chiasm and pituitary stalk. The circle of Willis is a structural adaptation that ensures a continuous blood supply in the event of occlusion of some major arteries supplying the brain.

## Coronary Arteries

Although intuitively one would expect the coronary arteries to arise as branches growing out from the aorta, experimental studies have shown instead that cellular precursors of the coronary arteries, arising in the same cellular primordium as the future epicardium, migrate toward the aorta and invade its wall (see Figure 6-16, *B*). The smooth muscle cells of the coronary vessels have a purely mesodermal origin instead of the mixed neural crest and mesodermal origin seen in the aortic arch derivatives. Studies involving the tagging of cells with retroviral markers confirm that progenitor cells of the coronary vessels penetrate the wall of the already beating heart as the epicardial layer envelops the myocardium and that after forming in situ, the coronary arteries secondarily enter the aorta.

## Development of Veins

Veins follow a morphologically complex pattern of development characterized by the formation of highly irregular networks of capillaries and the ultimate expansion of certain channels into definitive veins. Because of the multichanneled beginnings and the number of options (Figure 17-11), the adult venous system is characterized by a higher incidence of anatomical variations than the arterial system. A detailed description of the development of venous channels is beyond the scope of this text.

## *Cardinal Veins*

The cardinal veins form the basis for the intraembryonic venous circulation. Several sets of cardinal veins appear at different times and in different locations. Within any set of cardinal veins, some segments regress, and others persist, either as independent channels or as components of composite veins that also include portions of other cardinal veins.

The earliest pattern of cardinal veins consists of paired **anterior** and **posterior cardinal veins**, which drain blood

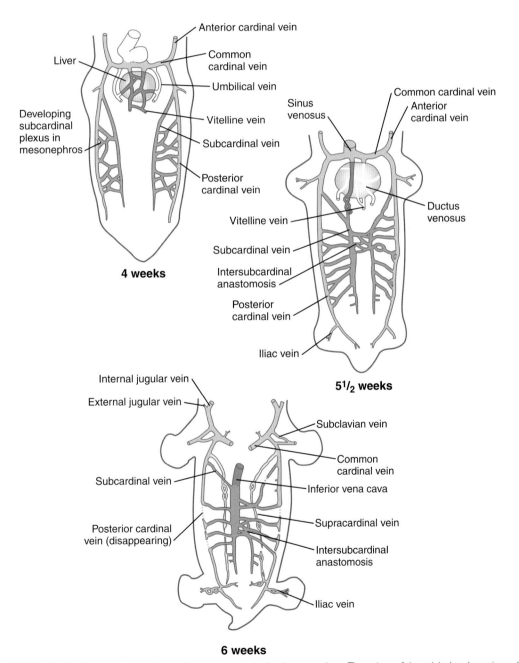

**FIGURE 17-11** Development of the cardinal vein system in the human embryo. The colors of the original embryonic cardinal veins are carried through in all drawings to facilitate an understanding of the derivations of the adult veins. (Based on McClure CFW, Butler EG: *Am J Anat* 35:331–383, 1925.)

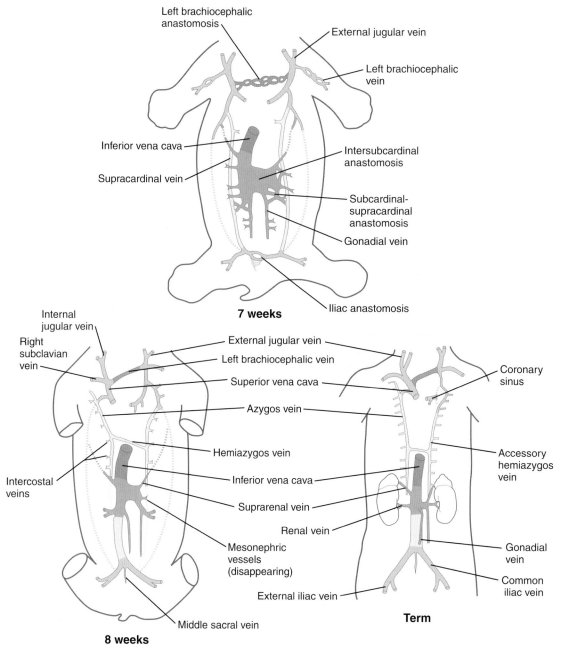

**FIGURE 17-11, CONT'D.**

from the head and body into a pair of short **common cardinal veins** (see Figure 17-11). The common cardinal veins in turn empty their blood into the **sinus venosus** of the primitive heart (see Figure 17-13).

In the cranial region the originally symmetrical anterior cardinal veins are transformed into the **internal jugular veins** (Figure 17-12). As the heart rotates to the right, the base of the left internal jugular vein is attenuated. At the same time a new anastomotic channel, which ultimately forms the **left brachiocephalic vein**, connects the left internal jugular vein to the right one. Through this anastomosis the blood from the left side of the head

is drained into the original right anterior cardinal vein, which ultimately becomes the **superior vena cava**, emptying into the right atrium of the heart. Meanwhile, the proximal part of the left common cardinal vein persists as a small channel, the **coronary sinus**, which is the final drainage pathway of many of the coronary veins, also into the right atrium of the heart.

In the trunk a pair of **subcardinal veins** arises in association with the developing mesonephros. The subcardinal veins are connected with the posterior cardinal veins and to each other through numerous anastomoses. Both the postcardinal and subcardinal veins drain the

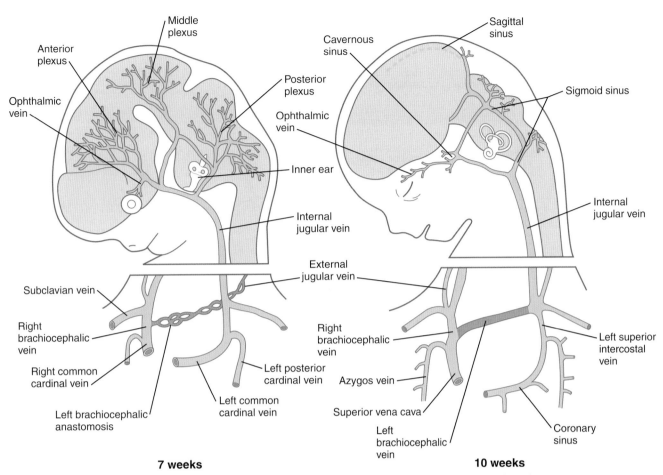

**FIGURE 17-12** Stages in the formation of the major veins that drain the head and upper trunk. At **7 weeks** an anastomosis *(purple)* between the left and right jugular vein forms the basis for establishment of the left brachiocephalic vein.

mesonephric kidneys through numerous small side branches. As the mesonephric kidneys start to regress, the veins draining them also begin to break up. At this point a pair of **supra-cardinal veins** appears in the body wall dorsal to the subcardinal veins. Over time, all three sets of cardinal veins in the body break up to varying degrees, with surviving remnants incorporated into the **inferior vena cava**. The inferior vena cava forms as a single asymmetrical vessel that runs parallel to the aorta on the right (see Figure 17-11). Most of the named veins of the thoracic and abdominal cavities are derived from persisting segments of the cardinal vein system.

### Vitelline and Umbilical Veins

The extraembryonic **vitelline** and **umbilical veins** begin as pairs of symmetrical vessels that drain separately into the sinus venosus of the heart (Figure 17-13). Over time, these vessels become intimately associated with the rapidly growing liver. The vitelline veins, which drain the yolk sac, develop sets of anastomosing channels both within and outside the liver. Outside the liver the two vitelline veins and their side-to-side anastomotic channels

become closely associated with the duodenum. Through the persistence of some channels and the disappearance of others, the **hepatic portal vein,** which drains the intestines, takes shape. Within the liver the vitelline plexus becomes transformed into a capillary bed, allowing the broad distribution of food materials absorbed from the gut through the functional parts of the liver. From the hepatic capillary bed the blood that arrives from the hepatic portal vein passes into a set of **hepatic veins,** which empty the blood into the sinus venosus.

The originally symmetrical umbilical veins soon lose their own hepatic segments and drain directly into the liver by combining with the intrahepatic vascular plexus of the vitelline veins. Soon, a major channel, the **ductus venosus,** forms and shunts much of the blood entering from the left umbilical vein directly through the liver and into the inferior vena cava. The ductus venosus is an important adaptation for maintaining a functional embryonic pattern of blood circulation. Soon, the right umbilical vein degenerates, leaving the left umbilical vein the sole channel for bringing blood that has been reoxygenated and purified in the placenta back to the embryonic body. The ductus venosus permits the incoming

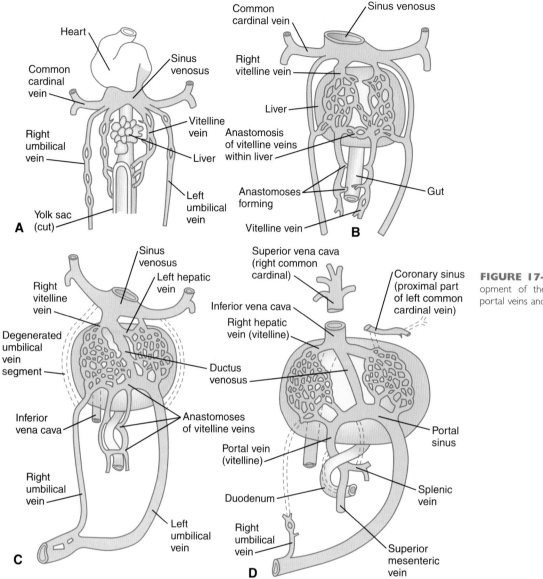

**FIGURE 17-13** Stages in the development of the umbilical and hepatic portal veins and intrahepatic circulation.

oxygenated placental blood to bypass the capillary networks of the liver and to distribute it to the organs (e.g., brain, heart) that need it most.

### Pulmonary Veins

The pulmonary veins are phylogenetically recent structures that form independently rather than taking over portions of the older cardinal vein systems. From each lung, venous drainage channels converge until they ultimately form a single large **common pulmonary vein,** which empties into the left atrium of the heart. As the atrium expands, the common pulmonary vein becomes incorporated into its wall (Figure 17-14). Ultimately the absorption passes the first and second branch points of the original pulmonary veins, resulting in the entrance of four independent pulmonary veins into the left atrium.

## Development of Lymphatic Channels

The origin of lymphatic channels has been poorly understood, but it now appears that the endothelial lining of many lymphatic vessels arises from the endothelium of the primary capillary plexus. Endothelial cells destined to become incorporated into the lymphatic channels express **VEGFR-3,** a form not seen in vascular endothelium, and they respond to two specific isoforms of VEGF, namely, VEGF-C and -D (see Figure 17-6). The lymphatic system first appears as six **primary lymph sacs** starting late in the sixth week of pregnancy (Figure 17-15). Two **jugular lymph sacs** appear at the angle between the precardinal (future internal jugular) veins and the subclavian veins. In the abdomen a **retroperitoneal lymph sac** forms on the posterior body wall at the root of the mesentery

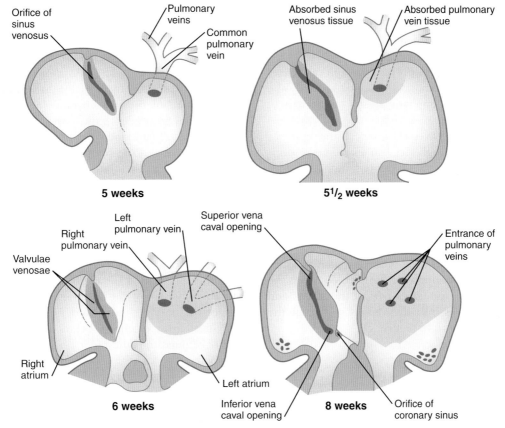

**FIGURE 17-14** Stages in the absorption of the common pulmonary vein and its branches into the wall of the left atrium and changes over time in the opening of the sinus venosus into the right atrium.

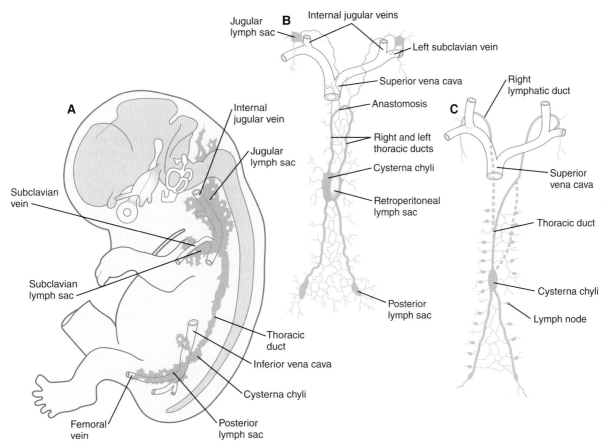

**FIGURE 17-15** Stages in the development of the major lymphatic channels. **A** and **B** show **9-week-old** embryos. **C** shows the fetal period. Between **B** and **C,** the transformation between the reasonably symmetrical disposition of the main lymphatic channels and the asymmetrical condition that is characteristic of the adult can be seen.

during the eighth week. Somewhat later a **cysterna chyli** forms at the same level but dorsal to the aorta. At about the same time a pair of **posterior lymph sacs** arises at the bifurcation of the femoral and sciatic veins. By the end of the ninth week, lymphatic vessels connect these lymph sacs.

Two major lymphatic vessels connect the cysterna chyli with the jugular lymph sacs. An anastomosis forms between these two channels. A single lymphatic vessel consisting of the caudal part of the right channel, the anastomotic segment, and the cranial part of the left channel ultimately becomes the definitive **thoracic duct** of the adult. The thoracic duct drains lymph from most of the body and the left side of the head into the venous system at the junction of the left internal jugular and sub-clavian veins. The right lymphatic duct, which drains the right side of the head and upper part of the thorax and right arm, also empties into the venous system at the original location of the right jugular sac.

## DEVELOPMENT AND PARTITIONING OF HEART

### Early Development of the Heart

#### Cellular Origins

The early tubular heart (see Figure 6-15) is derived from several tissue sources. The atrial and ventricular myocar-dial tissue arises from a horseshoe-shaped bilateral pri-mordium of splanchnic mesoderm (see Figure 6-13), which coalesces in the ventral midline to form the bulk of the early heart tube. The outflow tract has a quite different cellular origin, with endothelial components arising from cephalic paraxial and lateral mesoderm in the region of the otic placode. A major cellular component of the wall of the outflow tract is derived from cranial neural crest, specifically from the level between the midotic placode to the caudal end of the third somite (see Figure 12-5). These cranial components integrate with the bilateral cardiac primordia while in the cervical region. As the heart descends into the thoracic cavity, the cranially derived cells of the outflow tract accompany it.

#### Looping of the Heart

When the cardiac tube first forms late in the third week, it is bilaterally symmetrical (see Figure 6-15). Soon, it undergoes a characteristic dextral looping, making it the first asymmetrical structure to appear in the embryonic body. (The early molecular basis for asymmetry of the embryonic body is discussed on p. 95). In addition to these molecular cascades, certain heart-specific genes also appear to be involved in the early looping of the heart tube. Knockouts of three types of cardiac transcription

factors (Nkx2-5, MEF-2, HAND-1, and HAND-2) are all characterized by the blocking of heart development at the stage of looping. The first molecular indication of asymmetrical development of the heart tube is the shift in expression of the transcription factor, HAND-1 (e-Hand), from both sides to the left side of the caudal heart tube. HAND-2 (d-Hand) is expressed predominantly in the primordium of the right ventricle. The Hand mole-cules may play a role in interpreting earlier asymmetrical molecular signals and translating this information into cellular behavior that results in looping. Retinoids may also play a role in determining the asymmetry of the looping heart, as well as determining the level of the atrioventricular junction.

As the straight heart tube begins to undergo looping, the originally ventral surface of the heart tube becomes the outer border of the loop and the originally dorsal surface becomes the inner border of the loop. When the individual heart chambers begin to form, they arise as outpocketings from the outer border of the heart loop. Characterization of the cellular basis for cardiac looping has proven very difficult. Although it has been clearly demonstrated that looping is an intrinsic property of the developing heart tube, factors as diverse as microtubules, asymmetrically located bundles of actin, pressure of the cardiac jelly, and changes in the shape of individual myocardial cells have all been proposed as bases for looping.

The result of cardiac looping is an **S**-shaped heart in which the originally caudal inflow part of the heart (**atrium**) becomes positioned dorsal to the outflow tract. In the early heart the outflow tract is commonly called the **bulbus cordis** (Figure 17-16). In early looping the cranial limb of the **S** represents the bulbus cordis, and the middle limb represents the ventricular part of the heart, with the primordium of the right ventricle closest to the outflow tract and that of the left ventricle next to the caudal limb. The caudal limb represents a common atrium. Somewhat later the common atrium bulges on either side (Figure 17-17), and an internal septum begins to divide the common ventricle into right and left chambers. The outflow tract (bulbus cordis of the early heart) retains its gross tubular appearance. Its distal part, which leads directly into the aortic arch system, is called the **truncus arteriosus**. The shorter transitional segment between the truncus and the ventricle is called the **conus arteriosus**. The conus is separated from the ventricles by faint grooves.

### Early Atrioventricular Partitioning of the Heart

Early in heart development the atrium becomes partially separated from the ventricle by the formation of thick-ened **atrioventricular cushions**. A similar but less pro-nounced thickening forms at the junction between the

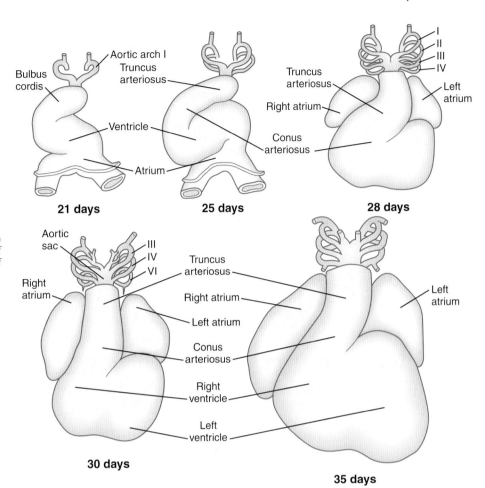

**FIGURE 17-16** Ventral views of human embryonic hearts, illustrating bending of the cardiac tube and the establishment of its regional divisions.

ventricle and the outflow tract (Figure 17-18). In these areas the cardiac jelly, which is organized like thick basement membrane, protrudes into the atrioventricular canal. The endocardial cushions function as primitive valves that assist in the forward propulsion of blood.

Acting in response to an inductive action by the underlying myocardium, certain antigenically distinct cells from the endocardium in two circumscribed areas lose their epithelial character and transform into mesenchymal cells, which migrate into the cardiac jelly. Only in the atrioventricular region and the proximal outflow tract do endocardial cells respond to the induction and transform into mesenchyme. Atrial and ventricular endocardial cells do not lose their epithelial character. The early heart is segmented molecularly. Segments of the endocardium that undergo a mesenchymal transformation express the *Msx-1* gene, whereas endocardial cells of the atrium and ventricle do not express it. Endocardial cells contain the cell adhesion molecule N-CAM on their surfaces. Those cells that transform into mesenchyme down-regulate the production of N-CAM. This presumably facilitates their production into motile cells.

In vivo studies have shown that just before transformation of the endocardial cells into mesenchyme, 20- to 50-nm particles appear in the cardiac jelly beneath these cells but not beneath other areas of endocardium (see Figure 17-18). Produced by the underlying myocardial cells, these particles, called **adherons**, contain a molecular complex of proteoglycan, fibronectin, and a number of matrix proteins. One of these proteins, **ES-130**, is also expressed in certain other tissues (e.g., notochord, neural tube ectoderm, apical ectodermal ridge), which are the only other tissues that can substitute for the myocardium in inducing the epithelial/mesenchymal transformation in the endocardium. These particles can induce atrioventricular endothelial cells to transform into mesenchyme in vitro. The induction of invasion of the cardiac jelly by atrioventricular endothelial cells is also accompanied by the activity of **TGF-β1** and **TGF-β3**. If this growth factor is inactivated, transformation fails to occur. The transformed mesenchymal cells secrete **proteases**, which destroy the inductively active adherons and restore morphogenetic stability to the endocardial cushion regions.

These cellular and molecular events form the basis for the early formation of the major heart valves. Disturbances in these processes can account for many malformations of the heart.

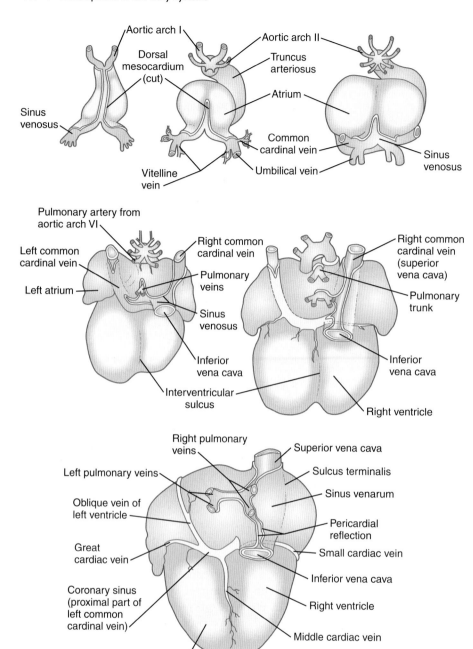

**FIGURE 17-17** Dorsal views of the development of the human heart, showing changes in the venous input channels into the heart.

## Later Partitioning of the Heart

### Separation of the Atria from the Ventricles

The endocardial cushions (see Figure 17-18), which ultimately become transformed into dense connective tissue, form on the dorsal and ventral walls of the atrioventricular canal. As they grow into the canal, the two cushions meet and separate the atrioventricular canal into right and left channels (Figures 17-19 and 17-20). The early endocardial cushions serve as primitive valves that assist in the forward propulsion of blood through the heart. Later in development, thin leaflets of anatomical valves take shape

in the atrioventricular canal. The definitive valve leaflets do not appear to come from endocardial cushion tissue as much as from invagination of superficial epicardially derived tissues of the atrioventricular groove. The valve that protects the right atrioventricular canal develops three leaflets (**tricuspid valve**), but the valve in the left canal (**mitral**, or **bicuspid, valve**) develops only two.

### Partitioning of the Atria

While the atrioventricular canals are taking shape, a series of structural changes divides the common atrium into separate left and right chambers. Partitioning begins in the

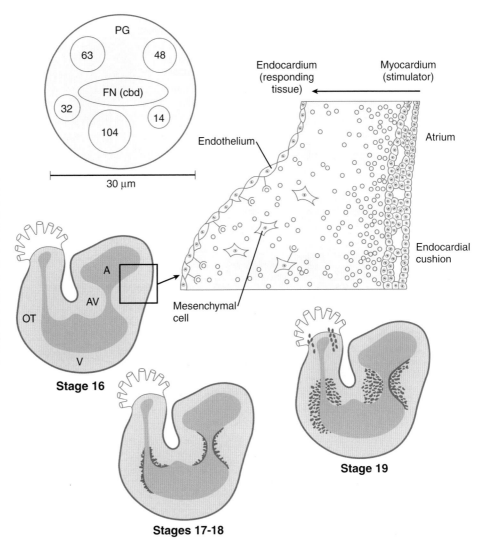

**FIGURE 17-18** Seeding of the endocardial cushions by mesenchymal cells in the developing avian heart. The higher-power drawing in the upper right shows details of the transformation of endocardial to mesenchymal cells. Also shown is a hypothetical model of the 30-nm adheron-like particle that appears to induce this transformation in the endocardial cells. *A,* Atrium; *AV,* atrioventricular canal; *FN (cbd),* fibronectin (cell-binding domain); *OT,* outlet tract; *PG,* proteoglycan; *V,* ventricle; *numbered circles,* other proteins. (Based on Bolender DL, Markwald RR. In Feinberg RN, Sherer GK, eds: *The development of the vascular system,* Basel, Switzerland, 1991, Karger, pp 109–124.)

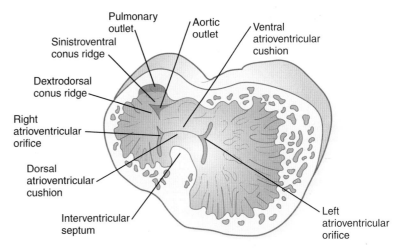

**FIGURE 17-19** Partitioning the atrioventricular canal from the ventricular aspect.

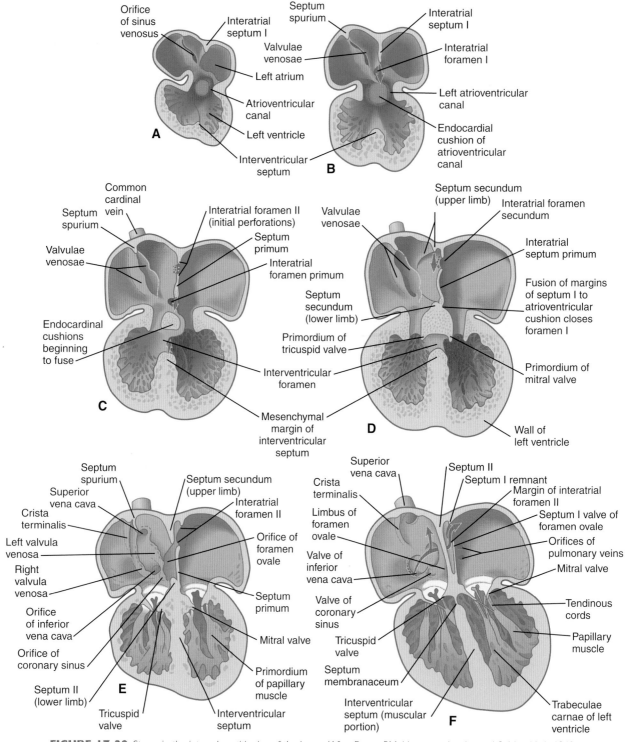

**FIGURE 17-20** Stages in the internal partitioning of the heart. (After Patten BM: *Human embryology,* ed 3, New York, 1968, McGraw-Hill.)

fifth week with the downgrowth of a crescentic **interatrial septum primum** from the cephalic wall of the common atrium (see Figure 17-20). The apices of the crescent of the septum primum extend toward the atrioventricular canal and merge with the endocardial cushions. The space between the leading edge of the septum primum and the endocardial cushions is called the **interatrial foramen primum.** This space serves as a shunt, permitting blood to pass directly from the right to the left atrium.

Circulatory shunts in the developing heart satisfy a very practical need. All incoming blood enters to the right side of the interatrial septum primum. However, because of the late development of the lungs and the poor carrying capacity of the pulmonary vessels during most of the fetal period, the pulmonary circulation cannot handle a full load of blood. If the heart were to form four totally separate chambers from the beginning, the pulmonary circulation would be overstressed, and the left side of the heart would not be pumping enough blood to foster normal development, especially in the early weeks.

The problem of maintaining a balanced circulatory load on all chambers of the heart is met by the existence of two shunts that allow most of the circulating blood to bypass the lungs. One shunt is a direct connection between the right and left atria, allowing blood entering the right atrium to bypass the pulmonary circulation completely by passing directly into the left atrium. This shunt permits the normal functional development of the left atrium. If all the blood entering the right atrium, however, passed directly into the left atrium, the right ventricle would have nothing to pump against and would become hypoplastic. In mid pregnancy more than 30% of the blood entering the right atrium is shunted directly into the left atrium; near term the percentage is reduced to somewhat less than 20%. With the arrangement of the openings of vascular channels into the right atrium, a significant amount of blood also enters the right ventricle and leaves that chamber through the pulmonary outflow tract. Most of the blood leaving the right ventricle, which is still far too much to be accommodated by the vasculature of the lungs, bypasses the lungs via the ductus arteriosus and empties directly into the descending aorta. By these two mechanisms, the heart is evenly exercised, and the pulmonary circulation is protected.

When the interatrial septum primum is almost ready to fuse with the endocardial cushions, an area of genetically programmed cell death causes the appearance of multiple perforations near its cephalic end (see Figure 17-20). As the leading edge of the septum primum fuses with the endocardial cushions, obliterating the foramen primum, the cephalic perforations in the septum primum coalesce and give rise to the **interatrial foramen secundum**. This new foramen preserves the direct connection between the right and left atria.

Shortly after the appearance of the foramen secundum, a crescentic **septum secundum** begins to form just to the right of the septum primum. This structure, which grows out from the dorsal to the ventral part of the atrium, forms a **foramen ovale**. The position of the foramen ovale allows most of the blood that enters the right atrium through the inferior vena cava to pass directly through it and the foramen secundum into the left atrium. However, the arrangement of the two interatrial septa allows them to act like a one-way valve, permitting blood to flow from the right to the left atrium but not in the reverse direction.

## Repositioning of the Sinus Venosus and the Venous Inflow into the Right Atrium

During the stage of the straight tubular heart, the sinus venosus is a bilaterally symmetrical chamber into which the major veins of the body empty (see Figure 17-13). As the heart undergoes looping and the interatrial septa form, the entrance of the sinus venosus shifts completely to the right atrium (see Figures 17-17 and 17-20). As this occurs, the right horn of the sinus venosus becomes increasingly incorporated into the wall of the right atrium, so the much reduced left horn, the **coronary sinus** (which is the common drainage channel for the coronary veins), opens directly into the right atrium (see Figure 17-14). Also in the right atrium, valvelike flaps of tissue (**valvulae venosae**) form around the entrances of the superior and inferior venae cavae. Because of the orientation of the orifice and its pressure, blood entering the right atrium from the inferior vena cava passes mostly through the interatrial shunt and into the left atrium, whereas blood entering from the superior vena cava and the coronary sinus flows through the tricuspid valve into the right ventricle.

## Partitioning of the Ventricles

When the interatrial septa are first forming, a muscular **interventricular septum** begins to grow from the apex of the common ventricle toward the atrioventricular endocardial cushions. The early division of the common ventricle is also reflected by the presence of a groove on the outer surface of the heart (Figure 17-21). Although an **interventricular foramen** is initially present, it is ultimately obliterated. This is accomplished by (1) further growth of the muscular interventricular septum, (2) a contribution by truncoconal ridge tissue that divides the outflow tract of the heart, and (3) a membranous component derived from endocardial cushion connective tissue.

## Partitioning of the Outflow Tract of the Heart

In the very early tubular heart the outflow tract is a single tube, the bulbus cordis. By the time the interventricular septum begins to form, the bulbus elongates and can be divided into a proximal conus arteriosus and a distal truncus arteriosus (see Figure 17-16). Although initially a single channel, the outflow tract is partitioned into separate aortic and pulmonary channels through the appearance of two spiral **truncoconal ridges**, which are derived largely from neural crest mesenchyme. These ridges bulge into the lumen and finally meet, separating it into two channels. The aortic sac, which is located distal to the truncoconal region, does not contain ridges. Partitioning of the outflow tract begins near the ventral aortic

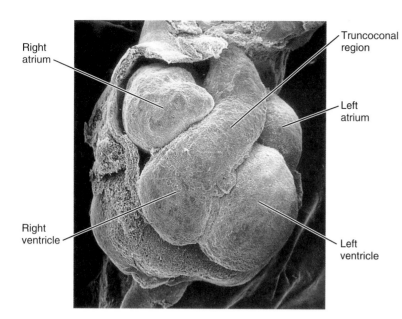

Right
atrium

Truncoconal
region

Left
atrium

Right
ventricle

Left
ventricle

**FIGURE 17-21** Scanning electron micrograph showing a right oblique view of the heart of a human embryo early in the sixth week. The pericardium has been dissected free from the heart. (From Jirásek J: *Atlas of human prenatal morphogenesis,* Boston, 1983, Martinus Nijhoff.)

root between the fourth and sixth arches and extends toward the ventricles, spiraling as it goes (Figure 17-22). This accounts for the partial spiraling of the aorta and the pulmonary artery in the adult heart.

Before and during the partitioning process, the neural crest–derived cells of the wall of the outflow tract begin to produce elastic fibers, which provide the resiliency required of the aorta and other great vessels. Elastogenesis follows a gradient, first through the outflow tract, then into the aorta itself, and ultimately into the smaller arterial branches off the aorta.

At the base of the conus, where endocardial cushion tissue is formed in the same manner as in the atrioventricular canal, two new sets of **semilunar valves** form (Figure 17-23). These valves, each of which has three leaflets, prevent ejected blood from washing back into the ventricles. Cranial neural crest cells and cardiac mesoderm contribute to the formation of the semilunar valves. As previously stated, the most proximal extensions of the truncoconal ridges contribute to the formation of the interventricular septum. Just past the aortic side of the aortic semilunar valve, the two coronary arteries join the aorta to supply the heart with blood.

### Innervation of the Heart

Although initial heart development occurs independently of nerves, three sets of nerve fibers ultimately innervate the heart (Figure 17-24). Sympathetic (adrenergic) nerve fibers, which act to speed up the heart beat, arrive as outgrowths from sympathetic ganglia of the trunk. These nerve fibers are derived from trunk neural crest. Parasympathetic (cholinergic) innervation is derived from the

cranial neural crest. Neurons of the cardiac ganglia, which are the second-order parasympathetic neurons, migrate directly to the heart from the cardiac neural crest. These synapse with axons of first-order parasympathetic neurons that gain access to the heart via the vagus nerve. Sensory innervation of the heart is also supplied via the vagus nerve, but the sensory neurons originate from placodal ectoderm (nodose placode) (see Figure 13-1). Thus the direct innervation of the heart has three separate origins.

If the cardiac neural crest is removed in the early chick embryo, cholinergic cardiac ganglia still form. Experiments have determined that the nodose placodes compensate for the loss of neural crest by supplying neurons that take the place of the normal parasympathetic ones.

### Conducting System of the Heart

The normal heart beat is a reflection of a complex of internal pacemakers and a conducting system that rapidly distributes the contractile stimulus throughout the heart. The input of the autonomic nerves, which modulate the heart beat to a faster (sympathetic) or slower (parasympathetic) rate, is also involved.

In very early heart development the location of the pacemaker shifts from the caudalmost end of the left tube of the unfused heart to the sinus venosus. As the sinus venosus is incorporated into the right atrium late in the fifth week, the pacemaker, now called the **sinoatrial node**, becomes situated high in the right atrium, close to the entrance of the superior vena cava. A few days later, an **atrioventricular node** forms in the interatrial septal area just above the endocardial cushion tissue. These two

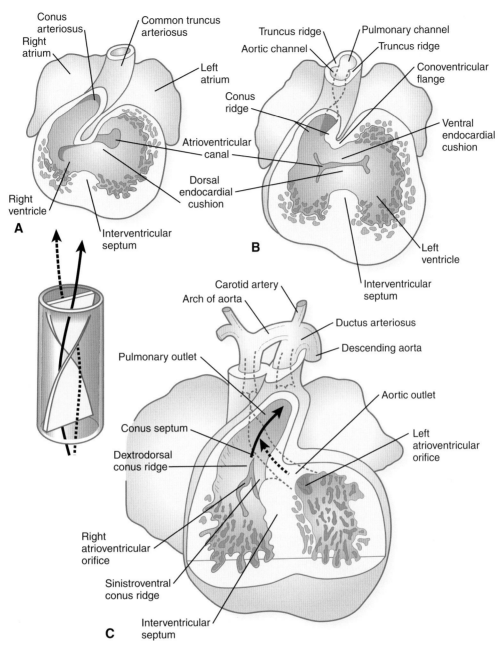

**FIGURE 17-22** Partitioning of the outflow tract of the developing heart. The truncoconal ridges undergo a 180-degree spiraling. (After Kramer TC: *Am J Anat* 71:343–370, 1942.)

nodes are connected by several strands of modified cardiac muscle cells that conduct the contractile stimulus from the sinoatrial node to the atrioventricular node. From the atrioventricular node a well-defined **atrioventricular bundle** passes from the atrium into the ventricle and splits into right and left branches. These branches then distribute conducting tissue (**Purkinje fibers**) throughout the ventricular myocardium.

Many aspects of the embryology of the conducting system have been poorly understood over the years, but recent research has begun to clarify some controversial points. Mature conducting bundles consist of highly modified cardiac myocytes that contain large amounts of glycogen. Research on chick embryos has shown that **endothelin-1**, secreted by the coronary arteries, stimulates cardiomyocytes to transform into cells of the conducting system. In mice, cells of the conducting system, which express **engrailed-2**, appear very early in development and may begin functioning before septation of the heart is completed. The atrioventricular node and bundle

**FIGURE 17-23** Formation of the semilunar valves in the outflow tract of the heart. Neural crest cells *(green)* contribute to the formation of the valvular leaflets.

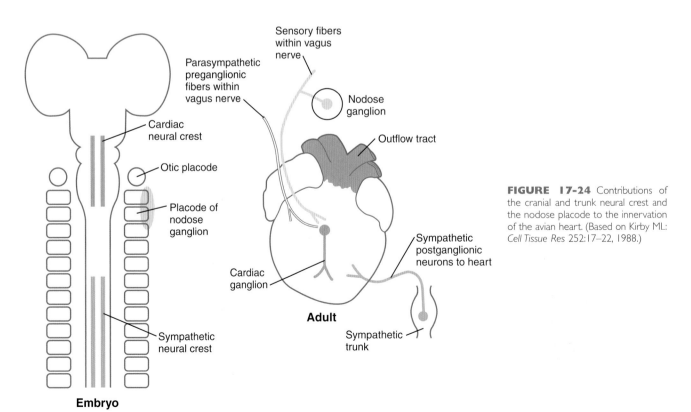

**FIGURE 17-24** Contributions of the cranial and trunk neural crest and the nodose placode to the innervation of the avian heart. (Based on Kirby ML: *Cell Tissue Res* 252:17–22, 1988.)

arise from a segment of a ring of myocardial cells that initially surround the interventricular foramen and later, in some species, become translocated to form a figure eight–shaped ring at the atrioventricular junction (Figure 17-25). Branches from this ring ultimately pass along either side of the interventricular septum and then arborize along the ventricular walls as the Purkinje fibers.

## INITIATION OF CARDIAC FUNCTION

Because of its accessibility, the chick embryo has taught scientists most of what is known about the earliest functions of the embryonic heart. In recent years the application of ultrasound techniques has allowed the investigation of some aspects of cardiac function in human embryos as young as 4½ to 5 weeks of age.

Bilateral regions of precardiac mesoderm in the chick embryo differentiate into right and left cardiac tubes with functional ventricular, atrial, and sinoatrial regions. Contraction of the embryonic heart begins as the right and left heart tubes begin to fuse, and circulation of the blood begins soon thereafter. In the human embryo, this occurs between 21 and 23 days' gestation.

As the heart tubes of the chick embryo first fuse in the ventricular region, the fused ventricles have an intrinsic beat of 25 per minute, and the unfused atria do not beat. A few hours later, when the atrial parts of the cardiac tubes have fused, the atrial region beats at a rate of 62 per minute. The atrial beat acts as a pacemaker, causing the ventricle to beat at the same rate. However, if the atrium is separated from the ventricle, the beat of the ventricle slows to an intrinsic rate of only 24 per minute. Finally, when the sinus venosus takes shape, its intrinsic beat of 140 per minute drives the overall heart beat.

In the early fusing heart a distinct pacemaker region is located in the left sinus venosus region. The pacemaker consists of an aggregation of approximately 60 to 150 cells rather than a signal arising from a single cell. The

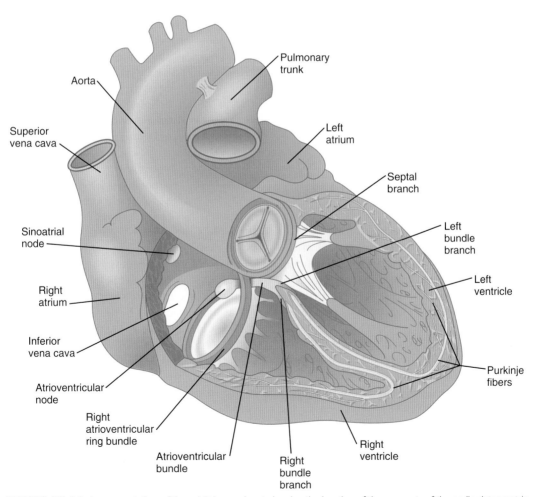

**FIGURE 17-25** A representation of the adult human heart showing the location of the remnants of the earlier interventricular myocardial ring *(green)* and the portion *(yellow)* that gives rise to the atrioventricular node and bundle. The left and right bundle branches emanate from this structure and ultimately spread out along the ventricular walls as the Purkinje fibers. (Based on Moorman A, Lamers WH. In Harvey RP and Rosenthal N: *Heart Development,* Academic Press, New York 1999.)

pacemaker initiates an excitation wave that is propagated through the early heart in about 0.5 second. As the heart matures and gets larger, the rate of propagation increases proportionally to the size of the heart. Thus the conduction velocity of the excitation stimulus increases by 100-fold, but the actual conduction time does not greatly change despite a 1000-fold increase in the mass of the heart in the chick embryo. Increasing numbers of gap junctions between developing cardiac myocytes may partly account for the increasing conduction velocity in the developing heart.

The mechanism by which the tubular heart is able to pump blood in the absence of valves is still not well understood. Once the atrium fills with blood from the sinus venosus, it contracts and sends the blood into the ventricle. A peristalsis-like contraction then moves the blood to the truncus region, from which it leaves the heart and enters the aortic sac. Active contraction of the truncus region prevents the reflux of blood into the heart from the aortic root. Even in the early heart the endocardial cushions of the atrioventricular canal and the outflow tract have a valvelike function. At times the patterns of blood flow in the early heart have been considered to be responsible for the patterns of internal septation of the heart. However, careful studies have shown that many aspects of cardiac morphogenesis are separate from its function.

The blood pressure of an early embryo is very low (0.61/0.43 mm Hg in the 3-day-old chick embryo). As the embryo grows, the blood pressure rises exponentially and then tapers off before birth.

## FETAL CIRCULATION

In many respects the overall plan of the embryonic circulation seems to be inefficient and more complex than needed to maintain the growth and development of the fetus. However, the embryo must prepare for the moment when it suddenly shifts to a totally different pattern of oxygenation of blood through the lungs rather than the placenta, making the modifications of the fetal plan of circulation essential.

Highly oxygenated blood from the placenta enters the umbilical vein in a large stream that is sometimes under increased pressure because of uterine contractions. Within the substance of the liver, blood from the umbilical vein under higher pressure passes directly into the ductus venosus, which allows it to bypass the small circulatory channels of the liver and flow directly into the inferior vena cava (Figure 17-26). Once in the vena cava, it has immediate access to the heart. Poorly oxygenated blood flowing in the inferior vena cava can be somewhat backed up because of the strength of the umbilical blood flow.

Functional evidence exists for a physiological sphincter in the ductus venosus, which forces much of the umbilical blood to pass through hepatic capillary channels and enter the inferior vena cava through hepatic veins when it tightens. This considerably reduces the pressure of the umbilical blood and allows poorly oxygenated systemic blood from the inferior vena cava to enter the right atrium at a lower pressure. Higher-pressure blood entering the umbilical vein from the placenta also tends to prevent blood from the hepatic portal vein from entering the ductus venosus. When the uterus is relaxed and the umbilical venous blood is under low pressure, poorly oxygenated portal blood mixes with the umbilical blood in the ductus venosus. More mixing of umbilical and systemic blood occurs in the inferior vena cava as well.

In the right atrium the orientation of the entrance of the inferior vena cava allows a stream of blood under slightly increased pressure to pass directly through the foramen ovale and foramen secundum into the left atrium (see Figure 17-26). This is the route normally taken by highly oxygenated umbilical blood entering the body under increased pressure. Because the interatrial shunt of the fetus is smaller than the opening of the inferior vena cava, some of the highly oxygenated caval blood eddies in the right atrium and enters the right ventricle. When low-pressure blood (typically poorly oxygenated systemic blood) enters the right atrium, it joins with the venous blood draining the head through the superior vena cava and the heart through the coronary sinus and is mostly directed through the tricuspid valve into the right ventricle.

All blood entering the fetal right ventricle leaves through the pulmonary artery and passes toward the lungs. Even in the relatively late fetus, the pulmonary vasculature is not ready to handle the full volume of blood that enters the pulmonary artery. The blood that cannot be accommodated by the pulmonary arteries is shunted to the aorta via the ductus arteriosus. This structure protects the lungs from circulatory overload, yet allows the right ventricle to exercise in preparation for its functioning at full capacity at birth. Only 12% of the right ventricular output passes through the lungs of the fetus. The control of patency of the ductus arteriosus has been subject to considerable speculation. Patency of both the ductus arteriosus and ductus venosus in the fetus is maintained actively through the action of prostaglandins (prostaglandin $E_2$ and prostaglandin $I_2$, respectively). Some of the effect of the prostaglandins is mediated by nitric oxide.

The left atrium receives a stream of highly oxygenated umbilical blood through the interatrial shunt and a small amount of poorly oxygenated blood from the pulmonary veins. This blood, which in aggregate is relatively highly oxygenated, passes into the left ventricle and leaves the

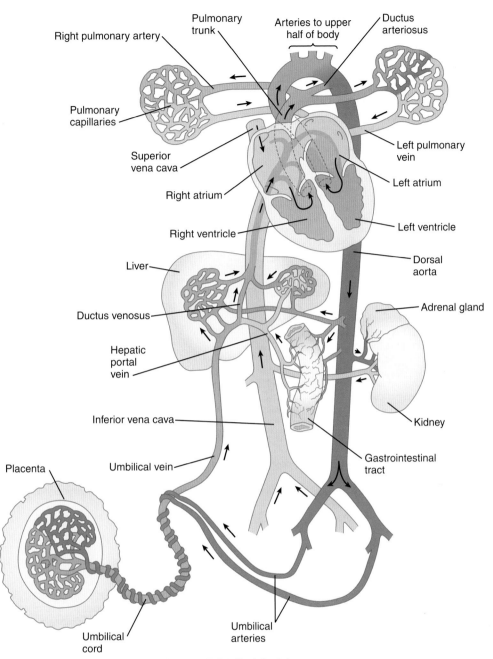

Right pulmonary artery

Pulmonary trunk

Arteries to upper half of body

Ductus arteriosus

Pulmonary capillaries

Superior vena cava

Right atrium

Right ventricle

Liver

Ductus venosus

Hepatic portal vein

Inferior vena cava

Placenta

Umbilical vein

Umbilical cord

Left pulmonary vein

Left atrium

Left ventricle

Dorsal aorta

Adrenal gland

Kidney

Gastrointestinal tract

Umbilical arteries

**FIGURE 17-26** Fetal circulation at term.

heart through the aorta. Some of the first arterial branches leaving the aorta supply the heart and brain, organs that require a high concentration of oxygen for normal development.

Where the aortic arch begins to descend, the ductus arteriosus empties poorly oxygenated blood into it. This mixture of well-oxygenated and poorly oxygenated blood is then distributed to the tissues and organs that are supplied by the thoracic and abdominal branches of the aorta. Near its caudal end the aorta gives off two large umbilical arteries, which carry blood to the placenta for renewal.

## SUMMARY

○ The vascular system arises from mesodermal blood islands in the wall of the yolk sac. Hemangioblasts give rise to either blood cells or vascular endothelial cells. Nucleated red blood cells produced in the blood islands are the first blood cells found in the embryo. Later, hematopoiesis shifts to the embryonic body, beginning in the paraaortic bodies, and then to the liver, and finally to the bone marrow.

**TABLE 17-5** *Timelines in Normal and Abnormal Cardiac Development*

| Normal time | Developmental events | Malformations arising during period |
|---|---|---|
| 18 days | Horseshoe-shaped cardiac primordium appears | Lethal mutants |
| 20 days | Bilateral cardiac primordia fuse<br>Cardiac jelly appears<br>Aortic arch is forming | Cardia bifida (experimental)<br>—<br>— |
| 22 days | Heart is looping into S shape<br>Heart begins to beat<br>Dorsal mesocardium is breaking down<br>Aortic arches I and II are forming | Dextrocardia<br>—<br>—<br>— |
| 24 days | Atria are beginning to bulge<br>Right and left ventricles act like two pumps in series<br>Outflow tract is distinguishable from right ventricle | —<br>—<br>— |
| Late fourth week | Sinus venosus is becoming incorporated into right atrium<br>Endocardial cushions appear<br>Early septum I appears between left and right atria<br>Muscular interventricular septum is forming<br>Truncoconal ridges are forming<br>Aortic arch I is regressing<br>Aortic arch III is formed<br>Aortic arch IV is forming | Venous inflow malformations<br>Persistent atrioventricular canal<br>Common atrium<br>Common ventricle<br>Persistent truncus arteriosus<br>—<br>—<br>Missing fourth aortic arch segment |
| Early fifth week | Endocardial cushions are coming together, forming right and left atrioventricular canals<br>Further growth of interatrial septum I and muscular interventricular septum occurs<br>Truncus arteriosus is dividing into aorta and pulmonary artery<br><br>Atrioventricular bundle is forming; possible neurogenic control of heart beat<br>Pulmonary veins are becoming incorporated into left atrium<br>Aortic arches I and II have regressed<br>Aortic arches III and IV have formed<br>Aortic arch VI is forming<br>Conduction system forms | Persistent atrioventricular canal<br><br>Muscular ventricular septal defects<br><br>Transposition of great vessels<br>Aortic and pulmonary stenosis or atresia<br><br>Aberrant pulmonary drainage<br>—<br>—<br>—<br>— |
| Late fifth to early sixth week | Endocardial cushions fuse<br>Interatrial foramen II is forming<br>Interatrial septum I is almost contacting endocardial cushion<br>Membranous part of interventricular septum starts to form<br>Semilunar valves begin to form | —<br>—<br>Low atrial septal defects<br>Membranous interventricular septal defects<br>Aortic and pulmonary valvular stenosis |
| Late sixth week | Interatrial foramen II is large<br>Interatrial septum II starts to form<br>Atrioventricular valves and papillary muscles are forming<br>Interventricular septum is almost complete<br>Coronary circulation is becoming established | High atrial septal defects<br>—<br>Tricuspid or mitral valvular stenosis or atresia<br>Membranous interventricular septal defects<br>— |
| Eighth to ninth week | Membranous part of interventricular septum is completed | Membranous interventricular septal defects |

○ During hematopoiesis, hemocytoblasts give rise to lymphoid and myeloid stem cells. Each of these stem cells further differentiates into the definitive lines of blood cells. Erythropoiesis involves the passage of precursor cells of red blood cells through a number of stages. The earliest stages are defined by behavioral, rather than morphological, characteristics. During later stages of differentiation, the precursor cells of erythrocytes gradually lose their RNA-producing machinery and accumulate increasing amounts of hemoglobin in their cytoplasm; at the same time the nucleus becomes more condensed and is eventually lost. Hemoglobin also undergoes isoform transitions during embryonic development.

*Text continued on page 472.*

## Malformations of the Heart

With an incidence of almost 1 per 100 live births, heart defects represent the most common class of congenital malformations. Because of the close physiological balance of the circulation, most malformations produce symptoms. Clinically, heart malformations are typically classified as those that are associated with cyanosis (**cyanotic defects**) in postnatal life and those that are not (**acyanotic defects**).

Cyanosis results when the blood contains more than 5 g/dl of reduced hemoglobin. Cyanosis is readily recognizable by a purplish to bluish tinge to the skin in areas with a dense superficial capillary circulation. It is associated with **polycythemia,** an increased concentration of erythrocytes in the blood resulting from the overall decreased oxygen saturation of the blood. Long-term cyanosis is associated with a prominent clubbing of the ends of the fingers (see Figure 17-37) and decreased growth. In severe cases of cyanosis, children often assume a squatting posture that may facilitate reoxygenation of the blood.

Postnatally, cyanosis is associated with the presence of a right-to-left shunt in which venous blood mixes with systemic blood. Some heart defects are acyanotic for many years but then become cyanotic. These defects are initially characterized by a left-to-right shunt in which oxygenated systemic blood refluxes into the right atrium or ventricle. The net result is an increased pumping load on the right ventricle, ultimately leading to right ventricular hypertrophy. Over a long period the increased blood flow through the lungs provokes a hypertensive reaction in the pulmonary vasculature, which effectively increases the pressure in the right ventricle and atrium. When the blood pressure on the right side of the heart exceeds that in the corresponding left chamber, the shunt reverses, and poorly oxygenated blood passes to the systemic circulation, leading to cyanosis. At this point the condition of the patient who has the cardiac lesion often rapidly worsens.

### CHAMBER-TO-CHAMBER SHUNTS

#### Interatrial Septal Defects

Several types of anatomical defects in the interatrial septum can result in a persisting shunt between the two atria. The most common varieties are caused by excessive resorption of tissue around the foramen secundum or hypoplastic growth of the septum secundum (Figure 17-27, *A*). A less common variety is a low septal

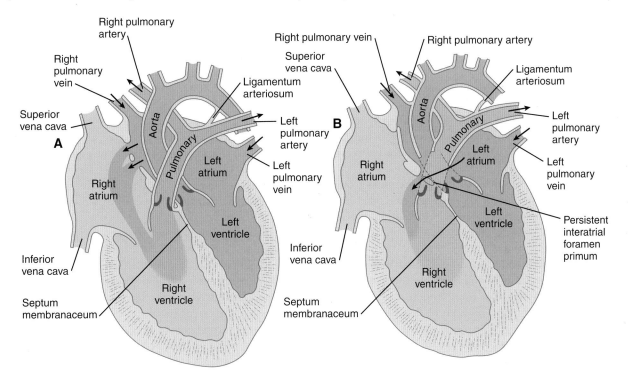

**FIGURE 17-27** High **(A)** and low **(B)** atrial septal defects in the heart. Red denotes well-oxygenated arterial blood, blue denotes poorly oxygenated venous blood, and purple denotes a mixture of arterial and venous blood.

*Continued*

defect, which is usually caused by the lack of union between the leading edge of the septum primum and the endocardial cushions (Figure 17-27, B). If the defect is the result of a deficiency of endocardial cushion tissue, associated defects of the atrioventricular valves can considerably complicate the lesion. Lack of septation of the atrium results in a **common atrium**, a serious defect that is usually associated with other heart defects. Atrial septal defects are among the most common heart malformations. Increasingly, atrial septal defects are being associated with chromosome 21. Individuals with Down syndrome (trisomy of chromosome 21) have a high incidence of defects of both the atrial and ventricular septa.

Individuals with autosomal dominant mutations of the *Nkx2-5* gene (see p. 446) have a high incidence of abnormalities of the septum secundum, resulting in atrial septal defects. Associated with the atrial septal defects is an equally high incidence of atrioventricular block, which can lead to sudden death in affected individuals whose hearts are not assisted by pacemakers. Before the discovery of this mutation, it was suspected that many of the cases of atrioventricular block were due to disruption of the atrioventricular bundle by the repair procedure. During the early days of cardiac surgery, before the anatomy of the atrioventricular bundle was precisely determined, surgically induced bundle branch block was a problem in the repair of low atrial septal defects.

Another condition that is strongly associated with atrial (and ventricular) septal defects, as well as limb anomalies, is the **Holt-Oram syndrome**. This syndrome is caused by a mutation in the *T-box* gene *Tbx-5*, the gene that is expressed in the upper limb, but not the lower limb (see p. 216).

Uncomplicated atrial septal defects are usually compatible with many years of symptom-free life. Even during the symptom-free period, blood from the left atrium, which is under slightly higher pressure than that in the right atrium, passes into the right atrium. This additional blood causes right atrial hypertrophy and results in increased blood flow into the lungs. Over many years, pulmonary hypertension can develop. This increases the blood pressure of the right ventricle and ultimately that of the right atrium. Only a few millimeters of increased right atrial pressure reverses the blood flow in the interatrial shunt and causes cyanosis.

A more serious condition is **premature closure of the foramen ovale**. In this situation the entire input of blood into the right atrium passes into the right ventricle, causing massive hypertrophy of the right side of the heart. The left side is severely hypoplastic because of the reduced blood that the left chambers carry. Although this defect is usually compatible with intrauterine life, infants typically die shortly after birth because the hypoplastic left heart cannot handle a normal circulatory load.

**Persistent Atrioventricular Canal**

The usual basis for persistent atrioventricular canal is underdevelopment of the endocardial cushions that results in a lack of division of the early atrioventricular canal into right and left channels. A number of specific causes of atrioventricular canal defects may exist, ranging from inappropriate expression of Msx-1 to defects in the production or reception of inductively active extracellular matrix components (e.g., subunits of adherons) by the endocardial cells (see Figure 17-18).

A persistent atrioventricular canal is often associated with major interatrial and interventricular septal defects (Figure 17-28). This severe defect leads to poor growth and a considerably shortened life. Interestingly, despite the potential for mixing of blood, the predominant shunt direction is left to right, and some patients have little cyanosis.

**Tricuspid Atresia**

In tricuspid atresia, the etiology of which is poorly understood, the normal valvular opening between the right atrium and right ventricle is completely occluded (Figure 17-29, B). Such a defect alone causes death because the blood cannot gain access to the lungs for oxygenation. However, children can survive with this malformation, illustrating an important point in cardiac embryology. Often a primary lesion is accompanied by one or more secondary lesions (usually shunts) that permit survival, although frequently at a poor functional level.

In this condition, secondary shunts must accomplish two things. First, a persisting atrial septal defect must shunt the blood that cannot pass through the atretic tricuspid valve into the left atrium. The left atrial blood then flows into the left ventricle. Second, one or more secondary shunts must allow blood to gain access to the lungs so that it can become oxygenated. Left ventricular blood could enter the right ventricle and pulmonary arterial system if a defect is present in the interventricular septum. Another possibility is for the blood in the left ventricle to pass into the systemic circulation, where it can gain access to the lungs by passing from the aorta

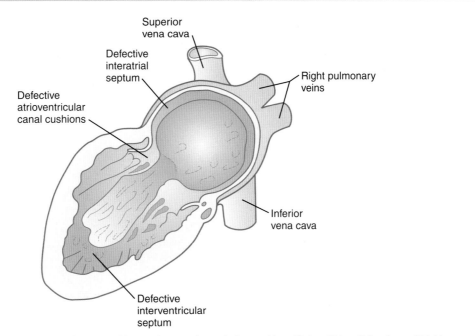

**FIGURE 17-28** Dissection of a heart with a persistent atrioventricular canal in a 12-day-old boy. (After Patten BM: *Human embryology*, ed 3, New York, 1968, McGraw-Hill.)

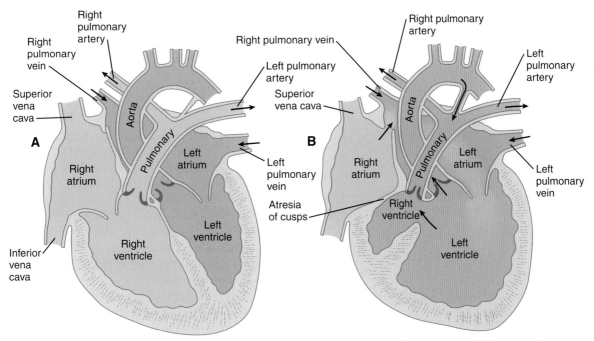

**FIGURE 17-29 A,** Normal postnatal heart. **B,** Tricuspid atresia, with compensating defects in the interatrial septum and interventricular septum *(arrows)*, which allow this patient to survive.

*Continued*

through a patent ductus arteriosus into the pulmonary arteries. From the lungs the oxygenated blood enters the left atrium, perhaps to be recycled through the lungs again before entering the systemic circulation.

**Mitral atresia** can also occur, but it is much rarer than tricuspid atresia. Secondary compensating defects again have to be present for survival. Infants with these lesions typically survive only a few months or years.

### Interventricular Septal Defect

Defects in the interventricular septum are the most common congenital cardiac defect in infants, but the vast majority of them close spontaneously before the age of 10. In the adult, they are not as common as atrial septal defects. Almost 70% of ventricular septal defects occur in the membranous part of the septum, where several embryonic tissues converge (Figure 17-30). Because the pressure of the blood in the left ventricle is higher than that in the right, this lesion is initially associated with a left-to-right acyanotic shunting of blood flow (Figure 17-31). However, the increased blood flow into the right ventricle produces right ventricular hypertrophy and can lead to pulmonary hypertension, ultimately causing reversal of the shunt. The basic pathological dynamics are similar to those for atrial septal defects.

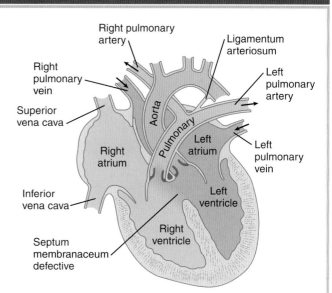

**FIGURE 17-31** Interventricular septal defect (membranous portion). Mixing of arterial and venous blood occurs in both outflow tracts but especially in the pulmonary artery.

## MALFORMATIONS OF THE OUTFLOW TRACT

The outflow tract of the heart (truncoconal region) is subject to a variety of malformations. Such malformations are responsible for about 20% to 30% of all congenital heart disease. Experimental studies have shown a prominent contribution of neural crest cells to this region. Extirpation and transplantation experiments have shown specific requirements for cardiac neural crest cells in the normal development of the cardiac outflow tract (Figure 17-32). If the cardiac neural crest is removed, ectodermal cells from the nodose placode populate the outflow tract, but septation of the outflow tract does not occur, leading to a persistent truncus arteriosus. If mesencephalic or truncal neural crest is grafted in place of cardiac neural crest or if foreign neural crest is grafted lateral to the cardiac neural crest, persistent truncus arteriosus consistently results. The last experiment shows that foreign neural crest interferes with the normal migration or function of the cardiac neural crest.

Although all malformations of this area cannot be attributed to defective neural crest development, circumstantial evidence suggests that this may be a significant factor. A number of defects of the outflow tract are associated with translocations or deletions in chromosome 22, and most of these involve the neural crest. Lesions of the outflow tract can be produced experimentally by interfering with the function of specific genes, often

**FIGURE 17-30** Ventricular septal defect (*arrow*) associated with tricuspid atresia. (Photo 147 from the Arey-DaPeña Pediatric Pathology Photographic Collection, Human Developmental Anatomy Center, National Museum of Health and Medicine, Armed Forces Institute of Pathology, Washington, DC.)

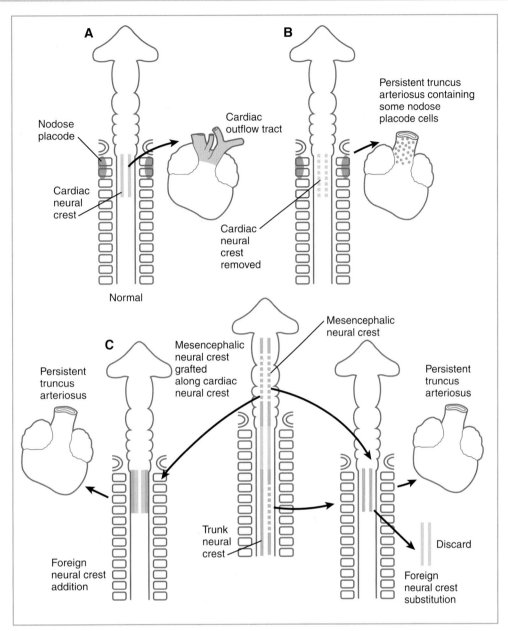

**FIGURE 17-32** Neural crest and morphogenesis of the outflow tract of the heart. **A,** Normal structure, showing cardiac neural crest contributing to the formation of the outflow tract in the avian heart. **B,** Removal of the cardiac neural crest leads to the formation of a persistent truncus arteriosus containing cells derived from the nodose placode. **C,** Experiments illustrating the importance of cardiac neural crest in the morphogenesis of the outflow tract. (Based on Kirby ML, Waldo KL: *Circulation* 82:332–340, 1990.)

genes located on chromosome 22 and genes that affect properties of cranial neural crest cells. For example, outflow-tract abnormalities are seen in mice deficient in **neurotrophin-3 (NT-3)**, a member of the nerve growth factor family. In addition, mutations of components of a cascade, starting with endothelin-1, HAND-2, and then neuropilin-1, a receptor for semaphorin in the nervous system and VEGF in the vascular system, all produce varying degrees of outflow-tract anomalies.

**Persistent Truncus Arteriosus**

Persistent truncus arteriosus is caused by the lack of partitioning of the outflow tract by the truncoconal ridges (Figures 17-33 and 17-34, *A*). Because of the contribution of the truncoconal ridges to the membranous part of the interventricular septum, this malformation is almost always accompanied by a ventricular septal defect. A large arterial outflow vessel overrides the ventricular

**FIGURE 17-33** Persistent truncus arteriosus *(arrow)*. (Photo 117 from the Arey-DaPeña Pediatric Pathology Photographic Collection, Human Developmental Anatomy Center, National Museum of Health and Medicine, Armed Forces Institute of Pathology, Washington, DC.)

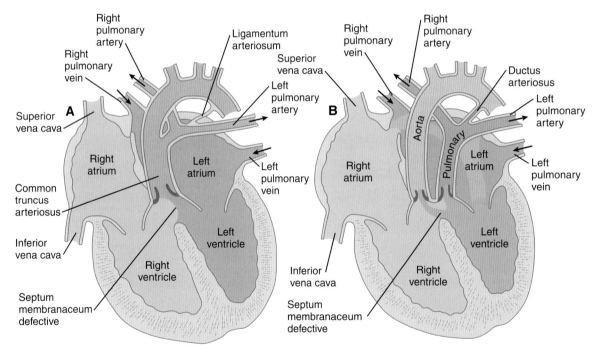

**FIGURE 17-34 A,** Persistent truncus arteriosus. A single outflow tract is fed by blood entering from the right and left ventricles. The membranous part of the interventricular septum is commonly defective. **B,** Transposition of the great vessels caused by lack of spiraling of the truncoconal ridges in the early embryo. The aorta arises from the right ventricle and the pulmonary artery from the left ventricle.

septum and receives blood that exits from each ventricle. As may be predicted, individuals with a persistent truncus arteriosus are highly cyanotic. Without treatment, 60% to 70% of infants born with this defect die within 6 months.

### Transposition of the Great Vessels

On rare occasions the truncoconal ridges fail to spiral as they divide the outflow tract into two channels. This results in two totally independent circulatory arcs, with the right ventricle emptying into the aorta and the left ventricle emptying into the pulmonary artery (Figure 17-34, *B*). If the condition were uncorrected, the left circulatory arc would continue pumping highly oxygenated blood through the left side of the heart and the lungs, whereas the right side of the heart would pump venous blood through the aorta into the systemic circulatory channels and back into the right atrium. This lesion, which is the most common cause of cyanosis in newborns, is compatible with life only if an atrial and a ventricular septal defect and an associated patent ductus arteriosus accompany it. Even with these anatomical compensations, the quality of blood reaching the body is poor.

### Aortic and Pulmonary Stenosis

If the septation of the outflow tract by the truncoconal ridges is asymmetrical, either the aorta or pulmonary artery is abnormally narrowed, resulting in **aortic** and **pulmonary stenosis** (Figures 17-35 and 17-36). The severity of symptoms is related to the degree of stenosis.

In the most extreme case, the stenosis is so severe that the lumen of the vessel is essentially obliterated. This condition is known as **aortic** or **pulmonary atresia**. A lesion reminiscent of pulmonary stenosis has been produced in mice bearing a null mutant of the gene for **connexin 43**, which encodes a protein component of the gap junction channel. Why such a genetic lesion would affect principally the pulmonary outlet of the heart is not yet known.

One of the best-known lesions of this type is the **tetralogy of Fallot**, which is characterized by (1) pulmonary stenosis, (2) a membranous interventricular septal defect, (3) a large aorta (overriding aorta, the opening of which extends into the right ventricle), and (4) right ventricular hypertrophy. The basic defect in tetralogy of Fallot is an asymmetrical fusion of the truncoconal ridges and a malalignment of the aortic and pulmonary valves. Because of the pulmonary stenosis and the wider-than-normal aortic opening, some poorly oxygenated right ventricular blood leaves via the enlarged aorta, causing cyanosis. Tetralogy of Fallot is the most common cyanotic heart lesion in young children. Patients with tetralogy of Fallot are highly cyanotic from birth and exhibit severe digital clubbing (Figure 17-37). When this condition is untreated, only 50% of patients survive past $2\frac{1}{2}$ years.

Pulmonary stenosis or tetralogy of Fallot is one of the conditions that characterizes the **Alagille syndrome**. This condition is caused by a mutation in **Jagged-1**, a ligand of the Notch receptor.

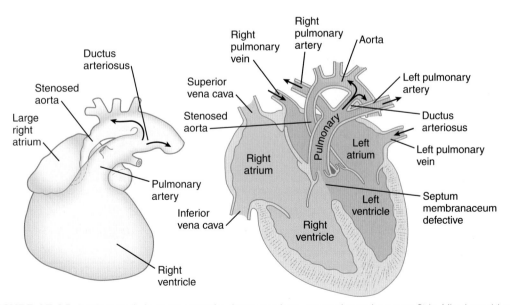

**FIGURE 17-35** Aortic stenosis. In severe cases the ductus arteriosus commonly remains patent. *Right,* Mixed arterial and venous blood in the pulmonary artery is shown in purple. Initially, blood from the pulmonary trunk *(purple)* goes through the ductus arteriosus into the aorta, often leading to cyanosis.

*Continued*

## Malformations of the Heart (Continued)

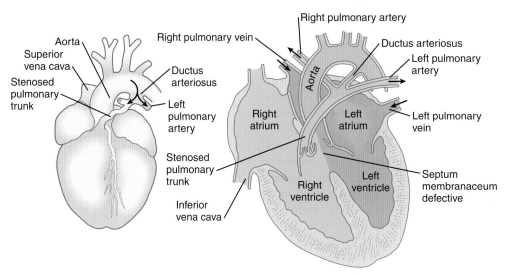

**FIGURE 17-36** Pulmonary stenosis. *Right,* Patterns of blood flow. In severe cases the ductus arteriosus remains patent, with blood flowing from the aorta into the pulmonary circulation *(arrows).*

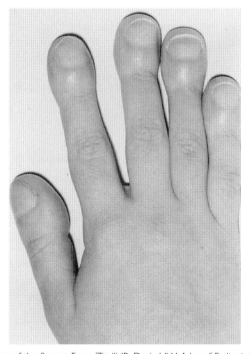

**FIGURE 17-37** Severe clubbing of the fingers. From Zitelli JB, Davis HW. *Atlas of Pediatric Physical Diagnosis,* ed 4, Mosby, St. Louis, 2002.

## Malformations of the Blood Vessels

Because of their mode of formation, in which one vascular channel is favored within a dense network, blood vessels (especially veins) are subject to numerous variations from normal. Most variations seen in the dissecting laboratory are of little functional significance. Animal experiments suggest that disturbances in the neural crest may be involved in the genesis of certain anomalies of the major arteries. When the cardiac neural crest is removed from early avian embryos, malformations involving the carotid arteries and arch of the aorta result. Certain malformations of the larger vessels can cause serious symptoms or be significant during surgery.

### DOUBLE AORTIC ARCH

Rarely, the segment of the right dorsal aortic arch between the exit of the right subclavian artery and its point of joining with the left aortic arch persists instead of degenerating. This results in a complete vascular ring surrounding the trachea and esophagus (Figures 17-38, A, and 17-39). A double aortic arch can cause **dyspnea** (difficulty breathing) in infants while they feed. Even if the condition is asymptomatic early in life, later growth typically narrows the diameter of the ring in relation to the size of the trachea and esophagus, causing symptoms in later years.

### RIGHT AORTIC ARCH

A right aortic arch arises from the persistence of the complete embryonic right aortic arch and the disappearance in the left arch of the segment caudal to the exit of the left subclavian artery (Figure 17-38, B). This condition is essentially a mirror image of normal development of the aortic arch, and it can occur as an isolated anomaly or as part of complete situs inversus of the individual. Symptoms are typically mild or absent unless an aberrant left subclavian artery presses against the esophagus or trachea.

### RIGHT SUBCLAVIAN ARTERY ARISING FROM THE ARCH OF THE AORTA

If the right fourth aortic arch degenerates between the common carotid artery and the exit of the right seventh thoracic intersegmental artery (see Figure 17-7, B and C) and if the segment between the exit of the right subclavian artery and the more distal segment of the right aortic arch (which normally disappears) persists, the right subclavian artery arises from the left aortic arch and passes behind the esophagus and trachea to reach the

right arm (Figure 17-38, C). As with a double aortic arch, this condition can cause difficulties in breathing and swallowing.

### INTERRUPTION OF THE LEFT AORTIC ARCH

Interruption of the left aortic arch is a relatively uncommon vascular malformation that usually results in a break proximal to the exit of the left subclavian artery (Figure 17-40). To be compatible with life, this lesion is usually accompanied by a patent ductus arteriosus, which allows blood flow to the lower part of the body. This lesion has been produced in mice that are lacking in the winged helix transcription factor **MFH-1** (mesenchyme fork head-1).

### PATENT DUCTUS ARTERIOSUS

One common vascular anomaly is failure of the ductus arteriosus to close after birth (Figure 17-41). This malformation occurs in a higher than normal incidence in pregnancies complicated by rubella or hypoxia. At least half of infants with this condition experience no symptoms, but over many years the strong flow of blood from the higher-pressure systemic (aortic) circulation into the pulmonary circulation overloads the vasculature of the lungs, resulting in pulmonary hypertension and ultimately heart failure. This causes a reversal of direction of blood flow through the persistent ductus and can result in lower-body cyanosis.

### COARCTATION OF THE AORTA

Another relatively common, nonlethal malformation of the vascular system is coarctation of the aorta, which occurs in two main variants. One consists of an abrupt narrowing of the descending aorta caudal to the entrance of the ductus arteriosus (Figure 17-42, B). The other variant, called **preductal coarctation**, occurs upstream from the ductus (Figure 17-42, A). The former variety (**postductal coarctation**) is by far the most common, accounting for more than 95% of all cases. The embryogenesis of coarctation is still not clear. Several underlying causes may lead to the same condition. In patients with both Down and Turner's syndromes, the incidence of coarctation of the aorta is increased.

In preductal coarctation of the aorta, which may be related to inadequate expression of MFH-1, the ductus arteriosus typically remains patent after birth. The blood supplying the trunk and limbs reaches the descending aorta through the ductus. This can lead to differential

*Continued*

**FIGURE 17-38** Aortic arch anomalies. *Left,* Configuration of embryonic vessels, *Right,* Postnatal appearance. **A,** Double aortic arch. **B,** Right aortic arch. **C,** Right subclavian artery from the arch of the aorta.

cyanosis, in which the head and upper trunk and arms have a normal color, but the lower trunk and limbs are cyanotic because of the flow of venous blood into the aorta through the patent ductus arteriosus.

The vasculature must compensate for a postductal coarctation in a different manner, since the location of the narrowing in this case effectively cuts off the arterial circulation of the head and arms from that of the trunk and legs. The body responds by opening up collateral circulatory channels and connections through normally relatively small arteries that lead from the upper to the lower body (Figure 17-38, C). Such channels are the internal

**FIGURE 17-39** Double aortic arch (*arrow*). (Photo 5992 from the Arey-DaPeña Pediatric Pathology Photographic Collection, Human Developmental Anatomy Center, National Museum of Health and Medicine, Armed Forces Institute of Pathology, Washington, DC.)

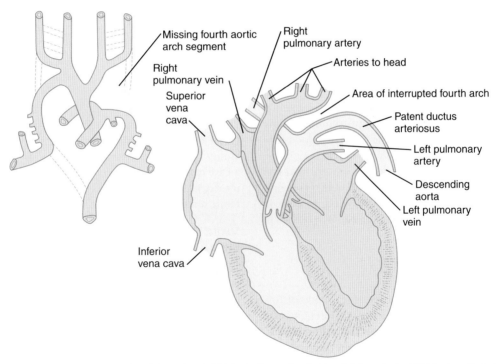

**FIGURE 17-40** Interruption of the left aortic arch. This lesion is associated with a deficiency in the MFH-1 winged helix transcription factor.

*Continued*

## Malformations of the Blood Vessels (Continued)

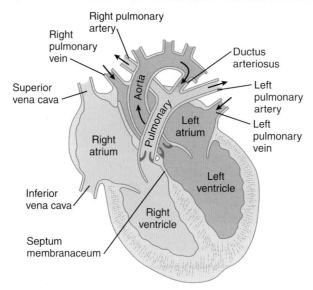

**FIGURE 17-41** Patent ductus arteriosus showing the flow of blood from the aorta into the pulmonary circulation. Later in life, pulmonary hypertension may result, causing the reversal of blood flow through the shunt and cyanosis.

thoracic arteries, the arteries associated with the scapula, and the anterior spinal artery. The unusually large flow of blood through these arteries passes through segmental branches (e.g., intercostal arteries) into the descending aorta caudal to the coarctation. The increased blood flow in the intercostal arteries causes a distinct notching in the posterior third of the third through eighth ribs that can be readily seen in radiological images. Despite these compensatory circulatory adaptations the blood pressure in patients with a postductal coarctation is much higher in the arms than in the legs.

### MALFORMATIONS OF THE VENAE CAVAE

As might be expected from their complex mode of formation (see Figure 17-11), the superior and inferior venae cavae are subject to a wide range of malformations. Common variants are duplications of the superior and inferior venae cavae or persistence of the left instead of the right segments of these vessels along with the absence of the normal vessel. In most cases, these malformations are asymptomatic.

### ANOMALOUS PULMONARY RETURN

Because of the way the individual pulmonary veins are joined and the later absorption of the distal part of the pulmonary venous system into the left atrial wall,

inappropriate connections of pulmonary veins to the heart can occur (Figure 17-43). One of the more common is for one or more branches of the pulmonary vein to enter the right instead of the left atrium. In other cases (**total anomalous pulmonary return**), all pulmonary veins empty into the right atrium or superior vena cava. Such a case must be accompanied by an associated shunt (e.g., interatrial shunt) to bring oxygenated blood into the systemic circulation.

### VASCULAR MALFORMATIONS AND HEMANGIOMAS

Localized abnormalities of the vasculature exist in a number of forms. One of the most dramatic is a **hemangioma** (Figure 17-44), which is actually a vascular tumor that typically appears within a few weeks of birth, rapidly expands, and then spontaneously regresses, usually before age 10. The endothelium of a hemangioma is mitotically very active. In contrast, **vascular malformations** are typically purplish, with a somewhat raised and irregular surface. Malformations of larger vessels consist of tangles of vessels that are relatively inactive mitotically, and their growth typically keeps pace with that of the rest of the body. They do not regress. Some familial cases occur because of mutations of Tie-2, the angiopoietin receptor. These mutations paradoxically result in a more active sprouting stimulus. **Capillary malformations,**

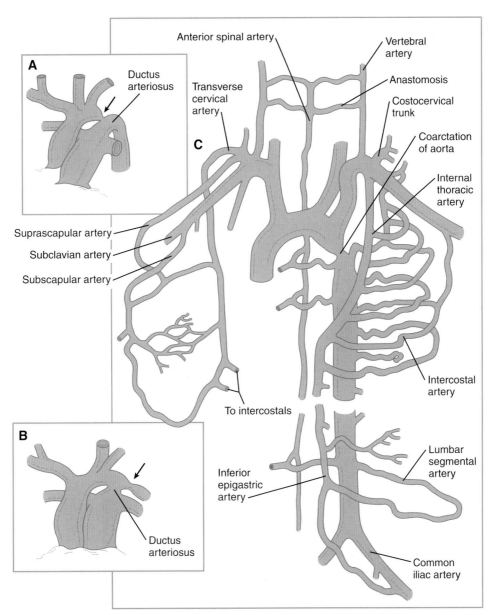

**FIGURE 17-42** Coarctation of the aorta. **A,** Preductal coarctation *(arrow)* with accompanying patent ductus arteriosus. **B,** Postductal coarctation *(arrow)* with an accompanying patent ductus arteriosus. **C,** Collateral circulation in postductal coarctation, with enlarged peripheral vessels carrying blood to the lower part of the body.

often called **port wine stains**, constitute the most common vascular anomaly of the skin. Typically reddish and later changing to purple, these are harmless, but do not disappear.

## MALFORMATIONS OF THE LYMPHATIC SYSTEM

Although minor anatomical variations of lymphatic channels are common, anomalies that cause symptoms are rare. These typically present as swelling caused by dilatation of major lymphatic vessels. By far the most common major lymphatic anomaly seen in fetuses is **cystic hygroma,** which manifests as large swellings, sometimes even collarlike, in the region of the neck (see Figure 8-1, *A*). Although the embryological basis for cystic hygroma is not certain, excessive local production and growth of lymphatic tissue, possibly originating as pinched off buds from the jugular lymph sacs, is probably the cause.

*Continued*

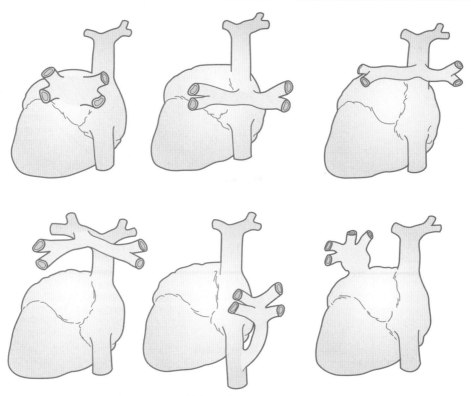

FIGURE 17-43 Variants of anomalous pulmonary drainage.

FIGURE 17-44 An oral hemangioma in a child. (Courtesy A. Burdi, Ann Arbor, Mich.)

## CLINICAL VIGNETTE

An 8-year-old boy is brought to the doctor with a complaint of excessive fatigue and uncomfortable legs when walking or running. On physical examination, the doctor notes a reduced dorsalis pedis pulse and some signs of cyanosis of the toes. The boy's hands show no signs of cyanosis.

On the basis of the physical examination the doctor suspects the presence of what malformation? Why?

○ The earliest blood and associated extraembryonic blood vessels arise from blood islands in the mesodermal wall of the yolk sac. Much of the vasculature of the embryonic body is derived from intraembryonic sources. Endothelial cell precursors (angioblasts) arise from most mesodermal tissues of the body except the notochord and prechordal mesoderm. Embryonic blood vessels form by three main mechanisms: (1) coalescence in situ (vasculogenesis), (2) migration of angioblasts into organs, and (3) sprouting from existing vessels (angiogenesis). Ingrowth of blood vessels into some organ primordia is stimulated by VEgf or other angiogenetic factors.

○ The first three pairs of aortic arches form arteries that supply the head. The fourth pair of arches develops asymmetrically, with the left arch forming part of the aortic arch of the adult. The fifth pair of arches never forms. A sixth pair of arches arises as a capillary plexus that connects with the fourth arch. The distal part of the left sixth arch forms the ductus arteriosus, a shunt that allows blood to bypass the immature lungs and directly enter the aorta. Many of the larger arteries of the adult arise from three sets of aortic branches: the dorsal intersegmental, the lateral segmental, and the ventral segmental. The coronary arteries arise from capillary plexuses associated with the epicardium. These plexuses are secondarily connected with the aorta.

○ The venous system arises from very complex capillary networks that initially develop into components of the cardinal vein system. Anterior and posterior cardinal veins drain the head and trunk, respectively. They then empty into the paired common cardinal veins and ultimately into the sinus venosus of the heart. Paired subcardinal veins are associated with the developing mesonephros. Paired extraembryonic umbilical and vitelline veins pass through the developing liver and directly into the sinus venosus. The pulmonary veins arise as separate structures and empty into the left atrium. The lymphatic system first appears as six primary lymph sacs. These become connected by lymphatic channels. Lymphatics from most of the body collect into the thoracic duct, which empties into the venous system at the base of the left internal jugular vein.

○ The heart arises from splanchnic mesoderm as a horseshoe-shaped primordium. Originally, bilateral endocardial tubes fuse in the midline. The fused cardiac tube then undergoes an **S**-shaped looping, and soon, specific regions of the heart can be identified. Starting with the inflow tract, these regions are the sinus venosus, the atria, the ventricles, and the outflow tract (bulbus cordis). The outflow tract later divides into the conus arteriosus and the truncus arteriosus.

○ Atrial endocardial cushions are thickenings between the atria and ventricles. The underlying myocardium induces cells from the endothelial lining of the endocardial cushion to leave the endocardial layer and transform into mesenchymal cells that invade the cardiac jelly. These events serve as the basis for the formation of the atrioventricular valves.

○ Internal partitioning of the heart begins with the separation of the atria from the ventricles and formation of the mitral and tricuspid valves. The left and right atria become separated by growth of the septum primum and septum secundum, but throughout embryonic life a shunt remains from the right to the left atrium via the foramen secundum and foramen ovale. The sinus venosus and the venae cavae empty into the right atrium, and the pulmonary veins drain into the left atrium. The ventricles are divided by the interventricular septum. Spiral truncoconal ridges partition the common outflow tract into pulmonary and aortic trunks. Semilunar valves prevent the reflux of blood in these vessels into the heart.

○ In addition to sensory innervation, the heart receives sympathetic and parasympathetic innervation. The conduction system distributes the contractile stimulus throughout the heart. The conduction system is derived from modified cardiac muscle cells. The heart begins to beat early in the fourth week of gestation. Physiological maturation of the heart beat follows maturation of the pacemaker system and the innervation of the heart.

○ The fetal circulation brings oxygenated blood from the placenta through the umbilical vein and into the right atrium, where much of it is shunted into the left atrium. Other blood entering the right atrium passes into the right ventricle. Blood leaving the right ventricle enters the pulmonary trunk, which supplies some blood to the lungs and the majority to the aorta via the ductus arteriosus. Blood in the left atrium empties into the left ventricle and aorta, where it supplies the body. Poorly oxygenated blood enters the umbilical arteries and is carried to the placenta for renewal.

○ Common malformations of the heart consist of atrial septal defects, which in postnatal life allow blood to pass from the left to the right atrium. Ventricular septal defects, which also result in a left-right shunting of blood, are more serious. Defects that block a channel for blood flow (e.g., tricuspid atresia) must be accompanied by secondary shunt defects to be compatible with life. A persistent atrioventricular canal can be attributed to a defect in the formation or further development of the atrioventricular endocardial cushions. Most malformations of the outflow tract of the heart appear to be related to inappropriate partitioning by the truncoconal ridges. The basis for this is frequently found in neural crest abnormalities.

○ Malformations of the major arteries often result from the inappropriate appearance or disappearance of specific components of the aortic arch system. Some, such as double aortic arch or right aortic arch, can interfere with swallowing or breathing because of pressure. Patent ductus arteriosus is caused by the failure of the ductus arteriosus to close properly after birth. Coarctation of the aorta must be compensated by either a patent ductus arteriosus or the opening of collateral vascular channels that allows blood to bypass the site of coarctation.

○ Because of their complex mode of origin, veins are commonly subject to considerable variation, but these malformations are frequently asymptomatic. Anomalous pulmonary return, which brings oxygenated blood into the right atrium, must be accompanied by a right-to-left shunt to be compatible with life. Malformations of the lymphatic system can cause local swellings such as cystic hygroma, which results in a collarlike swelling in the neck.

# Review Questions

1. Nucleated erythrocytes found circulating in the embryo are produced in the:
   A. Yolk sac
   B. Paraaortic clusters
   C. Liver
   D. Bone marrow
   E. None of the above

2. In a 7-month-old fetus, blood draining the left temporalis muscle enters the heart via the:
   A. Left anterior cardinal vein
   B. Coronary sinus
   C. Left common cardinal vein
   D. Superior vena cava
   E. None of the above

3. Adherons are inductive particles released by what structure in the endocardial cushion area?
   A. Endocardium
   B. Cardiac jelly
   C. Myocardium
   D. Epicardium
   E. None of the above

4. Neural crest contributes to the structure of which of the following?
   A. Truncus arteriosus
   B. Ascending aorta
   C. Pulmonary trunk
   D. All of the above
   E. None of the above

5. For which of these cardiovascular malformations is a patent ductus arteriosus necessary for survival of the individual?
   A. Atrial septal defect
   B. Ventricular septal defect
   C. Double aortic arch
   D. Right subclavian artery from arch of aorta
   E. None of the above

6. Five days after birth, an infant becomes cyanotic during a prolonged crying spell. The cyanosis is most likely caused by venous blood entering the systemic circulation through the:
   A. Interatrial septum
   B. Ductus arteriosus
   C. Ductus venosus
   D. Umbilical vein
   E. Interventricular septum

7. The internal carotid artery arises from aortic arch number:
   A. 1
   B. 2
   C. 3
   D. 4
   E. 5

8. A 12-year-old boy tells his doctor that over the past few months he has noticed some difficulty in swallowing when eating meat. The doctor performs a physical examination and then orders an upper gastrointestinal x-ray series. After examining the films, the doctor refers the boy for some vascular studies. What is the reasoning behind this decision?

9. An individual with atresia of the mitral valve could not survive after birth without other defects of the cardiovascular system that could compensate for the primary defect, in this case a complete blockage between the left atrium and ventricle. Construct at least one set of associated defects that could physiologically compensate for the disruption caused by the mitral atresia.

10. What is the embryological basis for a duplication of the inferior vena cava caudal to the kidneys?

## REFERENCES

Anderson RH: Simplifying the understanding of congenital malformations of the heart, *Int J Cardiol* 32:131–142, 1991.

Baron MH: Induction of embryonic hematopoietic and endothelial stem/progenitor cells by hedgehog-mediated signals, *Differentiation* 68: 175–185, 2001.

Bartelings MM, Gittenberger-de Groot AC: Morphogenetic considerations on congenital malformations of the outflow tract. I. Common arterial trunk and tetralogy of Fallot, *Int J Cardiol* 32:213–230, 1991.

Bartelings MM, Gittenberger-de Groot AC: Morphogenetic considerations on congenital malformations of the outflow tract. II. Complete transposition of the great arteries and double outlet right ventricle, *Int J Cardiol* 33:5–26, 1991.

Bergwerff M and others: Comparative anatomy and ontogeny of the ductus arteriosus, a vascular outsider, *Anat Embryol* 200:559–571, 1999.

Bernanke DH, Velkey JM: Development of the coronary blood supply: changing concepts and current ideas, *Anat Rec (New Anat)* 269:198–208, 2002.

Biben C, Harvey RP: Homeodomain factor Nkx2-5 controls left/right asymmetric expression of *bHLH* gene eHand during murine heart development, *Genes Dev* 11:1357–1369, 1997.

Bockman DE, Kirby ML, eds: Embryonic origins of defective heart development, *Ann NY Acad Sci* 588:1–464, 1990.

Brickner ME, Hillis LD, Lange RA: Congenital heart disease in adults, Parts I and II, *New Engl J Med* 342:256–263 & 334–342, 2000.

Brier G: Angiogenesis in embryonic development—a review, *Placenta*, Suppl. A Trophoblast Res 14:S11–S15, 2000.

Bristow J: The search for genetic mechanisms of congenital heart disease, *Cell Mol Biol Res* 41:307–319, 1995.

Coceani F, Olley PM: The control of cardiovascular shunts in the fetal and perinatal period, *Can J Physiol Pharmacol* 66:1129–1134, 1988.

Congdon ED: Transformation of the aortic-arch system during the development of the human embryo, *Carnegie Contr Embryol* 14:47–110, 1922.

Conte G, Pellegrini A: On the development of the coronary arteries in human embryos, stages 14–19, *Anat Embryol* 169:209–218, 1984.

Creazzo TL and others: Role of cardiac neural crest cells in cardiovascular development, *Annu Rev Physiol* 60:267–286, 1998.

Crossin KL, Hoffman S: Expression of adhesion molecules during the formation and differentiation of the avian endocardial cushion tissue, *Dev Biol* 145:277–286, 1991.

DeRuiter MC and others: The special status of the pulmonary arch artery in the branchial arch system of the rat, *Anat Embryol* 179:309–325, 1989.

Dettman RW and others: Common epicardial origin of coronary vascular smooth muscle, perivascular fibroblasts, and intermyocardial fibroblasts in the avian heart, *Dev Biol* 193:169–181, 1998.

Dieterlen-Lièvre F: Intraembryonic hematopoietic stem cells, *Hematol Oncol Clin North Am* 11:1149–1171, 1997.

Dieterlen-Lièvre F and others: Sites of hemopoietic stem cell production in early embryogenesis, *Colloque INSERM* 235:5–11, 1995.

Eichmann A and others: Ligand-dependent development of the endothelial and hematopoietic lineages from embryonic mesodermal cells expressing vascular endothelial growth factor receptor 2, *Proc Natl Acad Sci USA* 94:5141–5146, 1997.

Eisenberg LM, Markwald RR: Molecular regulation of atrioventricular valvuloseptal morphogenesis, *Circ Res* 77:1–6, 1995.

Evans SM and others: *Tinman*, a *Drosophila* homeobox gene required for heart and visceral mesoderm specification, may be represented by a family of genes in vertebrates: *Xnkx-2.3*, a second vertebrate homologue of tinman, *Development* 121:3889–3899, 1995.

Firulli AB, Thattaliyath BD: Transcription factors in cardiogenesis: the combinations that unlock the mysteries of the heart, *Internat Rev Cytol* 214:1–62, 2002.

Fisher SA and others: Forced expression of the homeodomain protein Gax inhibits cardiomyocyte proliferation and perturbs heart morphogenesis, *Development* 124:4405–4413, 1997.

Fishman MC, Chien KR: Fashioning the vertebrate heart: earliest embryonic decisions, *Development* 124:2099–2117, 1997.

Goor DA, Lillehei CW: *Congenital malformations of the heart: embryology, anatomy and operative considerations*, New York, 1975, Grune & Stratton.

Harvey RP, Rosenthal N, eds: *Heart Development*, San Diego, 1999, Academic Press.

Heuser CH: The branchial vessels and their derivatives in the pig, *Carnegie Contr Embryol* 15:121–139, 1923.

Ho E, Shimada Y: Formation of the epicardium studied with the scanning electron microscope, *Dev Biol* 66:579–585, 1978.

Hungerford JE, Little CD: Developmental biology of the vascular smooth muscle cell: building a multilayered vessel wall, *J Vasc Res* 36:2–27, 1999.

Icardo JM: Developmental biology of the vertebrate heart, *J Exp Zool* 275:144–161, 1996.

Iida K and others: Essential roles of the winged helix transcription factor MFH-1 in aortic arch patterning and skeletogenesis, *Development* 124:4627–4638, 1997.

Kanjuh VI, Edwards JE: A review of congenital anomalies of the heart and great vessels according to functional categories, *Pediatr Clin North Am* 11:55–105, 1964.

Kathiriya IS, Srivastava D: Left-right asymmetry and cardiac looping: implications for cardiac development and congenital heart disease, *Am J Med Genet* 97:271–279, 2000.

Kirby ML: Nodose placode provides ectomesenchyme to the developing chick heart in the absence of cardiac neural crest, *Cell Tissue Res* 252:17–22, 1988.

Kirby ML, Waldo KL: Role of neural crest in congenital heart disease, *Circulation* 82:332–340, 1990.

Kramer TC: The partitioning of the truncus and conus and the formation of the membranous portion of the interventricular septum of the human heart, *Am J Anat* 71:343–370, 1942.

Lawson ND and others: Notch signaling is required for arterial-venous differentiation during embryonic vascular development, *Development* 128:3675–3683, 2001.

Magovern JH, Moore GW, Hutchins GM: Development of the atrioventricular valve region in the human embryo, *Anat Rec* 215:167–181, 1986.

Männer J: Experimental study on the formation of the epicardium in chick embryos, *Anat Embryol* 187:281–289, 1993.

Männer J and others: The origin, formation and developmental significance of the epicardium: a review, *Cells Tiss Organs* 169:89–103, 2001.

Markwald RR and others: Epithelial-mesenchymal transformations in early avian heart development, *Acta Anat* 156:173–186, 1996.

McClure CFW, Butler EG: The development of the vena cava inferior in man, *Am J Anat* 35:331–383, 1925.

Mikawa T, Gourdie RG: Pericardial mesoderm generates a population of coronary smooth muscle cells migrating into the heart along with ingrowth of the epicardial organ, *Dev Biol* 174:221–232, 1996.

Milner LA, Bigas A: Notch as a mediator of cell fate determination in hematopoiesis: evidence and speculation, *Blood* 93:2431–2448, 1999.

Mohun T, Sparrow D: Early steps in vertebrate cardiogenesis, *Curr Opin Genet Dev* 7:628–633, 1997.

Mukouyama Y-S and other: Sensory nerves determine the pattern of arterial differentiation and blood vessel branching in the skin, *Cell* 109:693–705, 2002.

Nakajima Y and others: An autocrine function for transforming growth factor (TGF)-β3 in the transformation of atrioventricular canal endocardium into mesenchyme during chick heart development, *Dev Biol* 194:99–113, 1998.

Noden DM: Development of craniofacial blood vessels. In Feinberg RN, Sherer GK, Auerbach R, eds: *The development of the vascular system*, Basel, Switzerland, 1991, Karger, pp 1–24.

Oberlin E and others: Blood-forming potential of vascular endothelium in the human embryo, *Development* 129:4147–4157, 2002.

Olson EN, Srivastava D: Molecular pathways controlling heart development, *Science* 272:671–676, 1996.

Pardanaud L and others: Two distinct endothelial lineages in ontogeny, one of them related to hemopoiesis, *Development* 122:1363–1371, 1996.

Pexieder T: The tissue dynamics of heart morphogenesis. I. The phenomena of cell death, *Z Anat Entwickl-Gesch* 138:241–253, 1972.

Pexieder T and others: A suggested nomenclature for the developing heart, *Int J Cardiol* 25:255–264, 1989.

Rentschler S and other: Visualization and functional characterization of the developing murine cardiac conduction system, *Development* 128:1785–1792, 2001.

Rossant J, Howard L: Signaling pathways in vascular development, *Annu Rev Cell Devel Biol* 18:541–573, 2002.

Sabin FR: The origin and development of the lymphatic system, *Johns Hopkins Hosp Rep* 17:347–440, 1916.

Schott J-J and others: Congenital heart disease caused by mutations in the transcription factor NKX2-5, *Science* 108–111, 1998.

Sherer GK: Vasculogenic mechanisms and epitheliomesenchymal specificity in endodermal organs. In Feinberg RN, Sherer GK, Auerbach R, eds: *The development of the vascular system*, Basel, Switzerland, 1991, Karger, pp 37–57.

Sissman NJ: Developmental landmarks in cardiac morphogenesis: comparative chronology, *Am J Cardiol* 25:141–148, 1970.

Srivastava D: Genetic assembly of the heart: Implications for congenital heart disease, *Annu Rev Physiol* 63:451–469, 2001.

Srivastava D, Olson EN: Neurotrophin-3 knocks heart off Trk, *Nature Med* 2:1069–1071, 1996.

Srivastava D, Olson EN: Knowing in your heart what is right, *Trends Cell Biol* 7:447–453, 1997.

Steding G and others: Developmental aspects of the sinus valves and the sinus venosus septum of the right atrium in human embryos, *Anat Embryol* 181:469–475, 1990.

Takamura K and others: Association of cephalic neural crest cells with cardiovascular development, particularly that of the semilunar valves, *Anat Embryol* 182:263–272, 1990.

Thorsteinsdottir U, Sauvageau G, Humphries RK: Hox homeobox genes as regulators of normal and leukemic hematopoiesis, *Hematol Oncol Clin North Am* 11:1221–1237, 1997.

Tomanek RJ: Formation of the coronary vasculature: a brief review, *Cardiovasc Res* 31: E46–E51, 1996.

Van den Hoff MJB and others: Programmed cell death in the developing heart, *Cardiovasc Res* 45:603–620.

Vikkula M, Boon LM, Mulliken JB: Molecular genetics of vascular malformations, *Matrix Biol* 20:327–335, 2001.

Wilting J, Christ B: Embryonic angiogenesis: a review, *Naturwissenschaften* 83:153–164, 1996.

# CHAPTER 18

# Fetal Period
# and Birth

After the eighth week of pregnancy the period of organogenesis (embryonic period) is largely completed, and the fetal period begins. By the end of the embryonic period, almost all the organs are present in a grossly recognizable form. The external contours of the embryo show a very large head in proportion to the rest of the body and greater development of the cranial than of the caudal part of the body (Figures 18-1 and 18-2).

The fetal period has often been considered a time of growth and physiological maturation of organ systems, and it has not received much attention in traditional embryology courses. However, advances in imaging and other diagnostic techniques have provided considerable access to the fetus. Determining the fetus' pattern of growth and state of well-being with remarkable accuracy is now possible. Improved surgical techniques and the realization that surgical wounds in the fetus heal without scarring have led to a new field of fetal surgery.

This chapter emphasizes the functional development of the fetus and the adaptations that ensure a smooth transition to independent living once the fetus has passed through the birth canal and the umbilical cord is cut. Techniques that are used to monitor the functional state of the fetus are also described in Clinical Correlation 18-1 later in the chapter.

## GROWTH AND FORM OF FETUS

Despite the intense developmental activity that occurs during the embryonic period (3 to 8 weeks), the absolute

growth of the embryo in both length and mass is not great (Figure 18-3). The fetal period (9 weeks to birth), however, is characterized by rapid growth. The change in proportions of the various regions of the body during the prenatal and postnatal growth periods is as striking as the absolute growth of the embryo. The early dominance of the head is reduced as development of the trunk becomes a major factor in the growth of the early fetus. Even later, a relatively greater growth of the limbs changes the proportions of various regions of the body. During the early fetal period, the entire body is hairless and very thin because of the absence of subcutaneous fat (Figure 18-4). By midpregnancy the contours of the head and face approach those of the neonate, and the abdomen begins to fill out. Beginning at around week 27, the deposition of subcutaneous fat causes the body to round out. (Some of the major developmental landmarks during the fetal period are summarized in the table on pp. xiii and xiv.)

## FETAL PHYSIOLOGY

### Circulation

The circulation of the human embryo can be first studied at about 5 weeks by means of ultrasound. At that time the heart beats at a rate of approximately 100 beats per minute. This probably represents an inherent atrial rhythm. The pulse rate rises to about 160 beats per minute by 8 weeks and then drops to 150 beats per

**FIGURE 18-1** Drawings of fetuses from **8 to 25 weeks'** fertilization age. The fetuses from **8 through 17 weeks** are drawn actual size. Those **20 and 25 weeks** are drawn two-thirds actual size.

10 weeks

11 weeks

14 weeks

17 weeks

**9 weeks**

**8 weeks**

**25 weeks**

**20 weeks**

**FIGURE 18-1, CONT'D** For legend, see opposite page.

**FIGURE 18-2** A 37-mm crown-rump-length human fetus, approximately **9 weeks** old. (Courtesy A. Burdi, Ann Arbor, Mich.)

minute in the 15-week-old fetus, with a further slight decline near term. The pulse rate in utero is remarkably constant, and embryos exhibiting **bradycardia** (slow pulse rate) often die before term. Near term the pulse rate varies to some extent if conditions in the uterus change or if the embryo is stressed. This is probably the result of the functional establishment of the autonomic innervation of the heart (Figure 18-5).

The heart of the fetus has gross physiological properties quite different from those of the postnatal heart. For example, the myocardial force, the velocity of shortening, and the extent of shortening are all less in the fetal heart. Some gross functional characteristics of the fetal heart are related to the presence of fetal isoforms of contractile proteins in the cardiac myocytes. For example, in fetal heart cells the β-myosin heavy chain isoform predominates. This is advantageous because a lower oxygen requirement and less adenosine triphosphate are needed to develop the same amount of force as the α-myosin isoform in the adult heart.

The **stroke volume** (blood expelled with one heart beat) of the early (18 to 19 weeks' gestation) fetus is very small (less than 1 ml), but it increases rapidly with continued growth of the fetus. In the term human fetus the combined ventricular output is about 450 ml/kg/min. The right ventricle of the human fetus has a somewhat greater stroke volume than the left. This is correlated with an 8% greater diameter of the pulmonary artery than of the fetal aorta.

Quantitative studies have shown a good correlation between blood flow and functional needs of various regions of the embryo. Approximately 40% of the combined cardiac output goes to the head and upper body,

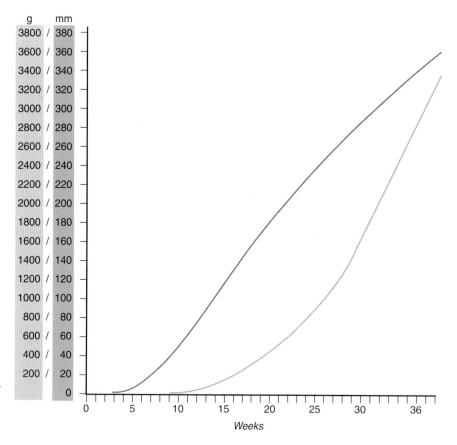

**FIGURE 18-3** Growth in crown-rump length (*green*) and weight (*orange*) of the human fetus. (Data from Patten BM: *Human embryology*, New York, 1968, McGraw-Hill.)

FIGURE 18-4 A **3¾-month-old** human fetus (130-mm crown-rump length). EH 902 from the Patten Embryological Collection at the University of Michigan. (Courtesy of A. Burdi, Ann Arbor, Mich.)

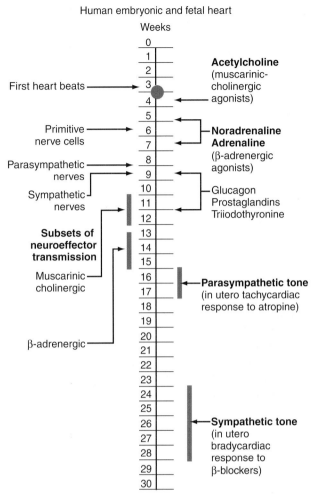

FIGURE 18-5 Sequence of events in the autonomic innervation of the heart. (Based on Papp JG: *Basic Res Cardiol* 83:2–9, 1988.)

thus supplying the relatively great needs of the developing brain. Another 30% of the combined cardiac output goes to the placenta via the umbilical arteries for replenishment. Figure 18-6 shows the relative amounts of blood that enter and leave the heart via various vascular channels. (The general qualitative pattern of blood flow in the human fetus is presented in Chapter 17.)

Differential streaming of blood within the heart results in different concentrations of oxygen in the chambers of the fetal heart. For example, blood in the left ventricle is 15% to 20% more saturated with oxygen than blood in the right ventricle (see Figure 17-26). This and the high volume of blood supplying the head via branches of the ascending aorta ensure that the developing heart and brain receive an adequate supply of oxygen.

A key factor in the maintenance of the fetal pattern of circulation is the patency of the ductus arteriosus and the ductus venosus. Patency of the fetal ductus venosus is maintained through the actions of prostaglandins $E_2$ and

$I_2$, whereas only prostaglandin $E_2$ is involved in maintaining patency of the ductus arteriosus.

Myocardial cells of the developing atrium gradually produce and store granules containing **atrial natriuretic peptide,** a hormone that has pronounced vasodilatory, natriuretic, and diuretic properties. This hormone is released after the atrial walls are stretched, normally a sign of increased blood volume. It has been detected in atrial cardiomyocytes as early as 8 to 9 weeks' gestation. After intrauterine blood transfusions during midgestation or later, blood levels of atrial natriuretic peptide increase significantly in response to the increased blood volume.

## Fetal Lungs and Respiratory System

The lungs develop late in the embryo and are not involved in respiratory gas exchange during fetal life. However, they must be prepared to assume the full

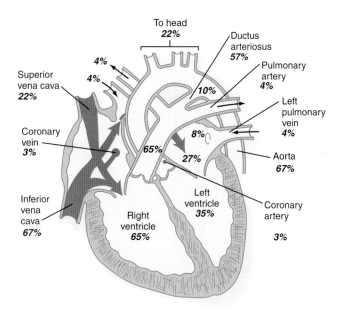

**FIGURE 18-6** Percentages of blood entering and leaving the fetal heart via various channels. (From Teitel DF. In Polin R, Rox W, eds: *Fetal and neonatal physiology,* vol 1, Philadelphia, 1992, WB Saunders, pp 609–619.)

burden of gas exchange as soon as the umbilical cord is cut.

The fetal lungs are filled with fluid, and the blood circulation to them is highly reduced. To perform normal postnatal breathing, the lungs must grow to an appropriate size, respiratory movements must be carried out continuously, and the air sacs (**alveoli**) must become appropriately configured for air exchange.

Normal growth of the fetal lungs depends on their containing an adequate amount of fluid. During the last trimester of pregnancy, fluid constitutes 90% to 95% of the total weight of the lung. The fluid filling the fetal lungs differs in composition from amniotic fluid, and it has been shown to be secreted by the pulmonary epithelial cells. Secretion begins with a net movement of chloride ions into the lumens of the pulmonary passages. Water movement then follows the chloride ions. A number of studies have shown a relationship between total fluid volume in the lungs and fetal breathing movements, with dilatation and constriction of the larynx serving a valvelike function. In vitro studies have shown that proliferation of lung epithelial cells is stimulated by mechanical stretching. In vivo the internal pressure of the lung fluid serves as the stretching agent. A reduced volume of lung fluid is associated with **pulmonary hypoplasia.**

Ultrasound analysis has shown that the fetus begins to make gross breathing movements as early as 11 weeks. These movements are periodic rather than continuous, and they take on two forms. One type of movement is rapid and irregular, with varying rate and amplitude. The

other form is represented by isolated, slow movements, almost like gasps. The former type is by far the most prominent and is associated with conditions of rapid eye movement (REM) sleep. Periods of rapid breathing (often for about 10 minutes) alternate with periods of **apnea** (cessation of breathing).

Much remains to be learned about the control of fetal breathing, but the breathing movements are known to be responsive to maternal factors, many of which remain to be identified. The amount of breathing (minutes of breathing per hour) is highest in the evening and lowest in the early morning. The fetal breathing rate increases after the mother has eaten. This is related to the concentration of glucose in the maternal blood. Maternal smoking causes a rapid decrease in the rate of fetal breathing for up to an hour.

Fetal breathing movements are essential for postnatal survival. One obvious function of fetal breathing is to condition the respiratory muscles so that they can perform regular postnatal contractions. Another important function is to stimulate the growth of the embryonic lungs. If intrauterine breathing movements are suppressed in fetal lambs, lung growth is retarded.

An important developmental adaptation of the fetal respiratory system is growth of the upper airway. Although a newborn is about 4% the weight of an adult, the diameter of its trachea is one third that of the adult trachea. Other components of the airway are similarly proportioned. If the trachea were narrower, the physical resistance to air flow would be so great that movement of air would be almost impossible. Even with these adaptations, the resistance of the neonate's airway is 5 to 6 times greater than that of the adult.

A functionally important aspect of fetal lung development is the secretion of **pulmonary surfactant** by the newly differentiating type II alveolar cells of the lung starting around 24 weeks' gestation. Surfactant is a mixture of phospholipids (about two-thirds phosphatidylcholine) and protein that lines the surface of the alveoli and lowers the surface tension. This reduces the inspiratory force required to inflate the alveoli and prevents the collapse of the alveoli during expiration.

Despite the relatively early initiation of surfactant synthesis, large amounts are not synthesized until a few weeks before birth. At this time the production of surfactant by the type II alveolar cells is higher than at any other period in an individual's life, an adaptation that is an important preparation for the newborn's first breath. A number of hormones and growth factors are involved in the synthesis of surfactant, and the effects of thyroid hormone and glucocorticoids are particularly strong.

Prematurely born infants are often afflicted with **respiratory distress syndrome,** which is manifested by rapid, labored breathing shortly after birth. This condition is related to a deficiency in pulmonary surfactant and can be ameliorated by the administration of glucocorticoids, which stimulate the production of surfactant by the alveolar epithelium.

## Fetal Movements and Sensations

Ultrasound analysis has revolutionized the analysis of fetal movements and behavior because the fetus can be examined virtually undisturbed (except for an increase in vascular activity induced by the ultrasound) for extended periods. Earlier studies of fetal movements were principally concerned with the development of reflex responses, and the information was obtained largely by the analysis of newly aborted fetuses (see Chapter 11). Although valuable information on maturation of reflex arcs was obtained in this manner, many of the movements elicited were not those normally made by the fetus in utero.

The undisturbed embryo does not show any indication of movement until about $7\frac{1}{2}$ weeks. The first spontaneous movements consist of slow flexion and extension of the vertebral column, with the limbs being passively displaced. Within a short time, a relatively large repertoire of fetal movements evolves. After study by a number of investigators, a classification of fetal movements has been suggested (Box 18-1). The first fetal movements are followed in a few days by startle and general movements. Shortly thereafter, isolated limb movements are added (Figure 18-7). Late in appearance are movements associated with the head and jaw (Figure 18-7). Toward the end of the fourth month the fetus begins a pattern of periods of activity followed by times of inactivity. Many women first become aware of fetal movements at this time. Between the fourth and fifth months, the fetus becomes capable of gripping firmly onto a glass rod. Although weak protorespiratory movements are possible, they cannot be sustained.

Continuous ultrasound monitoring for extended periods reveals patterns involving many types of movements (Figure 18-8). At different weeks of pregnancy, some movements are predominant, whereas others are in decline or are just beginning to take shape. Analysis of anencephalic fetuses has shown that although many movements take place, they are poorly regulated. They start abruptly, are maintained at the same force, and then stop abruptly. These abnormal patterns of movements are considered evidence for strong supraspinal modulation of movement in the fetus.

Human fetal activities, as reflected in breathing or general activity level, show distinct diurnal rhythms beginning at about 20 to 22 weeks' gestation. There is a strong negative correlation between maternal plasma glucocorticoid levels and fetal activity. Fetal activity is

---

### Box 18-1   Major Types of Fetal Movements

**Anteflexion of the head** Normally slow, forward bending of the head

**Fetal breathing movements** Paradoxical movements in which the thorax moves inward and the abdomen outward with each contraction of the diaphragm

**General movements** Slow gross movements involving the whole body lasting several seconds to a minute

**Hand-face contact** Contact that occurs any time the moving hand touches the face or mouth

**Hiccups** Repetitive phasic contractions of the diaphragm (A bout may last several minutes.)

**Isolated arm or leg movements** Movements of extremities that occur without movement of the trunk

**Lateral rotation of the head** Movement that involves isolated turning of the head from side to side

**Opening of mouth** Isolated movement that may be accompanied by protrusion of the tongue

**Retroflexion of the head** Slow to jerky backward bending of the head

**Startle movements** Quick (1 second), generalized movements that always start in the limbs and may spread to the trunk and neck

**Stretch** Complex movement that involves overextension of the spine, retroflexion of the head, and elevation of the arms

**Sucking** Burst of rhythmical jaw movements that is sometimes followed by swallowing (With this movement the fetus may be drinking amniotic fluid.)

**Yawn** Movement in which the mouth is slowly opened and rapidly closed after a few seconds

Based on studies by Prechtl HFR. In Hill A, Volpe J, eds: *Fetal neurology*, New York, 1989, Raven, pp 1–16.

---

highest in the early evening, when maternal blood glucocorticoid levels are lowest, and lowest in the early morning, when the concentration of maternal hormone peaks. Studies of women who have been given additional glucocorticoids or inhibitors have shown increased fetal activity when maternal corticoid levels are low. Usually when the overall fetal activity is low, the fetus is in a state of REM sleep, but definitions of sleep and wakefulness in the fetus need further clarification.

A number of sensory systems also begin to function during the fetal period. Near-term fetuses are responsive to 2000-Hz stimuli when in a state of wakefulness, but they are unresponsive during periods of sleep. Loud

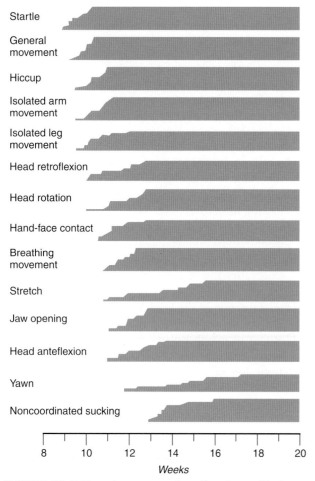

Startle

General
movement

Hiccup

Isolated arm
movement

Isolated leg
movement

Head retroflexion

Head rotation

Hand-face contact

Breathing
movement

Stretch

Jaw opening

Head anteflexion

Yawn

Noncoordinated sucking

8  10  12  14  16  18  20

*Weeks*

**FIGURE 18-7** Time of appearance of specific patterns of fetal motor movements. Each corner on the jagged edge at the left of the broad lines represents one fetus. (From Prechtl HFR. In Hill A, Volpe J, eds: *Fetal neurology*, New York, 1989, Raven, pp 1–16.)

vibroacoustic stimuli applied to the maternal abdomen produce a fetal response consisting of an eye blink, a startle reaction, and an increase in heart rate. Although the fetus is constantly in the dark, the **pupillary light reflex** can usually be elicited by 30 weeks.

## Fetal Digestive Tract

The fetal digestive tract is not functional in the standard sense because the fetus obtains its nutrition from the maternal blood via the placenta. However, the digestive tract must be prepared to assume the full responsibility for nutritional intake after birth. Once the basic digestive tube and glands have formed in the early embryo, the remainder of the intrauterine period is devoted to cellular differentiation of the epithelia of the gut and preparation of the numerous cells involved for their specific roles in the digestive process. Beneath the epithelium the walls of the digestive tube must become capable of propelling ingested food and liquid. Analysis of development

of the fetal digestive tract has concentrated on (1) the biochemical adaptations of the epithelium of the various regions for digestive function and (2) the development of motility of the digestive tube.

The development and differentiation of epithelia or specific regional characteristics of the gut lining typically follow gradients along the length of the segment of the gut specifically involved. In both the esophagus and stomach, differentiation of the mucosal epithelium is well under way starting around 4 months. Although **parietal cells** (hydrochloric acid producing) and **chief cells** (pepsinogen producing) are first seen at 11 and 12 weeks, respectively, there is little evidence of their secretions during fetal life. In fact, the contents of the stomach have a near-neutral pH until after birth, but then gastric acid production increases greatly within a few hours.

In the small intestine, villi begin to form in the upper duodenum at the end of the second month, and crypts appear 1 to 2 weeks later. The formation of villi and crypts spreads along the length of the intestine in a spatiotemporal gradient. By approximately 16 weeks, villi have formed along the entire length of the intestine, and crypts appear in the lower ileum by 19 weeks. Villi even form in the colon during the third and fourth months, but they then regress and are gone by the seventh or eighth month.

Individual epithelial cell types, including **Brunner's glands**, which protect the duodenal lining from gastric acid, appear in the small intestine early in the second trimester. Although the presence of most enzymes or proenzymes characteristic of the intestinal lining can be demonstrated histochemically during the midfetal period, their amounts are generally quite small. Activity of a number of the enzymes secreted by the exocrine pancreatic tissue can also be demonstrated between 16 and 22 weeks' gestation.

**Meconium,** a greenish mixture of desquamated intestinal cells, swallowed lanugo hair, and various secretions, begins to fill the lower ileum and colon late in the fourth month (Figure 18-9).

Differentiation of the neuromuscular complex of the digestive tract also follows a gradient, with the circular layer of smooth muscle forming in the esophagus at 6 weeks. **Myenteric plexuses** (parasympathetic neurons) take shape after the inner circular muscle layer is present but before the formation of the outer longitudinal layer of muscle a couple weeks later in any given region. Starting in the esophagus at 6 weeks, the final formation of myenteric plexuses throughout the length of the digestive tract is complete at 12 weeks. The first spontaneous rhythmical activity in the small intestine is seen in the seventh week at approximately the time of formation of the inner circular muscular layer. Recognizable peristaltic movements, however, do not begin until the fourth month. Fetuses older than 34 weeks are able to pass meconium in utero.

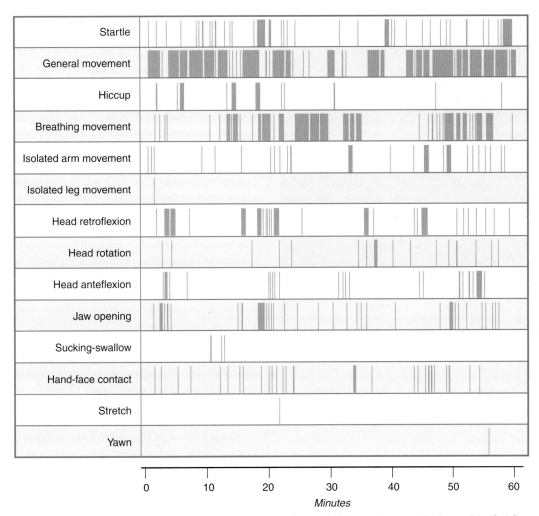

**FIGURE 18-8** Actogram record of types of movements of a **14-week-old** fetus taken over 60 minutes. (Modified from Prechtl HFR: *Fetal neurology*, New York, 1989, Raven.)

Another intrauterine preparation for feeding is the development of swallowing and the sucking reflex. Swallowing is first detected at 10 to 11 weeks, and then its incidence gradually increases. The function of fetal swallowing is unclear, but by term, fetuses swallow 200 to 750 ml or more of amniotic fluid per day. The amniotic fluid contains protein, and much of this is absorbed through the gut through a process of intracellular digestion, occurring by the uptake of macromolecules by fetal enterocytes. According to some estimates, 15% to 20% of total body protein deposition is derived from protein found in amniotic fluid. The swallowed amniotic fluid may contain growth factors that facilitate the differentiation of epithelial cells in the digestive tract. To a certain extent, taste seems to regulate fetal swallowing. Taste buds are seemingly mature by 12 weeks, and the amount of swallowing increases if saccharin is introduced into the amniotic fluid. Conversely, swallowing is reduced if noxious chemicals are added.

Cordinated sucking movements do not appear until late in fetal development. Although noncoordinated pre-

cursors of sucking movements occur as early as 18 weeks, it is not until 32 to 36 weeks that the fetus undertakes short bursts of sucking, but these are not associated with effective swallowing movements. Ineffective sucking is the main reason why premature infants of this age must be fed through a nasogastric tube. Mature sucking capability appears after 36 weeks.

## Fetal Kidney Function

Although the placenta carries out most excretory functions characteristic of the kidney during prenatal life, the developing kidneys also function by producing urine. As early as the fifth week of gestation, the mesonephric kidneys produce small amounts of very dilute urine, but the mesonephros degenerates late in the third month, after the metanephric kidneys have taken shape. Tubules of the metanephric kidneys begin to function between 9 and 12 weeks, and resorptive functions involving the loop of Henle occur by 14 weeks, even though new nephrons

**FIGURE 18-9** Meconium ileus (accumulation of fetal meconium [the greenish material]) in the fetal small intestine. (Photo 2536 from the Arey-DaPeña Pediatric Pathology Photographic Collection, Human Developmental Anatomy Center, National Museum of Health and Medicine, Armed Forces Institute of Pathology, Washington, DC.)

continue to form until birth. The urine produced by the fetal kidney is hypotonic to plasma throughout most of pregnancy. This is a reflection of immature resorptive mechanisms, which are manifested morphologically by short loops of Henle. As the neural lobe of the hypophysis produces antidiuretic hormone beginning at the eleventh week, another mechanism for the concentration of urine begins to be established.

Intrauterine renal function is not necessary for fetal life because embryos with bilateral renal agenesis survive in utero. Bilateral renal agenesis, however, is commonly associated with oligohydramnios (see Chapter 7), indicating that the overall balance of amniotic fluid requires a certain amount of fetal renal function.

## Endocrine Function in the Fetus

The development of prenatal endocrine function occurs in several phases. Most peripheral endocrine glands (e.g., thyroid, pancreatic islets, adrenals, gonads) form early in the second month as the result of epithelial-mesenchymal interactions. As these glands differentiate late in the second month or early in the third, they develop the intrinsic capacity to synthesize their specific hormonal products. In most cases the amount of hormone secreted

is initially very small; increased secretion often depends on the stimulation of the gland by a higher-order hormone produced in another gland.

The anterior pituitary gland develops like many other endocrine glands. Its hormonal products generally stimulate more peripheral endocrine glands such as the thyroid, adrenals, and gonads to produce or release their specific hormonal products. Pituitary hormones can be demonstrated immunocytochemically within individual pituitary epithelial cells as early as 8 weeks (adrenocorticotrophic hormone) or 10 weeks (luteinizing hormone and follicle-stimulating hormone). However, most pituitary hormones are typically not present in the blood in detectable quantities until a couple of months after they can be demonstrated in the cells that produce them. An exception is growth hormone, which can be detected in plasma as early as 10 weeks.

While the anterior pituitary is developing its intrinsic synthetic capacities, the hypothalamus also takes shape and develops its capacity to produce the various releasing and inhibitory factors that modulate the function of the pituitary gland. Regardless of its intrinsic capacities, the hypothalamus is limited in its influence on the embryonic pituitary gland until about 12 weeks, when the neurovascular links between the hypothalamus and pituitary become established.

At each level in the control hierarchy a generally low intrinsic level of hormone production can be stimulated by the actions of hormones produced by the next higher-order gland. For example, the amount of thyroid hormone released is considerably increased when thyroid-stimulating hormone, released by the anterior pituitary, acts on the thyroid gland. The release of this hormone by the pituitary is regulated by thyrotropin-releasing hormone, which is produced in the hypothalamus. Regardless of the nature of the upstream stimulation of the thyroid, the forms of thyroid hormone released by the fetal thyroid are largely biologically inactive because of enzymatic modifications or through sulfation. Late in gestation, thyroid hormone accelerates the development of brown fat in the fetus. Brown fat, much of which is stored in depots in the upper back, maintains body temperature in the neonate through a process of nonshivering thermogenesis. Studies on anencephalic fetuses have shown that the anterior pituitary can produce and release most of its hormones in the absence of hypothalamic input, although plasma concentrations of some are reduced.

Among the fetal endocrine glands the adrenal remains the most enigmatic. By 6 to 8 weeks of development, the inner cortex enlarges greatly to form a distinct fetal zone, which later in pregnancy occupies about 80% of the gland. By the end of pregnancy, the adrenal glands weigh 4 g each, the same mass as that of the adult glands (Figure 18-10). The fetal adrenal cortex produces 100 to 200 mg of steroids each day, an amount several times higher than

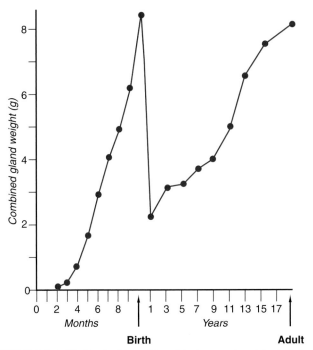

8

6

4

2

0

0 2 4 6 8 | 1 3 5 7 9 11 13 15 17

*Months* — **Birth** — *Years* — **Adult**

*Combined gland weight (g)*

**FIGURE 18-10** Graph of the weights of the human adrenal glands during prenatal and postnatal development. After birth, the weight of the gland decreases dramatically with the reorganization of the cortex of the gland. (Based on data from Neville AM, O'Hare MJ: *The human adrenal cortex*, Berlin, 1982, Springer-Verlag.)

precursor for estrogen biosynthesis by the placenta. Fetal adrenal hormones influence maturation of the lungs (as prolactin has also been postulated to do), liver, and epithelium of the digestive tract (Table 18-1). In sheep, products of the adrenal cortex prepare the fetus for independent postnatal life and influence the initiation of parturition, but the situation in primates is considerably less clear. Shortly after birth the fetal adrenal cortex rapidly involutes (see Figure 18-10). Within a month after birth the weight of each gland is reduced by 50%, and by 1 year of age each gland weighs only 1 g. Not until adulthood does the mass of the adrenal glands return to that of the late fetus.

Fetal endocrinology is complicated by the presence of the placenta, which can synthesize and release many hormones, convert hormones released from other glands to active forms, and potentially exchange other hormones with the maternal circulation. By 6 to 7 weeks, hormone production (e.g., progesterone) by the placenta is enough to maintain pregnancy even if the ovaries are removed.

One of the earliest placental hormones produced is human **chorionic gonadotropin (HCG)** (see Chapter 7). One later function of HCG is to stimulate steroidogenesis by the placenta. The synthesis of HCG by the syncytiotrophoblast of the placenta is regulated by the production of **gonadotropin-releasing hormone** by cells of the cytotrophoblast. Synthesis of this hormone by the placenta supplants its normal production by the hypothalamus and is probably an adaptation that allows earlier and more local control of HCG than could be accomplished by the hypothalamus.

that of the adult adrenal glands. The main hormonal products of the fetal adrenal are $\Delta^5$-3β-hydroxysteroids such as dehydroepiandrosterone, which are inactive alone but are converted to biologically active steroids (e.g., estrogens, especially estrone) by the placenta and liver. The fetal adrenal cortex depends on the presence of pituitary adrenocorticotrophic hormone; in its absence the fetal adrenal cortex is small. Conversely, if exogenous adrenocorticotrophic hormone is administered, the fetal adrenal cortex persists after birth.

Despite the prominence of the fetal adrenal cortex, its specific functions during pregnancy are still not clear. The large fetal zone of the adrenal cortex produces a steroid

**TABLE 18-1** *Maturation Processes That Are Affected by Fetal Cortisol*

Shift of the main hematopoietic site to bone marrow

Storage of glycogen by the liver

Final digestive enzymatic differentiation of intestinal absorptive cells

Stimulation of surfactant synthesis in the lung

Involvement in parturition

**Box 18-2 Uses for Ultrasonography during Pregnancy**

Estimation of age of fetus
Confirmation of multiple fetuses
Diagnosis of placental abnormalities, including hydatidiform mole
Localization of placenta in suspected placenta previa
Diagnosis of ectopic pregnancy
Documentation of follicular development
Adjunct to clinical procedures (e.g., amniocentesis, chorionic villus sampling, intrauterine transfusion, intrauterine surgical procedures)
Detection of congenital malformations of fetus
Detection of maternal uterine anomalies
Detection of oligohydramnios or polyhydramnios
Confirmation of fetal death
Confirmation of fetal position

## Clinical Study and Manipulation of the Fetus

New imaging and diagnostic techniques have revolutionized the study of the living fetus. Many congenital malformations can be diagnosed in utero with considerable accuracy. On the basis of this information the surgeon can treat some congenital malformations through fetal surgery much more efficiently than by traditional surgery on infants or older children.

### FETAL DIAGNOSTIC PROCEDURES

#### Imaging Techniques

Because of its safety, cost, and ability to look at the fetus in real time, **ultrasonography** is currently the most widely used obstetrical imaging technique (Figures 18-11 and 18-12). It is useful for the simple diagnosis of structural anomalies and can be used in real time to guide fetal invasive procedures such as chorionic villus sampling and intrauterine transfusions. The major uses of ultrasonography are summarized in Box 18-2.

Conventional **x-ray** testing continues to be used in certain circumstances, but because of the potential for radiation damage to the fetal and maternal gonads, its use is less common than in previous years. The use of x-ray testing is relatively limited by its inability to discriminate the details of soft tissues, including cartilaginous components of the skeleton. By injecting

**FIGURE 18-11** Ultrasound images of the normal fetal head. **A,** Lateral profile showing the nose *(arrowhead)*, mandible *(M)*, maxilla *(x)*, tongue *(t)*, and medial aspect of the bony orbit *(curved arrow)*. S, Sternocleidomastoid muscle. **B,** Frontal view of the face showing the nose *(white arrow)*, chin *(C)*, and corner of the mouth *(black arrow)*. **C,** Ear. *at,* Antitragus; *c,* antihelical crus; *h,* helix; *L,* earlobe; *black arrow,* antihelix; *white arrow,* scaphoid fossa. (**A** and **B** from Bowerman RA: *Atlas of normal fetal ultrasonographic anatomy,* ed 2, St Louis, 1992, Mosby. **C** from Nyberg DA and others: *Diagnostic ultrasound of fetal anomalies,* St Louis, 1990, Mosby.)

**FIGURE 18-12 A,** Ultrasound image of a fetus with trisomy 13 and a midline cleft lip *(L)* and palate. *N,* Nose; *curved arrow,* tongue. **B,** Post-natal photograph confirming the diagnosis. *L,* Lip; *N,* nose. **C,** Ultrasound image of facial profile showing marked micrognathia *(curved arrow)*. *A,* Anterior; *straight arrow,* nose. **D,** Postnatal photograph confirming the diagnosis. (**A** and **B** from Nyberg D, Mahony B, Pretorius D: *Diagnostic ultrasound of fetal anomalies,* St Louis, 1990, Mosby. **C** and **D** from Benson CB and others: *Ultrasound Med* 7:163–167, 1988.)

*Continued*

radiopaque substances into the amniotic cavity (**amniography, fetography**), clinicians can obtain outlines of the fetus and amniotic cavity. Other imaging techniques, such as **magnetic resonance imaging (MRI)**, **computed tomographic (CT) scans**, and **xeroradiography**, produce useful images of the fetus, but their use is limited because of factors such as cost and availability (Figures 18-13 and 18-14).

**Fetoscopy** is the direct visualization of the fetus through a tube inserted into the amniotic cavity. This is accomplished principally through the use of fiberoptic technology. Because of the risk of spontaneous abortion and infection, this technique is not normally used for purely diagnostic purposes but rather as an aid to intrauterine sampling procedures. Its use has been largely supplanted by other techniques that rely on ultrasonic guidance.

Sampling Techniques

The classical sampling technique is **amniocentesis**, which involves the insertion of a needle into the amniotic sac and removal of a small amount of amniotic fluid for analysis. Amniocentesis is normally not performed before the thirteenth week because of the relatively small amount of amniotic fluid.

Amniocentesis was originally used for detecting chromosomal anomalies (e.g., Down syndrome) in fetal cells found in the amniotic fluid and for the determination of levels of $\alpha$-fetoprotein, a marker for closure defects of the neural tube and certain other malformations. Analysis of the fetal cells in amniotic fluid is also the basis for determining the gender of embryos. This is typically accomplished by the use of a fluorescent dye that intensely stains the Y chromosome. At present, various analytic procedures on amniotic fluid and cells cultured from the fluid are used to detect many enzymatic and biochemical defects in embryos and to monitor the condition of the fetus.

Another widely used diagnostic technique is **chorionic villus sampling**. In this technique, ultrasonography is used as a guide to insert a biopsy needle into the placenta, where a small sample of the villi is removed for diagnostic purposes. This technique is typically used at earlier periods of pregnancy (6 to 9 weeks) than amniocentesis.

With increasing sophistication of fetal imaging techniques, especially ultrasonography, sampling fetal tissues directly is possible. Ultrasonography-guided sampling of fetal blood, mainly from umbilical vessels, is now rela-

tively common for the diagnosis of hereditary and pathological conditions such as immunodeficiencies, coagulation defects, hemoglobin abnormalities, and fetal infections. It is also possible to biopsy fetal skin and even the fetal liver for organ-specific abnormalities.

THERAPEUTIC MANIPULATIONS ON THE FETUS

Some conditions are better treated in the fetal period than after birth (Box 18-3). In some cases involving blockage, severe structural damage to the fetus can be prevented. In other cases the buildup of toxic waste products can be reduced. The recognition that fetal surgery produces essentially scarless results has stimulated some surgeons to consider corrective surgery in utero rather than waiting until after birth.

**Fetal shunts** can be applied to correct specific conditions in which major permanent damage would result before the time of birth. One such situation is a shunt into the urinary bladder to relieve the pressure and subsequent kidney damage caused by anatomical obstructions of the lower urinary tract. Figure 18-15 shows the consequence of nontreatment of a persistent cloacal plate, which results in **megacystitis** (enlarged bladder). Fetal shunts have also been used in attempts to relieve the cerebrospinal pressures that result in hydrocephaly (see Figure 11-38), but the results of these procedures have been equivocal.

**Fetal blood transfusions** are used for the treatment of fetal anemia and severe erythroblastosis fetalis (see Chapter 7). Earlier, the blood was introduced intraperitoneally. With the increasing sophistication of umbilical cord blood sampling techniques, direct intravascular transfusions are now possible.

**Open fetal surgery** can now be performed because of the diagnostic procedures that allow an accurate assessment of the condition of the fetus. This is still a new and highly experimental procedure, and its application has been confined to cases of fetal anomalies that would cause grave damage to the fetus if left uncorrected before birth. Currently, the principal indications for open fetal surgery are blockage of the urinary tract, severe diaphragmatic hernia, and some cases of hydrocephalus. Open fetal surgery entails a risk to the mother as well, and the advisability of such a procedure must be carefully considered. With future improvements in procedures, correcting other malformations such as cleft lip and palate or limb deformities in utero may be possible.

**FIGURE 18-13** High-resolution computed tomographic reconstructions of the skull of an **18-week-old** fetus. **A,** Focus on superficial bones of the skull. **B,** Deeper bones from the same skull. (Courtesy R.A. Levy, H. Maher, and A.R. Burdi, Ann Arbor, Mich.)

**FIGURE 18-14** Magnetic resonance image of a normal third-trimester fetus inside the uterus. The head of the fetus is near the point of the arrow from *I* (internal cervical os). *E,* External cervical os; *closed arrowheads,* placenta; *open arrowheads,* uterine wall. (From Friedman AC and others: *Clinical pelvic imaging,* St Louis, 1990, Mosby.)

*Continued*

**FIGURE 18-15** Fetus with great abdominal distention as a result of megacystis (large bladder) caused by a cloacal plate. (Courtesy M. Barr, Ann Arbor, Mich.)

## PARTURITION

**Parturition**, the process of childbirth, occurs approximately 38 weeks after fertilization (Figure 18-16). The process of childbirth consists of three distinct stages of labor. The first, the **stage of dilatation**, begins with the onset of regular, hard contractions of the uterus and ends with complete dilatation of the cervix. Although the contractions of the uterine smooth muscle may appear to be the dominant process in the first stage of labor, the most important component is the effacement and dilatation of the cervix. During the entire pregnancy the cervix functions to retain the fetus in the uterus. For the childbirth process to proceed, the cervix must change consistency from a firm, almost tubular structure to one that is soft,

distensible, and not like a canal. This change involves a reconfiguration and possibly removal of much of the cervical collagen. Although many of the factors underlying the reconfiguration of the cervix during the first stage of labor remain undefined, considerable evidence exists for an important role of prostaglandin $F_2\alpha$ in the process. Although variation is great, the average length of the first stage of labor is approximately 12 hours.

The second stage of labor (**stage of expulsion**) begins with complete dilatation of the cervix and ends with the passage of the baby from the birth canal. During this stage, which typically lasts 30 to 60 minutes depending on the number of previous deliveries of the mother, the baby still depends on a functioning umbilical circulation for survival.

## Box 18-3  Fetal Conditions Treatable in Utero

### SURGICAL TREATMENT

Urinary obstruction (urethral valves)
Diaphragmatic hernia
Sacrococcygeal teratoma
Chylothorax
Cystic adenomatoid malformation of lung
Twin-twin transfusion syndrome
Hydrocephalus caused by aqueductal stenosis
Complete heart block

### MEDICAL TREATMENT

Erythroblastosis fetalis
Adrenal hyperplasia
Hyperthyroidism and hypothyroidism
Fetal dysrhythmias
Diabetes
Agammaglobulinemia
Vitamin-responsive metabolic disorders
Idiopathic thrombocytic purpura

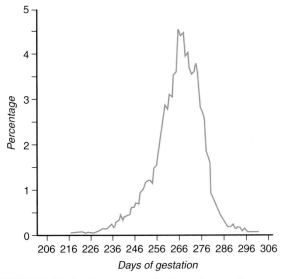

**FIGURE 18-16** Graph showing the distribution in days of normal pregnancy in 1336 spontaneous, full-term deliveries. (Modified from Wigglesworth J, Singer D: *Textbook of fetal and perinatal pathology,* London, 1991, Blackwell Scientific.)

The third stage of labor (**placental stage**) represents the period between delivery of the baby and expulsion of the placenta. Typically, the umbilical cord is cut within minutes of delivery, and the baby must then quickly adapt to independent living. During the next 15 to 30 minutes, continued contractions of the uterus separate the placenta from the maternal decidua and the intact placenta is delivered. After delivery of the placenta, major hemorrhage from the spiral uterine arteries is prevented naturally by continued contraction of the myometrium. In actual clinical practice the third stage is commonly abbreviated by the intramuscular injection of synthetic oxytocin and external manipulation of the uterus to reduce the amount of uterine blood loss.

The mechanisms underlying the initiation and progression of parturition in humans remain remarkably poorly understood, even though considerable progress has been made in uncovering the stimuli for parturition in certain domestic animals. In sheep, parturition is initiated by a sharp increase in the cortisol concentration in the fetal blood. As a result, placental enzyme activity changes, resulting in the conversion of placental progesterone to estrogen synthesis. This increase in estrogen stimulates the formation and release of prostaglandin $F_2\alpha$.

In humans, there is less dependence on activity of the pituitary-adrenal cortical axis for the initiation of parturition. Recent research on primate embryos has suggested that **corticotropin-releasing hormone (CRH)**, which is normally released by the hypothalamus, is produced in significant amounts by the placenta, starting at about 12 weeks of pregnancy. Some of the placental CRH stimulates the fetal adenohypophysis to release **adrenocorticotrophic hormone (ACTH)**. ACTH, in turn, stimulates the adrenal cortex to produce **cortisol**, which is necessary for many maturation processes in the fetus (see Table 18-1). Much of the CRH, however, acts directly upon the fetal adrenal cortex, stimulating it to produce dehydroepiandosterone sulfate, which the placenta uses directly as a substrate for the synthesis of estrogen. High levels of estrogen, accompanied by lowered levels of progesterone during late pregnancy tip the scales in favor of parturition, but the exact nature of the trigger for parturition remains obscure. Progesterone, as its name implies, acts to maintain pregnancy, increasing amounts of estrogen prepare the female reproductive tissues for parturition. For example, estrogen stimulates the production of **connexins**, which form junctions that electrically connect uterine smooth muscles to one another. It also stimulates the uterine smooth muscle cells to produce receptors for oxytocin, a major stimulus for the contraction of uterine smooth muscle during labor. Estrogen, through promoting the action of prostaglandins, stimulates the degradation of collagen fibers in the cervix to make them flexible enough to expand to accommodate the fetus during childbirth. The production of CRH by the placenta helps to explain why a fetus with pituitary or adrenal hypoplasia, or even anencephaly, is typically delivered within the normal time frame. In fact, spontaneous labor occurs in cases of pituitary or adrenal hypoplasia of the fetus or even in anencephaly, but the timing of parturition typically has a considerably wider range than normal. As in sheep, the local release of prostaglandin $F_2\alpha$ may be important in the initiation of labor in humans. In rare cases of human twins implanted in different horns of a double uterus, one member of the pair may not be born until several days or even weeks after the first delivery.

## ADAPTATIONS TO POSTNATAL LIFE

When the umbilical cord is clamped after birth, the neonate is suddenly thrust into a totally independent existence. The respiratory and cardiovascular systems must almost instantaneously assume a type and level of function quite different from those during the fetal period. Within hours or days of birth, the digestive system, immune system, and sense organs must also adapt to a much more complex environment.

### Circulatory Changes at Birth

Two major events drive the functional adaptations of the circulatory system immediately at birth. The first is the cutting of the umbilical cord, and the second is the changes in the lungs after the first breaths of the newborn. These events stimulate a series of sweeping changes that not only alter the circulatory balance but also result in major structural changes in the circulatory system of the infant.

Cutting the umbilical cord results in an immediate cessation of blood entering the body via the umbilical vein. This eliminates the major blood flow through the ductus venosus and greatly reduces the amount of blood that enters the right atrium via the inferior vena cava. A consequence of this is a reduction of the stream of blood that was directly shunted from the right to the left atrium via the foramen ovale during fetal life.

After just a few breaths, the pulmonary circulatory bed expands and can accommodate much greater blood flow than during the fetal period. Consequences of this change are a reduced flow of blood through the ductus arteriosus and a correspondingly greater return of blood into the left atrium via the pulmonary veins. Within minutes after birth, the ductus arteriosus undergoes a reflex closure. This shunt, which in prenatal life is actively kept open in great part through the actions of prostaglandin $E_2$, rapidly constricts after the oxygen concentration in the blood increases. The mechanism for constriction appears to involve the action of cytochrome P-450, but the way it is translated into contraction of the smooth musculature of the ductus is not entirely clear. The principal tissue involved in closure of the ductus is smooth muscle, and the shunt also experiences a breakdown of elastic fibers and a thickening of the inner intimal layer. Although initial closure of the ductus arteriosus is based upon a

reflex mechanism, over the next few weeks it is followed by a phase of anatomical closure, during which cell death and proliferation of connective tissue combine to reduce the ductus into a fibrous cord.

Because of closure of the ductus arteriosus, increased pulmonary venous flow, and loss of 25% to 50% of the peripheral vasculature (placental circulation) when the umbilical cord is cut, the blood pressure in the left atrium becomes slightly increased over that in the right atrium. This results in a physiological closure of the interatrial shunt, with the result that all the blood entering the right atrium empties into the right ventricle (Figure 18-17). Structural closure of the valve at the foramen ovale is prolonged, occurring over several months after birth. Before complete structural obliteration of the interatrial valve, it possesses the property of "probe patency," which allows a catheter inserted into the right atrium to pass freely through the foramen ovale into the left atrium. As structural fusion of the valve to the interatrial septum progresses, the property of probe patency is gradually reduced and ultimately disappears. In approximately 20% of individuals, structural closure of the interatrial valve is not completed, leading to the normally asymptomatic condition of **probe patent foramen ovale.**

Although the ductus venosus also loses its patency after birth, its closure is more prolonged than that of the ductus arteriosus. The tissue of the wall of the ductus venosus is not as responsive to increased oxygen saturation of the blood as that of the ductus arteriosus.

After the postnatal pattern of the circulation is fully established, obliterated vessels or shunts that were important circulatory channels in the fetus are either replaced by connective tissue strands, forming ligaments, or are represented by relatively smaller vessels (Figures 18-17 and 18-18). These changes are summarized in Table 18-2. In early postnatal life, the umbilical vein can still be used for exchange transfusions (in cases of hemolytic disease resulting from erythroblastosis fetalis) before its lumen becomes obliterated.

### Lung Breathing in the Perinatal Period

Immediately after birth, the baby must begin to breathe regularly and effectively with the lungs to survive. The initial breaths are difficult because the lungs are filled with fluid and the alveoli are collapsed at birth. On a purely mechanical basis, air breathing is facilitated by a proportionally large diameter of the trachea and major airways. This reduces resistance to airflow, which would be insurmountable if these passageways were proportionally as small as the lungs.

Just before birth, increased levels of both **arginine vasopressin** and **adrenalin** suppress the secretion of fetal lung fluid and stimulate its resorption by the pulmonary epithe-

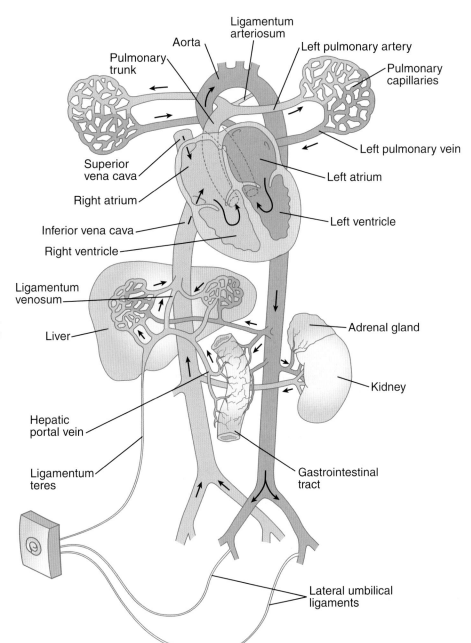

**FIGURE 18-17** Postnatal circulation showing the location of remnants of embryonic vessels.

lial cells. At birth the lungs contain about 50 ml of alveolar fluid, which must be removed for adequate air breathing. Approximately half of that volume enters the lymphatic system. Of the remainder, perhaps half may be expelled during birth. The remainder enters the bloodstream.

The alveolar sacs in the lungs begin to inflate on the first inspiration. The pulmonary surfactant, which was secreted in increasing amounts during the last few weeks of a term pregnancy, reduces the surface tension that would otherwise be present at the air-fluid interface on the alveolar surfaces and facilitates inflation of the lungs. With the rush of air into the lungs, the pulmonary vasculature opens, allowing a greatly increased flow of blood

through the lungs. This results in an increased oxygen saturation of the blood; the color of the newborn changes from a dusky purple to pink.

Breathing movements in the fetus are intermittent and irregular even after birth. Many factors can affect the frequency of breathing, but those responsible for the transition from intermittent to regular breathing remain poorly understood. Factors such as cold, touch, chemical stimuli, sleep patterns, and signals emanating from the carotid and aortic bodies have been implicated. During periods of wakefulness, breathing of the neonate soon stabilizes, but for several weeks after birth, short periods of apnea (5 to 10 seconds) are common during REM sleep.

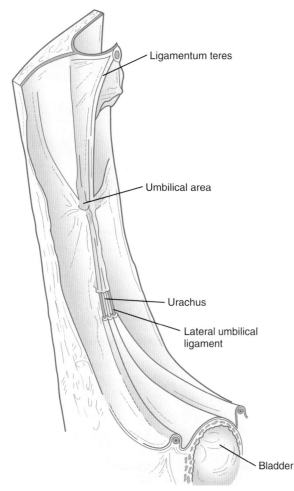

Ligamentum teres

Umbilical area

Urachus

Lateral umbilical
ligament

Bladder

**FIGURE 18-18** Posterior view of the umbilical region of the abdominal wall showing the two obliterated umbilical arteries flanking the urachus leading from the bladder to the umbilicus. The single strand at the top is the ligamentum teres (remnant of the umbilical vein) leading from the umbilicus to the liver.

**TABLE 18-2** *Postnatal Derivatives of Prenatal Circulatory Shunts or Vessels*

| Prenatal structure | Postnatal derivative |
| --- | --- |
| Ductus arteriosus | Ligamentum arteriosum |
| Ductus venosus | Ligamentum venosum |
| Interatrial shunt | Interatrial septum |
| Umbilical vein | Ligamentum teres |
| Umbilical arteries | Distal segments, lateral umbilical ligaments; proximal segments, superior vesical arteries |

## OVERVIEW

The story of prenatal development is complex but fascinating. Many generalizations can be extracted from the study of embryology, but one dominant theme is that of an overall coordination of a large number of very complex integrative processes that range from the translation of information encoded in structural genes, such as the homeobox-containing genes, to the influence of physical factors, such as pressure and tension, on the form and function of the developing embryo.

Sometimes, things go wrong. Studies on spontaneous abortions show that nature has provided a screening mechanism that eliminates many of the embryos least capable of normal development or independent survival. A simple base substitution in the DNA of an embryo can produce a defect that may be highly localized or have far-reaching consequences on the development of a variety of systems.

With ever greater insight into the molecular and cellular mechanisms underlying normal and abnormal development and with increasingly sophisticated technology, biomedical scientists and physicians can manipulate the embryo in ways that were unimaginable not long ago. It is an exciting era that is rapidly increasing in technological complexity and uncertain in many social and ethical aspects. It also has an economic impact that is difficult to predict.

## SUMMARY

○ The fetal period is characterized by intense growth in length and mass of the embryo. With time, the trunk grows relatively faster than the head, and later the limbs show the greatest growth. The early fetus is thin because of the absence of subcutaneous fat. By midpregnancy, subcutaneous fat is deposited.

○ At 5 weeks, the heart beats at 100 beats per minute; the heart rate rises to 160 beats per minute by 8 weeks and then declines slightly during the remainder of pregnancy. Some different physiological properties of the fetal heart can be explained by the presence of fetal isozymes in the cardiac muscle. The patency of the ductus arteriosus in the fetus is actively maintained through the actions of prostaglandin $E_2$.

○ The fetal lungs are filled with fluid, but they must be prepared for full respiratory function within moments after birth. The fetus begins to make anticipatory breathing movements as early as 11 weeks. Fetal breathing is affected by maternal physiological conditions such as eating and smoking. Disproportionate growth in diameter of the upper airway is important in allowing the newborn to take the first breath. The secretion of pulmonary surfactant begins at about 24 weeks, but large amounts are not synthesized until just a few weeks before birth. Premature infants with a deficiency of pulmonary surfactant often suffer from respiratory distress syndrome.

○ Fetal movements begin at about 7½ weeks and increase in complexity thereafter. The maturation of fetal move-

## CLINICAL VIGNETTE

A routine ultrasound examination of a woman in her eighth month of pregnancy shows a swelling of the abdomen of the fetus. A repeat examination a week later shows a further progression of the swelling. The woman is referred to an academic medical center and is told that without intrauterine surgery there is a very good chance that the fetus would undergo irreversible pathological changes before birth. She is informed that the condition affecting her fetus is one in which fetal surgery has produced a good record of success.

From this history, what is the likely type of condition, and what would be the nature of the surgical procedure?

ments mirrors the structural and functional maturation of the nervous system. Diurnal rhythms in fetal activity appear at 20 to 22 weeks. The fetus has alternating periods of sleep and wakefulness. Near term the fetus responds to vibroacoustic stimuli, and by 30 weeks the pupillary light reflex can be elicited.

○ The fetal digestive tract is nonfunctional in the usual sense, but maturation of enzyme systems for digestion and absorption occurs. Spontaneous rhythmical movements of the small intestine begin as early as 7 weeks. Meconium begins to fill the lower intestinal tract by mid-pregnancy. By term the fetus typically swallows more than $\frac{1}{2}$ L of amniotic fluid per day.

○ Fetal kidneys produce small amounts of dilute urine. Fetal endocrine glands produce small amounts of hormones that can be histochemically demonstrated in glandular tissue early in the fetal period, but several months often pass before the same hormones can be measured in the blood. The fetal adrenal cortex is very large and produces 100 to 200 mg of steroids per day. The exact functions of the fetal adrenal gland remain poorly understood, but fetal cortisol appears to prepare a number of organ systems for the transition to independent life after birth. The placenta continues to produce a variety of hormones throughout most of pregnancy.

○ Many new diagnostic techniques have considerably improved access to the fetus. Among the imaging techniques, ultrasonography has emerged as the most widely used in obstetrics. Through sampling techniques such as amniocentesis and chorionic villus sampling, fluids or cells of the embryo and fetus can be removed for analysis. These techniques allow certain manipulations on the fetus (e.g., fetal blood transfusions, fetal surgery for certain anomalies).

○ Parturition occurs in three stages of labor. The first is the stage of dilatation, which culminates with efface-

ment of the cervix. The second stage culminates with expulsion of the baby. The third stage represents the period between delivery of the baby and expulsion of the placenta. The mechanisms underlying the initiation of parturition in the human remain poorly understood.

○ After birth and cutting of the umbilical cord, the newborn must quickly adapt to an independent existence in terms of breathing and cardiac function. After the first breaths and severing of the umbilical cord, the pulmonary circulation opens. In response to increased flow into the left atrium, the interatrial shunt undergoes physiological closure, and the ductus arteriosus undergoes a reflex closure. Closure of the ductus venosus in the liver is more prolonged.

## Review Questions

1. The ligamentum teres is the postnatal remains of the:
   A. Ductus arteriosus
   B. Ductus venosus
   C. Umbilical vein
   D. Umbilical artery
   E. Urachus

2. Insufficient production of which of the following is a major cause of poor viability of infants born 24 to 26 weeks after conception?
   A. Pulmonary surfactant
   B. α-Fetoprotein
   C. Meconium
   D. Lanugo
   E. Urine

3. Meconium is formed in the fetal:
   A. Liver
   B. Ileum
   C. Lungs
   D. Amniotic fluid
   E. Kidneys

4. Which organ is much larger in the fetus than it is shortly after birth?
   A. Kidneys
   B. Heart
   C. Liver
   D. Urinary bladder
   E. Adrenal gland

5. Fetal movements can usually first be detected by ultrasound at how many weeks?
   A. 6
   B. 8
   C. 10
   D. 12
   E. 14

6. What blood vessel is commonly used for exchange transfusions in newborn infants?
   A. Umbilical artery
   B. Jugular vein
   C. Femoral artery
   D. Umbilical vein
   E. None of the above

7. A premature infant develops labored breathing and dies within a few days. What is the likely cause?

8. A rare condition that can persist even into adulthood is "caput medusae" (Medusa's head), in which a dark vascular ring with irregular radiations appears around the umbilicus with straining of the abdomen. What is an embryological basis for this condition?

9. A pregnant woman typically first feels fetal movements about 15 weeks into pregnancy. The movements become more noticeable during succeeding weeks but are commonly reduced during the last couple of weeks before parturition. What is the explanation for this?

10. List some recent medical advances that have allowed fetal surgery to become a reality.

## REFERENCES

Adzick NS, Harrison MR: Fetal surgical therapy, Lancet 343:897–902, 1994.

Avery ME, Wang N-S, Tacusch HW: The lung of the newborn infant, Sci Am 228:75–85, 1973.

Barclay AE, Franklin KJ, Prichard MML: The foetal circulation and cardiovascular system, and the changes that they undergo at birth, Oxford, England, 1944, Blackwell Scientific.

Barcroft J: Researches on prenatal life, vol 1, Oxford, 1946, Blackwell Scientific.

Barron DH: The changes in the fetal circulation at birth, Physiol Rev 24:277–295, 1944.

Bowerman RA: Atlas of normal fetal ultrasonographic anatomy, ed 2, St Louis, 1992, Mosby.

Busnel MC, Granier-Deferre C, LeCanuet JP: Fetal audition, Ann NY Acad Sci 662:118–134, 1992.

Coceani F, Olley PM: The control of cardiovascular shunts in the fetal and perinatal period, Can J Physiol Pharmacol 66:1129–1134, 1988.

Dawes GS: The development of fetal behavioural patterns, Can J Physiol Pharmacol 66:541–548, 1988.

Duenhoelter JH, Pritchard JA: Fetal respiration, Am J Obstet Gynecol 129:326–338, 1977.

Fuchs A-R, Fuchs F: Endocrinology of human parturition: a review, Br J Obstet Gynecol 91:948–967, 1984.

Fuse Y: Development of the hypothalamic-pituitary-thyroid axis in humans, Reprod Fertil Dev 8:1–21, 1996.

Grannum PA, Copel JA: Invasive fetal procedures, Radiol Clin North Am 28:217–226, 1990.

Harding R, Bocking AD, eds: Fetal growth and development, Cambridge, 2001, Cambridge University Press.

Hooker D: The prenatal origin of behavior, Lawrence, 1952, University of Kansas Press.

Hooper SB, Harding R: Fetal lung liquid: a major determinant of the growth and functional development of the fetal lung, Clin Exp Pharmacol Physiol 22:235–247, 1995.

Johnson P: The development of breathing. In Jones C, Nathanielsz P, eds: The physiological development of the fetus and newborn, London, 1985, Academic, pp 201–210.

Jones CT, Nathanielsz PW, eds: The physiological development of the fetus and newborn, London, 1985, Academic.

Kitterman JA: Physiological factors in lung growth, Can J Physiol Pharmacol 66:1122–1128, 1988.

Kline RM: Whose blood is it, anyway? Sci Am 284:42–49, 2001.

Lagercrantz H, Slotkin TA: The "stress" of being born, Sci Am 254:100–107, 1986.

Larsen T and others: Normal fetal growth evaluated by longitudinal ultrasound examinations, Early Hum Dev 24:37–45, 1990.

Lavery JP: The human placenta: clinical perspectives, Rockville, Md, 1987, Aspen.

Liggins GC: The role of cortisol in preparing the fetus for birth, Reprod Fertil Dev 6:141–150, 1994.

Liu M and others: Stimulation of fetal rat lung cell proliferation in vitro by mechanical stretch, Am J Physiol 263:L376–L383, 1992.

Manning FA: Fetal breathing movements, Postgrad Med 61:116–122, 1977.

Mastroiacovo P and others: Limb anomalies following chorionic villus sampling: a registry based case-control study, Am J Med Genet 44:856–864, 1992.

McArdle HJ, Ashworth CJ: Micronutrients in fetal growth and development, Brit Med Bull 55:499–510, 1999.

Naeye RL: Disorders of the placenta, fetus, and neonate: diagnosis and clinical significance, St Louis, 1992, Mosby.

Norgaard-Pedersen B, Christiansen M, Jensen SP: α-Fetoprotein in fetal pathology. In Pasqualini JR, Scholler R, eds: Hormones and fetal pathophysiology, New York, 1992, Marcel Dekker, pp 369–412.

Nyberg DA, Mahony BS, Pretorius DH: Diagnostic ultrasound of fetal anomalies: text and atlas, St Louis, 1990, Mosby.

Polin RA, Fox WW, eds: Fetal and neonatal physiology, vols 1 and 2, Philadelphia, 1992, WB Saunders.

Prechtl HFR: Fetal behavior. In Hill A, Volpe J, eds: Fetal neurology, New York, 1989, Raven, pp 1–16.

Rigatto H: Control of breathing in fetal life and onset and control of breathing in the neonate. In Polin, R, Fox W, eds: Fetal and neonatal physiology, vol 1, Philadelphia, 1992, WB Saunders, pp 790–801.

Semmekrot B, Guignard J-P: Atrial natriuretic peptide during early human development, Biol Neonate 60:341–349, 1991.

Siler-Khodr TM: Endocrine and paracrine function of the placenta. In Polin R, Fox W, eds: Fetal and neonatal physiology, vol 1, Philadelphia, 1992, WB Saunders, pp 74–86.

Smith BR: Visualizing human embryos, Sci Am 280:76–81, 1999.

Smith R: The timing of birth, Sci Am 280:68–75, 1999.

St. John Sutton M, Gill T, Plappert T: Functional anatomic development in the fetal heart. In Polin R, Fox W, eds: Fetal and neonatal physiology, vol 1, Philadelphia, 1992, WB Saunders, pp 598–609.

Stahlman MT, Gray ME, Whitsett JA: The ontogeny and distribution of surfactant protein B in human fetuses and newborns, J Histochem Cytochem 40:1471–1480, 1992.

Teitel DF: Physiologic development of the cardiovascular system in the fetus. In Polin R, Fox W, eds: Fetal and neonatal physiology, vol 1, Philadelphia, 1992, WB Saunders, pp 609–619.

Van Golde LMG and others: Synthesis of surfactant lipids in the developing lung. In Jones C, Nathanielsz P, eds: The physiological development of the fetus and newborn, London, 1985, Academic, pp 191–200.

Vanhatalo S, van Nieuwenhuizen O: Fetal pain? Brain Devel 22:145–150, 2000.

Wetzel GT, Klitzner TS: Developmental cardiac electrophysiology. Recent advances in cellular physiology, Cardiovasc Res 31:E52–E60, 1996.

Winter JSD: Fetal and neonatal adrenocortical physiology. In Polin R, Fox W, eds: Fetal and neonatal physiology, vol 2, Philadelphia, 1992, WB Saunders, pp 1829–1841.

# Answers to Clinical Vignettes and Review Questions

## CHAPTER 1

### Clinical Vignette

C. Although most tissues of the body are affected to some extent, the heart is not a primary target tissue of ovarian steroid hormones.

### Review Questions

1. D
2. E
3. B
4. A mediastinal teratoma, which is likely to have arisen from an aberrant primordial germ cell that became lodged in the connective tissue near the heart.
5. In the female, meiosis begins during embryonic life; in the male, meiosis begins at puberty.
6. At prophase (diplotene stage) of the first meiotic division and at metaphase of the second meiotic division.
7. Chromosomal abnormalities, such as polyploidy or trisomies of individual chromosomes.
8. Spermatogenesis is the entire process of sperm formation from a spermatogonium. It includes the two meiotic divisions and the period of spermiogenesis. Spermiogenesis, or sperm metamorphosis, is the process of transformation of a postmeiotic spermatid, which looks like an ordinary cell, to a highly specialized spermatozoon.
9. Estrogens, secreted by the ovary, support the preovulatory proliferative phase. From the time of ovulation, progesterone is secreted in large amounts by the corpus luteum and is responsible for the secretory phase, which prepares the endometrium for implantation of an embryo.
10. FSH produced by the anterior lobe of the pituitary gland and testosterone produced by the Leydig cells of the testis.

## CHAPTER 2

### Clinical Vignette

1. Before the plane crash, the issue is who is the "real" mother. After the crash, the issue is who gets the money—the surrogate mother who claims that she is the real mother or the aunt who claims a blood affinity. Although these present as legal issues that would likely be decided in a court, the concept of what is meant by surrogacy also involves psychological and religious issues.
2. This is a very important issue that hasn't been resolved. If the parents had been of a religion that strongly supports the rights of embryos to life, should the remaining embryos also be implanted into someone, and if so, whom? In a case where a considerable inheritance is involved, the financial implications could considerably cloud the issue. On the other hand, if there were no parental money, who would undergo both the risk and expense to prevent the frozen embryos from being simply thrown out? In many cases of in vitro fertilization and embryo transfer, the question of what to do with the "extra" frozen embryos when the first transfer is successful is a real one. Many frozen embryos are being stored at various sites around the world.

### Review Questions

1. E
2. D
3. The sharp surge of luteinizing hormone produced by the anterior lobe of the pituitary gland.
4. Capacitation is a poorly understood interaction between a spermatozoon and female reproductive tissues that increases the ability of the sperm to fertilize an egg. In some mammals, capacitation is obligatory, but in humans the importance of capacitation is less well established.

5. Fertilization usually occurs in the upper third of the uterine tube.

6. The ZP3 protein acts as a specific sperm receptor through its O-linked oligosaccharides; much of its polypeptide backbone must be exposed to stimulate the acrosomal reaction.

7. Polyspermy is the fertilization of an egg by more than one spermatozoon. It is prevented through the fast electrical block on the plasma membrane of the egg and by the later zona reaction, by which products released from the cortical granules act to inactivate the sperm receptors in the zona pellucida.

8. She had probably taken clomiphene for the stimulation of ovulation. Natural septuplets are almost never seen.

9. The introduction of more than one embryo into the tube of the woman is commonly done because the chance of any single implanted embryo surviving to the time of birth is quite small. The reasons for this are poorly understood. Extra embryos are frozen because if a pregnancy does not result from the first implantation, the frozen embryos can be implanted without the inconvenience and expense of obtaining new eggs from the mother and fertilizing them in vitro.

10. In cases of incompatibility between the sperm and egg, poor sperm motility, or deficient sperm receptors in the zona, introducing the sperm directly into or near the egg can bypass a weak point in the reproductive sequence of events.

# CHAPTER 3

## Clinical Vignette

She had an ectopic pregnancy in her right uterine tube. With the rapidly increasing size of the embryo and its extraembryonic structures, her right uterine tube had ruptured.

## Review Questions

1. D
2. E
3. A
4. C
5. The embryonic body proper arises from the inner cell mass.
6. Trophoblastic tissues.
7. They allow the trophoblast of the embryo to adhere to the uterine epithelium.
8. Cells derived from the cytotrophoblast fuse to form the syncytiotrophoblast.
9. In addition to the standard causes of lower abdominal pain such as appendicitis, the doctor should consider

ectopic pregnancy (tubal variety) as a result of stretching and possible rupture of the uterine tube containing the implanted embryo.

# CHAPTER 4

No Clinical Vignette.

## Review Questions

1. A homeobox is a highly conserved region consisting of 180 nucleotides that is found in many morphogenetically active genes. Homeobox gene products act as transcription factors.
2. B
3. In contrast to many receptors, the receptors for retinoic acid ($\alpha$, $\beta$, and $\gamma$) are, located in the nucleus.
4. A
5. D
6. D
7. E

# CHAPTER 5

## Clinical Vignette

C. Because of the respiratory problems associated with his situs inversus, this man probably has a mutation of a dynein gene. Commonly such individuals also have immotile spermatozoa, a condition that would lead to infertility.

## Review Questions

1. D
2. A
3. B
4. B
5. C
6. The epiblast.
7. The primitive node acts as the organizer of the embryo. Through it pass the cells that will become the notochord. The notochord induces the formation of the nervous system. The primitive node is also the site of synthesis of morphogenetically active molecules such as retinoic acid. If a primitive node is transplanted to another embryo, it stimulates the formation of another embryonic axis.
8. Hyaluronic acid and fibronectin.
9. Vg1 and activin.
10. Cell adhesion molecules are lost in a migratory phase. When the migratory cells settle down, they may reexpress cell adhesion molecules.

## CHAPTER 6

No Clinical Vignette.

## Review Questions

1. B
2. C
3. E
4. C
5. A
6. A change in cell shape at the median hinge point and pressures of the lateral ectoderm acting to push up the lateral walls of the neural plate.
7. Neuromeres provide the fundamental organization of parts of the brain in which they are present. Certain homeobox genes are expressed in a definite sequence along the neuromeres.
8. The somites. Axial muscles form from cells derived from the medial halves of the somites, and limb muscles arise from cellular precursors located in the lateral halves of the somites.
9. In blood islands that arise from mesoderm of the wall of the yolk sac.

## CHAPTER 7

### Clinical Vignette

D. α-Fetoprotein, which is produced principally by the fetal liver, is found in many tissues of the body, but normally, only small amounts are excreted into the amniotic fluid. With open neural tube defects, large quantities of α-fetoprotein escape through the opening and enter the amniotic fluid.

### Review Questions

1. A
2. E
3. B
4. D
5. E
6. C
7. Because the placental villi (specializations of the chorion) are directly bathed in maternal blood.
8. This depends on the age of the embryo. In an early fetus the molecule may have to pass through as many layers as the following: syncytiotrophoblast, cytotrophoblast, basal lamina underlying cytotrophoblast, villous mesenchyme, basal lamina of a fetal capillary, and endothelium of the fetal capillary. In a mature placenta the same molecule may pass from the maternal to the fetal circulation by traversing as few layers as syncytiotrophoblast, a fused basal lamina

of trophoblast and capillary endothelium, and the endothelium of a fetal capillary.
9. Human chorionic gonadotropin. This is the first distinctive embryonic hormone to be produced by the trophoblastic tissues. Early pregnancy tests involved injecting small amounts of urine of a woman into female African clawed toads (*Xenopus laevis*). If the woman was pregnant, the chorionic gonadotropin contained in the urine stimulated the frogs to lay eggs the next day. Contemporary pregnancy tests, which can be done using kits bought over the counter, give almost instantaneous results.
10. Many substances that enter a woman's blood are now known to cross the placental barrier. These include alcohol, many drugs (both prescribed and illicit), steroid hormones, and other low-molecular-weight substances. In general, molecules with molecular weights below 5000 daltons should be assumed to cross the placental barrier with little difficulty.

## CHAPTER 8

### Clinical Vignette

Although this woman's history suggests a number of risk factors, none of her children's problems could be definitely attributed to any specific cause. Nevertheless, there is a good likelihood that the spina bifida in the first child and the anencephaly of the third child could be related to overall poor nutrition and a specific deficiency in folic acid, since poor nutrition is not uncommon in alcoholics. The small stature of the middle child could possibly result from the mother's heavy smoking, but the behavior problem could be a consequence of the mother's cocaine use, smoking, or alcohol consumption. On the other hand, there could be no relation between any of the mother's risk factors and a prenatal influence on the child's later behavior. An important point is that despite a number of well-known risk factors, it is very difficult, if not impossible, to assign a given congenital anomaly to a specific cause. Realistically, one can only speak in terms of probabilities.

### Review Questions

1. E
2. C
3. E
4. B
5. A
6. B
7. The conditions that result in cleft palate occur during the second month of pregnancy. By the fourth month the palate is normally completely established. It is almost certain that this malformation had already been established by the time of the accident.

8. Although there may be a connection between the drug and the birth defect, proving a connection between an individual case and any drug, especially a new one, is very difficult. The woman's genetic background, other drugs that she may have taken during the same period, her history of illnesses during early pregnancy, her nutritional status, and so on should be investigated. Even in the best of circumstances, the probability of a specific malformation being caused by a particular factor can only be estimated in many cases.

9. A common cause of such malformations is an insufficiency of amniotic fluid (oligohydramnios), which can place exposed parts of fetuses under excessive mechanical pressure from the uterine wall and lead to deformations of this type.

10. Dysplasia of ectodermal derivatives is a likely cause.

## CHAPTER 9

### Clinical Vignette

1. B
2. A

### Review Questions

1. D
2. E
3. D
4. B
5. C
6. B
7. The dermis. Recombination experiments have clearly shown that the dermis confers regional morphogenetic information on the epidermis, instructing it to form, for example, cranial hair or abdominal hair.
8. They may be supernumerary nipples located along the caudal ends of the embryonic milk lines.
9. In the early embryo, brain tissue induces the formation of the surrounding membranous skeletal elements. If a significant region of the brain is missing, the inductive interaction does not occur.
10. In experiments involving the use of the quail nuclear marker, quail somites were grafted in place of the original somites in chick embryos. The muscles in the developing limbs all contained quail and not chick nuclei.

## CHAPTER 10

### Clinical Vignette

At a descriptive level, the mirror image asymmetry of the duplicated foot and digits is a classic example of Bateson's rule of symmetry in duplicated structures (see p. 56). The best explanation for this malformation would be the presence of a duplicated zone of polarizing activity (ZPA) in the anterior margin of the affected limb. Through the actions of sonic hedgehog, secreted by the duplicated ZPA, a secondary gradient of morphogenetic activity could have instructed the anterior mesoderm of the leg bud to form an additional set of posterior structures. This rare defect in humans parallels almost exactly the formation of supernumerary wing structures produced by ZPA transplant experiments on chickens (see Figure 10-11).

### Review Questions

1. B
2. D
3. A
4. C
5. E
6. D
7. A tear of the amnion during the chorionic villus sampling procedure could have resulted in an amniotic band wrapping around the digits and strangulating their blood supply, causing the tips to degenerate and fall off.
8. This defect is unlikely to be related to the amniocentesis procedure because the morphology of the digits is well established by the time such a procedure is undertaken (usually around 15 to 16 weeks). The most likely cause is a genetic mutation.
9. Muscle-forming cells arise from the somites.
10. The immediate cause is likely the absence of programmed cell death in the interdigital mesoderm. The cause of the disturbance in cell death is currently not understood.

## CHAPTER 11

### Clinical Vignette

The most immediate problems are surgery to deal with (1) the open spinal cord and (2) the developing hydrocephalus. The surgery for the rachischisis must first be directed toward closing the open lesion to prevent infection and to prevent the leakage of cerebrospinal fluid. Later, surgery will likely be necessary for problems associated with traction on the spinal cord and spinal nerves as the child grows. The hydrocephalus is typically treated by implantation of a shunt to lead excess cerebrospinal fluid from the ventricular system of the brain. Patency of the shunt must be maintained.

In addition to surgery, this infant will face many problems associated with impaired function of the lower spinal nerves. Impaired urinary bladder function is common among such infants, as is impaired mobility of the lower extremities. Infection is a constant threat because of the problem with both containment and circulation of the cerebrospinal fluid in the spinal cord lesion. Children with various forms of spina bifida typically require intensive physical therapy for a variety of problems. Clogging of the shunt leading from the ventricular system is a recurring threat. In this patient the thinning of the walls of the brain indicates that the brain tissue itself has been compromised. Some element of mental retardation and the associated educational and socialization problems represent another component of the problem.

In short, even relatively simple cases of spina bifida pose many chronic problems. The total annual medical, rehabilitation, and education costs of treatment for one individual are often significant. In addition to these are the stresses in the family, which is faced with a continuing need to care for the affected individual. There is a significantly higher than normal divorce rate among parents of children with chronic problems resulting from congenital malformations. A strong support network is important for successfully dealing with children with spina bifida conditions.

## Review Questions

1. E
2. A
3. D
4. B
5. D
6. C
7. C
8. B
9. Congenital megacolon (Hirschsprung's disease), in which a segment of large intestine develops without parasympathetic ganglia. Intestinal contents cannot actively move through such an aganglionic segment.
10. The nerves would be hypoplastic (much smaller than normal), and the spinal cord would be thinner than normal in the area from which the nerves supplying the affected limb arise. The likely cause is excessive neuronal cell death because of the absence of an end organ for many of the axons that normally supply the limb.

## CHAPTER 12

### Clinical Vignette

With the diagnosis of immune deficiency along with the infant's outflow tract defect of the heart, the pediatrician's differential diagnosis included the DiGeorge syndrome. This was confirmed when the blood levels of parathyroid

hormone were found to be low. The cause of the infant's problem probably goes back to the fourth week of pregnancy or possibly earlier, when the cranial neural crest supplying the outflow tract of the heart and pharynx was migrating or preparing to migrate into the affected regions.

## Review Questions

1. E
2. B
3. C
4. D
5. A
6. B
7. C
8. D
9. Along the length of the spinal cord, migrating neural crest cells are funneled into the anterior sclerotomal region of the somites and are excluded from the posterior half. This results in the formation of a pair of ganglia for each vertebral segment and space between ganglia in the craniocaudal direction.
10. Cranial crest cells can form skeletal elements; trunk crest cells cannot. Migrating cranial neural crest cells have more morphogenetic information encoded in them than trunk crest cells do. (For example, craniocaudal levels are specified in cranial crest, whereas they are not fixed in trunk crest cells.) Cranial crest cells form large amounts of dermis and other connective tissues, whereas trunk crest cells do not.

## CHAPTER 13

### Clinical Vignette

The common embryological denominator is a deficit in neural crest associated with the first pharyngeal arch. The first arch gives rise to the lower jaw, much of the middle ear complex, and a significant part of the external ear. Because of the statistical association between abnormalities of the external ear and kidney defects, the doctor wants to be sure that there are no underlying abnormalities of the urinary system.

### Review Questions

1. D
2. B
3. A
4. D
5. C
6. Coloboma of the iris is caused by failure of the choroid fissure to close during the sixth week of pregnancy. Because the area of the defect remains open

when the rest of the iris constricts in bright light, excessive unwanted light can enter the eye through the defect.

7. Some of the secretions of the lacrimal glands enter the nasolacrimal ducts, which carry the lacrimal fluid into the nasal cavity.

8. Hyaluronic acid. Migration of neural crest cells into the developing cornea occurs during a period when large amounts of hyaluronic acid have been secreted into the primary corneal stroma.

9. During the fetal period the middle ear cavity is filled with a loose connective tissue that dampens the action of the middle ear ossicles. After birth the connective tissue is resorbed.

10. Like the lower jaw, much of the external ear arises from tissue of the first arch bordering the first pharyngeal cleft.

## CHAPTER 14

### Clinical Vignette

The woman had a hormone-secreting thyroid adenoma that gave her the symptoms of hyperthyroidism. Because the radioactivity was concentrated at the base of her tongue, its location suggested that the tumor formed within a remnant of thyroid tissue left behind at the beginning of the pathway of thyroid tissue migration from its site of origin at the midline base of the future tongue.

### Review Questions

1. B
2. B
3. C
4. E
5. A
6. One option is simply acne. Another more significant possibility is a branchial cyst. Branchial cysts are typically located along the anterior border of the sternocleidomastoid muscle. One possible reason for its late manifestation is that the same conditions that resulted in the boy's acne caused a simultaneous reaction in the epidermis lining the cyst.

7. First, all epithelium lining the cyst must be removed, or the remnants could reform into a new cyst and the symptoms could recur. The surgeon must also determine that the cyst is isolated and not connected to the pharynx via a sinus, which would result from an accompanying persistence of the corresponding pharyngeal pouch.

8. Some of the secretions of the lacrimal glands enter the nasolacrimal ducts, which carry the lacrimal fluid into the nasal cavity.

9. By 10 weeks, all the processes of fusion of facial primordia have already been completed. The cause of the defects could almost certainly be attributed to something that influenced the embryo long before the time when the anticonvulsant therapy was initiated, probably before the seventh week of pregnancy.

10. These defects could be a manifestation of fetal alcohol syndrome. They would represent a relatively mild form of holoprosencephaly, which in this case would relate to defective formation of the forebrain (prosencephalon). The defects in olfaction and in the structure of the upper lip could be secondary effects of a primary defect in early formation of the prosencephalon.

## CHAPTER 15

### Clinical Vignette

The girl had a Meckel's diverticulum that contained ectopic endometrial tissue. When she had menstrual periods, the reaction of the ectopic endometrial tissue gave her upper abdominal cramps. After surgery, her symptoms disappeared.

### Review Questions

1. E
2. A
3. C
4. C
5. B
6. A
7. Esophageal atresia or a tracheoesophageal fistula. In the former, the milk fills the blind esophageal pouch and then spills into the trachea via the laryngeal opening. In the latter, milk may pass directly from the esophagus into the trachea depending on the type of fistula.

8. Congenital pyloric stenosis. Projectile vomiting is a common symptom of this condition, and palpation of the knotted pyloric opening of the stomach confirmed the diagnosis.

9. The most likely diagnosis is a vitelline duct fistula connecting the midgut with the umbilicus. This allows some contents of the small intestine to escape through the umbilicus. Another possibility is a urachal fistula (see Chapter 16), which connects the urinary bladder to the umbilicus through a persistent allantoic duct. In this case, however, the escaping fluid would be urine and would likely not be accompanied by mucus.

10. Imperforate anus. When examining a newborn, clinicians must ensure that there is an anal opening.

# CHAPTER 16

## Clinical Vignette

1. To be diagnosed as a male by the sex chromatin test, none of the cells that were examined should have exhibited Barr bodies (condensed X-chromosomes).
2. The most likely cause for her female phenotype is a lack of testosterone receptors (androgen insensitivity syndrome).
3. Her gonads would be male (internal testes). Because in the embryo her testes produced müllerian inhibitory substance, her paramesonephric ducts regressed. Hence, she formed no uterus, uterine tubes, or upper vagina. This, of course, is also the reason for her amenorrhea, although amenorrhea is common in female athletes who train intensively. Although her testes produce abundant testosterone, the lack of receptors resulted in the lack of differentiation of male genital duct structures or external genitalia that would normally be dependent on testosterone.

## Review Questions

1. A
2. D
3. B
4. A
5. A
6. D
7. B
8. The most likely cause is a urachal fistula connecting the urinary bladder to the umbilicus and allowing the leakage of urine. This is caused by the persistence of the lumen in the distal part of the allantois.
9. Bilateral renal agenesis. The first clue was the mother's low weight gain, which could have been the result of oligohydramnios (although this is not the only cause for low weight gain during pregnancy). The infant's appearance showed many of the characteristics of Potter's syndrome, which is caused by intrauterine pressures on the fetus when the amount of amniotic fluid is very low.
10. In normal development the caudal ends of the paramesonephric ducts swing toward the midline and fuse. In this patient's case the point of fusion probably occurred more caudally than normal. This condition is not incompatible with a normal pregnancy and delivery, although in some cases, pain or problems with delivery can occur.

# CHAPTER 17

## Clinical Vignette

The doctor suspected a high coarctation of the aorta with an accompanying patent ductus arteriosus. In both high and low coarctation of the aorta, the pulse in the lower part of the body is commonly reduced. The cyanosis of the feet resulted from the spillage of venous blood into the systemic circulation through the patent ductus arteriosus.

## Review Questions

1. A
2. D
3. C
4. D
5. E
6. A
7. C
8. The doctor suspected that the boy had a double aortic arch or a right aortic arch, either of which can cause difficulty in swallowing (dysphagia) during childhood, especially when growth spurts are occurring. Another possibility for an embryologically based dysphagia is esophageal stenosis.
9. To survive, an individual with this defect would have to have a means for draining blood entering the left atrium and a means of getting blood into the left ventricle or the systemic circulation. One combination that would compensate is an atrial septal defect, which allows incoming blood to escape from the left atrium, and an associated ventricular septal defect, which allows blood from the right ventricle to pass into the left ventricle. A patent ductus arteriosus added to the first two compensatory defects could also help to balance the circulation by adding blood to the systemic side of the circulation. This would not be very helpful in the physiological sense, however, because the added blood would be unoxygenated blood entering the aorta from the pulmonary artery.
10. Persistence of the caudal segment of the left supracardinal vein. Normally the caudal segment of the right supracardinal vein persists and becomes incorporated into the inferior vena cava, and the corresponding segment of the left supracardinal vein disappears (see Figure 17-11). A wide variety of anomalous patterns of the abdominal veins exists.

# CHAPTER 18

## Clinical Vignette

The fetus likely had an obstruction of the lower urinary tract (perhaps urethral valves) leading to megacystis (see Figure 18-15). This condition is treated by inserting a shunt into the bladder, allowing the urine to escape into the amniotic fluid. If the shunt functions during the remainder of pregnancy, the actual problem with the urinary outlet can be treated surgically after birth. The placement of shunts into the fetal bladder is one of the more successful types of intrauterine surgery practiced to date.

## Review Questions

1. C
2. A
3. B
4. E
5. B
6. D
7. Hyaline membrane disease of the newborn. If the baby was born prematurely, the fetal lungs had not produced sufficient pulmonary surfactant to support normal breathing.
8. This condition is the result of persistence of a patent ductus venosus and umbilical vein. When the individual strains, venous blood fills these vessels and small venous branches radiating from the umbilical area. This is reminiscent of the head of Medusa, with snakes taking the place of hairs.
9. One simple explanation is that with continued growth of the fetus the extremities become so tightly packed in the uterus that there is little room for movement.
10. More refined imaging techniques, such as ultrasonography, that allow more accurate diagnosis in utero of congenital malformations; recognition of the exceptional healing powers of the fetus; improved intrauterine and extrauterine surgical techniques, some assisted by ultrasonographic visualization, that allow direct surgery on the fetus; and increased ability to forestall or prevent premature labor after surgery on the uterus.

# Index

Page numbers in *italics* indicate figures. Page numbers followed by "b" indicate boxes and "t", tables.